FISH AND FISH OIL IN HEALTH AND DISEASE PREVENTION

FISH AND FISH OIL IN HEALTH AND DISEASE PREVENTION

Edited by

SUSAN K. RAATZ
Research Nutritionist
United States Department of Agriculture
Agricultural Research Service
Grand Forks Human Nutrition Research Center
Grand Forks, North Dakota
United States

DOUGLAS M. BIBUS
The Center for Spirituality and Healing
The University of Minnesota, and
Lipid Technologies, LLC
Austin, Minnesota
United States

ELSEVIER

AMSTERDAM • BOSTON • HEIDELBERG • LONDON • NEW YORK
OXFORD • PARIS • SAN DIEGO • SAN FRANCISCO • SINGAPORE
SYDNEY • TOKYO

Academic Press is an imprint of Elsevier

Academic Press is an imprint of Elsevier
125 London Wall, London EC2Y 5AS, United Kingdom
525 B Street, Suite 1800, San Diego, CA 92101-4495, United States
50 Hampshire Street, 5th Floor, Cambridge, MA 02139, United States
The Boulevard, Langford Lane, Kidlington, Oxford OX5 1GB, United Kingdom

Library of Congress Cataloging-in-Publication Data
A catalog record for this book is available from the Library of Congress

British Library Cataloguing-in-Publication Data
A catalogue record for this book is available from the British Library

ISBN: 978-0-12-802844-5

For information on all Academic Press publications
visit our website at https://www.elsevier.com/

Publisher: Nikki Levy
Acquisition Editor: Megan Ball
Editorial Project Manager: Karen Miller
Production Project Manager: Nicky Carter
Designer: Victoria Pearson

Typeset by Thomson Digital

Contents

9. Fish Oil and The Retinopathy of Prematurity

S. BEKEN, E.U. KABATAŞ

10. Fish Oil for Physical Performance in Athletes

G.E. PEOPLES, P.L. McLENNAN

11. Fish Intake and Strength in the Elderly

L.C. FERNANDES

12. Fish and Fish Oil for the Aging Brain

C.M. BUTT, N. SALEM JR.

III

FISH AND FISH OILS IN HEALTH PROMOTION AND DISEASE PREVENTION AND TREATMENT

13. Farmed Fish: A Valuable Source of Lipid Based Nutrients

M.J. PICKLO

14. Fish and Fish Oil and the Metabolic Syndrome

C. TØRRIS

15. Dietary and Supplemental Long-Chain N3 Fatty Acids and Incident Type 2 Diabetes

L.M. STEFFEN, B.T. STEFFEN

16. Seafood Consumption and Fasting Leptin and Ghrelin in Overweight and Obese

B.E. BIRGISDOTTIR, I. THORSDOTTIR

List of Contributors

N.A. Babenko Department of Physiology of Ontogenesis, Institute of Biology, Kharkov Karazin National University, Kharkov, Ukraine

S. Beken Department of Neonatology, Acıbadem University School of Medicine, Istanbul, Turkey

N. Bernoud-Hubac CarMeN Laboratory, INRA UMR1397, INSERM U1060, Université de Lyon, INSA-Lyon, Villeurbanne, France

B.E. Birgisdottir Unit for Nutrition Research, Faculty of Food Science and Nutrition, University of Iceland, Reykjavik; Landspitali University Hospital, Reykjavík, Iceland

C.M. Butt HNH-Biological Models, DSM Nutritional Products, Boulder, Colorado, United States

T.C. Chen Clinical Translational Science Institute, Boston University, Massachusetts, United States

A. Daschner Allergy Department, Health Research Institute, University Hospital La Princesa, Madrid, Spain

A. Erkkilä Institute of Public Health and Clinical Nutrition, University of Eastern Finland, Kuopio, Finland

G.L. Fell Department of Surgery and Vascular Biology Program, Boston Children's Hospital, Boston, Massachusetts, United States

L.C. Fernandes Physiology Department, University Federal of Paraná, Curitiba, Paraná, Brazil

C. Genot Biopolymères Interactions Assemblages, INRA, Nantes, France

B. Grung Department of Chemistry, University of Bergen, Bergen, Norway

K.M. Gura Department of Pharmacy, Boston Children's Hospital, Boston, Massachusetts, United States

A.L. Hansen Department of Clinical Psychology, University of Bergen, Bergen; Centre for Research and Education in Forensic Psychiatry, Haukeland University Hospital, Bergen, Norway

M.A. Harris Department of Food Science and Human Nutrition, College of Health and Human Sciences, Colorado State University, Fort Collins, Colorado, United States

W.S. Harris Department of Internal Medicine, Sanford School of Medicine, University of South Dakota, Sioux Falls, South Dakota; OmegaQuant Analytics, LLC, Sioux Falls, South Dakota, United States

K. Hintze Department of Nutrition, Dietetics and Food Sciences, Utah State University, Logan, Utah, United States

A. Ismail Global Organization for EPA and DHA Omega-3s (GOED), Salt Lake City, Utah, United States

J. Jaczynski Division of Animal and Nutritional Sciences, West Virginia University, Morgantown, West Virginia, United States

L. Jahns United States Department of Agriculture, Agricultural Research Service, Grand Forks Human Nutrition Research Center, Grand Forks, North Dakota, United States

E.U. Kabataş Department of Ophthalmology, Dr Sami Ulus Maternity and Children Training and Research Hospital, Ankara, Turkey

M.W. Khan DST-INSPIRE Faculty, Cell Biology & Physiology Division, CSIR-Indian Institute of Chemical Biology, Kolkata, India

S.A. Khan SVKMs Mithibai College, Bhakti Vedanta Swami Marg, Mumbai, India

P.M. Kris-Etherton Department of Nutritional Sciences, The Pennsylvania State University, University Park, Pennsylvania, United States

C.J. Lammi-Keefe School of Nutrition and Food Sciences, Louisiana State University, Baton Rouge, Louisiana; Pennington Biomedical Research Center, Baton Rouge, Louisiana, United States

B. Lands American Society for Nutrition, College Park, Maryland, United States

M. Lankinen Institute of Public Health and Clinical Nutrition, University of Eastern Finland, Kuopio, Finland

J. Lara Department of Applied Sciences, Faculty of Health and Life Sciences, Northumbria University, Newcastle upon Tyne, United Kingdom

M. Lean School of Medicine, University of Glasgow, Glasgow Royal Infirmary, Glasgow, Scotland

M.D. Lewis Brain Health Education and Research Institute, Potomac, Maryland, United States

P.L. McLennan School of Medicine, University of Wollongong, Wollongong, New South Wales, Australia

A. Meynier Biopolymères Interactions Assemblages, INRA, Nantes, France

M-C. Michalski CarMeN Laboratory, INRA UMR1397, INSERM U1060, Université de Lyon, INSA-Lyon, Villeurbanne, France

G.E. Peoples School of Medicine, University of Wollongong, Wollongong, New South Wales, Australia

M.J. Picklo United States Department of Agriculture, Agricultural Research Service, Grand Forks Human Nutrition Research Center, Grand Forks, North Dakota, United States

S. Priyamvada Division of Gastroenterology and Hepatology, Department of Medicine, University of Illinois at Chicago, Chicago, Illinois, United States

M. Puder Department of Surgery and Vascular Biology Program, Boston Children's Hospital, Boston, Massachusetts, United States

R. Ramón Bonache Life-course Health Promotion and Prevention Department, General Directorate of Public Health, Valencia; Spanish Consortium for Research on Epidemiology and Public Health (CIBERESP), Spain

H.B. Rice Global Organization for EPA and DHA Omega-3s (GOED), Salt Lake City, Utah, United States

C.K. Richter Department of Nutritional Sciences, The University of Arizona, Tucson, Arizona, United States

N. Salem Jr. Nutritional Lipids, DSM Nutritional Products, Columbia, Maryland, United States

M. Seelaender Department of Cell and Developmental Biology, Institute of Biomedical Sciences and Department of Surgery, Faculdade de Medicina, University of São Paulo, São Paulo, Brazil

A.P. Simopoulos The Center for Genetics, Nutrition and Health, Washington, District of Columbia, United States

A.C. Skulas-Ray Department of Nutritional Sciences, The Pennsylvania State University, University Park, Pennsylvania, United States

B.T. Steffen Department of Laboratory Medicine and Pathology, University of Minnesota, Minneapolis, Minnesota, United States

L.M. Steffen Division of Epidemiology and Community Health, University of Minnesota School of Public Health, Minneapolis, Minnesota, United States

C. Tørris Department of Behavioural Sciences, Faculty of Health Sciences, Oslo and Akershus University of Applied Sciences, Oslo, Norway

R. Tahergorabi Department of Family and Consumer Sciences, North Carolina Agricultural and Technical State University, Greensboro, North Carolina, United States

I. Thorsdottir School of Health Sciences, University of Iceland, Háskóli Íslands, Iceland

S.M. Ulven Department of Nutrition, University of Oslo, Oslo, Norway

C. von Schacky Preventive Cardiology, Medical Clinic I, Ludwig Maximilians-University, Munich; Omegametrix, Martinsried, Germany

R. Ward Department of Nutrition, Dietetics and Food Sciences, Utah State University, Logan, Utah, United States

A.N.K. Yusufi Department of Biochemistry, Faculty of Life Sciences, Aligarh Muslim University, Aligarh, UP, India

F.N. Khan Yusufi Department of Statistics and Operations Research, Faculty of Science, Aligarh Muslim University, Aligarh, UP, India

S. Zheng Division of Nutrition and Food Sciences, Department of Health Sciences, California Baptist University, Riverside, California, United States

Preface

Fish is an important dietary component due to its contribution of valuable nutrients. In addition to the high quality protein and micronutrients provided, fish is the primary source of long chain omega-3 fatty acids which are found in oils of "fatty" cold water fish. Biomedical evidence supports the importance of nutrients in fish and fish oil in promoting normal nutrition for growth, development, and health maintenance. In addition, fish and fish oil have been shown to lower the risk of progressive chronic disorders (eg, cardiovascular, metabolic, and inflammatory diseases) and may be useful in disease treatment. The intention of this book is to provide current and indepth information on these topics. Additional important information is included regarding the availability of fish for consumption as well as other issues relevant to the inclusion of fish in the diet. The book, written by an international group of experts in human nutrition, medicine, and fish biology, provides current up to date information on these topics and more. The structure of the text includes main topics covering fish and fish oil intake, fish and fish oil nutrition in the lifecycle, fish and fish oil in health promotion and disease prevention, and the wild and farmed fish supply.

Our goal for this book is to clearly describe what is currently known about fish and fish oil intake in nutrition and health. The included chapters explore the current literature surrounding their primary topic and provide the authors' view on each subject. Readers will gain knowledge ranging from the current state of fish and fish oil intake; their health promoting effects and influences on individual response; how they influence development and health maintenance through the life cycle; and their role in disease prevention and treatment. This book will be an invaluable resource for basic and clinical researchers working to understand the relationship between fish and human health. It will be a valuable reference for physicians, nutritionists, dietitians, and other health care providers. The text may also be an important for students in nutrition, food science, and other biologic sciences.

Although there is much scientific literature and a number of books devoted to the role of fish oil and omega-3 fatty acids in health and disease treatment, our book is unique in that it also includes scientific assessment of the role of fish consumption. Having long been interested in the role of diet in health promotion, it was a pleasure to work on this text focused on fish. As this topic continues to intrigue, it has been a satisfying endeavor to have the opportunity to conceptualize and then follow through to completion of this text.

Susan K. Raatz
Douglas M. Bibus

Acknowledgment

We are grateful to the authors who have participated in putting this work together by their outstanding contributions. Their effort has made this book a possibility. We would also like to thank Mr Jordan Sprecher from the University of North Dakota, Grand Forks, ND for editorial assistance.

This work was partially supported by USDA-ARS project 3062-51000-053-00D. Any opinions, findings, conclusions, or recommendations expressed in this publication are those of the author(s) and do not necessarily reflect the view of the United States Department of Agriculture. The United States Department of Agriculture, Agricultural Research Service, Plains Area is an equal opportunity/affirmative action employer and all agency services are available without discrimination. Mention of trade names or commercial products in this article is solely for providing specific information and does not imply recommendation or endorsement by the United States Department of Agriculture.

PART I

FISH AND FISH OIL INTAKE AND RECOMMENDATIONS

CHAPTER

1

Fish Intake in the United States

L. Jahns

United States Department of Agriculture, Agricultural Research Service, Grand Forks Human Nutrition Research Center, Grand Forks, North Dakota, United States

Worldwide, fish has an increasingly important role in the health of both developed and developing nations. Demand for sustainability has increased production capacity through aquaculture; in fact, aquaculture now provides half of all seafood in the world (FAO, 2014). In developing countries struggling with undernutrition, fish provide a valuable source of protein (FAO, 2014). In countries where overnutrition is endemic, such as the United States of America (US), seafood consumption can lower energy intake when used to replace protein foods high in saturated fats. Fish is also the best food source of the omega 3 (n–3) long chain polyunsaturated fatty acids eicosapentaenoic acid (EPA; 20:5n3) and docosahexaenoic acid (DHA; 22:6n3). Fish consumption is strongly associated with decreased risk of cardiovascular disease (Raatz et al., 2013; Virtanen et al., 2008). Depending upon the species, fish can also be a rich source of iodine, selenium, potassium, vitamin D and B vitamins (Health Canada, 2010; NDL, 2015; Table 1.1).

Unlike many other countries, the US has no formal recommendations for intake of EPA or DHA. The American Heart Association recommends at least two 3.5 oz servings per week of fish, particularly oily fish (Lloyd–Jones et al., 2010). In the US, the *Dietary Guidelines for Americans, 2010* (DGA, 2010) recommend that Americans over two years of age consume at least 8 oz of seafood each week, which provides an average of 250 mg EPA and DHA per day. Seafood should provide approximately one-fifth of the protein food group intake recommendation, so the amount increases along with energy needs, up to 12 oz/week. No further information as to type of seafood recommended is specified, but high n–3 seafood is encouraged. The most often consumed high n–3, low mercury fish in the US are salmon, anchovies, herring, sardines, Pacific oysters, trout, and Atlantic and Pacific mackerel. Limitations to seafood consumption are also outlined in the recommendations. Because of mercury content, the recommendation for albacore (white) tuna is no more than 6 oz/week for pregnant and breastfeeding women and the following fish should not be eaten at all by pregnant or breastfeeding women: shark, swordfish, tilefish, and king mackerel. Suggestions by the 2015 Dietary Guidelines Advisory Committee are for a diet rich in seafood and that intake can be from both farmed and wild caught sources. (DGAC, 2015).

The US Food and Drug Administration and Environmental Protection Agency (EPA) have also drafted recommendations about fish consumption for women who are or might become pregnant or are breastfeeding, and for young children. The guidelines are consistent with the *Dietary Guidelines for Americans, 2010*, but also include a recommendation that young children should eat 2–3 age appropriate servings per week. Recreational fishers should be aware of and follow any advisories about eating fish from local rivers, streams and lakes. In the absence of advisories, individuals are encouraged to limit caught fish to 6 oz/week and 1–3 oz/week for young children and to consume no other fish that week (FDA, 2014).

IMPORTS AND PRODUCTION

The Fisheries of the US 2013 report states that Food and Agriculture Organization (FAO) calculations indicate that the United States is the 3rd largest consumer of seafood in the world after China and Japan (FUS, 2014). By edible weight, over 90% of US seafood consumed is imported (NOAA, 2015) and the United States is the 2nd largest importer of seafood, after Japan (FAO, 2014), however, the import numbers are somewhat inflated as much imported seafood is caught domestically, shipped overseas for processing, and reimported. In 2013, 5.4 billion pounds of

Fish and Fish Oil in Health and Disease Prevention. http://dx.doi.org/10.1016/B978-0-12-802844-5.00001-4

TABLE 1.1 Nutrient Content of Common Fish per 100 g Portion[a]

Name	Shrimp (mixed, raw)	Atlantic salmon farmed (raw)	Atlantic salmon wild (raw)	Salmon canned	Tuna canned in water	Tilapia (raw)	Alaska pollock (raw)	Atlantic cod (raw)	Fish sticks (frozen, prepared)
Energy (kJ)	297	871	594	576	361	400	233	343	1160
Energy (kcal)	71	208	142	138	86	96	56	82	277
Protein (g)	13.61	29.42	19.84	23.10	19.44	20.08	12.19	17.81	11.01
Total Fat (g)	1.01	13.42	6.34	5.02	0.96	1.70	0.41	0.67	16.23
Calcium (mg)	54	9	12	283	17	10	15	16	16
Iron (mg)	0.21	0.34	0.80	0.77	1.63	0.56	0.22	0.38	0.84
Magnesium (mg)	22	27	29	32	23	27	16	32	25
Phosphorous (mg)	244	240	200	379	139	170	284	203	191
Potassium (mg)	113	363	490	333	179	302	160	413	185
Selenium (μg)	29.6	24.0	36.5	39.5	70.6	41.8	15.9	33.1	15.7
Sodium (mg)	566	59	44	381	247	52	333	54	402
Zinc (mg)	0.97	0.36	0.64	0.96	0.69	0.33	0.31	0.45	0.42
Thiamin (mg)	0.020	0.207	0.226	0.027	0.030	0.041	0.030	0.076	0.122
Riboflavin (mg)	0.015	0.155	0.380	0.202	0.084	0.063	0.080	0.065	0.116
Niacin (mg)	1.778	8.672	7.860	7.409	10.136	3.903	0.653	2.063	1.536
Vitamin B6 (mg)	0.161	0.636	0.818	0.105	0.319	0.162	0.069	0.245	0.078
Vitamin B–12 (μg)	1.11	3.23	3.18	4.95	2.55	1.58	1.63	0.91	0.96
Folate (μg)	19	26	25	4	4	24	3	7	24
Vitamin E (mg)	1.32	3.55	N/A	1.28	0.33	0.40	0.49	0.64	6.88
Vitamin D (mcg)	0.1	[b]6.033	[b]6.370	14.5	1.2	3.1	0.2	0.9	0.0
EPA	0.068	0.862	0.321	0.334	0.028	0.005	0.049	0.064	0.050
DHA	0.070	1.104	1.115	0.743	0.196	0.086	0.116	0.120	0.088

[a] *Values from the USDA National Nutrient Database, Standard Reference release 27.*
[b] *Values from the Canadian Nutrient File, 2010.*

seafood was imported. Over a billion pounds of shrimp was imported in 2013, making it the most highly imported of all seafood; most coming from India, Thailand, and Indonesia. The next highest imported fish was salmon, mostly in the form of fillets, at 600 million pounds. Canned tuna imports were nearly 350 million (FUS, 2014), and tilapia imports over 500 million pounds (ERS, 2015), unsurprising as tilapia has gained popularity in the United States in the past decade. Domestic production of edible fish and shellfish included over 8 billion pounds of commercial landings and nearly 600 million pounds produced by aquaculture. The recreational fish harvest was an estimated 240 million pounds (FUS, 2014).

INDIVIDUAL INTAKE

It is difficult to measure individual fish consumption. This chapter will discuss fish intake from the perspective of four levels of the food supply; (1) disappearance data; (2) self-reported intake at the national level, (3) the retail level; and (4) recreational fishing and subpopulations of the US. All methods suffer from biases, and examples of disparate results from using different data sources are discussed.

Disappearance data

Disappearance, or food availability data, is derived by adding domestic landing and import supplies then subtracting exports and amounts used for industrial purposes such as fish meal to estimate edible weight amounts. This amount is divided by the population number to arrive at a per capita consumption amount. Disappearance data are used in various ways. Often it is used as a proxy for food consumption. Economists use it to track and predict price changes. Market researchers use the data to study market shares for commodity foods. Food availability data can be used to estimate changes in food commodity consumption in response to public health initiatives or changes in the composition of nutrients available for consumption. In the US, the National Marine Fisheries Service of the US Department of Commerce collects data on supply and disappearance of fishery products; the most recent data can be found on their website (http://www.st.nmfs.noaa.gov/). Based upon their disappearance statistics, US per capita intake was 14.5 pounds in 2013, or about 18 g/day (FUS, 2014).

This method is not without limitations. Domestic landings are often sent overseas for further processing and return as imports, potentially inflating the estimates of imported fish and shellfish. Data may be acquired from a number of sources, and error can be introduced at each step of the estimation procedures. Using disappearance data as a proxy for consumption data of seafood may overestimate intake. The USDA Economic Research Service estimates the amounts and value of food loss at the retail and consumer level. Food loss refers to edible food that is not consumed for any reason. At the retail level this includes discarding spoiled or unattractive foods and at the individual level includes spoilage before cooking and plate waste after cooking. In 2010, the food supply provided approximately 15.8 lbs of seafood per capita. Of that, retail loss consisted of about 8% and loss at the consumer level was 31%, or about 6 lbs total (Buzby et al., 2014).

Self-Reported Intake at the National Level

Self-report is another way of measuring intakes. National information on fish consumption in the US comes from the Centers for Disease Control and Prevention, National Center for Health Statistics (NCHS), National Health and Nutrition Examination Survey (NHANES) and its dietary intake component, the USDA, Agricultural Research Service (ARS), What We Eat in America (WWEIA) survey. NHANES is a continuous crosssectional survey of the civilian, noninstitutionalized US population. The survey uses a complex, multistage probability sampling design with oversampling of selected sociodemographic subgroups of public health interest. Sample weights are provided to produce nationally representative estimates. Dietary intake data are collected by two interviewer assisted 24 h dietary recalls administered approximately 10 days apart. As another way of collecting fish intake information, individuals also complete a questionnaire that asks how often different species of seafood were consumed during the past 30 days (NHANES, 2015). Fish intake has been reported using these data during different time periods and with different analytic methodologies, which will be discussed below. Both 24 h recall and questionnaire data have a number of limitations. When an individual completes a 24 h recall, they are prompted to report everything they ate or drank the previous day. Responses are subject to errors such as forgetting or reporting foods incorrectly, particularly with foods considered to be healthy. Importantly, an individual may not know the type of fish they ate, particularly if consumed out of the home. Another limitation is the survey instrument itself. For instance, the current questionnaire asking people to report the number of times a specific fish was consumed in the past 30 days does not list tilapia. Therefore, when using NHANES, tilapia consumption can only be reported by 24 h recall by those who consumed it the previous day, and in the United States, most people do not eat fish every day.

Differences in the top 10 species consumed estimated by disappearance data, 24 h recall self-report and 30 day questionnaire self-report can be seen in Table 1.2. All 3 estimates show shrimp to be the most consumed seafood, followed by tuna. However, discrepancies soon become apparent. Although the third most consumed fish is salmon according to the disappearance and questionnaire data, it is listed as number four using the recall data. Individuals' confusion about what fish they are eating during recalls is apparent as 11% of fish consumed is reported as "unspecified". As the questionnaire did not ask about tilapia specifically, it is possible that tilapia makes up a large part of the "other" fish category. Alaska pollock and pangasius, both listed in the top 10 by disappearance data, are not reported as consumed in the recall data. The questionnaire does not include pangasius but does include pollock. As the 5th most commonly consumed fish in the US by disappearance estimates, pollock is often used to make breaded fish products (Facts.org), most likely making up a large part of the "unspecified" fish category reported by consumers and the "breaded fish" category reported by the questionnaire. In fact, one of the largest fast food chains in the US uses wild-caught pollock in their fish sandwiches (McDonalds, 2015). Pangasius, the 6th most consumed fish, is a catfish produced almost exclusively by aquaculture, but the name is unfamiliar to much of the US population.

TABLE 1.2 Top 10 Consumed Seafood Species by Disappearance Data,[a] Self-Report by 24-h Recall, and Self-Report by 30-day Questionnaire

	Disappearance data per capita in 2012		24-h recall data adults[b] in 2005–2012		30 day questionnaire adults[b] in 2005–2012	
	Species	**lbs**	**Species**	**Percentage of seafood reported**	**Species**	**Times reported consumed in past 30 days**
1.	Shrimp	3.800	Shrimp	26.16	Shrimp	23023
2.	Canned tuna	2.400	Canned tuna	13.75	Tuna	18288
3.	Salmon	2.020	Unspecified fish	10.92	Salmon	13033
4.	Tilapia	1.476	Salmon	8.62	Other fish	8690
5.	Pollock	1.167	Cod	5.77	Catfish	5043
6.	Pangasius	0.726	Flatfish	5.09	Crab	4806
7.	Crab	0.523	Crab	3.87	Breaded fish	3946
8.	Cod	0.521	Tilapia	3.55	Unknown	3671
9.	Catfish	0.500	Catfish	3.53	Cod	3247
10.	Clams	0.347	Unspecified shellfish	2.28	Clams	2483

[a] *https://www.aboutseafood.com/about/about-seafood/top-10-consumed-seafoods*
[b] *Data from National Health and Nutrition Examination Surveys 2005–2012.*

TABLE 1.3 Estimated Amounts (g/day) of Seafood, Fish, and Shellfish Consumed Using National Health and Nutrition Examination Surveys (NHANES) and the Continuing Survey of Food Intakes of Individuals (CSFII)

	Years	Seafood, fish, shellfish	Men and women Mean (SE) (g/day)	Men	Women
Wang et al. (2010)	1988–94	Seafood[b,c]	17.1 (1.3)	20.2 (1.8)	14.4 (1.5)
	1999–04	Seafood[a,c]	14.2 (0.7)	16.5 (1.0)	12.1 (0.7)
Tran et al. (2013)	2003–04	Seafood[a]		18.4	
		Fish[a,c]		13.5 (0.51)	9.2 (0.33)
		Shellfish[a,c]		4.9 (0.27)	3.2(0.15)
		Fish[a,d]		17.9 (0.20)	12.3 (0.14)
		Shellfish[a,d]		8.7 (0.12)	6.0 (0.09)
Papanikolaou et al. (2014)	2003–08	Seafood[a,c]	17.3 (0.8)	20.1 (1.1)	14.5 (0.8)
Jahns et al. (2014)	2005–10	Seafood[a,d]	22.6 (0.8)	25.6 (1.3)	19.8 (0.8)
		Fish[a,d]	18.4 (0.7)	20.3 (1.1)	16.6 (0.8)
		Shellfish[a,d]	9.0 (0.7)	10.8 (1.0)	7.2 (0.6)

[a] *National Health and Nutrition Examination Survey. http://www.cdc.gov/nchs/nhanes/*
[b] *Continuing Survey of Food Intakes by Individuals (http://www.ars.usda.gov/Services/docs.htm?docid=14531).*
[c] *per capita.*
[d] *Seafood consumers only.*

As NHANES has been used to estimate intake amounts at different times and using different methods, reported amounts by 24 h recall data are shown in Table 1.3 (Jahns et al., 2014; Papanikolaou et al., 2014; Tran et al., 2013; Wang et al., 2010). Per capita estimates are similar to that of the most recent disappearance data, ~17 g/day compared to ~18 g/day. Amounts estimated as consumed only by people who report eating seafood are higher, around 20 g/day. Although the single most highly consumed seafood is shrimp, almost twice as much total fish is eaten.

Increasing seafood intake, either by public health interventions or by marketing efforts, requires a segmented approach as the reasons for low consumption may vary by subpopulations of Americans. Facing the underlying factors influencing seafood intake requires an understanding of various interrelated sociodemographic and cultural factors involved. However, the paucity of data (Leung et al., 2012, 2014; Mahaffey et al., 2009; Nayga and Capps, 1995; Wang et al., 2010) within the past 20 years regarding sociodemographic characteristics of those who consume seafood compared to those who do not and the quantity and type of seafood eaten by consumers complicates this issue. Using NHANES data from 2005 to 2010, we combined questionnaire data and 24 h recall data to examine the prevalence of any seafood (fish or shellfish) consumers and the amounts consumed by sociodemographic subgroups (age, income and education level, and race ethnicity).

Eighty-four percent of Americans reported eating any seafood at least once in the past 30 days. Of those, 74% reported eating fish and 54% reported eating shellfish. Since many people ate both fish and shellfish, the percentage of seafood consumers is less than the sum of the two types of seafood. Mean consumption was 23 g/day; and more fish (18 g/day) than shellfish (9 g/day) was eaten. Differences were observed by sociodemographic group (Jahns et al., 2014).

The percentage of women and men who reported eating seafood was not significantly different. Men ate more seafood than women (26 versus 20 g/day). As men generally have higher energy needs and consume more food than women, this is unsurprising. When stratified by sex, there were few differences in either the proportion of consumers or amount consumed in each sociodemographic category (Jahns et al., 2014). Thus, we conclude that it would be less effective to segment public health and marketing interventions by sex than to focus on other characteristics.

Young adults aged 19–30 reported the lowest percentage of seafood consumption (75%) of all age groups compared to adults aged 31–50 (84%), 51–70 (88%), and 71+ (85%). Even among young adults who reported eating seafood, intake was low. Compared to the youngest age group, adults aged 31–50 years and 51–70 consumed more seafood (23 and 25 g/day, respectively, versus 20 g/day). The intake of adults 71+ years (21 g/day) was not different from that of young adults (Jahns et al., 2014). The lower intake observed among adults aged 71+ years may reflect lower energy needs. This observed pattern may indicate a future decline in seafood consumption in the United States if young adults continue their current low intake levels as they age. In the United Kingdom, younger adults also consumed less fish than older adults as reported in a recent review (Weichselbaum et al., 2013). The bulk of research on characteristics of seafood sassociated with seafood intake (Olsen, 2003), even within limited age ranges (Myrland et al., 2000; Trondsen et al., 2004). Olsen examined the reasons for discrepancies in seafood intakes by different age groups (Olsen, 2003). Older individuals reported consuming seafood more frequently than younger individuals. Greater age was associated with having positive attitudes towards seafood, such as saying that it tastes good. The perception that fish is convenient to prepare was also significant, as was consumption of seafood for perceived health benefits. However, whether the pattern identified in Norway is consistent in other countries and cultures remains to be seen. Twenty years earlier, using nationally representative data, researchers in the US also reported a positive relationship of age with fish intake (Nayga and Capps, 1995), and a recent internet survey also reported that individuals aged 45 years or older were more likely than younger age groups to report frequent seafood consumption (Hicks et al., 2008). Using data from 2007 to 2010, Nielsen and coworkers found that of the 83% of men and women who reported eating any seafood in the past 30 days, half reported eating it at least 5 times/month and using data from 2009 to 2012, found that 62% of children aged 1–19 years reported consuming seafood in the previous month, with half consuming it at least three times each month (Nielsen et al., 2015). Although there is little research on fish intake in children, it is somewhat alarming that a large percentage of children do not consume any fish given the beneficial health effects of n–3 fatty acids. It is possible that as people age, they begin to eat more seafood than they did when they were younger. Longitudinal studies beginning in young adulthood would be needed to parse out the question of whether people change their fish intake as they age. Alternatively, as fish and shellfish are discrete foods that are most likely well-remembered, asking older people if they consume more seafood currently than they did in their early adulthood and reasons for any change (or continuation) in consumption habits may yield useful information. Regardless of whether observed differences are due to age or generation effects, further research is needed to identify modifiable factors associated with seafood consumption among young adults.

We stratified household income by those eligible for federal food assistance and those who are not. A smaller percentage of individuals from lower than higher income households reported consuming seafood (81% versus 86%, respectively). However, when seafood was consumed, there was not a significant difference in the amount consumed (Jahns et al., 2014). These results are in line with previous research showing that at greater income levels, the number of times seafood is consumed in the past month is greater. In this study, women with the greatest income consumed fish more often than the lowest income women (5.23 versus 3.65 days, respectively, Mahaffey et al., 2009). Interestingly, low-income participants in federal food assistance programs consumed less seafood and were only about half as likely to meet recommended intakes as income-eligible individuals who did not participate (Leung et al., 2012). However, when including consumers and non-consumers into the estimate, there was no difference in intake by food security status, although the types of fish consumed may differ (Leung et al., 2014). An internet survey of seafood consumption and attitudes towards seafood among almost 1000 individuals also found that individuals with greater income were more likely to report eating seafood at least twice per week (Hicks et al., 2008). Own price elasticity for fish is relatively inelastic compared to other meats, meaning that it is less sensitive to price changes, but this has not yet been studied at different income levels. Individuals with post-secondary education were more likely to consume any seafood and to report the consumption of more seafood than those with lower education levels. A greater percentage of adults with postsecondary education reported intake of seafood (87%) in the past 30 days when compared with those with a high school diploma (82%) or less than a high school degree (78%). Compared to individuals with postsecondary education, those with a high school degree (21 versus 24 g/day or lower (20 versus 24g/day) consumed less of any seafood (Jahns et al., 2014). A study from Belgium reported that individuals at the lowest income level consumed fish the least frequently, but found no association between frequency of fish consumption and education level. Income and education are highly correlated in the US, and both were found to be positively associated with being a seafood consumer (Jahns et al., 2014), suggesting that the disparities in fish consumption may be due to perceived or real cost. However, the greater intake in individuals with postsecondary education indicates that knowledge may also play a role in fish consumption.

There is little information on seafood intake by race-ethnic group. Wang et al. (2010) described trends in amounts of seafood consumption and reported that, in 1999–2004, Non-Hispanic black men and women consumed nearly twice as much seafood as Non-Hispanic whites and Mexican Americans. However, in our analysis we found no differences by race ethnicity in reported seafood intake (Jahns et al., 2014). This discordance may be due to analytic reasons; in our models we controlled for the effects of all other sociodemographic factors examined.

We also compared intakes to the *Dietary Guidelines* recommendations for individuals. The amount recommended varies by energy needs, so while a person with energy needs of 2,000 kcal/day (8,374 kJ/day) has a recommended intake amount of 8 oz (227 g) seafood/week, a person who requires 3,000 kcal/day (12,560 kJ/day) has a recommended intake of 11 oz (312 g) seafood/week. When adjusted for energy needs and activity level (sedentary or active), 80–90% of people did not meet the recommendations (Jahns et al., 2014). Our estimates approximate the proportion of people who do not meet recommendations as reported by recent National Cancer Institute (NCI, 2014) data in which 84% of men and 90% of women did not meet recommended intake amounts. Though simple information in public health messaging is useful, such as recommending a minimum of 8 oz/week, public health researchers and clinicians need to ensure that recommendations are individualized when assessing the adequacy of seafood intake.

Retail Availability and Consumption Patterns

Americans spent $86 billion dollars on seafood in 2013. Of that, $58 billion was spent away from home and $28 billion on food for home consumption (FUS, 2014). At the retail level, half of all supermarket seafood department sales are finfish and three-fourths of fish sold consist of salmon, tilapia, and catfish. Of these, salmon is the largest seller, with 38% of the market share. One-fourth of fish sold is tilapia. The third greatest is catfish at 10%, with cod coming in at 7% (Seafood International, 2015). These figures echo the disappearance data more closely than the self-reported intake. As nearly two-thirds of the money spent on seafood was on away-from-home consumption, it is important to identify patterns of seafood consumption away from home. The USDA Economic Research Service used NHANES data to estimate the amount of fish consumed by retail weight at home and away from home and by different sociodemographic groups. Total per capita consumption was 17 g/day and 45% was consumed away from home. Lower-income individuals consumed the least seafood (15 g/day) and only 38% was consumed outside the home compared to higher-income people who consumed 19 g/day, half of which was outside the home. Contrary to our findings, Non-Hispanic blacks consumed the most fish of all race-ethnic groups (27 g/day), with twice as much consumed at home than away from home (18 versus 9 g/day). Non-Hispanic whites consumed approximately 16 g/day; half away from home. Hispanics consumed the least amount of fish (12 g/day) with slightly more consumed at home than away (7 versus 5 g/day) (ERS, 2014). Again, these findings may differ from our own due to differing analytical methods or the reporting of retail amounts of fish only, not seafood. Although slightly less than half of the fish reported was consumed at home, the majority of money spent on seafood was away from home. In the US, the majority of caloric intake (65%) is from home sources. To increase consumption, research is needed to identify and facilitate determinants of the choice to eat fish at home.

Regional and Subpopulation Consumption

In 2013, approximately 8% of the total fish harvest came from recreational fishing, and the amount of fish caught and kept (not thrown back) was an estimated 240 million pounds. Most of the catch occurred on the Atlantic coast states (51%), the Gulf states (45%), and the Pacific coast (4%), primarily in inland waters. Fifty-seven percent of the harvest occurred in inland areas (FUS, 2014). People fish recreationally for a variety of reasons including relaxation, being outdoors, being with friends, and having fish to eat (Burger, 2002). Subsistence anglers may rely on or supplement their food supply by fishing. Individual fishing for the purpose of having fish to eat can vary by race-ethnicity and by geographic location. Subgroups of Americans, such as some American Indians and Alaska Natives, recent immigrants, and Asians and Pacific Islanders may view fishing as a link to traditional culture.

Much of the extant literature focusing on recreational anglers, geographic differences and population subgroups in the United States is designed in terms of risk assessment. While national estimates are useful for public health messaging about exposure to the general pool of commercially available fish in the food supply, some populations may have very different intake levels, putting them at higher risk for exposure to fish contaminated with dioxin and polychlorobiphenyls (PCBs), mercury and/or arsenic. Small, local studies with targeted populations are needed to describe intake for risk assessment, and as studies assess fish consumption in a variety of ways, making comparisons across studies or to national intake data challenging. For instance, intake of fish and crabs by fishing habits and reasons was investigated on the Newark Bay Complex, a series of waterways between New Jersey and New York State (Burger, 2002). The Newark Bay Complex is considered polluted and advisories are in place about consuming fish from this source, including a total ban on consumption of crabs. Individuals found fishing in this waterway were interviewed and asked about their consumption behavior, knowledge of the health advisories, and reasons for fishing. Most people reported that relaxation or recreation was the main reason they fished, not consumption. Lower income people consumed more of their catch than did higher income individuals, and consumption was positively associated with age for fish, but not for crab. There were also differences by race-ethnicity, with a lower percentage of whites consuming high levels of seafood from their catch than blacks or Hispanics. The authors concluded that while most people did not fish for subsistence reasons, the high amounts of crab and fish eaten by some individuals suggested that tailored messages regarding consumption risk should be targeted to recreational fishers. (Burger, 2002). More information is needed about the reasons people fish and consume their catch to develop effective risk and benefit advisories.

The EPA reviews studies about regional and recreational fishing practices and consumption (EPA, 2011) to make recommendations for fish to be consumed. Recommendations for specific age groups based upon body weight are made using the NHANES data at per capita levels and for consumers at the national level. Recommended values are also set for recreational marine fish intake from the Atlantic, Gulf coast, and Pacific oceans. The mean EPA recommendation for adults over 18 years of age for fish consumption from recreational or subsistence fishing is greatest for products caught from the Gulf coast; 7.2 g/day. The next greatest is for Atlantic fish at 5.6 g/day. The recommended value for Pacific fish is 2.0 g/day. Due to limitations of the available data and heterogeneity of exposure, no recommendations are made for recreational fishers for freshwater fish or for Native Americans specifically (EPA, 2011).

In a recent study, individuals living within 50 miles of a coast reported consuming seafood 5–6 times each month while those in inland areas reported consumption 3–4 times a month. The type of fish also varied; individuals living on the Gulf coast reported consuming shrimp most often and those living close to the Atlantic coast reported consuming the most salmon. Individuals living on the coast also consumed more fish that contain ≥ 0.2 μg/g mercury (Fig. 1.1). Women living in these areas also had greater blood mercury levels. However, within all geographic regions, greater income and being an Asian or Pacific Islander was associated with greater risk of high blood mercury concentrations (Mahaffey et al., 2009).

Asian American and Pacific Islander (AAPI) immigrants may be at risk for exposure to contaminants through subsistence fishing practices and high intakes. In the state of Washington, on the Northwestern Pacific coast of the US, a study described seafood intakes among recent and second generation immigrants from 10 AAPI ethnic groups. All individuals consumed seafood. They found that the average seafood intake was 117 g/kg per day, far greater than the US consumer mean of approximately 23 g/day. Heterogeneity among the ethnic groups was pronounced; Vietnamese and Japanese individuals consumed the most seafood and Hmong, Mien, and Samoan individuals the least. Women, older people, and first-generation immigrants consumed the most seafood. However, most seafood was purchased, either at grocery stores or from street vendors and one-fifth or less was caught, depending upon the ethnic group. These intake rates indicate that, at least in this geographic area, culturally appropriate community based risk messaging is warranted to reduce exposure to contaminants (Sechena et al., 2003).

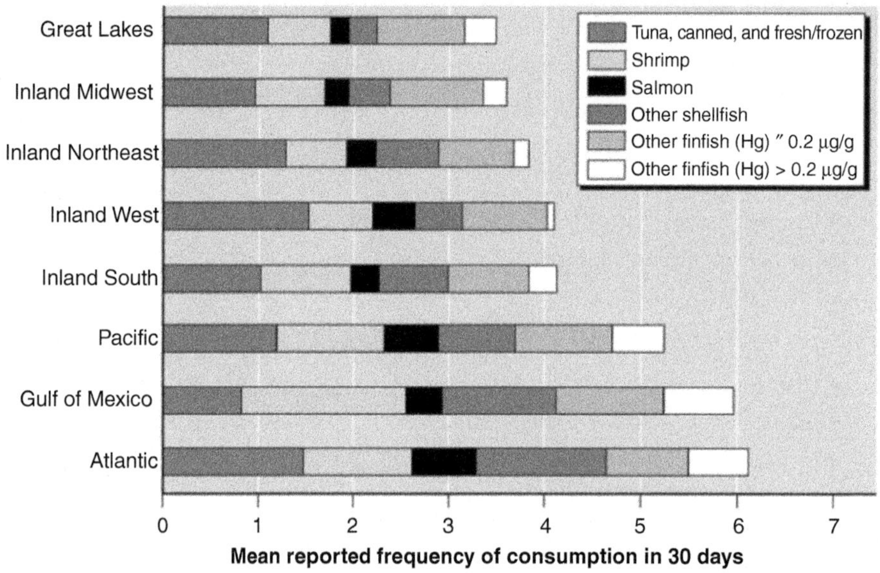

FIGURE 1.1 **Species and frequency of meals consumed by geographic residence.** *Source: Reproduced from Mahaffey K.R., Clickner R.P., and Jeffries R.A., 2009. Adult women's blood mercury concentrations vary regionally in the United States: association with patterns of fish consumption (NHANES 1999–2004). Environ. Health Persp. 117(1), 47–53.*

The term Native American encompasses both American Indian and Alaska Native peoples. There are vast differences between tribal groups and geographic location in the amount and types of fish harvested and consumed, but intake of harvested fish is thought to be greater than that of the general population. This generalization makes the assumption that all Native Americans fish locally, although the literature contains specific groups chosen for their known greater fishing and intake rates. A 2004 review of the literature of fish consumption in the US found that consumption rates for marine recreational fishers were 18–48 g/day, freshwater fishers consumed 5–70 g/day, and Native Americans ate even greater amounts; 57–271 g/day. The author highlights the difficulties in measuring fish intake, especially in vulnerable subpopulations, in a comparable, meaningful way. In addition, there is considerable heterogeneity of fishing practices and dietary intake, making generalizations difficult. The author urges caution and a careful examination of the data from smaller, localized studies in formulating risk advisories (Moya, 2004). Other issues in measuring fish intake and making advisories in Native Americans are data collection methods that are not culturally competent, lack of understanding of tribal values and health beliefs, and bypassing of issues of cultural heritage (Donatuto and Harper, 2008). The limitations of self-reported intake found in national surveys apply to smaller studies as well. In an assessment of fish consumption in Ojibwa tribal members living in the North-Central US and fishing in the Great Lakes Region, fish intake by self-reported food frequency questionnaire was 60 g/day. When individuals were asked to record their catch and weigh it during preparation the amounts were far lower. Amongst the tribe with the greatest consumption by weighed record, the mean intake was only 11 g/day, and the average was 8 g/day, lower than the national average. Another potential bias identified was a seasonal effect; far more individuals reported consuming fish in the spring and summer than the fall and winter. Therefore the time span of selfreported intake could either over- or underestimate intake levels, depending on the season of data collection (Dellinger, 2004).

The Alaska Native population has traditionally relied heavily upon harvested fish in the diet. In the 1980s, fish was the 4th most frequently consumed food after coffee, sugar, and bread and Alaska Natives consumed fish six times more than the general population (Nobmann et al., 1992). Bersamin et al., in a study among Yup'ik Eskimos in Western Alaska, found that the largest source of energy for adults aged 20–39 and 40–81 years was fish and fish roe (15.5% and 19.9% of energy, respectively). Among younger individuals aged 14–19, fish contributed only 8.1% of energy. However, fish was the main source of protein for all age groups (Bersamin et al., 2006). The age disparity has been found in other studies. Another study in two regions of Alaska reported that 10% of total energy came from fish and seafood, but did not examine age groupings (Johnson et al., 2009). Nobmann et al., in a different Alaska Native group, found that younger individuals (aged 17–39 years) consumed less energy from traditional foods than older people aged 40–92 years. The authors also speculate that it is unknown whether younger people will age into increasing the consumption of traditional foods or continue with a more Western diet. In this population, soda was the largest contributor to energy intake and all traditional foods accounted for only 15% of energy, highlighting that generalization about fish intake of Alaska Native peoples must be made cautiously (Nobmann et al., 2005).

BARRIERS TO SEAFOOD CONSUMPTION

Little research has examined the reasons why most Americans do not consume enough fish. The American palate tends to prefer mild "non-fishy" tasting fish; therefore the stronger taste of fatty fish is not as desirable as white fish. Fish is also perceived as expensive and difficult to prepare (Bloomingdale et al., 2010). The majority of money spent on seafood is for consumption outside the home (FUS, 2014), suggesting that handling and preparation of seafood is challenging for many consumers. A national survey found that 46% of individuals listed taste preference as the main reason for not consuming fish, followed by affordability (45%, Hicks et al., 2008). Perceived cost is a barrier to fish consumption for many people. Mozaffarian and Rimm however, describe how consumption of enough fish to obtain 250 mg of EPA and DHA can be achieved at low cost (Mozaffarian and Rimm, 2006), particularly by the use of canned salmon and tuna. Another large study found that among the 16% of people who reported not eating any fish in the past year, the major reason was not liking the taste (65%). Six percent reported having a fish allergy, although another study found that only about 2.5% of Americans report having an allergy to fish or shellfish (Lando and Zhang, 2011; McGowan and Keet, 2013).

Another barrier to fish consumption is conflicting messaging through the media about the benefits and risks associated with eating fish. A qualitative study of fish consumption among pregnant women identified several barriers, including that fish consumption messages were "conflicting and confusing" (Bloomingdale et al., 2010). Consumers report getting most of their information about seafood from the media, more of which is negative than positive (Hicks et al., 2008). Media messages conveying risk far outnumber those reporting the benefits of eating fish. A 15-year study of television and print messages found that 80% of all coverage relating to fish was about health risks, not benefits (Greiner et al., 2010). Amberg and Hall analyzed news coverage of farmed salmon in a 5-year period around two scientific publications in 2003 and 2004 that described risks of farmed salmon consumption. Half of text in articles was about health risks while only 7% reported health benefits. They found that after the 2004 article, over 80% of articles that mentioned health benefits did so in the context of health risk (Amberg and Hall, 2010).

With special advisories for pregnant women, nursing mothers, and young children for specific fish, an overwhelming body of evidence suggests that fish consumption, particularly fatty fish, is important for optimal health for all individuals and benefits outweigh risk (Mozaffarian and Rimm, 2006). It is challenging to communicate both health risks and benefits to the population in a way that is balanced and understandable. Public health officials must be cognizant of unintended shifts in fish intake in response to either effort to increase fish consumption or to decrease contaminant exposure (Cohen et al., 2005). A nationally representative survey found that after a federal advisory in 2001 about specific fish to be avoided by pregnant women, the prevalence of consumer awareness of mercury as a hazard in fish rose from 69% to 80% in 2006. In this study, few individuals could identify specific fish to avoid. Older and better educated individuals with greater income, were more likely to report being aware of recommendations, as were whites compared to other race-ethnic groups. Unfortunately, women of childbearing age did not report greater awareness. In response to an open-ended question, 84% of respondents said they ate fish in the past year. Of those, 17% reported knowledge of the health benefits of fish only, 9% heard only risks from eating fish and 58% reported hearing both. Troublingly, 17% had not heard either message. Those individuals who heard only concerns consumed less fish than those who heard only the benefits (Lando and Zhang, 2011). A study in 2005 found that compared to a control group (nonpregnant and nonpostpartum) pregnant and postpartum women were more likely to report awareness of mercury as a problem in fish. Pregnant women also reported consuming less fish compared to postpartum and control women, although very few reached 12 oz/week. Greater income and education were positively associated with awareness of mercury in food and Non-Hispanic white women were least likely to consume fish, as were younger women (Lando et al., 2012). From 2001 to 2002 another study found that pregnant women decreased intake of all fish, including canned tuna, by approximately 1.4 servings per month. In addition, the number of women consuming fish more than three times a month decreased from 15% to 11% (Oken et al., 2003). Clearly, public messaging about the benefits of fish consumption including recommended intake amounts, and fish to avoid needs to include balanced information that reaches vulnerable subpopulations while not negatively impacting the general population (Hughner et al., 2008).

CONCLUSION

Research is needed to identify not only barriers but facilitators to increasing seafood consumption in the US. It is likely that factors that limit seafood intake by those who do not consume enough seafood will be different from factors that lead people to not eat any seafood. With ~20% of Americans not eating seafood and fewer than

20% of seafood consumers eating recommended amounts, much work remains to move Americans toward seafood consumption at recommended levels while reducing risk of contaminants. To attain that goal, public health intervention is needed at three levels: first, to shift nonseafood eaters to adoption of regular consumption; second, to increase the amount of seafood consumed in those already consuming some seafood; and third, ensure that consumers include n–3 rich seafood in their diets while helping vulnerable subgroups to follow advisories to avoid or limit intake of fish that may pose health risks due to mercury content or other contaminants. The seafood industry can play a role in the promotion of fish in the diet by transmitting health messaging as part of their marketing and by developing products acceptable to consumers that are easy to prepare and at competitive costs with other protein sources. Improvements in aquaculture by selective breeding and feed products to increase the amount of n–3 in fish that are popular in the US will also help increase the healthiness of the fish supply. Adequate production and delivery infrastructure must be in place to ensure the availability of fresh, affordable seafood to support increased demand if recommendations are to be met.

Acknowledgments

This work was supported by the US Department of Agriculture (USDA) and the Agricultural Research Service project USDA 3062-51000-051-00D. The contents of this article do not necessarily reflect the views or policies of the USDA or the Agricultural Research Service. The mention of trade names, commercial products, or organizations does not imply endorsement by the US government.

References

Amberg, S., Hall, T.E., 2010. Precision and rhetoric in media reporting about contamination in farmed salmon. Sci. Comm. 32, 489–513.

Bersamin, A., Luick, B.R., Ruppert, E., Stern, J.S., Zidenberg-Cherr, S., 2006. Diet quality among Yup'ik Eskimos living in rural communities is low: the Center for Alaska Native Health Research Pilot Study. J. Am. Diet Assoc. 106, 1055–1063.

Bloomingdale, A., Guthrie, L.B., Price, S., Wright, R.O., Platek, D., Haines, J., Oken, E., 2010. A qualitative study of fish consumption during pregnancy. Am. J. Clin. Nutr. 92, 1234–1240.

Burger, J., 2002. Consumption Patterns and Why People Fish. Environ. Res. 90, 125–135.

Cohen, J.T., Bellinger, D.C., Connor, W.E., Kris-Etherton, P.M., Lawrence, R.S., Savitz, D.A., Shaywitz, B.A., Teutsch, S.M., Gray, G.M., 2005. A quantitative risk-benefit analysis of changes in population fish consumption. Am. J. Prev. Med. 29, 325–334.

Dellinger, J.A., 2004. Exposure assessment and initial intervention regarding fish consumption of tribal members of the Upper Great Lakes Region in the United States. Environ. Res. 95, 325–340.

Dietary Guidelines Advisory Committee Scientific Report (DGAC), 2015. http://health.gov/dietaryguidelines/2015-scientific-report/14-appendix-e2/e2-38.asp

Dietary Guidelines for Americans (DGA), 2010. U.S. Department of Agriculture and U.S. Department of Health and Human Services, seventh ed. U.S. Government Printing Office, Washington, DC.

Donatuto, J., Harper, B.L., 2008. Issues in evaluating fish consumption rates for Native American tribes. Risk Anal. 28, 1497–1506.

Economic Research Service (ERS), 2015. Aquaculture Data, Aquaculture Trade: Recent Years and Top Countries. http://www.ers.usda.gov/datafiles/Aquaculture/Trade/aquaculturetraderecent.pdf

Economic Research Service (ERS), 2014. Commodity Consumption by Population Characteristics. http://www.ers.usda.gov/data-products/commodity-consumption-by-population-characteristics.aspx

Environmental Protection Agency (EPA), 2011. Exposure Factors Handbook, National Center for Environmental Assessment, EPA/600/R-09/052F, Washington, DC http://www.epa.gov/ncea/efh

FAO. 2014. The State of the World Fisheries and Aquaculture. Food and Agriculture Organization of the United Nations, Rome.

Fisheries of the United States 2013 (FUS), 2014. Current Fishery Statistics No. 2013, National Marine Fisheries Service. https://www.st.nmfs.noaa.gov/Assets/commercial/fus/fus13/FUS2013.pdf

Food and Drug Administration (FDA), 2014. http://www.fda.gov/Food/FoodborneIllnessContaminants/Metals/ucm393070.htm

Greiner, A., Clegg Smith, K., Guallar, E., 2010. Something fishy? News media presentation of complex health issues related to fish consumption guidelines. Public Health Nutr. 13, 1786–1794.

Health Canada, Canadian Nutrient File, 2010. http://webprod3.hc-sc.gc.ca/cnf-fce/index-eng.jsp

Hicks, D., Pivarnik, L., McDermott, R., 2008. Consumer perceptions about seafood -an Internet survey. J. Foodservice 19, 213–226.

Hughner, R.S., Maher, J.K., Childs, N.M., 2008. Review of food policy and consumer issues of mercury in fish. J. Am. Coll. Nutr. 27, 185–194.

Jahns, L., Raatz, S.K., Johnson, L.K., Kranz, S., Silverstein, J.T., Picklo, M.J., 2014. Intake of seafood in the US varies by age, income, and education level but not by race-ethnicity. Nutrients 6, 6060–6075.

Buzby, J.C., Wells, H.F., Hyman, J., 2014. The estimated amount, value, and calories of postharvest food losses at the retail and consumer levels in the United States. Economic Research Service. Economic Information Bulletin No. 121.

Johnson, J.S., Nobmann, E.D., Asay, E., Lanier, A.P., 2009. Dietary intake of Alaska Native people in two regions and implications for health: the Alaska Native Dietary and Subsistence Food Assessment Project. Int. J. Circumpol. Health 68, 109–122.

Lando, A.M., Fein, S.B., Choinière, C.J., 2012. Awareness of methylmercury in fish and fish consumption among pregnant and postpartum women and women of childbearing age in the United States. Environ. Res. 116, 85–92.

Lando, A.M., Zhang, Y., 2011. Awareness and knowledge of methylmercury in fish in the United States. Environ. Res. 111, 442–450.

Leung, C.W., Ding, E.L., Catalano, P.J., Villamor, E., Rimm, E.B., Willett, W.C., 2012. Dietary intake and dietary quality of low-income adults in the Supplemental Nutrition Assistance Program. Am. J. Clin. Nutr. 96, 977–988.

Leung, C.W., Epel, E.S., Ritchie, L.D., Crawford, P.B., Laraia, B.A., 2014. Food insecurity is inversely associated with diet quality of lower-income adults. J. Acad. Nutr. Diet 114, 1943–1953, e1942.

Lloyd–Jones, D.M., Hong, Y., Labarthe, D., Mozaffarian, D., Appel, L.J., Van Horn, L., Greenlund, K., Daniels, S., Nichol, G., Tomaselli, G.F., Arnett, D.K., Fonarow, G.C., Ho, P.M., Lauer, M.S., Masoudi, F.A., Robertson, R.M., Roger, V., Schwamm, L.H., Sorlie, P., Yancy, C.W., Rosamond, W.D., 2010. Defining and setting national goals for cardiovascular health promotion and disease reduction: the American Heart Association's strategic impact goal through 2020 and beyond. Circulation 121, 586–613.

Mahaffey, K.R., Clickner, R.P., Jeffries, R.A., 2009. Adult women's blood mercury concentrations vary regionally in the United States: association with patterns of fish consumption (NHANES 1999–2004). Environ. Health Persp. 117, 47–53.

McDonalds, 2015 http://www.mcdonalds.com/content/us/en/your_questions/our_food/what-type-of-fish-do-you-use-in-the-filet-o-fish.html

McGowan, E.C., Keet, C.A., 2013. Prevalence of self-reported food allergy in the National Health and Nutrition Examination Survey (NHANES) 2007–2010. J. Allergy Clin. Immunol. 132, 1216–1219, e1215.

Moya, J., 2004. Overview of fish consumption rates in the United States. Human Ecol. Risk Assess.Int. J. 10, 1195–1211.

Mozaffarian, D., Rimm, E.B., 2006. Fish intake, contaminants, and human health: evaluating the risks and the benefits. JAMA 296, 1885–1899.

Myrland, O., Trondsen, T., Johnston, R.S., Lund, E., 2000. Determinants of seafood consumption in Norway: lifestyle, revealed preferences, and barriers to consumption. Food Quality Prefer. 11, 169–188.

National Cancer Institute (NCI), 2014. http://appliedresearch.cancer.gov/diet/usualintakes/pop/2007-10/table_b12.html

National Health and Nutrition Examination Survey (NHANES), 2015. About the National Health and Nutrition Examination Survey. National Center for Health Statistics; CDC; US Department of Health and Human Services, Hyattsville, MD. http://www.cdc.gov/nchs/nhanes/about_nhanes.htm

National Oceanic and Atmospheric Administration (NOAA), 2015. http://www.st.nmfs.noaa.gov/Assets/commercial/fus/fus13/materials/FUS2013_FactSheet_FINAL.pdf

Nayga, J.R., Capps, J., 1995. Factors affecting the probability of consuming fish and shellfish in the away from home and at home markets. J. Agr. Appl. Econ. 27, 161–171.

Nielsen, S.J., Aoki, Y., Kit, B.K., Ogden, C.L., 2015. More than half of US youth consume seafood and most have blood mercury concentrations below the EPA reference level 2009–2012. J. Nutr. 145, 322–327.

Nobmann, E.D., Byers, T., Lanier, A.P., Hankin, J.H., Jackson, M.Y., 1992. The diet of Alaska Native adults: 1987–1988. Am. J. Clin. Nutr. 55, 1024–1032.

Nobmann, E.D., Ponce, R., Mattil, C., Devereux, R., Dyke, B., Ebbesson, S.O., Laston, S., MacCluer, J., Robbins, D., Romenesko, T., Ruotolo, G., Wenger, C.R., Howard, B.V., 2005. Dietary intakes vary with age among Eskimo adults of Northwest Alaska in the GOCADAN study 2000–2003. J. Nutr. 135, 856–862.

Nutrient Data Laboratory (NDL), 2015. US Department of Agriculture, Agricultural Research Service, National Nutrient Database for Standard Reference, Release 27. http://www.ars.usda.gov/ba/bhnrc/ndl

Oken, E., Kleinman, K.P., Berland, W.E., Simon, S.R., Rich–Edwards, J.W., Gillman, M.W., 2003. Decline in fish consumption among pregnant women after a national mercury advisory. Obstet. Gynecol. 102, 346–351.

Olsen, S.O., 2003. Understanding the relationship between age and seafood consumption: the mediating role of attitude, health involvement and convenience. Food Qual. Prefer. 14, 199–209.

Papanikolaou, Y., Brooks, J., Reider, C., Fulgoni, 3rd., V.L., 2014. U.S. adults are not meeting recommended levels for fish and omega-3 fatty acid intake: results of an analysis using observational data from NHANES 2003–2008. Nutr. J. 13(31), 1–6.

Raatz, S.K., Silverstein, J.T., Jahns, L., Picklo, M.J., 2013. Issues of fish consumption for cardiovascular disease risk reduction. Nutrients 5, 1081–1097.

Seafood International, 2015. http://seafoodinternationaldigital.com/

Sechena, R., Liao, S., Lorenzana, R., Nakano, C., Polissar, N., Fenske, R., 2003. Asian American and Pacific Islander seafood consumption-a community-based study in King County, Washington. J. Expo. Anal. Environ. Epidemiol. 13, 256–266.

Tran, N.L., Barraj, L.M., Bi, X., Schuda, L.C., Moya, J., 2013. Estimated long-term fish and shellfish intake-national health and nutrition examination survey. J. Expo. Sci. Environ. Epidemiol. 23, 128–136.

Trondsen, T., Braaten, T., Lund, E., Eggen, A.E., 2004. Health and seafood consumption patterns among women aged 45–69 years. A Norwegian seafood consumption study. Food Qual. Prefer. 15, 117–128.

Virtanen, J.K., Mozaffarian, D., Chiuve, S.E., Rimm, E.B., 2008. Fish consumption and risk of major chronic disease in men. Am. J. Clin. Nutr. 88, 1618–1625.

Wang, Y., Beydoun, M.A., Caballero, B., Gary, T.L., Lawrence, R., 2010. Trends and correlates in meat consumption patterns in the US adult population. Public Health Nutr. 13, 1333–1345.

Weichselbaum, E., Coe, S., Buttriss, J., Stanner, S., 2013. Fish in the diet: a review. Nutr. Bull. 38, 128–177.

CHAPTER

2

Fish and Fish Oil in the Mediterranean Diets

A.P. Simopoulos

The Center for Genetics, Nutrition and Health, Washington, District of Columbia, United States

INTRODUCTION

The beneficial effects of Mediterranean diets have been studied for many years, beginning with the Seven Countries Study and continuing today (Keys, 1970). Although some authors refer to the "Mediterranean Diet" there is not "one" Mediterranean diet (Simopoulos and Visioli, 2000; Simopoulos and Visioli, 2006) and in fact the term "Mediterranean diet" may be considered a misnomer. The populations around the Mediterranean basin have different cultures, religions, economic prosperity, and educational profiles. In epidemiological studies it has been customary to compare health statistics and poorly defined dietary patterns of people in Southern Europe (Mediterranean) and Northern Europe without taking into consideration the different types of fats (monounsaturated (MUFA), omega-6 (n–6), omega-3 (n–3), and *trans* fatty acids), or genetic differences in the populations, such as the genotypic frequencies of APOE4 and factor VII between Northern and Southern Europe. This approach led to conclusions that are; (1) the major dietary factors contributing to the development of coronary heart disease (CHD) were due to saturated fat (SFA) and cholesterol intake and (2) to the dominance of the lipid hypothesis in the causation of CHD. What is distressing is the fact that the over emphasis on replacing SFA with polyunsaturated (PUFA) oils to lower serum cholesterol levels led to an unprecedented experiment in Western societies, namely the introduction of large amounts of vegetable oils (corn oil, sunflower, safflower, cottonseed, and soybean) rich in n–6 fatty acids (Figure 2.1). Omega-6 fatty acids increase the tendency to inflammation, thrombus, and tumor formation. This Chapter reviews the importance of the composition of the Mediterranean diets, focusing on the diet of Crete as the best representative diet consistent with the diet of evolution being balanced in the n–6/n–3 fatty acid ratio. The review focuses on n–3 fatty acids both from terrestrial-alpha-linolenic acid (ALA) and marine sources eicosapentaenoic acid (EPA), docosapentaenoic acid (DPA), and docosahexaenoic acid (DHA) as significant biomarkers for the Mediterranean diet adherence score and major contributors to health.

THE MEDITERRANEAN DIET

Historical Aspects and the Seven Countries Study

Although Greece and the Mediterranean countries are usually considered as areas of medium high death rates (14.0–18.0 per 1000 inhabitants), death rates on the island of Crete have been below this level continuously since before 1930 (Allbaugh, 1953). No other area in the Mediterranean basin has had as low a death rate as the island of Crete, according to data compiled by the United Nations in their Demographic Yearbook for 1948 (Allbaugh, 1953). It was 11.3–13.7 prewar and about 10.6 in 1946–48 (Allbaugh, 1953). Cancer and heart disease caused almost three times as many deaths proportionally in the USA as in Crete (Allbaugh, 1953). The diet of Crete represents the traditional diet of Greece prior to 1960.

Fish and Fish Oil in Health and Disease Prevention. http://dx.doi.org/10.1016/B978-0-12-802844-5.00002-6

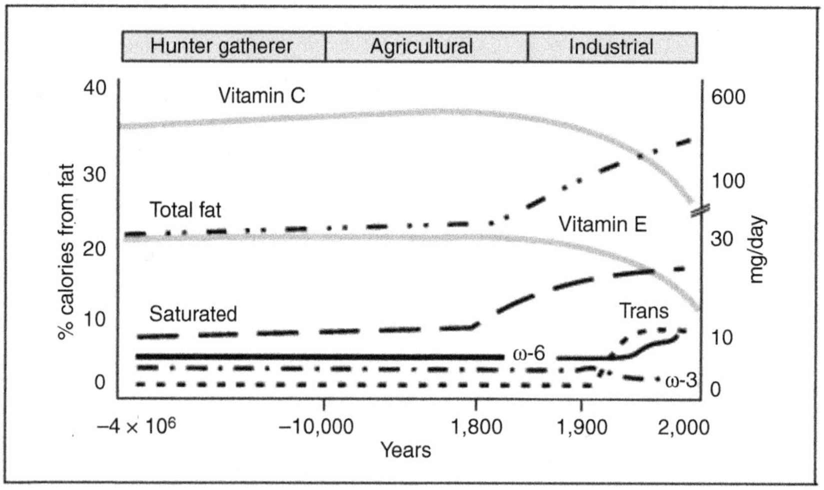

FIGURE 2.1 Hypothetical scheme of fat, fatty acid (w–3, w–6, trans, and total) intake (as percent of calories from fat) and intake of vitamins E and C (mg/day). Data were extrapolated from crosssectional analyses of contemporary hunter–gatherer populations and from longitudinal observations and their putative changes during the preceding 100 years.

The first survey on diet and health in Crete took place in the fall of 1948 by Leland G. Allbaugh, who was the Field Director of the Crete survey. The survey was sponsored by the Rockefeller Foundation and was published in 1953 by Princeton University Press (Allbaugh, 1953). In 1948, the Cretan diet consisted chiefly of foods of vegetable origin, with cereals, vegetables, fruits, and olive oil predominating. Pulses and nuts were eaten in appreciable quantities, especially during the winter, and potatoes were used quite extensively, whereas meat, fresh fish, milk, eggs and sweets were consumed in relatively small amounts. Butter was seldom used. Slightly more cheese per person was consumed in Crete than in the USA. The frequent use of braising and boiling and the commendable habit of dipping bread into the sauce saved nutrients, particularly minerals and vitamins.

Olive oil, olives, cereal grains, pulses, wild greens, herbs, and fruits, together with limited quantities of goat meat and milk, snails, game, and fish were the basic Cretan foods for forty centuries (Allbaugh, 1953). Such evidence is substantiated from the agricultural products, storage facilities, equipment, and artwork found in the Minoan ruins. Additional indications of the food patterns of the past and the changes, which have taken place, are found in Homer and in the writings of others down through the centuries. Except for the addition of citrus fruit and tomatoes during the past millennium, and of apples, grapes, wine, pomegranates, and sheep during the Doric era, almost three millenniums ago, the basic foods for the modern Cretan diet are probably much the same as during the Minoan period about 2000 BC that is 4500 years ago (Allbaugh, 1953).

The Seven Countries Study was the first to establish credible data on cardiovascular disease prevalence rates in contrasting populations (United States, Finland, The Netherlands, Italy, former Yugoslavia, Japan, and Greece), with differences found on the order of 5- to 10-fold in coronary heart disease (Keys, 1970). In 1958, the fieldwork started in Dalmatia in the former Yugoslavia. From the inception of the research program an important focus was on the diet and its possible relationship to the etiology of coronary heart disease. The five-year follow-up found favorable all-cause death rates in Greece, Japan, and Italy compared with the other areas, as well as a lower incidence rate of coronary disease (Keys, 1970). The Seven Countries Study was designed to investigate relations between diet and cardiovascular diseases, primarily described in terms of the fatty acid composition of the diet.

Thus interest in the Mediterranean diets derives directly from the results in the Seven Countries Study. After 5–15 years of follow-up, the study demonstrated that the mortality rate from coronary heart disease in southern Europe was two- to three-fold lower than in northern Europe or the United States (Keys, 1970). The mortality from coronary heart disease and all causes, in the cohort from Crete, was much lower than that among the nine other cohorts from southern Europe. These findings suggested that the population of Crete could be considered to have the greatest life expectancy in the Western world, even though average serum cholesterol concentrations in the population of Crete were similar to those in the other Mediterranean cohorts. What are the components in the diet of Crete that are responsible for longer life expectancy? They certainly could not be those that influence serum cholesterol concentrations. We embarked on a series of studies to evaluate the nutritional composition of the diet of Crete in terms of the antioxidant content and n–6 and n–3 fatty acids (Simopoulos, 2001).

TABLE 2.1 Fatty Acid Content of Plants[a]

Fatty acid	Purslane	Spinach	Mustard	Red leaf lettuce	Buttercrunch lettuce
14:0	0.16	0.03	0.02	0.03	0.01
16:0	0.81	0.16	0.13	0.10	0.07
18:0	0.20	0.01	0.02	0.01	0.02
18:1n–9	0.43	0.04	0.01	0.01	0.03
18:2n–6(LA)	0.89	0.14	0.12	0.12	0.10
18:3n–3(LNA)	4.05	0.89	0.48	0.31	0.26
18:5n–3(EPA)	0.01	0.00	0.00	0.00	0.00
18:6n–3(DHA)	0.00	0.00	0.001	0.002	0.001
Other	1.95	0.43	0.32	0.12	0.11
Total fatty acid content	8.50	1.70	1.101	0.702	0.60

Values are expressed as mg/g of wet weight.
[a] *Modified from Simopoulos and Salem (1986).*

The Composition of the Diet of Crete

In the past, major emphasis was put on the low SFA content of the Mediterranean diets while more recent evidence has emphasized the importance of plant foods (including carbohydrates and nondigestible fiber) rich in antioxidants, phytochemicals, and of the regular use of olive oil (Simopoulos, 2001). There is growing evidence that classic risk factors such as serum cholesterol and blood pressure are not much different in the populations of southern Europe when compared to other Western countries, suggesting that other unexplored risk factors in addition to the classical ones, may be favorably affected by their diets (Simopoulos, 2001).

Although the investigators of the Seven Countries Study emphasized the low SFA intake and the high MUFA fat intake from olive oil as the major factors responsible for the biological health effects of the diet of Crete being associated with the lowest rate of coronary heart disease and the longest life expectancy (Keys, 1970), there is good evidence that foods rich in n–3 fatty acids both from terrestrial and marine sources and antioxidants could account for the decreased death rate of the people of Crete (Renaud et al., 1986; de Lorgeril et al., 1994; Renaud et al., 1995; de Lorgeril et al., 1998; de Lorgeril and Salen, 2000). The Cretans obtained alpha-linolenic acid (ALA) by eating wild plants (Table 2.1) (Simopoulos and Salem, 1986; Simopoulos et al., 1992; Simopoulos et al., 1995), snails, nuts, fruit (figs), and eggs (Table 2.2) (Simopoulos and Salem, 1989; Simopoulos and Salem, 1992); and EPA and DHA from fresh fish and dry or canned sardines and herring, and from eggs (Simopoulos and Salem, 1989; Simopoulos and Salem, 1992), game (Crawford, 1968), and snails. Grazing animal's meat contains n–3 fatty acids whereas grain-fed animal's meat does not (Crawford, 1968). Since sheep, swine, and goats graze, they obtain n–3 fatty acids from grass, moss, purslane (Simopoulos and Salem, 1986; Simopoulos et al., 1992; Simopoulos et al., 1995), and in general from the leaves and stems of green leafy vegetables. They also feed on dry fruits and nuts. In some areas the swine feed on acorns. The livestock obtain a mixture of n–6 and n–3 fatty acids from the foods they eat, and the same mixture is found in their meat and in the milk and the cheese and all other dairy products made from the milk (Simopoulos, 1991; Simopoulos, 1999a). This balance of n–6:n–3 fatty acids is lost in the Western diets (Fig. 2.1, Table 2.3) (Simopoulos, 1999b). Due to agribusiness, the grain-fed animals have higher amounts of n–6 fatty acids in their meat unlike animals in the wild. The vegetable oils such as corn, sunflower, safflower, and cottonseed oil are all very rich in n–6 fatty acids and the margarines made from them contain *trans* fatty acids that behave like SFAs in terms of raising blood cholesterol while lowering HDL (Simopoulos, 1994). Eggs from chickens eating wild greens, worms and insects produce eggs balanced in n–6 and n–3 fatty acids with a ratio of 1.3 whereas the USA supermarket egg has a ratio of about 20 (Simopoulos and Salem, 1989; Simopoulos and Salem, 1992, Table 2.2). Studies of the serum cholestery1 esters of the people in Crete showed a three-fold increase of ALA versus the population of Zutphen (Table 2.4, Sandker et al., 1993). Wine, fruits, vegetables, and olive oil provide high amounts of vitamin C, vitamin E, lycopene, beta-carotene, polyphenols, and other antioxidants (Slater and Block, 1991; Hertog et al., 1992; Mazur et al., 1998; Joseph et al., 1999; Weisburger, 1999). The importance of a Cretan-type diet rich in ALA, fish, fruits, and vegetables has been demonstrated in the Diet and Reinfarction Trial (DART) (Burr et al., 1989), the Lyon Heart Study (de

TABLE 2.2 Fatty Acid Levels in Chicken Eggs Yolks[a] (mg of Fatty Acids[b])

Fatty acid	Greek egg	Supermarket egg
Saturated fats		
Total	100.66	80.65
Monounsaturated fats		
16:1n–7	21.70	4.67
18:1	120.50	109.97
20:1n–9	0.58	0.68
22:1n–9	–	–
24:1n–9	–	0.04
Total	142.78	115.36
n–6 Fatty acids		
18:2n–6	16.00	26.14
18:3n–6	–	0.25
18:2n–6	0.17	0.36
18:3n–6	0.46	0.47
18:4n–6	5.40	5.02
18:4n–6	0.70	0.37
18:5n–6	0.29	1.20
Total	23.02	33.81
n–3 Fatty acids		
18:3n–3	6.90	0.52
18:3n–3	0.16	0.03
18:5n–3	1.20	–
18:5n–3	2.80	0.09
18:6n–3	6.60	1.09
Total	17.66	1.73
Ratio of fatty acids to saturated fats	0.4	0.44
Ratio of n–6 to n–3	1.3	19.4

[a] *The eggs were hard-boiled, and their fatty acid composition and lipid content were assessed.*
[b] *Per gram of egg yolk.*

TABLE 2.3 The n–6:n–3 Ratios in Various Populations

Population	n–6:n–3	Reference
Paleolithic	0.79[a,b]	Eaton et al. (1998)
Greece prior to 1960	1.00-2.00	Simopoulos (1998)
Current United States	16.74	Eaton et al. (1998)
United Kingdom and northern Europe	15.00	Sanders (2000)
Japan	4.00	Sugano and Hirahara (2000)
India rural	5-6.1	Pella et al. (2003)
India urban	38-50	Pella et al. (2003)

[a] *Data from Eaton et al. (1998) Dietary intake of long-chain polyunsaturated fatty acids during the paleolithic. World Rev. Nutr. Diet 1998; 83:12–23.*
[b] *Assuming an energy intake of 35:65 of animal: plant sources.*

TABLE 2.4 Mean Fatty Acid Composition of Cholesteryl Esters in Serum of 92 Elderly Men from Crete and 97 Elderly Men from Zutphen[a,b]

	Percentage (%) methylesters		
Fatty acids	**Crete**	**Zutphen**	***P* value**
16:0	11.1 ± 1.0	11.9 ± 1.3	<0.001
16:1	3.2 ± 1.1	2.9 ± 1.6	0.213
18:0	0.7 ± 0.3	1.1 ± 0.5	<0.001
18:1	31.0 ± 2.7	21.4 ± 3.9	<0.001
18:2n–6	41.9 ± 3.7	53.1 ± 6.5	<0.001
18:3n–3	0.9 ± 0.5	0.3 ± 0.4	<0.001
18:4n–6	6.5 ± 1.6	4.5 ± 1.5	<0.001
Others	4.6 ± 3.3	4.7 ± 3.7	0.891
Ratio 18:2/18:1	1.37 ± 0.20	2.60 ± 0.75	<0.001

[a] *Results are expressed as mean % (by weight) methylesters ±SD.*
[b] *Modified from Sandker et al., 1993.*

Lorgeril et al., 1994), the study by Singh et al. (1992, 1997) and the Gruppo Italiano per lo Studio della Sopravivenza nell'Infarto miocardico (GISSI)-Prevenzione trial (GISSI, 1999).

Olive oil being high in MUFA and low in SFA and n–6 fatty acids does not compete with the desaturation and elongation of ALA nor with the incorporation of n–3 fatty acids into the red cell membrane phospholipids (Simopoulos, 1991). Furthermore, the n–6:n–3 ratio in the Greek diet is between 2–1:1 which is very close to the dietary ratio of the Paleolithic diet (Eaton et al., 1998) (Table 2.3). The beneficial effects of such a ratio and their importance in normal growth and development (Birch et al., 1993; Uauy et al., 1994; Birch et al., 1998) and in the prevention and management of cardiovascular disease, hypertension, diabetes, arthritis, and possibly cancer have been extensively reviewed (Leaf and Weber, 1988; Simopoulos, 1991; Simopoulos et al., 1991; GISSI, 1999; Lagarde et al., 1999; Simopoulos, 1999c; Simopoulos et al., 1999).

Since the Greeks have a cultural dislike for animal fats, the SFA intake of the Greek diet is lower than other Western diets (Allbaugh, 1953). The Greek diet as exemplified by the diet of Crete is characterized by being moderate in fat (about 35%), low in SFA (7%–8%), high in MUFA, and balanced in the n–6:n–3 essential fatty acids. The antioxidant and phytoestrogen content, and other phytochemicals is much higher than in other diets of the people around the Mediterranean basin because Greeks continue to eat wild greens which are rich sources of ALA, vitamin C, vitamin E, glutathione, and melatonin (Simopoulos and Salem, 1986; Simopoulos et al., 1992; Simopoulos et al., 1995; Simopoulos et al., 2005). The beneficial effects of the various compounds found in the vegetables and fruits eaten by Greeks have been shown to have euglycemic, hypocholesterolemic, and antitumor properties in animal experiments (Slater and Block, 1991). Even today the mortality from breast cancer is lower in Greece than in the USA, Japan and Europe (Levi et al., 1995). Finally, the Lyon Heart Study based on the modified diet of Crete described by de Lorgeril et al. (1994) clearly showed cardioprotective and anticancer effects in a French population indicating that such a diet is not only palatable but can be adapted to other populations. Furthermore, one could consider that the traditional diet of Greece even in its present form is the diet that is closer, than the diets of other developed countries, to the diet on which humans evolved (Fig. 2.1).

What appears to be so special about the Greek diet relative to the other Mediterranean diets is the content of bioprotective nutrients, specifically: (1) a balanced intake of essential fatty acids from vegetable, animal and marine sources, (2) an n–6:n–3 ratio of about 2:1 instead of 10–20:1 as in Europe and the US, respectively, and (3) a high antioxidant intake from fruits and vegetables from both cultivated and wild sources.

MEDITERRANEAN DIET AND OMEGA-3 FATTY ACIDS

Healthy Mediterranean Seafood and the Omega-3 Fatty Acid Intake

The Mediterranean Sea is characterized by a variety of fish. It has been estimated that more than 8500 species of fish live in the Mediterranean Sea, which is considered to be between 4% and 18% of the world marine species.

Compared to the world oceans, the Mediterranean Sea is only 0.82% in surface area and 0.32% in volume (Bianchi and Morri, 2000). About 84% of the marine species are animals, of which 77% invertebrates and 7% vertebrates, while the 16% left are algae and sea grasses (Bianchi and Morri, 2000).

Lloret states that, "Biological and chemical investigations have shown that Mediterranean seafood species are a good dietary source of n–3 fatty acids, particularly the pelagic fish species such as sardine (*Sardina pilchardus*), anchovy (*Engraulis encrasicolus*), mackerel (*Scomber scomber*) and bluefin tuna (*Thunnus thynnus*), and crustaceans such as lobster (*Palinurus elephas*) and crabs (*Liocarcinus* spp). The muscle (ie, the edible part) of these pelagic fishes and crustaceans can contain up to 10 times more total lipids and n–3 fatty acids than that of demersal fish species such as angler (*Lophius* spp.) or hake (*Merluccius merluccius*), or mollusks such as squid (*Loligo vulgaris*) and cuttlefish (*Sepia officinalis*) (Tornaritis et al., 1993; Soriguer et al., 1997; Imre and Saglik, 1998; Saglik and Imre, 2001; Mourente et al., 2001; Sirot et al., 2008). Pelagic species tend to concentrate the lipid reserves in their muscle whereas demersal species tend to concentrate lipids in their livers or mesenteries (Lloret et al., 2008). Pelagic species contribute the most to the total Mediterranean landings, representing about 67% of the total landings (compared to 59% in the Pacific, 51% in the Atlantic, 45% in the Indian Oceans according to FAO, 1995). Thus, marine resources of the Mediterranean represent a particularly important stock of n–3 fatty acids."

In Mediterranean countries, the traditional diet has been consistently shown to be associated with favorable health outcomes and a better quality of life (reviewed by Sofi et al., 2008; Sofi, 2009). Several epidemiological and observational studies suggest that this type of diet traditionally followed by Mediterranean people may protect against chronic diseases and mortality, with Mediterranean nations presenting lower rates of cardiovascular disease and cancer in comparison to other nations. Cardiovascular diseases and cancer are the two most important causes of disease in the world. According to the (World Health Organization, 2009a,b), cardiovascular diseases and cancer accounted for an estimated 17- and 8 million deaths in 2004 and 2007 respectively, representing 29% and 13% of all global deaths in those years, respectively. Greater adherence to this diet has been also associated with longevity in the elderly (Trichopoulou, 2004), a reduction of depressive disorders (Sánchez-Villegas et al., 2009), and prevention of iron deficiency (Mesias et al., 2009).

The long chain n–3 fatty acids (EPA, DPA, and DHA) found in seafood, is an important component of the "Mediterranean diet" (Simopoulos, 2001). The relatively high intake of essential n–3 fatty acids by Mediterranean people contributes to a healthy diet in several ways. First, fish consumption has been shown to reduce coronary heart disease mortality because n–3 fatty acids from fish oil help to improve cardiovascular health by decreasing risk factors such as triglyceride concentrations, blood pressure, platelet aggregation, and heart arrhythmias (Fung et al., 2009; Chrysohoou et al., 2007). Second, fish-derived n–3 fatty acid consumption protects against the development of certain cancers, eg, mammary (Stoll, 2002) and prostate cancer (Itsiopoulos et al., 2009). In addition to the cardiovascular and cancer protective effects of fish consumption, fish intake in the Mediterranean has been also associated with less severe depressive symptoms in adults (Bountziouka, 2009; Simopoulos, 2011) and less development of asthma and respiratory allergies in children (Biltagi et al., 2009; Olsen et al., 2008). Omega-3 fatty acids also mediate the inflammatory process and influence the general health status of the skeletal system throughout the body (Watkins et al., 2001; Benito et al., 2005).

Despite fish-derived n–3 fatty acid consumption being an important determinant of the health of Mediterranean people, some authors have suggested that the role of the overall Mediterranean dietary pattern may be more important than the effect of single components (Sánchez-Villegas et al., 2009). Thus, there may be a fair degree of protection from the combination of the n–3 fatty acids found in fish with other natural ingredients in olive oil, nuts, fruit and plant foods, which are also common in the Mediterranean diet (Sánchez-Villegas et al., 2009).

Seafood is a major component of the Mediterranean diets as is olive oil. Infact olive oil accounts for more energy in the Mediterranean diets than any other single food. Olive oil increases the incorporation of EPA and DHA into cell membrane phospholipids and prevents the oxidation of LDL, whereas n–6 rich oil such as corn oil (66% LA), sunflower and safflower (77% LA) increase the oxidation of LDL and interfere with the incorporation of EPA and DHA into the health membrane phospholipids (Cleland et al., 1992). Determination of fatty acids in plasma or red cell membrane phospholipids should be carried out in all clinical studies, as well as randomized clinical intervention studies because they are a biomarker of fish intake. However in the presence of APOE4 carriers the absorption of EPA is decreased (Plourde et al., 2009), whereas in the presence of genetic variants of FADS1 and FADS2 (Simopoulos, 2010) there could be an increase of 30% of endogenous production of EPA, whereas a high LA intake decreases the desaturation and elongation of ALA to EPA (Wood et al., 2015). Exercise and moderate alcohol intake are associated with higher levels (plasma and red blood cell membrane phospholipids) of EPA and DHA.

Following the results of the Lyon Heart Study a number of studies have been carried out in various parts of the world on the modification of their traditional diets to that of a Mediterranean diet with similar results. The traditional diet of Crete was the beginning of the recognition of the importance of both terrestrial and marine sources of n–3 fatty acids which along with high antioxidant intake from fruits and vegetables, have led to the importance of a dietary pattern for health and to the importance of the nutrient composition of the diet in the maintenance of health and the prevention and management of chronic diseases.

Adherence to Mediterranean-type Diet Score, Plasma Fatty Acids and the Omega-6/Omega-3 Fatty Acid Ratio

The traditional diet of Crete, prior to 1960, was the diet that was shown in the Seven Countries Study to have the lowest rate of CHD, cancer, and the greatest longevity. The diet of Crete, as well as the other diets of Southern Europe have changed significantly over the years, due to high intake of vegetable oils high in n–6 fatty acids, processed foods, sugary drinks, less fish, and more meat consumption. In epidemiological studies a Mediterranean type diet score is being used in order to compare the effects of the Mediterranean type diet to various diseases and conditions in various populations outside the Mediterranean region. Recently a further effort was made by Sofi et al. (2014) to improve on the use of the score, by using data from cohort studies, and proposed a literature-based adherence score that can represent an easy tool for the estimation of adherence to the Mediterranean type diet at the individual level.

The adherence score to a Mediterranean type diet is based on food groups and food patterns and has been widely used for epidemiological research. Trichopoulou et al. (2003) based the score on median amounts of consumption of food groups that are characteristic of the traditional diet of Greece in the sample investigated. However the score does not give the amount of consumption for food groups composing the score that can be used in everyday clinical practice at an individual level and it is only applicable to the group under study. Others (Panagiotakos et al., 2007) attempted to correct these inadequacies by creating a simple questionnaire based on recommendations of the guidelines for a healthy diet and characterized by a few questions used for estimating the frequency of consumption (monthly or daily) of food groups more or less characteristic of the diet of Greece. Another example is the questionnaire developed in the SUN (Segiomiento Universidad de Navarra) cohort (Domínguez et al., 2013). Both of these questionnaires have the advantage of being feasible for assessing adherence to a Mediterranean like diet at an individual level.

Greater adherence to a Mediterranean type diet has long been reported to be protective against the occurrence of chronic degenerative diseases (Martinez-Gonzalez et al., 2009). Sofi et al. (2008, 2010) carried two meta-analyses and reported the Mediterranean diet to be the optimal diet for preserving good health status. Recently the protective role of the Mediterranean type diet has been also demonstrated in a dietary intervention study conducted in Spanish middle-aged subjects. Over a follow-up period of 4–8 years the subjects who followed a Mediterranean type diet reported to have a reduction of 30% compared to the incidence of CVD in a primary prevention setting (Estruch et al., 2013).

The Mediterranean diet score is based on foods instead of the nutrient composition of the diet. Therefore it assumes incorrectly that all Mediterranean type diet foods have the same nutritional composition. The first data addressing this issue date back to the analysis of data from the Seven Countries Study in 1993 when Sandker et al. (1993) compared blood fatty acids profile of participants of the Greek and Dutch cohorts showing that the Greeks had 33% more ALA ($P < 0.001$) and 20% lower LA ($P < 0.001$) in their plasma (Sandker et al., 1993) which indicates that the traditional Greek Mediterranean diet was rich in ALA but low in LA and n–6 fatty acids in general, which is exactly the opposite of what one finds in Western diets that have high amounts of n–6 fatty acids due to the intake of vegetable oils rich in LA. This is not surprising, since ALA is present in a large number of plant-derived foods (purslane, other wild green leafy vegetables, and walnuts) (Simopoulos, 2004) that are consumed by the people along the Mediterranean basin. Although the total fat content of vegetables and legumes is rather low, their relative abundance in ALA, associated with the large size of the average portions and the high frequency of consumption results in significant amounts of ALA (Galli and Marangoni, 2006). ALA is the precursor of EPA and DHA and may have beneficial properties for health on its own, as well as through its metabolism to EPA and DHA (Stark et al., 2015). The consumption of fish and fish products in the Mediterranean region is not geographically uniform. In certain countries and regions, such as coastal Spain and Portugal the intake of fish is very high, where it is low in Italy (Galli and Marangoni, 2006; FAO, 1987). Since the concentrations of EPA and DHA vary from one fish species to another (Lloret, 2010) fish consumption data provides only a crude estimate of the actual intake of marine n–3 fatty acids.

Since computation of the Mediterranean type diet score is based on foods, which may not accurately reflect the bioavailability of nutrients (Trichopoulou et al., 2003) plasma fatty acid determinations, in particular n–3 PUFA biomarkers are more precise risk predictors than dietary intake estimates (Harris, 2009). Plasma fatty acids have largely been used to validate nutrient intake but less frequently to characterize food patterns. Hence, data on the association between Mediterranean type diet score adherence and fatty acid status are scarce. However, a single observational study conducted in Greece reported an association between Mediterranean type diet score adherence and plasma fatty acids in adults (Panagiotakos et al., 2009). It is possible that several dietary patterns corresponding to similar Mediterranean like diet adherence score may differ in other countries not close to the Mediterranean Sea. Feart et al. (2011) showed that indeed, the Mediterranean type diet adherence score was associated with plasma fatty acids in a large population based sample of older people in France. The study population (mean age 75.9 years) consisted of 1050 subjects from Bordeaux (France) included in the Three-City cohort. Adherence to the Mediterranean type diet (scored as 0–9) was computed from a FFQ and 24 h recall. The proportion of each plasma fatty acid was determined. Cross-sectional analysis of the association between plasma fatty acids and Mediterranean type diet adherence score was performed by multi-linear regression. After adjusting for age, sex, energy intake, physical activity, smoking status, BMI, plasma triglycerides, and apoE-4 genotype, plasma palmitoleic acid was significantly inversely associated with Mediterranean type diet adherence score, whereas plasma DHA, the EPA + DHA index and total n–3 PUFA were positively associated with Mediterranean type diet adherence score. The n–6:n–3 PUFA, AA:EPA, AA:DHA and AA:(EPA + DHA) ratios were significantly inversely associated with Mediterranean diet adherence score. Plasma EPA was positively associated with Mediterranean diet adherence score only in apoE-4 noncarriers (Plourde et al., 2009). There was no association between Mediterranean diet adherence score and SFA and total MUFA. The results of this study suggest that the protective effect of the Mediterranean diet on cognitive functions might be mediated by higher plasma DHA and lower n–6:n–3 PUFA ratios which can serve as biomarkers for the Mediterranean type diet adherence score.

In the intervention study carried out by Ambring et al. (2006) the administration of a Mediterranean type diet to healthy subjects for 4 weeks resulted in a 47% increase in DHA plasma concentrations ($P < 0.001$) compared to their ordinary Swedish diet. All these studies demonstrate that a Mediterranean type diet low in LA assures higher n–3 fatty acid bioavailability than the common Western diets; therefore at least part of the protective effects exerted by Mediterranean diets may be attributed to both ALA from vegetables and the EPA and DHA from marine sources in the presence of low LA.

CONCLUSIONS

The Mediterranean diets consist of a dietary pattern first described from observational studies, which have reported low all-cause and coronary heart disease death rates in cohorts of the Mediterranean basin, with olive oil as the main dietary fat. There is no single Mediterranean diet but several definitions, since populations living in countries bordering the Mediterranean Sea have various dietary habits. Nevertheless, a high consumption of vegetables, legumes, fruits and cereals, a moderate-to-high intake of fish, a high MUFA:SFA ratio and a low intake of dairy products and meat, along with a low-to-moderate intake of wine, define the common aspect of this dietary pattern (Willett et al., 1995; Trichopoulou et al., 2003; Bach et al., 2006).

The diet of Crete prior to 1960 was associated with the lowest rate of cardiovascular disease, cancer, and highest longevity. The Cretan diet had higher amounts of ALA and lower amounts of LA than the other Mediterranean diets. Both plant ALA and marine-derived n–3 fatty acids (EPA, DPA, and DHA) should be considered as valuable mediators of protection provided by traditional Mediterranean diets.

The Mediterranean-style diets represent an optimal dietary strategy for health since a greater adherence to the Mediterranean type diets, as evaluated by the Mediterranean type diet score, has been associated with longer survival, reduced risk for cardiovascular mortality and cancer incidence and mortality (Sofi et al., 2008; Trichopoulou et al., 2009; Sofi et al., 2010).

Biological and chemical investigations have shown that Mediterranean seafood species are a good dietary source of n–3 fatty acids, particularly the pelagic fish species such as sardine, anchovy, mackerel, and bluefin tuna, and crustaceans such as lobster and crabs. The muscle (ie, the edible part) of these pelagic fishes and crustaceans can contain up to 10 times more total lipids and n–3 fatty acids than that of demersal fish species such as angler or hake, or mollusks such as squid and cuttlefish.

References

Allbaugh, L.G., 1953. Crete: A Case Study of an Undeveloped Area. Princeton University Press, Princeton, NJ.

Ambring, A., Johansson, M., Axelsen, M., Gan, L., Strandvik, B., Friberg, P., 2006. Mediterranean inspired diet lowers the ratio of serum phospholipid n-6 to n-3 fatty acids, the number of leukocytes and platelets, and vascular endothelial growth factor in healthy subjects. Am. J. Clin. Nutr. 83, 575–581.

Bach, A., Serra-Majem, L., Carrasco, J.L., Roman, B., Ngo, J., Bertomeu, I., Obrador, B., 2006. The use of indexes evaluating the adherence to the Mediterranean diet in epidemiological studies: a review. Public Health Nutr. 9 (1A), 132–146.

Benito, M.J., Veale, D.J., FitzGerald, O., van den Berg, W.B., Bresnihan, B., 2005. Synovial tissue inflammation in early and late osteoarthritis. Annal. Rheum. Dis. 64, 1263–1267.

Bianchi, C.N., Morri, C., 2000. Marine biodiversity of the Mediterranean Sea: situation, problems, and prospects for future research. Marine Pol. Bull. 40 (5), 367–376.

Biltagi, M.A., Baset, A.A., Bassiouny, M., Kasrawi, M.A., Attia, M., 2009. Omega-3 Fatty Acids, vitamin C and Zn supplementation in asthmatic children: a randomized self-controlled study. Acta Paediatr. 98 (4), 737–742.

Birch, E., Birch, D., Hoffman, D., Hale, L., Everett, M., Uauy, R., 1993. Breast-feeding and optimal visual development. J. Pediatr. Ophthalmol. Strab. 30, 33–38.

Birch, E.E., Hoffman, D.R., Uauy, R., Birch, D.G., Prestidge, C., 1998. Visual acuity and the essentiality of docosahexaenoic acid and arachidonic acid in the diet of term infants. Pediatr. Res. 44, 201–209.

Bountziouka, V., 2009. Long-term fish intake is associated with less severe depressive symptoms among elderly men and women. J. Aging Health 21 (6), 864–880.

Burr, M.L., Fehily, A.M., Gilbert, J.F., Rogers, S., Holliday, R.M., Sweetnam, P.M., Elwood, P.C., Deadman, N.M., 1989. Effect of changes in fat, fish and fibre intakes on death and myocardial reinfarction: Diet and reinfarction trial (DART). Lancet 2, 757–761.

Chrysohoou, C., Panagiotakos, D.B., Pitsavos, C., Skoumas, J., Krinos, X., Chloptsios, Y., Nikolaou, V., Stefanadis, C., 2007. Long-term fish consumption is associated with protection against arrhythmia in healthy persons in a Mediterranean region – the ATTICA study. Am. J. Clin. Nutr. 85 (5), 1385–1391.

Cleland, L.G., James, M.J., Neumann, M.A., D'Angelo, M., Gibson, R.A., 1992. Linoleate inhibits EPA incorporation from dietary fish-oil supplements in human subjects. Am. J. Clin. Nutr. 55, 395–399.

Crawford, M.A., 1968. Fatty acid ratios in free-living and domestic animals. Lancet 1, 1329–1333.

de Lorgeril, M., Salen, P., 2000. Modified Cretan Mediterranean diet in the prevention of coronary heart disease and cancer. Simopoulos, A.P., Visioli, F. (Eds.), Mediterranean Diets. World Review Nutrition Diet, vol. 87, Karger, Basel, pp. 1–23.

de Lorgeril, M., Renaud, S., Mamelle, N., Salen, P., Martin, J.L., Monjaud, I., Guidollet, J., Touboul, P., Delaye, J., 1994. Mediterranean alpha-linolenic acid-rich diet in the secondary prevention of coronary heart disease. Lancet 343, 1454–1459.

de Lorgeril, M., Salen, P., Martin, J.-L., Monjaud, I., Boucher, P., Mamelle, N., 1998. Mediterranean dietary pattern in a randomized trial. Prolonged survival and possible reduced cancer rate. Arch. Int. Med. 158, 1181–1187.

Domínguez, L.J., Bes-Rastrollo, M., de la Fuente-Arrillaga, C., Toledo, E., Beunza, J.J., Barbagallo, M., Martínez-González, M.A., 2013. Similar prediction of total mortality, diabetes incidence and cardiovascular events using relative- and absolute-component Mediterranean diet score: the SUN cohort. Nutr. Metabol. Cardiovascul. Dis. 23 (5), 451–458.

Eaton, S.B., Eaton, III, S.B., Sinclair, A.J., Cordain, L., Mann, N.J., 1998. Dietary intake of long-chain polyunsaturated fatty acids during the Paleolithic. Simopoulos, A.P. (Ed.), The Return of x3 Fatty Acids Into The Food Supply. I. Land-Based Animal Food Products and Their Health Effects. World Review Nutrition Diet, vol. 83, Karger, Basel, pp. 12–23.

Estruch, R., Ros, E., Salas-Salvadó, J., Covas, M.I., Corella, D., Arós, F., Gómez-Gracia, E., Ruiz-Gutiérrez, V., Fiol, M., Lapetra, J., Lamuela-Raventos, R.M., Serra-Majem, L., Pintó, X., Basora, J., Muñoz, M.A., Sorlí, J.V., Martínez, J.A., Martínez-González, M.A., 2013. Predimed Study Investigators, Primary prevention of cardiovascular disease with a Mediterranean diet. New England J. Med. 368 (14), 1279–1290.

Food and Agriculture Organization of United Nations (FAO), 1987. Fish consumption and production in Mediterranean countries. Corporate document, repository.

FAO, 1995. Chronicles of Marine Fishery Landings (1950–94): Trend Analysis and Fisheries Potential FAO Fisheries Technical Paper 359.

Feart, C., Torrès, M.J., Samieri, C., Jutand, M.A., Peuchant, E., Simopoulos, A.P., Barberger-Gateau, P., 2011. Adherence to a Mediterranean diet and plasma fatty acids: data from the Bordeaux sample of the Three-City study. Br. J. Nutr. 106 (1), 149–158.

Fung, T., Rexrode, K.M., Mantzoros, C.S., Manson, J.E., Willett, W.C., Hu, F.B., 2009. Mediterranean diet and incidence of and mortality from coronary heart disease and stroke in women. Circulation 119 (8), 1093–1100.

Galli, C., Marangoni, F., 2006. N-3 fatty acids in the Mediterranean diet. Prostagland. Leukotr. Essen. Fatty Acid. 75, 129–133.

GISSI-Prevenzione Investigators, 1999. Dietary supplementation with n-3 polyunsaturated fatty acids and vitamin E after myocardial infarction: Results of the GISSI-Prevenzione trial. Lancet 354, 447–455.

Harris, W.S., 2009. The Omega-3 Index: from biomarker to risk marker to risk factor. Curr. Atheroscler. Rep. 11, 411–417.

Hertog, M.G.L., Hollman, P.C.H., Katan, M.B., 1992. Content of potentially anticarcinogenic flavonoids of 28 vegetables and 9 fruits commonly consumed in The Netherlands. J. Agric. Food Chem. 40, 2379–2383.

Imre, S., Saglik, S., 1998. Fatty acid composition and content cholesterol of some Turkish fish species. Turkish J. Chem. 22 (4), 321–324.

Itsiopoulos, C., Hodge, A., Kaimakamis, M., 2009. Can the Mediterranean diet prevent prostate cancer? Molec. Nutr. Food Res. 53, 227–239.

Joseph, J.A., Shukitt-Hale, B., DenisovaNA, BielinskiD, Martin, A., McEwen, J.J., Bickford, P.C., 1999. Reversals of age-related declines in neuronal signal transduction, cognitive, and motor behavioral deficits with blueberry, spinach, or strawberry dietary supplementation. J. Neuroscience 19, 8114–8121.

Keys, A., 1970. Coronary heart disease in seven countries. Circulation 41 (suppl.), 1–211.

Lagarde, M., Spector, A.A., Galli, C., Hamazaki, T., Knapp, H.R. (Eds), 1999. Fatty acids and lipids from cell biology to human disease. Proceedings of the Thirdrd Congress of International Society for the Study of Fatty Acids and Lipids (ISSFAL). Lipids 43 (Suppl.), S1–S350.

Leaf, A., Weber, P.C., 1988. Cardiovascular effects of n-3 fatty acids. New England J. Med. 318, 549–557.

Levi, F., La Vecchia, C., Lucchini, F., Negri, E., 1995. Cancer mortality in Europe, 1990–1992. Eur. J. Can. Prev. 4, 389–417.

Lloret, J., 2010. Human health benefits supplied by Mediterranean marine biodiversity. Mar. Pollut. Bull. 60, 1640–1646.

Lloret, J., Demestre, M., Sanchez-Pardo, J., 2008. Lipid (energy) reserves of Europe hake (*Merluccius merluccius*) in the North-western Mediterranean. Vie et milieu Life Environ. 58 (1), 75–85.

Martinez-Gonzalez, M.A., Bes-Rastrollo, M., Serra-Majem, L., Lairon, D., Estruch, R., Trichopoulou, A., 2009. Mediterranean food pattern and the primary prevention of chronic disease: recent developments. Nutr. Rev. 67 (Suppl. 1), S111–S1116.

Mazur, W.M., Duke, J.A., Wahala, K., Rasku, S., Adlercreutz, H., 1998. Isoflavonoids and lignans in legumes – Nutritional and health aspects in humans. J. Nutr. Biochem. 9, 193–200.

Mesias, M., Seiquer, I., Muñoz-Hoyos, A., Galdó, G., Navarro, M.P., 2009. The beneficial effect of Mediterranean dietary patterns on dietary iron utilization in male adolescents aged 11–14 years. Int. J. Food Sci. Nutr. 60 (Suppl. 7), 355–368.

Mourente, G., Megina, C., Diaz-Salvago, E., 2001. Lipids in female northern Bluefin tuna (*Thunnus thynnus* thynnus L) during sexual maturation. Fish Physiol. Biochem. 24 (4), 351–363.

Olsen, S.F., Østerdal, M.L., Salvig, J.D., Mortensen, L.M., Rytter, D., Secher, N.J., Henriksen, T.B., 2008. Fish oil intake compared with olive oil intake in late pregnancy and asthma in the offspring: 16 y of registry-based follow-up from a randomized controlled trial. Am. J. Clin. Nutr. 88 (1), 167–175.

Panagiotakos, D.B., Pitsavos, C., Arvaniti, F., Stefanadis, C., 2007. Adherence to the Mediterranean food pattern predicts the prevalence of hypertension, hypercholesterolemia, diabetes and obesity, among healthy adults; the accuracy of the MedDietScore. Preven. Med. 44 (4), 335–334.

Panagiotakos, D., Kalogeropoulos, N., Pitsavos, C., Roussinou, G., Palliou, K., Chrysohoou, C., Stefanadis, C., 2009. Validation of the MedDietScore via the determination of plasma fatty acids. Int. J. Food Sci. Nutr. 60 (Suppl. 5), 168–180.

Pella, D., Dubnov, G., Singh, R.B., Sharma, R., 2003. Effects of an Indo-Mediterranean diet on the omega-6/omega-3 ratio in patients at high risk of coronary artery disease: the Indian paradox. World Rev. Nutr. Diet. 92, 74–80.

Plourde, M., Vohl, M.C., Vandal, M., Couture, P., Lemieux, S., Cunnane, S.C., 2009. Plasma n-3 fatty acid response to an n-3 fatty acid supplement is modulated by apoE epsilon4 but not by the common PPAR-alpha L162V polymorphism in men. Br. J. Nutr. 102, 1121–1124.

Renaud, S., Godsey, F., Dumont, E., Thevenon, C., Ortchanian, E., Martin, J.L., 1986. Influence of long-term diet modification on platelet function and composition in Moselle farmers. Am. J. Clin. Nutr. 43, 136–150.

Renaud, S., de Lorgeril, M., Delaye, J., Guidollet, J., Jacquard, F., Mamelle, N., Martin, J.L., Monjaud, I., Salen, P., Touboul, P., 1995. Cretan Mediterranean diet for prevention of coronary heart disease. Am. J. Clin. Nutr. 61 (Suppl.), 1360S–1367S.

Saglik, S., Imre, S., 2001. Omega-3 Fatty Acids in some fish species from Turkey. J. Food Sci. 66 (2), 210–212.

Sánchez-Villegas, A., Delgado-Rodríguez, M., Alonso, A., Schlatter, J., Lahortiga, F., Serra Majem, L., Martínez-González, M.A., 2009. Association of the Mediterranean dietary pattern with the incidence of depression. Archiv. Gen. Psychiatr. 66 (10), 1090–1098.

Sanders, T.A., 2000. Polyunsaturated fatty acids in the food chain in Europe. Am. J. Clin. Nutr. 71, 176S–178S.

Sandker, G.W., Kromhout, D., Aravanis, C., Bloemberg, B.P., Mensink, R.P., Karalias, N., Katan, M.B., 1993. Serum cholesteryl ester fatty acids and their relation with serum lipids in elderly men in Crete and The Netherlands. Eur. J. Clin. Nutr. 47 (3), 201–208.

Simopoulos, A.P., 1991. Omega-3 fatty acids in health and disease and in growth and development. Am. J. Clin. Nutr. 54, 438–463.

Simopoulos, A.P., 1994. Fatty Acids, chap 16. In: Goldberg, I. (Ed.), Functional Foods. Designer Foods, Pharmafoods, Nutraceuticals. Chapman & Hall, New York, pp. 355–392.

Simopoulos, A.P., 1998. Overview of evolutionary aspects of ω-3 fatty acids in the diet. World Rev. Nutr. Diet. 83, 1–11.

Simopoulos, A.P., 1999a. New products from the agri-food industry: The return of n-3 fatty acids into the food supply. Lipids 34 (Suppl.), S297–S301.

Simopoulos, A.P., 1999b. Genetic variation and evolutionary aspects of diet. In: Papas, A.M. (Ed.), Antioxidant Status, Diet, Nutrition and Health. CRC Press, Boca Raton, pp. 65–88.

Simopoulos, A.P., 1999c. Essential fatty acids in health and chronic disease. Am. J. Clin. Nutr. 70 (Suppl.), 560S–569S.

Simopoulos, A.P., 2001. Mediterranean diets: what is so special about the diet of Greece? The scientific evidence. J. Nutr. 131, 3065S–3073S.

Simopoulos, A.P., 2004. Omega-3 fatty acids and antioxidants in edible wild plants. Biol. Res. 37, 263–277.

Simopoulos, A.P., 2010. Genetic variants in the metabolism of omega-6 and omega-3 fatty acids: their role in the determination of nutritional requirements and chronic disease risk. Exp. Biol. Med. 235 (7), 785–795.

Simopoulos, A.P., 2011. Evolutionary aspects of diet: the omega-6/omega-3 ratio and the brain. Mol. Neurobiol. 44 (2), 203–215.

Simopoulos, A.P., Salem, Jr., N., 1986. Purslane: a terrestrial source of omega-3 fatty acids. New England J. Med. 315, 833.

Simopoulos, A.P., Salem, Jr., N., 1989. n–3 fatty acids in eggs from range-fed Greek chickens (letter). New England J. Med. 321, 1412.

Simopoulos, A.P., Salem, Jr., N., 1992. Egg yolk as a source of long-chain polyunsaturated fatty acids in infant feeding. Am. J. Clin. Nutr. 55, 411–414.

Simopoulos, A.P., Visioli, F. (Eds.), 2000. Mediterranean Diets. World Review Nutrition Diet, vol. 87, Karger, Basel.

Simopoulos, A.P., Visioli, F. (Eds.), 2006. More on Mediterranean Diets. World Review Nutrition Diet, vol. 97, Karger, Basel.

Simopoulos, A.P., Kifer, R.R., Martin, R.E., Barlow, S.M. (Eds.), 1991. Health Effects of w3 Polyunsaturated Fatty Acids in Seafoods. World Review Nutrition Diet, vol. 66, Karger, Basel.

Simopoulos, A.P., Norman, H.A., Gillaspy, J.E., Duke, J.A., 1992. Common purslane: a source of omega–3 fatty acids and antioxidants. J. Am. College Nutr. 11, 374–382.

Simopoulos, A.P., Norman, H.A., Gillaspy, J.E., 1995. Purslane in human nutrition and its potential for world agriculture. World Review Nutrition Diet, Plants in Human Nutrition. Basel, Karger, vol. 77, 7–74.

Simopoulos, A.P., Leaf, A., Salem, Jr., N., 1999. Essentiality of and recommended dietary intakes for omega-6 and omega-3 fatty acids. Ann. Nutr. Metabol. 43, 127–130.

Simopoulos, A.P., Tan, D.-X., Manchester, L.C., Reiter, R.J., 2005. *Commentary purslane*: a plant source of omega-3 fatty acids and melatonin. J. Pineal Res. 39, 331–332.

Singh, R.B., Rastogi, S.S., Verma, R., Laxmi, B., Singh, R., Ghosh, S., Niaz, M.A., 1992. Randomized controlled trial of cardioprotective diet in patients with recent acute myocardial infarction: results of one year follow-up. BMJ 304, 1015–1019.

Singh, R.B., Niaz, M.A., Sharma, J.P., Kumar, R., Rastogi, V., Moshiri, M., 1997. Randomized, double-blind, placebo-controlled trial of fish oil and mustard oil in patients with suspected acute myocardial infarction: The Indian experiment of infarct survival – 4. Cardiovasc. Drug. Ther. 11, 485–491.
Sirot, V., Oseredczuk, M., Bemrah-Aouachria, N., Volatier, J.L., Leblanc, J., 2008. Lipid and fatty acid composition of fish and seafood consumed in France. CALIPSO study. J. Food Compos. Anal. 21, 8–16.
Slater, T.F., Block, G. (Eds), 1991. Antioxidant vitamins and b-carotene in disease prevention. Proceedings of a conference. London, UK, October 2–4, 1989. Am. J. Clin. Nutr. 53 (Suppl. 1), 189S–396S.
Sofi, F., 2009. The Mediterranean diet revisited: evidence of its effectiveness grows. Curr. Opin. Cardiol. 24 (5), 442–446.
Sofi, F., Cesari, F., Abbate, R., Gensini, G.F., Casini, A., 2008. Adherence to Mediterranean diet and health status: meta-analysis. Br. Med. J. 337, a1344.
Sofi, F., Abbate, R., Gensini, G.F., Casini, A., 2010. Accruing evidence on benefits of adherence to the Mediterranean diet on health: an updated systematic review and meta-analysis. Am. J. Clin. Nutr. 92 (5), 1189–1196.
Sofi, F., Macchi, C., Abbate, R., Gensini, G.F., Casini, A., 2014. Mediterranean diet and health status: an updated meta-analysis and a proposal for a literature-based adherence score. Public Health Nutr. 17 (12), 2769–2782.
Soriguer, F., Serna, S., Valverde, E., Hernando, J., Martín-Reyes, A., Soriguer, M., Pareja, A., Tinahones, F., Esteva, I., 1997. Lipid, protein and caloric content of different Atlantic and Mediterranean fish, shellfish, and mollusks, commonly eaten in the south of Spain. Eur. J. Epidemiol. 13, 451–463.
Stark, A.H., Reifen, R., Crawford, M.A., 2015. Past and Present Insights on Alpha-Linolenic Acid and the Omega-3 Fatty Acid Family. Critic. Rev. Food Sci. Nutr. (Epub ahead of print).
Stoll, B.A., 2002. N-3 Fatty Acids and lipid peroxidation in breast cancer inhibition. Br. J. Nutr. 87 (3), 193–198.
Sugano, M., Hirahara, F., 2000. Polyunsaturated fatty acids in the food chain in Japan. Am. J. Clin. Nutr. 71, 189S–196S.
Tornaritis, M., Peraki, E., Georgulli, M., et al.,1993. Fatty acid composition and total fat content of eight species of Mediterranean fish. Int. J. Food Sci. Nutr. 45, 135–139.
Trichopoulou, A., 2004. Traditional Mediterranean diet and longevity in the elderly: a review. Public Health Nutr. 7, 943–947.
Trichopoulou, A., Bamia, C., Trichopoulos, D., 2009. Anatomy of health effects of Mediterranean diet: Greek EPIC prospective cohort study. Br. Med. J. 338, b2337.
Trichopoulou, A., Costacou, T., Bamia, C., Trichopoulos, D., 2003. Adherence to a Mediterranean diet and survival in a Greek population. New England J. Med. 348, 2599–2608.
Uauy, R., Hoffman, D., Birch, E., Birch, D., Jameson, D., Tyson, J., 1994. Safety and efficacy of x-3 fatty acids in the nutrition of very low birth weight infants: soy oil and marine oil supplementation of formula. J. Pediatr. 124, 612–620.
Watkins, B.A., Lippman, H.E., Le Bouteiller, L., Li, Y., Seifert, M.F., 2001. Bioactive fatty acids: role in bone biology and bone cell function. Prog. Lipid Res. 40, 125–148.
Weisburger, J.H., 1999. Mechanisms of action of antioxidants as exemplified in vegetables, tomatoes and tea. Food Chem. Toxicol. 37, 943–948.
Willett, W.C., Sacks, F., Trichopoulou, A., Drescher, G., Ferro-Luzzi, A., Helsing, E., Trichopoulos, D., 1995. Mediterranean diet pyramid: a cultural model for healthy eating. Am. J. Clin. Nutr. 61 (Suppl. 6), 1402S–1406S.
Wood, K.E., Mantzioris, E., Gibson, R.A., Ramsden, C.E., Muhlhausler, B.S., 2015. The effect of modifying dietary LA and ALA intakes on omega-3 long chain polyunsaturated fatty acid (n-3 LCPUFA) status in human adults: A systematic review and commentary. Prostagland. Leukotrien. Essen. Fatty Acid. 95, 47–55.
World Health Organization, 2009a. WHO Facsheet number 317. http://www.who.int/mediacentre/factsheets/fs317/en/index.html
World Health Organization, 2009b. WHO Facsheet number 297. http://www.who.int/mediacentre/factsheets/fs297/en/index.html

CHAPTER

3

Recommended Intake of Fish and Fish Oils Worldwide

C.K. Richter, A.C. Skulas-Ray**, P.M. Kris-Etherton***

*Department of Nutritional Sciences, The University of Arizona, Tucson, Arizona, United States; **Department of Nutritional Sciences, The Pennsylvania State University, University Park, Pennsylvania, United States

INTRODUCTION

The relationship between long-chain (LC) omega-3 (n–3) polyunsaturated fatty acid (PUFA) intake and reduced cardiovascular disease (CVD) mortality was first discovered decades ago and the cardiovascular health benefits of the LC n–3 PUFAs, eicosapentaenoic acid (EPA, 20:5n3) and docosahexaenoic acid (DHA, 22:6n3), have been extensively studied (Mozaffarian and Wu, 2012; Mozaffarian and Wu, 2011; Mozaffarian and Rimm, 2006). In a pooled analysis of prospective studies and randomized clinical trials, modest consumption of fish or fish oil (eg, 1–2 servings/week providing ~250 mg/day of EPA + DHA) lowered the relative risk of CHD mortality by 36% when compared to little or no intake (Mozaffarian and Rimm, 2006). EPA and DHA also lower plasma triglycerides, resting heart rate, and blood pressure, and may improve endothelial function (Mozaffarian and Wu, 2011); however, the effect of these changes on clinical events (ie, CHD death) tend to have varying time courses and depend on the dose of EPA + DHA (Mozaffarian and Rimm, 2006). For instance, at intakes <750 mg/day, antiarrhythmic effects predominate and can reduce clinical events within weeks. Conversely, a reduction in triglycerides is hypothesized to require a longer period of time to reduce clinical events (ie, months or years) and has a stronger effect at higher doses of EPA + DHA (Mozaffarian and Rimm, 2006). Oily fish are the primary dietary source of EPA and DHA, and LC n–3 PUFA supplements (eg, fish oil) are also widely available. Based on the evidence for their role in cardiovascular health and other disease outcomes, multiple authoritative organizations worldwide have issued recommendations for fish and/or LC n–3 PUFA intake.

Despite appreciation for the health-promoting effects of LC n–3 PUFAs, there is wide variation in global intake and many populations consume well below the amounts associated with beneficial health outcomes. For instance, the diet of Greenland Eskimos is much higher in LC n–3 PUFAs than the typical Danish diet because of their reliance on whale, seal, and fish meat (Bang et al., 1976; 1980). Similarly, daily fish and shellfish consumption in Japan is also relatively high and was estimated to be ≈ 80 g/day in 2000 (Sugano and Hirahara, 2000). Conversely, fish and LC n–3 PUFA intake is generally very low in the United States. The most recent analysis of National Health and Nutrition Examination Survey (NHANES) data (2003–08) found that the mean intake of total fish and fish high in omega-3 fatty acids was 0.61 and 0.15 oz/day, respectively (Papanikolaou et al., 2014). Since the data are skewed by a very small percentage of high fish consumers, median intakes were even lower at 0.43 and 0.07 oz/day, respectively (Papanikolaou et al., 2014). With respect to EPA and DHA, average intake from dietary sources (18 and 50 mg/day, respectively) and foods plus supplements (41 and 72 mg/day, respectively) were also far below recommended amounts (Papanikolaou et al., 2014). This is similar to previously reported averages for EPA and DHA intake from 1999–2000 NHANES data (30 and 70 mg/day, respectively, Ervin et al., 2004), as well as the 1994–96 and 1998 Continuing Survey of Food Intakes by Individuals (28 and 57 mg/day, respectively; Institute of Medicine, 2005). Other countries with relatively low LC n–3 PUFA intake include Australia (Howe et al., 2006), Belgium (Sioen et al., 2006), Germany (Linseisen et al., 2003), the United Kingdom (Givens and Gibbs, 2006), and Canada (Dewailly et al., 2001).

Fish and Fish Oil in Health and Disease Prevention. http://dx.doi.org/10.1016/B978-0-12-802844-5.00003-8

This chapter will discuss the recommendations for fish and/or LC n–3 PUFA intake issued by organizations worldwide. The omega-3 content of common fish and seafood varieties will be provided to demonstrate the number of servings that need to be consumed per week to meet recommendations for LC n–3 PUFA. With respect to fish consumption, concerns about potential contaminants and differences between wild-caught versus farmed species will be discussed. Fish oil and other types of supplements are also available. The potential benefits and drawbacks of using supplements as a source of LC n–3 PUFA will be discussed, including considerations about the amount and type of LC n–3 PUFA provided per capsule, as well as possible side effects. Although fish and fish oil are the primary sources of LC n–3 PUFA, other dietary sources and supplements are likely to become increasingly important contributors to LC n–3 PUFA intake and will be discussed in the chapter. Special attention should also be given to the LC n–3 PUFA needs of specific life stages (ie, pregnant and/or lactating women) and populations (ie, vegetarians). Emerging evidence has indicated that a third LC n–3 PUFA species—docosapentaenoic acid (DPA, 22:5n3)—may contribute to the beneficial health effects previously attributed solely to EPA and DHA. The sustainability of fish and fish oil is also a primary concern and the chapter will conclude with a brief discussion about this and the potential alternatives for meeting LC n–3 PUFA needs in the future.

INTAKE RECOMMENDATIONS

Recommendations Issued by Worldwide Authorities

LC n–3 PUFA were first considered for inclusion in nutrition recommendations by a North Atlantic Treaty Organization (NATO) workshop that was convened in 1988, based on earlier pioneering research with Greenland Eskimos. Although the members could not agree on a recommendation for n–3 fatty acid intake, it was recognized that 300–400 mg/day of LC n–3 PUFA was likely needed to prevent a deficiency in adults (Simopoulos, 1989). In 2002, the Institute of Medicine (IoM) concluded that there was insufficient data to determine dietary reference intakes for EPA and/or DHA. However, an Adequate Intake (AI), which is a recommended daily intake based on the nutrient intake of apparently healthy people that is assumed to be adequate, was established for alpha-linolenic acid (ALA) as 1.6 g/day for men and 1.1 g/day for women. It was recommended that up to 10% of this AI for ALA could be provided by EPA and/or DHA (Institute of Medicine, 2005). Since then, substantial evidence has accumulated demonstrating a clear, inverse relationship between EPA + DHA intake and the risk of fatal CHD and possibly other disease states (Harris et al., 2009). Recommendations have evolved to reflect this growing evidence-base, and numerous authorities have issued recommendations that now incorporate more specific guidelines for fish consumption and/or EPA + DHA intake to promote health and reduce the risk of CVD and other chronic diseases.

The most up-to-date recommendations for fish and/or specific LC n–3 PUFA intake issued by selected dietary and health authorities are provided in Table 3.1. A range of EPA + DHA intakes are recommended by different authorities. For instance, whereas the European Food Safety Authority (EFSA) and Food and Agriculture Organization (FAO) recommend 250 mg/day, the Japanese Ministry of Health recommends a minimum consumption of 1000 mg/day (Table 3.1; EFSA Panel on Dietetic Products, 2010; Joint FAO/WHO Expert Consulation, 2010a; Ezaki et al., 2012). However, there is general consensus among the majority of expert bodies for 250–500 mg of EPA + DHA per day, which can be provided by 2–3 servings of oily fish per week. Of the health organizations listed in Table 3.1, only the Australia & New Zealand National Health and Medical Research Council specifically refer to the LC n–3 PUFA docosapentaenoic acid (DPA, 22:5 n3). Comparatively, little is known about DPA, but current evidence indicates that it may provide a significant amount of LC n–3 PUFA intake in populations that consume meat from grass-fed ruminants and may provide similar health benefits (further discussion of DPA is provided later in the chapter). Further research on the role of DPA is warranted and future recommendations may need to consider including specific reference to DPA.

The recommendations issued by many organizations are intended to reduce the risk of chronic diseases (especially CHD) and promote the general health of the adult population as a whole. However, the optimal intake of LC n–3 PUFAs and/or fish may depend on the specific population and outcome of interest; thus, some organizations also provide recommendations to reduce the risk of specific chronic conditions/diseases, such as, secondary prevention of CHD and treatment of hypertriglyceridemia. For instance, the American Heart Association (AHA) recommends the equivalent of 500 mg EPA + DHA per day (provided by two servings/week of preferably oily fish) for primary prevention, 1 g/day for secondary prevention in individuals with established CHD (preferably from oily fish, or using EPA+DHA supplements in consultation with a physician), and 2–4 g/day for the treatment of high triglycerides.

TABLE 3.1 Current Fish and/or LC n-3 PUFA Intake Recommendations for Adults from Selected National and International Authorities

Country/ region	Authority (year)	Target	Recommendation
Global	FAO/WHO Expert Consultation (2010) (Joint FAO/WHO Expert Consulation, 2010a)	Healthy adults	250 mg EPA + DHA per day
		Pregnant/lactating women	300 mg EPA + DHA per day with at least 200 mg from DHA
	International Society for the Study of Fatty Acids and Lipids (Cunnane et al., 2004)	Reduce CHD risk in healthy adults	*Minimum* of 500 mg EPA + DHA per day
	Perinatal Lipid Intake Working Group (2008) (Koletzko et al., 2007)	Pregnant and lactating women	At least 200 mg per day of DHA Consume 1–2 portions of sea fish, including oily fish, per week
Europe	European Food Safety Authority (EFSA Panel on Dietetic Products, 2010)	Healthy adults	250 mg EPA + DHA per day 1–2 fatty fish meals per week
		Pregnancy and lactation	General 250 mg per day of EPA + DHA recommendation plus additional 100 mg per day of DHA
United States	American Heart Association (Kris-Etherton et al., 2002; Lloyd-Jones et al., 2010)	Healthy adults	500 mg EPA + DHA per day At least two 3.5 ounce servings of (preferably oily) fish per week
		Secondary CHD prevention	1 g EPA + DHA per day
		Treatment of hypertriglyceridemia	2–4 g EPA + DHA per day
		Pregnant/lactating women	Up to 12 ounces per week of a variety of fish that are low in mercury (avoid shark, swordfish, king mackerel, and tilefish; limit consumption of albacore "white" tuna to six ounces per week)
	Dietary Guidelines for Americans U.S. Department of Health and Human Services and U.S. Department of Agriculture. 2015–2020 Dietary Guidelines for Americans. 8th ed, 2015.	General health of adults	Consume at least 8 ounces of seafood per week, which provides on average 250 mg/day EPA+DHA
		Pregnant/lactating women	Consume at least 8 and up to 12 ounces of seafood per week from a variety of seafood types that are lower mercury
	New 2015 Dietary Guidelines for Americans have been issued, which supplants the Dietary Guidelines Advisory Committee Report		
	Academy of Nutrition and Dietetics (Vannice and Rasmussen, 2014)	General adult population	Consume two or more servings of fatty fish per week to provide at least 500 mg EPA + DHA per day
	National Lipid Association (2014)	Treatment of hypertriglyceridemia	2–4 g/d LC n-3 fatty acids Jacobson T.A., et al., 2014. National Lipid Association recommendations for patient-centered management of dyslipidemia: Part 1 - executive summary. J. Clin. Lipidol. 8 (5), 473–88.
United Kingdom	NICE (National Institute for Health and Care Excellence, 2014)	Secondary prevention and/or people at high risk of CVD	Eat at least two portions of fish per week, including a portion of oily fish

(*Continued*)

TABLE 3.1 Current Fish and/or LC n-3 PUFA Intake Recommendations for Adults from Selected National and International Authorities (*cont.*)

Country/ region	Authority (year)	Target	Recommendation
Australia and New Zealand	National Heart Foundation of Australia (2008; updated in 2015) (Sugano and Hirahara, 2000; Papanikolaou et al., 2014)	Adults	2–3 servings of fish (including oily fish) per week to provide 250–500 mg EPA + DHA per day
		Secondary CHD prevention	1000 mg EPA + DHA per day
		Treatment of hypertriglyceridemia	Starting dose of 1200 mg EPA + DHA per day, increasing to 4000 mg per day until TG target is reached
	Australia & New Zealand National Health and Medical Research Council (Australian National Health and Medical Research Council, 2006)	Reduce chronic disease risk	Combined EPA + DPA + DHA intake of 610 mg per day for men and 430 mg per day for women
Netherlands	Health Council of the Netherlands (Health Council of the Netherlands, 2001)	General health of adults	200 mg per day of n–3 fatty acids in fish
France	French Food Safety Agency (ANSES, 2010)	General health of adults	250 mg per day of DHA and 250 mg per day of EPA for a combined intake of 500 mg per day of EPA + DHA
Canada	Dietitians of Canada (Kris-Etherton et al., 2007)	General health of adults	Two servings of fish per week, preferably fatty fish
			~8 ounces of cooked fish per week provides ~500 mg per day EPA and DHA
Japan	Japanese Ministry of Health (2010) (Ezaki et al., 2012)	Preventing lifestyle-related disease	More than 1 g per day of EPA and DHA (lower boundary; no upper boundary set)

Although these recommendations have existed for many years, only select populations consistently consume the recommended amount of fish and/or EPA + DHA. Therefore, strategies to increase consumption need to be devised and implemented. One such strategy may be improving messages to the public and increasing awareness of how these recommendations can be met by either dietary sources or supplements.

DIETARY SOURCES

Meeting Recommendations with Fish and/or Other Dietary Sources

Seafood, particularly oily fish, is the primary dietary source of LC n–3 PUFA. However, the LC n–3 PUFA content of fish varies by species and can also be influenced by how the fish were raised (ie, wild-caught or farm-raised). The EPA, DPA, and DHA content of common fish/seafood varieties is presented in Table 3.2 along with the number of servings needed per week to meet the daily EPA + DHA recommendation. Compared to oily fish, white fish, or non-oily fish tends to provide much less LC n–3 PUFA. For instance, whereas the recommended daily intake of 500 mg of EPA + DHA can be met by consuming approximately 2 servings of salmon or herring over the course of a week, it would require over 10 servings of canned light tuna and ~30 servings of tilapia to provide a similar amount of EPA and DHA (Table 3.2). In general, the best sources of LC n–3 PUFA include Atlantic, Chinook, Coho, or Sockeye varieties of salmon; Pacific or Atlantic herring; anchovies; sardines; and rainbow trout (Table 3.2).

Although all seafood provides EPA and DHA, it is important for consumers to recognize that not all varieties are rich sources of LC n–3 PUFA (Weaver et al., 2008; Harris, 2008). Large differences in the fatty acid profile within species can also occur due to many factors, including diet (Hardy and Lee, 2010; Theophilus Olayiwola et al., 2011) and the location or time of year that wild fish are harvested (Jobling and Bendiksen, 2003; Gallagher et al., 1989; Zlatanos and Laskaridis, 2007). In 2013, the most commonly consumed fish/seafood varieties in the United States were shrimp, salmon, canned tuna, tilapia, pollock, pangasius, cod, catfish, crab, and clams (National Fisheries Institute, 2013). Unfortunately, the majority of these species are very low in fat and therefore contain little LC n–3 PUFAs. Without a clear understanding of which types of fish provide the most LC n–3 PUFA content, consumers are likely to base their seafood choices on availability and cost—which in many cases will result in the consumption of predominantly low LC n–3 PUFA varieties, such as, farmed tilapia. However, fish are also a good source of

TABLE 3.2 Omega-3 Content (Milligrams per 3 Ounce Serving) Provided by Common Fish/Seafood Varieties and the Number of Servings Required per Week to Meet the 500 mg/day Recommendation for EPA + DHA[a]

	EPA	DPA	DHA	EPA+DHA	Servings/week to meet 500 mg/day recommendation[b]
SALMON					
Atlantic, farmed	586	NA	1238	1824	2
Atlantic, wild	349	313	1215	1564	2
Chinook	858	252	618	1476	2.5
Coho	462	250	706	1168	3
Sockeye	353	145	690	1043	3.5
Chum	254	86	429	683	5
Pink	185	48	339	524	6.5
HERRING					
Pacific	1056	187	751	1807	2
Atlantic	773	60	939	1712	2
Anchovies (raw)	457	25	774	1231	3
Sardines[c]	402	0	433	835	4
TROUT (RAINBOW)					
Wild	398	NA	442	840	4
Farmed	220	93	524	744	4.5
BASS					
Striped	184	NA	638	822	4.5
Sea	175	82	473	648	5.5
Freshwater	259	92	389	648	5.5
POLLOCK					
Atlantic	77	24	383	460	7.5
Alaska	73	23	360	433	8
TUNA					
Bluefin	309	136	970	1279	3
White, canned[d]	198	15	535	733	5
Skipjack	77	14	201	278	12.5
Light, canned[d]	40	8	190	230	15
Yellowfin	13	4	89	102	34
MACKEREL					
Atlantic	428	90	594	1022	3.5
King[e]	148	19	193	341	10
OYSTER (RAW)					
Pacific	372	17	212	584	6
Farmed	160	NA	173	333	10.5
Eastern	149	8	114	263	13.5

(Continued)

TABLE 3.2 Omega-3 Content (Milligrams per 3 Ounce Serving) Provided by Common Fish/Seafood Varieties and the Number of Servings Required per Week to Meet the 500 mg/day Recommendation for EPA + DHA[a] (*cont.*)

	EPA	DPA	DHA	EPA+DHA	Servings/week to meet 500 mg/day recommendation[b]
CRAB					
Alaska king	251	26	100	351	10
Dungeness	239	11	96	335	10.5
Blue	86	8	57	143	24.5
HALIBUT					
Greenland	573	97	428	1001	3.5
Atlantic and Pacific	68	17	132	200	17.5
COD					
Pacific	36	4	100	136	25.5
Atlantic	3	11	131	134	26
CATFISH					
Wild	85	NA	116	201	27.5
Farmed	17	15	59	76	46
OTHER					
Swordfish[e]	108	143	656	764	4.5
Tilefish[e]	146	122	623	769	4.5
Shark (mixed species; raw)[e]	269	93	448	717	5
Walleye (pink)	94	42	245	339	10.5
Flounder/Sole	143	29	112	255	13.5
Clam	117	88	124	241	14.5
Shrimp	115	10	120	235	15
Grouper	30	14	181	211	16.5
Lobster	99	5	66	165	21
Scallop	61	4	88	149	23.5
Haddock	43	5	93	136	25.5
Mahi mahi (dolphinfish)	22	10	96	118	29.5
Tilapia	4	52	113	117	30
Orange roughy	5	1	21	26	134.5

NA, not available.
[a] *Data from USDA National Nutrient Database for Standard Reference Release 27. All values are based on cooked varieties unless otherwise specified.*
[b] *Servings rounded to nearest 0.5 value.*
[c] *Atlantic, canned in oil, drained solids with bone.*
[d] *Canned in water, without salt, drained solids.*
[e] *Species with highest mercury content (≈1 ppm).*

high-quality protein, are low in total and saturated fat, and are a good source of other nutrients, including iodine, vitamin D, zinc, magnesium, phosphorus, selenium, and potassium (Ruxton, 2011). Thus, although they contribute very little to LC n–3 PUFA intake, these types of seafood can remain healthful choices if they are baked or broiled (not breaded or fried; Harris, 2008).

Aquaculture production has risen dramatically since the early 1990s in response to declining wild fish stocks (FAO, 2014). Salmon, tilapia, catfish, and trout are the most commonly consumed farm-raised fish (Weaver et al., 2008). For some species, it is important to distinguish between wild caught and farmed varieties due to differences in LC n–3 PUFA content and concerns about environmental sustainability (discussed in the following sections). For instance, farmed versus wild Atlantic salmon typically has higher EPA + DHA content, whereas wild rainbow trout may contain more EPA + DHA than its farmed counterparts (Table 3.2). A recent analysis of the fatty acid composition of farmed and wild species concluded that, in general, farmed species have equivalent or greater amounts of EPA and DHA compared to their wild-caught comparators (Cladis et al., 2014). However, farm-raised fish also tend to be higher in total fat, largely due to saturated fatty acids (SFA), monounsaturated fatty acids (MUFA), and n–6 fatty acids (Weaver et al., 2008; Cladis et al., 2014; Gebauer et al., 2006). These differences in the fatty acid profile are likely influenced by the composition of the diet consumed by farmed fish. Diets high in SFA, MUFA, and n–6 obtained from plant or animal sources are inexpensive, readily available, and thus are often used to reduce costs. Certain species, such as tilapia, can also be cultured intensively with feeds that contain less protein, more carbohydrates, and a wide range of fat sources, which influences tissue fatty acid concentrations (Weaver et al., 2008).

Concerns have also been raised about environmental toxins in fish, such as, methylmercury, polychlorinated biphenyls (PCBs), and dioxins. Most fish contain trace amounts of methylmercury from natural sources (eg, erosion of geologic deposits and volcanic emissions), but this can be exacerbated by environmental contamination from industrial practices. Methylmercury is readily absorbed by tissues and thus tends to bioaccumulate. Therefore, larger, older, and higher-trophic-level species generally have higher methylmercury content. However, methylmercury content can vary greatly between and within species because it reflects the concentration of methylmercury in their prey species, the level of contamination in their environment, and species-specific physiological factors related to metabolism and growth rate (Mahaffey et al., 2011). In general, shark, tilefish, swordfish, and king mackerel contain the highest methylmercury content. At-risk population groups (ie, women who are pregnant, could become pregnant, or are lactating, and infants and young children) should avoid consuming these species (US Food and Drug Administration and Environment Protection Agency, 2004). The health effects of low-level methylmercury exposure in adults who are not considered at-risk are not well established. However, methylmercury may modestly decrease the benefits of fish intake (Mozaffarian and Rimm, 2006). Although regulatory efforts have effectively reduced the use and emission of PCBs and dioxins, both compounds persist in the environment and remain present in low concentrations in many foods. However, commercially sold fish—whether wild-caught or farm-raised—contain very little PCBs and dioxins and are responsible for only ≈ 9% of total dietary exposure in the United States (Mozaffarian and Wu, 2011; Joint FAO/WHO Expert Consulation, 2010b). Cooking as well as removing the skin and fat of fish can also substantially reduce PCB and dioxin concentrations. Unfortunately, preparation methods have little impact on methylmercury content. Overall, the health benefits of fish intake outweigh the potential risks and consuming a variety of seafood will minimize exposure to environmental toxins while still maximizing the health benefits of consuming fish (Mozaffarian and Rimm, 2006).

Although oily fish are the most concentrated source of LC n–3 PUFA, many non–fish sources of EPA and DHA are now available and can be used to fortify foods. Numerous food products have been enriched with LC n–3 PUFAs from fish or microalgae (Mahaffey et al., 2011; Whelan and Rust, 2006). Enriching chocolates, instant oats, milk, dips, salad dressings, breads, and other products with ≈ 125 mg EPA + DHA per serving (to provide ≈ 1 g/day) has been shown to increase LC n–3 PUFA status (Murphy et al., 2007). Eggs can also provide a substantial source of LC n–3 PUFA if laying hens are fed supplemental fish oil or algae oil because the fatty acid composition of the egg yolk reflects the lipid content of the hen's diet(Leskanich and Noble, 1997). For instance, eggs containing 56 mg EPA and 211 mg DHA have been produced from hens supplemented with fish oil (Elkin et al., 2015). Algae oil supplementation has resulted in similar increases in the total n–3 fatty acid and DHA content of egg yolks (Herber and Van Elswyk, 1996). Supplementing animal feeds with fish oil or fishmeal can similarly increase the LC n–3 PUFA content of poultry and pork products, although this requires the development of feeding strategies that maximize LC n–3 PUFA enrichment without compromising consumer palatability (Leskanich and Noble, 1997; Howe et al., 2002). For instance, a tuna fishmeal supplement has been used to increase the total LC n–3 PUFA content of pork and chicken products to ≈ 60–200 mg per 100 g serving, while maintaining consumer acceptance (Howe et al., 2002). However, this strategy has proven less promising in ruminant species that typically consume a smaller amount of dietary fat and usually biohydrogenate unsaturated fatty acids unless they are protected (ie, with an enteric coating) (Wachira et al., 2002; Ashes et al., 1992; Mandell et al., 1997). Producing plant and animal products enriched with LC n–3 PUFA by genetic engineering may also provide an alternative (Whelan, 2009; Kang et al., 2004; Lai et al., 2006). Based on the historic reluctance of Western populations to increase fatty fish intake, fortification of commonly consumed foods with LC n–3 PUFA may offer a feasible solution (Harris, 2007a).

SUPPLEMENTAL SOURCES

Meeting Recommendations with Fish Oil or Other Supplements

LC n–3 PUFA can also be obtained from a variety of supplements, including fish oil and non fish-based products. Some individuals may prefer supplements due to personal preferences, such as, ethical or environmental concerns, disliking the taste of fish, unfamiliarity with seafood preparation and cooking methods, cost, food allergies, and a perceived risk of pollutants. Others may require a supplement to achieve higher recommended LC n–3 PUFA intakes that are not attainable by dietary means alone (ie, those with established CHD or elevated triglycerides). The EPA and DHA content of prescription products and dietary supplements is provided in Table 3.3. The EPA + DHA content provided by a 1 g capsule is typically 200–800 mg (Chee et al., 1990; Tatarczyk et al., 2007). Supplements are not subject to the same regulatory standards as pharmaceutical preparations (ie, Lovaza, Vascepa, and Epanova) and thus may have more variation in their LC n–3 PUFA content. However, multiple quality assessments of common brands have confirmed that the actual LC n–3 PUFA content of fish oil supplements is generally consistent with that reported on the manufacturers' label (Chee et al., 1990; Tatarczyk et al., 2007; ConsumerLab.com, 2014). Additionally, fish oil supplements contain little to no mercury (Foran et al., 2003) and low absolute quantities of other contaminants (ie, dioxins and PCBs; Mozaffarian and Wu, 2011; Food Safety Authority of Ireland, 2002; Jacobs et al., 2002).

LC n–3 PUFA supplements are available in a variety of formulations [ie, natural triglycerides (TG), ethyl esters (EE), free fatty acids (FFA), and reesterified triglycerides (rTG)]. In foods and standard fish body oils (ie, menhaden or cod liver oils), LC n–3 PUFAs are naturally found in the TG form (Rubio-Rodríguez et al., 2010). However, crude fish body oil supplements contain only ≈ 18% EPA and ≈ 12% DHA (Schuchardt and Hahn, 2013). This requires that a relatively large number of capsules be taken to meet recommended LC n–3 PUFA intake, creating significant challenges for compliance (Dyerberg et al., 2010). Refining processes—referred to as molecular distillation—have been developed to deodorize and concentrate fish oils, resulting in products with 50%–85% EPA + DHA content (Rubio-Rodríguez et al., 2010). This manufacturing process involves hydrolysis of the TG-bound LC n–3 PUFA from the glycerol backbone, releasing FFAs that are then bound to ethanol, creating an EE fatty acid. This concentrates the

TABLE 3.3 EPA and DHA Content of Common Supplements and the Number of Capsules Required to Meet the 1 g/day Recommendation.

Prescription omega-3 products[a]	Formulation	EPA	DHA	EPA + DHA	Capsules required to meet ≈ 1 g/day EPA + DHA recommendation
VascEPA[b] (Bays et al., 2011)	Ethyl esters	≥960	0	≥960	1 (960 mg/day EPA only)
EPAnova (Kastelein et al., 2014)	Free fatty acids	550	200	750	1 (750 mg/day)
Lovaza[c] (Bays, 2006)	Ethyl esters	465	375	840	1 (840 mg/day)
Dietary Supplements					
Standard menhaden fish body oil[d] (Kris-Etherton et al., 2002)	Triglycerides	180	120	300	3 (900 mg/day)
Omega-3 fatty acid concentrate[d] (Kris-Etherton et al., 2002)	Triglycerides	300	200	500	2 (1000 mg/day)
Cod liver oil[e]	Triglycerides	80	100	180	5 (900 mg/day)
Microalgae oil[f]	Triglycerides	90	160	250	4 (1000 mg/day)
Krill oil[g]	Phospholipids, free fatty acids, and triglycerides	128	60	~190	5 (950 mg/day)

[a] *Approved by the FDA for the treatment of hypertriglyceridemia (fasting serum triglycerides ≥500 mg/dL).*

[b] *Also referred to as AMR101 (Amarin) or Icosapent ethyl, and is marketed as Epadel in Japan.*

[c] *Previously known as Omacor.*

[d] *The United States Pharmacopeial Convention (USP) has verified supplements made by Berkley & Jensen, Equaline, Kirkland Signature, and Nature Made. ConsumerLab.com has also performed quality testing on 53 supplements containing omega-3 fatty acids and verified their contents of EPA and DHA, as well as freshness, purity, and cost (ConsumerLab.com, 2014).*

[e] *EPA and DHA content may vary by brand. Values in table represent labeled EPA and DHA content of Carlson cod liver oil gems super 1000 mg (http://www.carlsonlabs.com/p-109-cod-liver-oil-gems-super-1000-mg.aspx).*

[f] *EPA and DHA content may vary by brand. Values in table represent labeled EPA and DHA content of Nordic Naturals Algae Omega 650 mg softgels (http://www.nordicnaturals.com/en/Products/Product_Details/514/?ProdID = 1654).*

[g] *EPA and DHA content may vary by brand. Values in table represent labeled EPA and DHA content of Schiff MegaRed Ultra Strength Omega-3 Krill Oil 1000 mg softgels (http://www.megared.com/our-products/megared-ultra-strength-1000-mg-omega-3-krill-oil/).*

fatty acids and removes any contaminants. Once the desired concentration is achieved, EEs can be chemically converted back to triglycerides, forming rTG. Since the production of EEs is less costly, the majority of fish oil concentrate supplements and the two of the three FDA-approved pharmaceutical preparations (ie, Lovaza and Vascepa) are in the EE form. FFAs, which are susceptible to autooxidation and more likely to cause gastrointestinal side effects when administered orally (Lawson and Hughes, 1988), were traditionally removed during the refining process (Schuchardt and Hahn, 2013). However, these effects can be reduced by encapsulation (Lawson and Hughes, 1988) and coating with a polyacrylate material that facilitates a delayed release in the small intestine rather than the stomach (Davidson et al., 2012). FFA formulations using these technologies have become commercially available (ie, Epanova).

There is much debate regarding potential differences in the bioavailability of these different LC n–3 PUFA formulations and how different factors, such as taking capsules with a fat-containing meal, may affect digestion and absorption. In general, there seems to be some indication that bioavailability is highest for the FFA form (Ghasemifard et al., 2014), with TG-bound and rTG-bound forms being more bioavailable than the EE form (Schuchardt and Hahn, 2013; Ghasemifard et al., 2014). However, these conclusions are limited by differences in sample size, length of supplementation, and the outcome measure used to assess bioavailability (ie, red blood cell [RBC] or plasma/serum fatty acid concentrations; Schuchardt and Hahn, 2013; Ghasemifard et al., 2014). Most importantly, equal amounts of LC n–3 PUFA were not provided by the different formulations in many studies (Ghasemifard et al., 2014). Other studies have also found no differences in bioavailability among the different formulations (Nordoy et al., 1991; Krokan et al., 1993). Thus, at this time, there is not scientific consensus about the bioavailability of different preparations of LC n–3 fatty acids. It is generally recommended that fish oil supplements be taken with a meal; however, the fat content of the meal can substantially alter bioavailability, particularly for EE preparations. Thus, whether a lipid-rich meal was incorporated into the supplementation design may have substantially influenced bioavailability results (Schuchardt and Hahn, 2013; Dyerberg et al., 2010; Ghasemifard et al., 2014). It is also unclear whether potential differences in bioavailability translate into significant differences in physiological effects. Although current evidence indicates that EE preparations may have the lowest bioavailability, the key randomized trials demonstrating the cardioprotective effects of EPA and DHA used EE preparations (GISSI-Prevenzione Investigators, 1999; Tavazzi et al., 2008; Yokoyama et al., 2007). EE-based supplements also consistently increase the n–3 index, a robust marker of EPA and DHA intake (Skulas-Ray et al., 2011; Neubronner et al., 2011; Harris, 2007b). In addition, there is extensive evidence for the triglyceride-lowering effect of each form of supplement (Skulas-Ray et al., 2008; Bays, 2006; Kastelein et al., 2014; Ballantyne et al., 2012). Thus, bioavailability is not typically an important consideration for selecting a LC n–3 PUFA supplement.

Other types of LC n–3 PUFA supplements are also available, including EPA- or DHA-only supplements, cod liver oil, krill oil, and microalgae oil. Purified EPA-only and DHA-only supplements have been used to investigate potential differential effects of the two fatty acids on CVD risk factors. It is beyond the scope of this chapter to provide an in-depth discussion of these findings; however, reviews have concluded that EPA and DHA have shared and complementary effects, although further investigation is warranted as studies of individual fatty acids are relatively limited (Mori and Woodman, 2006; Wei and Jacobson, 2011; Jacobson et al., 2012). However, it may be more practical to continue focusing on their combined consumption as this is how LC n–3 PUFA are consumed in dietary sources, evidence for their individual effects remains limited, and increasing consumption of either would be beneficial (Mozaffarian and Wu, 2012). Cod liver oil is a less concentrated source of EPA and DHA but also provides substantial amounts of vitamins A, D, and E (Lentjes et al., 2014). Although cod-liver oil supplementation is more often associated with traditional "folk" medicine approaches (ie, prevention of rickets), it has been shown to reduce total cholesterol (Kingsbury et al., 1961), as well as triglycerides, while increasing HDL-C (Sanders et al., 1981). Oil can also be extracted from cultivated microalgae (Adarme-Vega et al., 2012), with different varieties producing varying concentrations of EPA, DHA, and other LC n–3 PUFA (Doughman et al., 2007; Ward and Singh, 2005; Patil et al., 2007); however, the microalgae strains that have been developed for commercial use (ie, *Crypthecodinium cohnii, Schizochytrium* species, and *Ulkenia* species) produce DHA-rich oil (≈ 40% DHA w/ ≤ 2.5% EPA; Doughman et al., 2007; Bernstein et al., 2012). Microalgae oil is very low in contaminants (Doughman et al., 2007), can be a nutritionally equivalent source of DHA as cooked salmon (Arterburn et al., 2008), and lowers triglycerides to a similar extent as fish oil supplementation (Bernstein et al., 2012). Krill oil has recently gained a great deal of attention as an alternative to fish oil. It is processed from Antarctic krill (*Euphausia superba*) and also provides astaxanthin—an antioxidant responsible for the pink coloration of krill, salmon, trout, shrimp, and other crustaceans. Compared to fish oil, krill oil has a much lower concentration of LC n–3 PUFA (Tou et al., 2007; Ulven et al., 2011) with a higher EPA to DHA ratio (2:1 versus 1.5:1; Berge et al., 2014) [99]. Krill oil also provides EPA and DHA in the phospholipid rather than TG form (Berge et al., 2014) and many claims have been made about greater bioavailability due to the provision of fatty acids in this form. However, this has yet to be conclusively demonstrated as no direct comparisons of krill oil and fish oil supplements have been conducted (Salem and Kuratko, 2014). Commercial krill oil products can also vary in phospholipid content (19–81%) and contain di- and triglycerides (13–34%), as well as free fatty acids (3.5–36%; Salem and Kuratko, 2014; Araujo et al., 2014). Limited evidence demonstrates that krill oil supplementation has been shown to lower serum triglycerides (Ulven et al., 2011; Berge et al., 2014; Bunea et al., 2004). Compared to standard fish oil supplements, microalgae and krill oil supplements are more expensive.

Although fish oil supplements offer a viable alternative to consuming fish and effectively increase LC n–3 PUFA intake, there is some risk of mild, predominately gastrointestinal, side effects. With respect to prescription LC n–3 PUFAs, the most commonly reported side effects are: (1) diarrhea, nausea, abdominal pain or discomfort, and burping with Epanova (AstraZeneca, 2014); (2) burping, upset stomach, and a change in the sense of taste with Lovaza (GlaxoSmithKline, 2014); and (3) joint pain with Vascepa (Amarin Corporation, 2015). Like other lipid-lowering medications, both Lovaza and Epanova can also transiently increase liver function enzymes in some individuals and should be periodically monitored by a medical practitioner (AstraZeneca, 2014; GlaxoSmithKline, 2014). Gastrointestinal side effects can often be resolved by switching to a different formulation or taking the capsule with meals or at a different time of day (Mozaffarian and Wu, 2011). EE preparations should not be frozen but for other formulations, taking the capsule frozen may help to reduce gastrointestinal side effects. Some supplements are provided as enteric-coated capsules designed to release the oils in the intestine rather than the stomach to prevent a fishy aftertaste or fishy burps. Both prescription and dietary supplement formulations containing DHA have been shown to increase LDL-C (Mozaffarian and Wu, 2012; Mori and Woodman, 2006; Bernstein et al., 2012). However, increases in LDL-C were typically associated with greater reductions in TG (Wei and Jacobson, 2011; Jacobson et al., 2012) and were primarily due to an increase in LDL particle size, thereby resulting in a less atherogenic lipid/lipoprotein profile (Mozaffarian and Wu, 2012; Mori and Woodman, 2006). The magnitude of this response also typically depends on the TG and LDL-C concentrations of individuals prior to supplementation (Wei and Jacobson, 2011; Jacobson et al., 2012).

Additional Considerations Regarding LC n–3 PUFA

Special attention should also be given to the LC n–3 PUFA needs of specific life stages and population groups, the emerging role of docosapentaenoic acid (DPA, 22:5n3), and the sustainability of fish and fish oil supplements as the primary source of LC n–3 PUFA.

SPECIFIC LIFE STAGES AND POPULATION GROUPS

Pregnant or Lactating Women

DHA is an essential nutrient required for proper growth and development of the brain and retina (Innis, 2004; Koletzko and Rodriguez-Palmero, 1999). Both observational studies and intervention trials have demonstrated that greater maternal LC n–3 PUFA consumption during pregnancy is associated with better visual and neural development (Mahaffey et al., 2011; Innis, 2007), whereas reduced DHA in these brain and retinal tissues can result in decreased visual and psychomotor development (Innis, 2004). The DHA content of the maternal diet is the primary determinant of the amount of DHA transferred to the fetus via the placenta and the amount of DHA secreted in breastmilk (Innis, 2004; Innis, 2008). Uptake of DHA into these tissues is greatest during the third trimester and the first 2 years of life, making the pre- and postnatal periods of critical importance for maternal DHA consumption (Mahaffey et al., 2011; Koletzko and Rodriguez-Palmero, 1999). Therefore, women should consume adequate quantities of seafood high in LC n–3 PUFA or supplement their diet during pregnancy and lactation to ensure that they can meet the needs of the fetus in addition to their own physiological needs. Recommendations for LC n–3 PUFA intake have been issued specifically for women who are pregnant, may become pregnant, or are lactating (Table 3.1). In many cases, these recommendations specify the amount of DHA that should make up the total LC n–3 PUFA intake (Joint FAO/WHO Expert Consulation, 2010a) or advocate additional DHA intake beyond that suggested for the general population (EFSA Panel on Dietetic Products, 2010).

Awareness of the benefits of DHA intake for fetal development coexists with concerns about environmental toxins in fish/seafood. Women who are pregnant, women who may become pregnant, lactating women, and children are considered at-risk groups due to the potential for detrimental neurodevelopmental effects of pre- and postnatal methylmercury exposure. Three long-term studies have been conducted in populations with frequent maternal fish consumption (New Zealand, the Faroe Islands, and the Seychelles) to evaluate the effects of prenatal methylmercury exposure (Crump et al., 1998; Grandjean et al., 1997; Myers et al., 2003). In some cases, higher maternal methylmercury exposure was associated with poorer scores on subsets of neurodevelopmental assessments in children (Crump et al., 1998; Grandjean et al., 1997). These studies provided the basis for the Environmental Protection Agency's (EPA) methylmercury reference dose (RfD), which is defined as the amount that can be consumed daily over the course of the lifetime without any expectation of adverse effects, and is set at 0.1 μg of mercury per kg of body weight per day. The mercury content in selected fish/seafood species is provided in Table 3.4. In June 2004, the United States Food and Drug Administration (FDA) and EPA jointly issued an advisory on seafood consumption for pregnant and nursing women (US Food and

TABLE 3.4 Average Mercury Content of Selected Species of Fish/Seafood Compared to the EPA + DHA Content of These Species (per Three Ounce Serving)[a]

Species	Mercury (μg)	EPA + DHA (mg)
Varieties with highest mercury content[b]		
Tilefish (Gulf of Mexico)	123	770
Swordfish	84.6	760
Shark	83.2	720
King mackerel	62.1	340
Commonly consumed varieties		
Salmon	1.87	520–1820
Herring	7.14	1710–1810
Anchovies	1.45	1230
Atlantic mackerel	4.25	1020
Sardines	1.11	840
Trout (freshwater)	6.04	740–840
Bass (saltwater, black, striped)	12.9	650–820
Pollock	2.64	430–460
Tuna, canned, light	10.9	230
Tuna, canned, white	29.8	730
Tuna, yellowfin	30.1	100
Tuna, Skipjack	12.2	280
Oyster	1.02	260–580
Crab	5.53	140–350
Halibut	20.5	200–1000
Cod	9.44	130–140
Catfish	2.13	80–200
Flatfish (includes flounder, plaice, sole)	4.76	260
Clam	0.77	240
Shrimp	0.77	240
Grouper	38.1	210
Lobster (Northern/American)	9.1	170
Scallop	0.26	150
Haddock	4.68	140
Tilapia	1.11	120
Orange roughy	48.5	30

[a] *Data from United States Food and Drug Administration, "Mercury Levels in Commercial Fish and Shellfish (1990–2010)" (available at: http://www.fda.gov/food/foodborneillnesscontaminants/metals/ucm115644.htm) and USDA National Nutrient Database for Standard Reference Release 27.*
[b] *Should be avoided by at-risk population groups (ie, pregnant or lactating women, women of child-bearing potential, and children).*

Drug Administration and Environment Protection Agency, 2004). It recommended that species with the highest methylmercury content (ie, shark, swordfish, king mackerel, and tilefish) be avoided entirely by at-risk groups. Women and young children were advised to "eat up to 12 ounces or 2 average meals a week of a variety of fish and shellfish that are lower in mercury,", such as, shrimp, canned light tuna, salmon, pollock, and catfish (US Food and Drug Administration and Environment Protection Agency, 2004). Although the advisory acknowledges the nutritional benefits of consuming a variety of fish/shellfish, of the examples of commonly consumed low-mercury species given in the advisory, salmon is the only option that would provide the recommended EPA + DHA intake within the 12 ounce per week restriction (Table 3.2). The advisory additionally restricts consumption of albacore ("white") tuna to 6 ounces per week due to its higher methylmercury content. Conversely, canned light tuna does not need to be restricted in this way, although it contains lesser amounts of EPA and DHA. Unfortunately, many pregnant women and their health-care providers likely do not make this distinction, resulting in complete avoidance of tuna (and likely other seafood, as well).

While the neurodevelopmental harm associated with excessive methylmercury consumption should not be ignored, most authorities agree that the benefits of fish consumption far outweigh the potential risk from consuming small amounts of contaminants (Mozaffarian and Rimm, 2006; Joint FAO/WHO Expert Consulation, 2010b). Unfortunately, this message has not always been effectively conveyed to the public (Verbeke et al., 2005). Messages about risk often predominate in the news media (Greiner et al., 2010) and concerns about prenatal methylmercury exposure and developmental impairments can quickly overtake the message that greater fish consumption is beneficial for fetal development (Bloomingdale et al., 2010). This may create an unnecessarily negative perception of fish and cause pregnant women to further reduce their already insufficient fish intake. For instance, following well-publicized national advisories about the risks of mercury in fish in 2001, total fish consumption decreased in a cohort of pregnant Massachusetts women (Oken et al., 2003). A risk assessment of the effects of the 2001 advisory also demonstrated that consumers tend to reduce consumption of all types of fish species, resulting in reduced intake of LC n–3 PUFA as well as methylmercury (Shimshack and Ward, 2010). Additionally, although the FDA/EPA advisory is intended for at-risk groups (ie, women of child-bearing age and children), there are likely spill-over effects in low-risk groups and reduced consumption in the general population (Shimshack et al., 2007).

The FDA and EPA have issued a 2014 draft revision of their 2004 advisory, although it has yet to be finalized (US Food and Drug Administration, 2014). The new advisory is intended to encourage women to eat the recommended amount and types of fish and now includes a minimum of 8 ounces per week (US Food and Drug Administration, 2014), in accordance with the DGA2015 recommendation that "women who are pregnant or breastfeeding consume at least 8 ounces and up to 12 ounces of a variety of seafood per week, from choices lower in methyl mercury" (USDA, HSS, 2010). Other countries, such as Japan, offer less restrictive guidance and highlight the nutritional value of fish consumption. For instance, the Japanese Ministry of Health urges pregnant women not to stop eating fish or reduce their intake but to pay attention to which species may contain high mercury levels (Ser and Watanabe, 2012).

Fish consumption advisories require careful formulation to ensure that the benefits and risks of fish consumption are communicated effectively and are accessible to both high- and low-risk groups (Mahaffey et al., 2011; Oken et al., 2012). It is possible to select species that will minimize methylmercury exposure while providing the benefits associated with fish consumption (Bellinger, 2014; Del Gobbo et al., 2010; Dewailly et al., 2008); for instance, Atlantic mackerel, salmon, and sardines contain substantial LC n–3 PUFA content with low-to-moderate methylmercury (Mahaffey et al., 2011). However, there are currently no clear guidelines for consumers to select an appropriate combination of fish to obtain the recommended amount of LC n–3 PUFA without exceeding the methylmercury reference dose. Many consumers may also be overwhelmed by the number and complexity of factors that must be considered (Oken et al., 2012). The difficulty of conveying this message is likely somewhat responsible for pregnant and lactating women in Canada, Australia, Europe, and the United States consuming far below the recommended amount of fish and/or DHA (Cosatto et al., 2010; Sioen et al., 2010; Denomme et al., 2005; Innis and Elias, 2003; Jia et al., 2015). Ultimately, the best long-term solution for reducing methylmercury concentrations in fish is controlling global mercury sources. Unfortunately, despite the progress that has been made in this regard, it will take many years for these changes to become apparent in the food system. In the interim, clearer and more effective messages are needed to ensure that pregnant and lactating women consume adequate amounts of fish and LC n–3 PUFA while remaining protected from undue methylmercury exposure.

Vegetarian and Vegan Populations

As LC n–3 PUFA are primarily obtained from the consumption of fish and/or fish oil, vegetarian and vegan populations tend to have very low or no LC n–3 PUFA intake and may benefit from alternative dietary and/or supplement options. Vegetarians consume minimal EPA (<5 mg/day) and varying amounts of DHA (typically ≈20 mg/day), depending on dairy and egg consumption (Davis and Kris-Etherton, 2003; Sanders, 2009; Geppert et al., 2005). Vegans consume negligible amounts of both EPA and DHA (Davis and Kris-Etherton, 2003). Even if vegetarians/vegans consume adequate amounts of ALA—the precursor of LC n–3 PUFA—this is not a viable substitute for preformed EPA and DHA due to poor conversion. Conversion of ALA to LC n–3 PUFA requires a series of alternating desaturation and elongation reactions, and conversion efficiency tends to vary considerably among individuals. General consensus is that conversion to EPA is limited (≈8% in adult men; Burdge and Calder, 2005). Further conversion to DHA is estimated to be even lower, with the majority of studies reporting estimates of less than 0.05% in adult men (Burdge and Calder, 2005). Premenopausal women tend to exhibit higher conversion rates, particularly for the production of DHA (≈2.5-fold greater conversion rates for EPA and >200-fold greater for DHA; Burdge and Calder, 2005), possibly as a means of ensuring that the DHA needs of the fetus/neonate can be met (Burdge and Calder, 2005; Burdge et al., 2002). However, greater dietary intake of n–6 fatty acids and/or LC n–3 PUFA may inhibit ALA conversion (Burdge and Calder, 2005). In general, vegetarians and vegans tend to have substantially lower plasma, blood cell, tissue, and breastmilk concentrations of EPA and DHA compared to omnivores (Sanders, 2009; Harris, 2014), indicating that in vivo ALA conversion rates may be insufficient to achieve EPA and DHA concentrations equivalent to those achieved by consuming fish. Therefore, vegetarian/vegan dietary sources and/or supplements are needed to ensure that this portion of the population has the means to meet LC n–3 PUFA recommendations.

A limited number of vegetarian dietary sources and supplements are now available and are likely to become increasingly accessible in the future as demand for these products grows. Individuals who consume eggs can obtain a reasonable amount of DHA (up to 100–150 mg DHA/egg from chicken fed microalgae), but very little EPA (Davis and Kris-Etherton, 2003). Seaweed, or macroalgae, is even lower in fat than most vegetables, but does contain small amounts of LC n–3 PUFA (≈100 mg EPA per 100 g serving; Davis and Kris-Etherton, 2003). As previously noted, microalgae oil is a viable supplement option but still remains more expensive compared to fish body oil supplements. Supplementation with microalgae has been shown to significantly increase the n–3 index, an established marker of LC n–3 PUFA intake, to concentrations associated with the lowest cardiovascular risk (Geppert et al., 2005). However, the algae oils currently commercially available are DHA-rich and provide much less EPA (Doughman et al., 2007). There is some evidence to suggest that retroconversion of supplemental DHA occurs at physiologically meaningful rates (Conquer and Holub, 1997), but additional sources of EPA may also be required.

Stearidonic acid (SDA; 18:4 n–3), the metabolic intermediate of ALA and EPA, may provide a viable plant-based alternative for obtaining EPA (Whelan, 2009). Although SDA is not a major component of the diet, it is a minor constituent in fish/seafood and is found in relatively high amounts in seeds from the Boraginaceae family, such as, echium oil (12–14% SDA; Walker et al., 2013; Surette, 2013; Guil-Guerrero et al., 2001; Kuhnt et al., 2012). Few SDA-containing seed oils are commercially available, but growing interest in alternative LC n–3 PUFA sources has led to development of genetically modified varieties of canola and soybean enriched in SDA (SDA soybean, 20–30% SDA; Lemke et al., 2010; Ursin, 2003). SDA-enriched soybean oil is also relatively oxidatively stable, increasing its potential integration into a wide range of food products (Decker et al., 2012), and has been predicted to be a less costly source of EPA than seafood or fish oil supplements (Kennedy et al., 2012). Interest in SDA is largely due to the fact that it is more efficiently converted to EPA than ALA. SDA does not appear to accumulate in tissues; when preformed SDA is consumed it is rapidly converted to EPA resulting in significant increases in tissue EPA and the n–3 index (Lemke et al., 2010; Harris et al., 2008; Krul et al., 2012; James et al., 2003). However, compared to dietary EPA, dietary SDA is ≈ 17% as effective at raising EPA concentrations in plasma phospholipids and RBC membranes and has no effect on DHA concentrations (Harris et al., 2008). Despite the evidence that SDA can increase tissue EPA concentrations, it remains unclear whether SDA can impart health benefits for CVD risk factors or outcomes. Randomized controlled trials have found no effect of SDA supplementation on lipid biomarkers (ie, TG, TC, LDL-C, and HDL-C; Whelan et al., 2012) in healthy (Krul et al., 2012), overweight, or obese populations (Lemke et al., 2010; Harris et al., 2008; Pieters and Mensink, 2015). However, the lack of effect in these trials may be due to the wide range of BMI and lipid levels of participants as the EPA-supplementation comparator group employed by many of these studies also did not experience reductions in TG (Walker et al., 2013; Lemke et al., 2010; Harris et al., 2008; Krul et al., 2012). Additionally, the duration of these trials may have been too short, they may have been underpowered with too few participants, or used doses of SDA that were too low as an SDA dose of 9 g/day may be required to detect health effects (Walker et al., 2013). Thus, further investigation into the potential health effects of SDA is warranted. Although they remain many years away from commercial production, transgenic varieties of canola, soybean, and safflower have also been developed to produce seed oils enriched in EPA and/or DHA (Surette, 2013; Truksa et al., 2006; Sayanova and Napier, 2011; Napier et al., 2015; Petrie et al., 2014; Damude and Kinney, 2007). However, any genetically modified crops are likely to face some degree of consumer resistance due to the negative perception of transgenic products.

Additional research is needed to clarify the benefits of LC n–3 PUFA supplementation in vegetarian and vegan populations. Vegetarian and vegan dietary patterns tend to be associated with better health (Harris, 2014), and it remains unclear whether LC n–3 PUFA supplementation can further reduce the risk of chronic disease in these populations (Sanders, 2009; Harris, 2014). However, the EPA and DHA status of vegetarians and vegans is generally well below that considered to be cardioprotective (Harris, 2014). At this point in time, increasing ALA and SDA consumption, combined with supplementation of preformed DHA from algae oil, offers the best means of increasing EPA and DHA in people who do not consume any animal products.

Docosapentaenoic Acid (DPA, 22:5n3)

Emerging evidence suggests that docosapentaenoic acid (DPA, 22:5n3), the intermediate fatty acid species between EPA and DHA, may also play a role in imparting the health benefits previously attributed solely to EPA and DHA. Although evidence remains limited, a lower serum concentration of n–3 DPA has been associated with greater risk of myocardial infarction (Oda et al., 2005). Furthermore, plasma n–3 DPA has been inversely associated with total mortality (particularly from stroke-related deaths; Mozaffarian et al., 2013), nonfatal myocardial infarction (Sun et al., 2008), and incident CVD in some ethnic groups (de Oliveira Otto et al., 2013). An inverse relationship between RBC n–3 DPA and triglycerides has been documented in two studies (Dai et al., 2016; Skulas-Ray et al., 2015), and this may have important implications for the management of atherogenic dyslipidemia. An inverse association with the inflammatory marker C-reactive protein (CRP) has also consistently been reported for plasma, serum, and RBC n–3 DPA concentrations (de Oliveira Otto et al., 2013; Skulas-Ray et al., 2015; Reinders et al., 2012; Mozaffarian et al., 2011; Micallef et al., 2009; Labonte et al., 2014) whereas no association between CRP and RBC EPA or DHA content has been found in many of these same study populations (Skulas-Ray et al., 2011; Labonte et al., 2014; Flock et al., 2014). Like EPA and DHA, n–3 DPA is also converted into unique specialized pro-resolving mediators (ie, resolvins, protectins, and maresins) that promote the resolution of inflammation (Dangi et al., 2009; Dalli et al., 2013). Based on their differing associations with inflammatory markers and the structural differences among n–3 DPA, EPA, DHA, and their metabolites, it is possible that they may influence different aspects of the innate immune system.

A better understanding of how n–3 DPA stores respond to LC n–3 PUFA supplementation is needed to clarify the role of n–3 DPA in health outcomes. Cell-based studies have demonstrated that interconversion of EPA and n–3 DPA occurs readily (Benistant et al., 1996; Kaur et al., 2011; Norris and Dennis, 2012), while conversion of n–3 DPA to DHA is limited (Kaur et al., 2010). In clinical trials, supplementation with EPA + DHA (Skulas-Ray et al., 2015; Cao et al., 2006; Meyer et al., 2009; Katan et al., 1997) and purified EPA (Krul et al., 2012; Mori et al., 2000; von Schacky and Weber, 1985) has also been shown to increase RBC and plasma n–3 DPA. Prior to supplementation, EPA and n–3 DPA levels in the body are also commonly associated whereas there is no relationship between n–3 DPA and DHA concentrations (Mozaffarian et al., 2013; Sun et al., 2008; Skulas-Ray et al., 2015; Mozaffarian et al., 2011). Therefore, endogenous production from EPA may be an important means of increasing tissue n–3 DPA reserves.

Endogenous n–3 DPA stores may also serve as a source of EPA, which could have important implications for disease states related to LC n–3 PUFA intake. EPA and n–3 DPA are highly interconvertible and EPA concentrations have been increased by DPA supplementation in both cell-based (Benistant et al., 1996) and clinical studies (Miller et al., 2013). LC n–3 PUFA also tend to exhibit cell/tissue specificity. Plasma EPA appears to serve as a more dynamic and readily available pool of LC n–3 fatty acids that increases and decreases more quickly than DHA (Sun et al., 2008; Katan et al., 1997; Brown et al., 1991). Furthermore, DHA is enriched in myocardial and neuronal membranes (Harris et al., 2004), and the EPA content of RBCs is lower than that of n–3 DPA and DHA (Dai et al., 2016; Cao et al., 2006; Katan et al., 1997; Miller et al., 2013). Thus, 22-carbon fatty acids may be preferentially stored in specific tissue compartments, and in the case of n–3 DPA, may serve to replenish plasma EPA that has been utilized.

Less research has been conducted on n–3 DPA compared to EPA and DHA, and consequently the contribution of n–3 DPA to total LC n–3 PUFA intake has not been a focus of nutrition information messaging. Supplement labels typically do not quantify the amount of n–3 DPA provided and intervention studies rarely report the n–3 DPA content of supplements. Nutrient databases may also be similarly limited and inaccuracies in the DPA content of foods have been found in both Canadian and Australian nutrient databases, resulting in substantial underestimations of intake (Howe et al., 2006; Jia et al., 2015). For example, when the 1995 Australian National Nutrition Survey was reanalyzed using a database with updated fatty acid composition data, 30% greater estimates for LC n–3 PUFA intake were found, largely due to inaccuracies in preexisting data regarding the DPA content of meats (Howe et al., 2006). Whereas DPA is a much smaller component of most fish and fish oil supplements compared to EPA and DHA (Howe et al., 2007), grass-fed red meat (particularly beef and lamb) is a modest source of n–3 DPA (and to a lesser extent, EPA; Howe et al., 2006). In Australians, the category of meat, poultry, and game is often the 2nd largest contributor to LC n–3 PUFA intake (following fish and seafood) due to its DPA content (Howe et al., 2006; Rahmawaty et al., 2013). Conversely, United States nutrient databases typically report very little, if any, LC n–3 PUFA content in meat. This may reflect lack of available fatty acid composition data or differences in the PUFA composition of meat from pasture-fed versus grain-fed livestock. Studies comparing the effect of different feeding systems on the fatty acid composition of beef have demonstrated that grass-based feeding can significantly increase EPA, DPA, and DHA content, although the increase in these fatty acids is modest (Ponnampalam et al., 2006; Nuernberg et al., 2005; Scollan et al., 2006; Turner et al., 2015). Therefore, Australian cattle, which are predominantly pasture-fed, tend to have higher LC n–3 PUFA concentrations than grain-fed cattle, which is a common feeding system in the United States (Howe et al., 2007; Ponnampalam et al., 2006). Thus, additional research is needed to better quantify the amount of n–3 DPA in supplements and foods, and identify factors that may influence n–3 DPA concentrations (ie, farming practices). However, current evidence indicates that n–3 DPA is a physiologically important LC n–3 PUFA and should be included in future investigations of the health benefits of individual n–3 fatty acid species, analyses of LC n–3 PUFA intakes, and dietary recommendations.

SUSTAINABILITY

Even at current levels of fish and fish oil consumption—which are far below recommendations—the sustainability of fish production is uncertain (Jenkins et al., 2009). In the 1950s and 1960s, global production from wild fisheries increased ~6% per year but average rates of increase had declined to ≈2% by the 1970s and 1980s (FAO, 2000). By the 1990s, despite increasing fishing effort, global catches had plateaued and the majority of fish stocks were fully exploited or had already collapsed (Jenkins et al., 2009; FAO, 2000). The proportion of fish stocks being harvested at a biologically sustainable amount has declined from 90% in 1974 to 71.2% in 2011 (FAO, 2014). Furthermore, in 2011, 28.8% of fish stocks were considered overfished (FAO, 2014). Global marine capture has remained relatively stable at ≈80–90 million tons from 1990–2014 (FAO, 2014, 2012, 2012). To meet the growing demand for seafood, which could no longer be met by increasing wild catches, aquaculture production has steadily risen since the 1970s. In 2014, aquaculture production contributed a record 42.2% of total fish production, compared to just 25.7% in 2000 (FAO, 2014). However, annual growth rates have declined from 10.8% over 1990–2000 to 6.2% during the 2000–12 period (FAO, 2014). Per capita fish consumption has increased from 10 kg in the 1960s to over 19 kg in 2012 and is projected to continue increasing (FAO, 2014). If the global population were to begin following intake recommendations, for each individual, the 500 mg EPA + DHA per day recommendation would translate to 182.5 g/year (Salem and Eggersdorfer, 2015); assuming a worldwide population of 7.2 billion, total global intake requirements would be ≈1.3 billion kg/year (Salem and Eggersdorfer, 2015). In terms of fish servings, this would require over 100 three-ounce servings of wild Atlantic salmon per person per year—and even greater quantities for species with less LC n–3 PUFA (Table 3.2). Thus, pressures on both wild fish stocks and aquaculture systems is unlikely to subside and the development of more sustainable harvesting practices or alternative sources of LC n–3 PUFA will likely be required.

Although aquaculture is often perceived as a potential solution to reduce pressure on wild fish stocks, certain types of aquaculture may actually contribute to the collapse of global fisheries (Naylor et al., 2000). Farming carnivorous fish (eg, salmon, Bluefin tuna, and sea bass) and marine shrimp can further deplete wild fishery stocks through habitat destruction, pollution from waste disposal, exotic species and pathogen invasions (Krkosek et al., 2007), and requirements for high-protein diets that contain substantial amounts of fish meal from wild-caught fish (Jenkins et al., 2009; Naylor et al., 2000; Naylor et al., 1998). Many intensive aquaculture systems rely heavily on added feeds because fish are stocked at a density beyond the capacity of natural food sources (Naylor et al., 2000). In these systems, carnivorous fish require 2.5–5 times more fish protein in fish meal than is ultimately produced by the farmed product (Tacon, 1997). Many of the species typically used for fish meal are already over-fished, which may have ramifications throughout the food web for their larger predator species (Pauly et al., 2005). Conversely, farming herbivorous species or filter feeders (ie, carp and mollusks) reduces the need for fish meal/oil in feed and thus is a greater contributor to the net global fish supplies (Naylor et al., 2000). By integrating the production of multiple trophic levels, polyculture systems utilize resources more efficiently and reduce environmental contamination compared to typical intensive monoculture methods, and may offer a practical solution for continued, sustainable expansion of the industry (Naylor et al., 2000; Neori et al., 2004; Chopin et al., 2001; Granada et al., 2015). For instance, seaweed (Neori et al., 1996; Troell et al., 1999) (Troell et al., 1999; Samocha et al., 2015), oysters (Jones and Iwama, 1991), and mussels (Soto and Mena, 1999; Handå et al., 2012) can be grown in wastewater from salmon and/or shrimp farming, using effluent output from one system as a resource for others. Ultimately, aquaculture sustainability will likely require greater regulation and enforcement of management techniques to reduce habitat destruction, prevent the escape of pathogens or farmed fish, and ensure proper treatment of wastewater (Naylor et al., 2000).

Identifying and developing alternative LC n–3 PUFA sources will also help to alleviate pressures on wild fisheries and allow aquaculture systems to grow sustainably. Microalgae oil, krill oil, and genetically modified plants and/or animals are currently the most promising alternatives but still encounter some limitations. Algae oil has been commercially produced since the 1990s to fortify infant formula with DHA (to achieve amounts similar to those found in human breastmilk; Kuratko and Salem, 2013; Spolaore et al., 2006). There is likely considerable room for growth and marketing to consumer niches as algae oil is considered environmentally friendly, free of ocean-borne contaminants, vegetarian, and can be manufactured under kosher and halal conditions (Salem and Eggersdorfer, 2015); however, algae oil remains more expensive than fish oil supplements and the development of new production facilities continues to be capital-intensive. Supplementation with algae oil may increase LDL-C (Bernstein et al., 2012), an effect that can also be caused by fish oil supplementation, and which may be due to the DHA and/or saturated fat content of commercially available algae oil (Geppert et al., 2005). Despite krill oil recently becoming a larger contributor to the supplement market, the present krill oil harvest is estimated to be below 0.1% of the over 300 million tons of available biomass in the Antarctic Ocean (Kwantes and Grundmann, 2015). The Commission for the Conservation of Antarctic Living Resources has estimated sustainable harvest rates (Kwantes and Grundmann, 2015; Nicol et al., 2012), but concerns have been raised about the fragility of the Antarctic ecosystem (Kwantes and Grundmann, 2015), negative effects of climate change in krill populations (Nicol et al., 2012; Flores et al., 2012), possible declines in krill stocks (Atkinson et al., 2004), and potential ramifications for species higher on the food chain (Atkinson et al., 2004; Trivelpiece et al., 2011). Krill oil is much more expensive than fish oil and contains a lower concentration of LC n–3 PUFA, requiring that more krill oil be consumed to achieve the same dose of LC n–3 PUFA (Kwantes and Grundmann, 2015). Genetically modified plants and/or animals capable of producing LC n–3 PUFA may offer a more efficient alternative, but are likely to face consumer resistance in some markets. Soybeans that have been genetically modified to produce SDA may offer an alternative to preformed EPA, but additional research is needed to determine if SDA can impart health benefits similar to those of EPA and DHA. Progress has been made in developing transgenic crops enriched in EPA and/or DHA, but they are not yet commercially available. Transgenic pigs that can endogenously synthesize LC n–3 PUFA have also been successfully produced (Lai et al., 2006) but likely face the greatest degree of consumer resistance and regulatory hurdles. Although these alternatives are likely to remain relatively minor contributors to LC n–3 PUFA intake for the immediate future, the increasingly limited supply of fish and fish oil may ultimately require that these barriers be overcome.

CONCLUSION

Despite substantial evidence that health benefits are associated with higher intake of fish and/or LC n–3 PUFA, many populations consume very little. Numerous expert authorities have issued recommendations for amounts of fish and/or LC n–3 PUFA intake to promote health and reduce CVD risk, with the general consensus specifying intake of 250–500 mg of EPA + DHA per day or 2–3 servings of oily fish per week. These recommendations can be met by consuming a variety of different fish species. However, many commonly consumed fish contain relatively low concentrations of LC n–3 PUFA and some are a source of environmental toxins. For individuals who cannot or prefer not to eat fish and those who require a higher intake of LC n–3 PUFA, supplementation may offer a viable alternative. Many varieties of fish and nonfish-based supplements are now available. Important considerations regarding supplements include: the amount of EPA + DHA provided in each capsule, the supplement formulation, potential side effects, cost, and sustainability. Although fish oils are the predominant source of LC n–3 PUFA, alternative supplement options include krill oil, algae oil, and SDA-enriched oils that can be converted to EPA. In addition to recommendations for the general population, special consideration should be given to the DHA needs of pregnant/lactating women and the LC n–3 PUFA needs of vegetarian/vegan populations. Emerging evidence also indicates that in addition to EPA and DHA, a third LC n–3 PUFA, DPA, may confer health benefits. Therefore, the amount of DPA in foods and supplements should be better quantified and additional research is needed to determine the effect of DPA supplementation and better characterize how DPA stores respond to n–3 supplementation. Although global LC n–3 PUFA intake remains well below recommendations, the sustainability of worldwide fish production is a significant concern. Careful management of wild-capture fisheries, implementation of more sustainable aquaculture systems, as well as identification and development of alternative LC n–3 PUFA sources, will be essential to ensuring the continued availability of LC n–3 PUFA to meet global recommended intakes.

References

Adarme-Vega, T.C., et al., 2012. Microalgal biofactories: a promising approach towards sustainable omega-3 fatty acid production. Microb. Cell Fact 11, 96.
Amarin Corporation, 2015. Highlights of prescribing information, Vascepa.
ANSES, 2010. Avis de l'Agence francaise de securite sanitaire des aliments relatif a l'actualisation des apports ntritionnels conseilles pour les acides gras.
Araujo, P., et al., 2014. Determination and structural elucidation of triacylglycerols in krill oil by chromatographic techniques. Lipids 49 (2), 163–172.
Arterburn, L.M., et al., 2008. Algal-oil capsules and cooked salmon: nutritionally equivalent sources of docosahexaenoic acid. J. Am. Diet Assoc. 108 (7), 1204–1209.
Ashes, J.R., et al., 1992. Incorporation of n-3 fatty acids of fish oil into tissue and serum lipids of ruminants. Lipids 27 (8), 629–631.
AstraZeneca, 2014. Highlights of prescribing information: Epanova.
Atkinson, A., et al., 2004. Long-term decline in krill stock and increase in salps within the Southern Ocean. Nature 432 (7013), 100–103.
Australian National Health and Medical Research Council, 2006. Nutrient reference values for Australia and New Zealand including recommended dietary intakes.
Ballantyne, C.M., et al., 2012. Efficacy and safety of eicosapentaenoic acid ethyl ester (AMR101) therapy in statin-treated patients with persistent high triglycerides (from the ANCHOR study). Am. J. Cardiol. 110 (7), 984–992.
Bang, H.O., Dyerberg, J., Hjoorne, N., 1976. The composition of food consumed by Greenland Eskimos. Acta. Med. Scand. 200 (1–2), 69–73.
Bang, H.O., Dyerberg, J., Sinclair, H.M., 1980. The composition of the Eskimo food in north western Greenland. Am. J. Clin. Nutr. 33 (12), 2657–2661.
Bays, H., 2006. Clinical overview of Omacor: a concentrated formulation of omega-3 polyunsaturated fatty acids. Am. J. Cardiol. 98 (4A), 71i–76i.
Bays, H.E., et al.,2011. Eicosapentaenoic acid ethyl ester (AMR101) therapy in patients with very high triglyceride levels (from the Multi-center, plAcebo-controlled, Randomized, double-blINd, 12-week study with an open-label Extension [MARINE] trial). Am. J. Cardiol. 108 (5), 682–690.
Bellinger, D.C., 2014. Mercury and pregnancy. Birth Defects Res. A: Clinical and Molecular Teratology 100 (1), 1–3.
Benistant, C., et al., 1996. Docosapentaenoic acid (22:5,n-3): metabolism and effect on prostacyclin production in endothelial cells. Prostagland. Leukot. Essent. Fatty Acid 55 (4), 287–292.
Berge, K., et al., 2014. Krill oil supplementation lowers serum triglycerides without increasing low-density lipoprotein cholesterol in adults with borderline high or high triglyceride levels. Nutr. Res. 34 (2), 126–133.
Bernstein, A.M., et al., 2012. A meta-analysis shows that docosahexaenoic acid from algal oil reduces serum triglycerides and increases HDL-cholesterol and LDL-cholesterol in persons without coronary heart disease. J. Nutr. 142 (1), 99–104.
Bloomingdale, A., et al., 2010. A qualitative study of fish consumption during pregnancy. Am. J. Clin. Nutr. 92 (5), 1234–1240.
Brown, A.J., Pang, E., Roberts, D.C., 1991. Persistent changes in the fatty acid composition of erythrocyte membranes after moderate intake of n-3 polyunsaturated fatty acids: study design implications. Am. J. Clin. Nutr. 54 (4), 668–673.
Bunea, R., El Farrah, K., Deutsch, L., 2004. Evaluation of the effects of Neptune Krill Oil on the clinical course of hyperlipidemia. Altern. Med. Rev. 9 (4), 420–428.
Burdge, G.C., Calder, P.C., 2005. Conversion of alpha-linolenic acid to longer-chain polyunsaturated fatty acids in human adults. Reprod. Nutr. Dev. 45 (5), 581–597.
Burdge, G.C., Jones, A.E., Wootton, S.A., 2002. Eicosapentaenoic and docosapentaenoic acids are the principal products of alpha-linolenic acid metabolism in young men. Br. J. Nutr. 88 (4), 355–363.
Cao, J., et al., 2006. Incorporation and clearance of omega-3 fatty acids in erythrocyte membranes and plasma phospholipids. Clin. Chem. 52 (12), 2265–2272.
Chee, K.M., et al., 1990. Fatty acid content of marine oil capsules. Lipids 25 (9), 523–528.
Chopin, T., et al., 2001. Integrating seaweeds into marine aquaculture systems: a key toward sustainability. J. Phycol. 37 (6), 975–986.
Cladis, D.P., et al., 2014. Fatty acid profiles of commercially available finfish fillets in the United States. Lipids 49 (10), 1005–1018.
Conquer, J.A., Holub, B.J., 1997. Dietary docosahexaenoic acid as a source of eicosapentaenoic acid in vegetarians and omnivores. Lipids 32 (3), 341–345.
ConsumerLab.com, 2014. Product review: fish oil and omega-3 fatty acid supplements review (including krill, algae, calamari, green-lipped mussel oil).
Cosatto, V.F., Else, P.L., Meyer, B.J., 2010. Do pregnant women and those at risk of developing post-natal depression consume lower amounts of long chain omega-3 polyunsaturated fatty acids? Nutrients 2 (2), 198–213.
Crump, K.S., et al., 1998. Influence of prenatal mercury exposure upon scholastic and psychological test performance: benchmark analysis of a New Zealand cohort. Risk Anal. 18 (6), 701–713.
Cunnane, S., et al., 2004. Recommendations for intakes of polyunsaturated fatty acids in healthy adults. ISSFAL Newsl. 11 (2), 12–25.
Dai, X.W., et al., 2016. Association between n-3 polyunsaturated fatty acids in erythrocytes and metabolic syndrome in Chinese men and women. Eur. J. Nutr. 55 (3), 981–9.
Dalli, J., Colas, R.A., Serhan, C.N., 2013. Novel n-3 immunoresolvents: structures and actions. Sci. Rep. 3, 1940.
Damude, H.G., Kinney, A.J., 2007. Engineering oilseed plants for a sustainable, land-based source of long chain polyunsaturated fatty acids. Lipids 42 (3), 179–185.
Dangi, B., et al., 2009. Biogenic synthesis, purification, and chemical characterization of anti-inflammatory resolvins derived from docosapentaenoic acid (DPAn-6). J. Biol. Chem. 284 (22), 14744–14759.
Davidson, M.H., et al., 2012. A novel omega-3 free fatty acid formulation has dramatically improved bioavailability during a low-fat diet compared with omega-3-acid ethyl esters: the ECLIPSE (Epanova((R)) compared to Lovaza((R)) in a pharmacokinetic single-dose evaluation) study. J. Clin. Lipidol. 6 (6), 573–584.

Davis, B.C., Kris-Etherton, P.M., 2003. Achieving optimal essential fatty acid status in vegetarians: current knowledge and practical implications. Am. J. Clin. Nutr. 78 (3 (Suppl.)), 640S–646S.

de Oliveira Otto, M.C., et al., 2013. Circulating and dietary omega-3 and omega-6 polyunsaturated fatty acids and incidence of CVD in the multi-ethnic study of atherosclerosis. J. Am. Heart Assoc. 2 (6), pe000506.

Decker, E.A., Akoh, C.C., Wilkes, R.S., 2012. Incorporation of (n-3) fatty acids in foods: challenges and opportunities. J. Nutr. 142 (3), 610S–613S.

Del Gobbo, L.C., et al., 2010. Risks and benefits of fish consumption for childbearing women. Can. J. Diet Pract. Res. 71 (1), 41–45.

Denomme, J., Stark, K.D., Holub, B.J., 2005. Directly quantitated dietary (n-3) fatty acid intakes of pregnant Canadian women are lower than current dietary recommendations. J. Nutr. 135 (2), 206–211.

Dewailly, E.E., et al., 2001. Relations between n-3 fatty acid status and cardiovascular disease risk factors among Quebecers. Am. J. Clin. Nutr. 74 (5), 603–611.

Dewailly, E., et al., 2008. Balancing the risks and the benefits of local fish consumption in Bermuda. Food Addit. Contam. Part A 25 (11), 1328–1338.

Dietary Guidelines Advisory Committee, 2015. Scientific Report of the 2015 Dietary Guidelines Advisory Committee.

Doughman, S.D., Krupanidhi, S., Sanjeevi, C.B., 2007. Omega-3 fatty acids for nutrition and medicine: considering microalgae oil as a vegetarian source of EPA and DHA. Curr. Diab. Rev. 3 (3), 198–203.

Dyerberg, J., et al., 2010. Bioavailability of marine n-3 fatty acid formulations. Prostagland. Leukot. Essen. Fatty Acid. 83 (3), 137–141.

EFSA Panel on Dietetic Products, 2010. Nutrition, and Allergies (NDA), Scientific Opinion on Dietary Reference Values for fats, including saturated fatty acids, polyunsaturated fatty acids, monounsaturated fatty acids, trans fatty acids, and cholesterol. EFSA J., 83.

Elkin, R.G., Ying, Y., Harvatine, K.J., 2015. Feeding laying hens stearidonic acid-enriched soybean oil, as compared to flaxseed oil, more efficiently enriches eggs with very long-chain n-3 polyunsaturated fatty acids. J. Agric. Food Chem. 63 (10), 2789–2797.

Ervin, R.B., et al., 2004. Dietary intake of fats and fatty acids for the United States population: 1999-2000. Adv. Data 348, 1–6.

Ezaki, O., et al., 2012. Dietary Reference Intakes for Japanese 2010: Fat. J. Nutr. Sci. Vitaminol. 59 (Supplement), S44–S52.

FAO, 2000. The State of World Fisheries and Aquaculture - 2000: Rome.

FAO, 2012. The state of world fisheries and aquaculture - 2012: Rome.

FAO, 2014. The state of the world fisheries and aquaculture - 2014: Rome.

Flock, M.R., et al., 2014. Effects of supplemental long-chain omega-3 fatty acids and erythrocyte membrane fatty acid content on circulating inflammatory markers in a randomized controlled trial of healthy adults. Prostagland. Leukot. Essen. Fatty Acid. 91 (4), 161–168.

Flores, H., et al., 2012. Impact of climate change on Antarctic krill. Mar. Ecol. Prog. Ser. 458, 1–19.

Food Safety Authority of Ireland, 2002. Dioxins, Furans and PCBs in Farmed and Wild Salmon, Farmed Trout and Fish Oil Capsules - Summary of Investigation.

Foran, S.E., Flood, J.G., Lewandrowski, K.B., 2003. Measurement of mercury levels in concentrated over-the-counter fish oil preparations: is fish oil healthier than fish? Arch. Pathol. Lab. Med. 127 (12), 1603–1605.

Gallagher, M.L., McLeod, S.H., Rulifson, R., 1989. Seasonal variations in fatty acids of striped bass Morone saxatilis. J. World Aquaculture Soc. 20 (2), 38–45.

Gebauer, S.K., et al., 2006. n-3 fatty acid dietary recommendations and food sources to achieve essentiality and cardiovascular benefits. Am. J. Clin. Nutr. 83 (6 (Suppl.)), 1526S–1535S.

Geppert, J., et al., 2005. Docosahexaenoic acid supplementation in vegetarians effectively increases omega-3 index: a randomized trial. Lipids 40 (8), 807–814.

Ghasemifard, S., Turchini, G.M., Sinclair, A.J., 2014. Omega-3 long chain fatty acid "bioavailability": a review of evidence and methodological considerations. Prog. Lipid Res. 56, 92–108.

GISSI-Prevenzione Investigators, 1999. Dietary supplementation with n-3 polyunsaturated fatty acids and vitamin E after myocardial infarction: results of the GISSI-Prevenzione trial. The Lancet 354 (9177), 447–455.

Givens, D., Gibbs, R., 2006. Very long chain n-3 polyunsaturated fatty acids in the food chain in the UK and the potential of animal-derived foods to increase intake. Nutr. Bull. 31 (2), 104–110.

GlaxoSmithKline, 2014. Lovaza: highlights of prescribing information.

Granada, L., et al., 2015. Is integrated multitrophic aquaculture the solution to the sectors' major challenges?–a review. Rev. Aquacult. 6, 1–18.

Grandjean, P., et al., 1997. Cognitive deficit in 7-year-old children with prenatal exposure to methylmercury. Neurotoxicol. Teratol. 19 (6), 417–428.

Greiner, A., Clegg Smith, K., Guallar, E., 2010. Something fishy? News media presentation of complex health issues related to fish consumption guidelines. Public Health Nutr. 13 (11), 1786–1794.

Guil-Guerrero, J.L., García Maroto, F.F., Giménez Giménez, A., 2001. Fatty acid profiles from forty-nine plant species that are potential new sources of γ-linolenic acid. J. Amer Oil Chem. Soc. 78 (7), 677–684.

Handå, A., et al., 2012. Incorporation of fish feed and growth of blue mussels (*Mytilus edulis*) in close proximity to salmon (*Salmo salar*) aquaculture: Implications for integrated multi-trophic aquaculture in Norwegian coastal waters. Aquaculture 356–357, 328–341.

Hardy, R.W., Lee, C., 2010. Aquaculture feed and seafood quality. Bull. Fish Res. Agen. 31, 43–50.

Harris, W.S., 2007a. n-3 Fatty acid fortification: opportunities and obstacles. Br. J. Nutr. 97 (04), 593–595.

Harris, W.S., 2007b. Omega-3 fatty acids and cardiovascular disease: a case for omega-3 index as a new risk factor. Pharmacol. Res. 55 (3), 217–223.

Harris, W.S., 2008. You are what you eat applies to fish, too. J. Am. Dietetic Assoc. 108 (7), 1131–1133.

Harris, W.S., 2014. Achieving optimal n–3 fatty acid status: the vegetarian's challenge… or not. Am. J. Clin. Nutr. 100 (1 (Suppl.)), 449S–452S.

Harris, W.S., et al., 2004. Omega-3 fatty acids in cardiac biopsies from heart transplantation patients: correlation with erythrocytes and response to supplementation. Circulation 110 (12), 1645–1649.

Harris, W.S., et al., 2008. Stearidonic acid-enriched soybean oil increased the omega-3 index, an emerging cardiovascular risk marker. Lipids 43 (9), 805–811.

Harris, W.S., et al., 2009. Towards establishing dietary reference intakes for eicosapentaenoic and docosahexaenoic acids. J. Nutr. 139 (4), 804S–819S.

Health Council of the Netherlands, 2001. Dietary reference intakes: energy, proteins, fats, and digestible carbohydrates. Health Council of the Netherlands: The Hague.

Herber, S.M., Van Elswyk, M.E., 1996. Dietary marine algae promotes efficient deposition of n-3 fatty acids for the production of enriched shell eggs. Poult. Sci. 75 (12), 1501–1507.

Howe, P.R., et al., 2002. Tuna fishmeal as a source of DHA for n-3 PUFA enrichment of pork, chicken, and eggs. Lipids 37 (11), 1067–1076.

Howe, P.R., et al., 2006. Dietary intake of long-chain omega-3 polyunsaturated fatty acids: contribution of meat sources. Nutrition 22 (1), 47–53.

Howe, P.R., Buckley, J., Meyer, B., 2007. Long-chain omega-3 fatty acids in red meat. Nutr. Dietetic. 64, S135–S139.

Innis, S.M., 2004. Polyunsaturated fatty acids in human milk: an essential role in infant development. Adv. Exp. Med. Biol. 554, 27–43.

Innis, S.M., 2007. Dietary (n-3) fatty acids and brain development. J. Nutr. 137 (4), 855–859.

Innis, S.M., 2008. Dietary omega 3 fatty acids and the developing brain. Brain Res. 1237, 35–43.

Innis, S.M., Elias, S.L., 2003. Intakes of essential n-6 and n-3 polyunsaturated fatty acids among pregnant Canadian women. Am. J. Clin. Nutr. 77 (2), 473–478.

Institute of Medicine, 2005. Food and Nutrition Board, Dietary Reference Intakes for Energy, Carbohydrate, Fiber, Fat, Fatty Acids, Cholesterol, Protein, and Amino Acids. Washington, DC.

Jacobs, M.N., Covaci, A., Schepens, P., 2002. Investigation of selected persistent organic pollutants in farmed Atlantic salmon (Salmo salar), salmon aquaculture feed, and fish oil components of the feed. Environ. Sci. Technol. 36 (13), 2797–2805.

Jacobson, T.A., et al., 2012. Effects of eicosapentaenoic acid and docosahexaenoic acid on low-density lipoprotein cholesterol and other lipids: a review. J. Clin. Lipidol. 6 (1), 5–18.

James, M.J., Ursin, V.M., Cleland, L.G., 2003. Metabolism of stearidonic acid in human subjects: comparison with the metabolism of other n-3 fatty acids. Am. J. Clin. Nutr. 77 (5), 1140–1145.

Jenkins, D.J., et al., 2009. Are dietary recommendations for the use of fish oils sustainable? CMAJ 180 (6), 633–637.

Jia, X., et al., 2015. Women who take n-3 long-chain polyunsaturated fatty acid supplements during pregnancy and lactation meet the recommended intake. Appl. Physiol. Nutr. Metab. 40 (5), 474–481.

Jobling, M., Bendiksen, E.Å., 2003. Dietary lipids and temperature interact to influence tissue fatty acid compositions of Atlantic salmon, *Salmo salar* L., parr. Aquaculture Res. 34 (15), 1423–1441.

Joint FAO/WHO Expert Consulation, 2010. Fats and fatty acids in human nutrition - Report of an expert consulation: Geneva, Switzerland.

Joint FAO/WHO Expert Consulation, 2010. Risks and Benefits of Fish Consumption: Rome.

Jones, T.O., Iwama, G.K., 1991. Polyculture of the Pacific oyster, *Crassostrea gigas* (Thunberg), with chinook salmon *Oncorhynchus tshawytscha*. Aquaculture 92, 313–322.

Kang, J.X., et al., 2004. Transgenic mice: fat-1 mice convert n-6 to n-3 fatty acids. Nature 427 (6974), 504.

Kastelein, J.J., et al., 2014. Omega-3 free fatty acids for the treatment of severe hypertriglyceridemia: the EpanoVa fOr Lowering Very high triglyceridEs (EVOLVE) trial. J. Clin. Lipidol. 8 (1), 94–106.

Katan, M.B., et al., 1997. Kinetics of the incorporation of dietary fatty acids into serum cholesteryl esters, erythrocyte membranes, and adipose tissue: an 18-month controlled study. J. Lipid Res. 38 (10), 2012–2022.

Kaur, G., et al., 2010. Short-term docosapentaenoic acid (22:5 n-3) supplementation increases tissue docosapentaenoic acid, DHA and EPA concentrations in rats. Br. J. Nutr. 103 (1), 32–37.

Kaur, G., et al., 2011. Docosapentaenoic acid (22:5n-3): a review of its biological effects. Prog. Lipid Res. 50 (1), 28–34.

Kennedy, E.T., Luo, H., Ausman, L.M., 2012. Cost implications of alternative sources of (n-3) fatty acid consumption in the United States. J. Nutr. 142 (3), 605S–609S.

Kingsbury, K.J., et al., 1961. Effects of ethyl arachidonate, cod-liver oil, and corn oil on the plasma-cholesterol level. A comparison in normal volunters. Lancet 1 (7180), 739–741.

Koletzko, B., Rodriguez-Palmero, M., 1999. Polyunsaturated fatty acids in human milk and their role in early infant development. J. Mammary Gland Biol. Neoplasia 4 (3), 269–284.

Koletzko, B., Cetin, I., Brenna, J.T., 2007. Dietary fat intakes for pregnant and lactating women. Br. J. Nutr. 98 (5), 873–877.

Kris-Etherton, P.M., Harris, W.S., Appel, L.J., 2002. Fish consumption, fish oil, omega-3 fatty acids, and cardiovascular disease. Circulation 106 (21), 2747–2757.

Kris-Etherton, P.M., Innis, S.M., 2007. Position of the American Dietetic Association and Dietitians of Canada: dietary fatty acids. J. Am. Diet Assoc. 107 (9), 1599–1611.

Krkosek, M., et al., 2007. Declining wild salmon populations in relation to parasites from farm salmon. Science 318 (5857), 1772–1775.

Krokan, H.E., Bjerve, K.S., Mork, E., 1993. The enteral bioavailability of eicosapentaenoic acid and docosahexaenoic acid is as good from ethyl esters as from glyceryl esters in spite of lower hydrolytic rates by pancreatic lipase in vitro. Biochem. Biophys. Acta 1168 (1), 59–67.

Krul, E.S., et al., 2012. Effects of duration of treatment and dosage of eicosapentaenoic acid and stearidonic acid on red blood cell eicosapentaenoic acid content. Prostagland. Leukot. Essen. Fatty Acid. 86 (1-2), 51–59.

Kuhnt, K., et al., 2012. Searching for health beneficial n-3 and n-6 fatty acids in plant seeds. Eur. J. Lipid Sci. Technol. 114 (2), 153–160.

Kuratko, C.N., Salem, N., 2013. Docosahexaenoic acid from algal oil. Eur. J. Lipid Sci. Technol. 115 (9), 965–976.

Kwantes, J.M., Grundmann, O., 2015. A brief review of krill oil history, research, and the commercial market. J. Dietary Suppl. 12 (1), 23–35.

Labonte, M.E., et al., 2014. Association of red blood cell n-3 polyunsaturated fatty acids with plasma inflammatory biomarkers among the Quebec Cree population. Eur. J. Clin. Nutr. 68 (9), 1042–1047.

Lai, L., et al., 2006. Generation of cloned transgenic pigs rich in omega-3 fatty acids. Nat. Biotechnol. 24 (4), 435–436.

Lawson, L.D., Hughes, B.G., 1988. Human absorption of fish oil fatty acids as triacylglycerols, free acids, or ethyl esters. Biochem. Biophy. Res. Commun. 152 (1), 328–335.

Lemke, S.L., et al., 2010. Dietary intake of stearidonic acid-enriched soybean oil increases the omega-3 index: randomized, double-blind clinical study of efficacy and safety. Am. J. Clin. Nutr. 92 (4), 766–775.

Lentjes, M.A., et al., 2014. Cod liver oil supplement consumption and health: cross-sectional results from the EPIC-Norfolk cohort study. Nutrients 6 (10), 4320–4337.

Leskanich, C., Noble, R., 1997. Manipulation of the n-3 polyunsaturated fatty acid composition of avian eggs and meat. World's Poultry Sci. J. 53 (02), 155–183.

Linseisen, J., et al., 2003. Quantity and quality of dietary fat, carbohydrate, and fiber intake in the German EPIC cohorts. Ann. Nutr. Metab. 47 (1), 37–46.
Lloyd-Jones, D.M., et al., 2010. Defining and setting national goals for cardiovascular health promotion and disease reduction: the American Heart Association's strategic Impact Goal through 2020 and beyond. Circulation 121 (4), 586–613.
Mahaffey, K.R., et al., 2011. Balancing the benefits of n-3 polyunsaturated fatty acids and the risks of methylmercury exposure from fish consumption. Nutr. Rev. 69 (9), 493–508.
Mandell, I.B., et al., 1997. Effects of fish meal in beef cattle diets on growth performance, carcass characteristics, and fatty acid composition of longissimus muscle. J. Anim. Sci. 75 (4), 910–919.
Meyer, B.J., Lane, A.E., Mann, N.J., 2009. Comparison of seal oil to tuna oil on plasma lipid levels and blood pressure in hypertriglyceridaemic subjects. Lipids 44 (9), 827–835.
Micallef, M.A., Munro, I.A., Garg, M.L., 2009. An inverse relationship between plasma n-3 fatty acids and C-reactive protein in healthy individuals. Eur. J. Clin. Nutr. 63 (9), 1154–1156.
Miller, E., et al., 2013. A short-term n-3 DPA supplementation study in humans. Eur. J. Nutr. 52 (3), 895–904.
Mori, T.A., Woodman, R.J., 2006. The independent effects of eicosapentaenoic acid and docosahexaenoic acid on cardiovascular risk factors in humans. Curr. Opin. Clin. Nutr. Metab. Care 9 (2), 95–104.
Mori, T.A., et al., 2000. Purified eicosapentaenoic and docosahexaenoic acids have differential effects on serum lipids and lipoproteins, LDL particle size, glucose, and insulin in mildly hyperlipidemic men. Am. J. Clin. Nutr. 71 (5), 1085–1094.
Mozaffarian, D., Rimm, E.B., 2006. Fish intake, contaminants, and human health: evaluating the risks and the benefits. JAMA 296 (15), 1885–1899.
Mozaffarian, D., Wu, J.H., 2011. Omega-3 fatty acids and cardiovascular disease: effects on risk factors, molecular pathways, and clinical events. J. Am. Coll. Cardiol. 58 (20), 2047–2067.
Mozaffarian, D., Wu, J.H., 2012. (n-3) fatty acids and cardiovascular health: are effects of EPA and DHA shared or complementary? J. Nutr. 142 (3), 614S–625S.
Mozaffarian, D., et al., 2011. Circulating long-chain omega-3 fatty acids and incidence of congestive heart failure in older adults: the cardiovascular health study: a cohort study. Ann. Intern Med. 155 (3), 160–170.
Mozaffarian, D., et al., 2013. Plasma phospholipid long-chain omega-3 fatty acids and total and cause-specific mortality in older adults: a cohort study. Ann. Intern Med. 158 (7), 515–525.
Murphy, K.J., et al., 2007. Impact of foods enriched with n-3 long-chain polyunsaturated fatty acids on erythrocyte n-3 levels and cardiovascular risk factors. Br. J. Nutr. 97 (4), 749–757.
Myers, G.J., et al., 2003. Prenatal methylmercury exposure from ocean fish consumption in the Seychelles child development study. The Lancet 361 (9370), 1686–1692.
Napier, J.A., et al., 2015. Transgenic plants as a sustainable, terrestrial source of fish oils. Eur. J. Lipid Sci. Technol. 117 (9), 1317–24.
National Fisheries Institute, 2013. Top 10 Consumed Seafoods. https://www.aboutseafood.com/about/about-seafood/top-10-consumed-seafoods
National Institute for Health and Care Excellence, 2014. Lipid modification: cardiovascular risk assessment and the modification of blood lipids for the primary and secondary prevention of cardiovascular disease, in NICE clinical guideline 181.
Naylor, R.L., et al., 1998. Nature's subsidies to shrimp and salmon farming. Science 282 (5390), 883.
Naylor, R.L., et al., 2000. Effect of aquaculture on world fish supplies. Nature 405 (6790), 1017–1024.
Neori, A., et al., 1996. Seaweed biofilters as regulators of water quality in integrated fish-seaweed culture units. Aquaculture 141 (3-4), 183–199.
Neori, A., et al., 2004. Integrated aquaculture: rationale, evolution and state of the art emphasizing seaweed biofiltration in modern mariculture. Aquaculture 231 (1-4), 361–391.
Neubronner, J., et al., 2011. Enhanced increase of omega-3 index in response to long-term n-3 fatty acid supplementation from triacylglycerides versus ethyl esters. Eur. J. Clin. Nutr. 65 (2), 247–254.
Nicol, S., Foster, J., Kawaguchi, S., 2012. The fishery for Antarctic krill–recent developments. Fish Fisher. 13 (1), 30–40.
Nordoy, A., et al., 1991. Absorption of the n-3 eicosapentaenoic and docosahexaenoic acids as ethyl esters and triglycerides by humans. Am. J. Clin. Nutr. 53 (5), 1185–1190.
Norris, P.C., Dennis, E.A., 2012. Omega-3 fatty acids cause dramatic changes in TLR4 and purinergic eicosanoid signaling. Proc. Natl. Acad. Sci. USA 109 (22), 8517–8522.
Nuernberg, K., et al., 2005. Effect of a grass-based and a concentrate feeding system on meat quality characteristics and fatty acid composition of longissimus muscle in different cattle breeds. Livestock Prod. Sci. 94 (1), 137–147.
Oda, E., et al., 2005. A case-control pilot study on n-3 polyunsaturated fatty acid as a negative risk factor for myocardial infarction. Int. Heart J. 46 (4), 583–591.
Oken, E., et al., 2003. Decline in fish consumption among pregnant women after a national mercury advisory. Obstet. Gynecol. 102 (2), 346–351.
Oken, E., et al., 2012. Which fish should I eat? Perspectives influencing fish consumption choices. Environ. Health Perspect. 120 (6), 790–798.
Papanikolaou, Y., et al., 2014. U.S. adults are not meeting recommended levels for fish and omega-3 fatty acid intake: results of an analysis using observational data from NHANES 2003-2008. Nutr. J. 13, 31.
Patil, V., et al., 2007. Fatty acid composition of 12 microalgae for possible use in aquaculture feed. Aquaculture Int. 15 (1), 1–9.
Pauly, D., Watson, R., Alder, J., 2005. Global trends in world fisheries: impacts on marine ecosystems and food security. Philos. Trans. R Soc. London B 360 (1453), 5–12.
Petrie, J.R., et al., 2014. Metabolic engineering Camelina sativa with fish oil-like levels of DHA. PLoS One 9 (1), e85061.
Pieters, D.J., Mensink, R.P., 2015. Effects of stearidonic acid on serum triacylglycerol concentrations in overweight and obese subjects: a randomized controlled trial. Eur. J. Clin. Nutr. 69 (1), 121–126.
Ponnampalam, E.N., Mann, N.J., Sinclair, A.J., 2006. Effect of feeding systems on omega-3 fatty acids, conjugated linoleic acid and trans fatty acids in Australian beef cuts: potential impact on human health. Asia Pac. J. Clin. Nutr. 15 (1), 21–29.
Rahmawaty, S., et al., 2013. Dietary intake and food sources of EPA, DPA and DHA in Australian children. Lipids 48 (9), 869–877.
Reinders, I., et al., 2012. Association of serum n-3 polyunsaturated fatty acids with C-reactive protein in men. Eur. J. Clin. Nutr. 66 (6), 736–741.

Rubio-Rodríguez, N., et al., 2010. Production of omega-3 polyunsaturated fatty acid concentrates: a review. Innovativ. Food Sci. Emerg. Technol. 11 (1), 1–12.
Ruxton, C.H.S., 2011. The benefits of fish consumption. Nutr. Bull. 36 (1), 6–19.
Salem, Jr., N., Eggersdorfer, M., 2015. Is the world supply of omega-3 fatty acids adequate for optimal human nutrition? Curr. Opin. Clin. Nutr. Metab. Care 18 (2), 147–154.
Salem, Jr., N., Kuratko, C.N., 2014. A reexamination of krill oil bioavailability studies. Lipids Health Dis. 13 (1), 1–5.
Samocha, T.M., et al., 2015. Growth and nutrient uptake of the macroalga *Gracilaria tikvahiae* cultured with the shrimp *Litopenaeus vannamei* in an Integrated Multi-Trophic Aquaculture (IMTA) system. Aquaculture 446, 263–271.
Sanders, T.A., 2009. DHA status of vegetarians. Prostagland. Leukotrien. Essen. Fatty Acid. 81 (2), 137–141.
Sanders, T.A., Vickers, M., Haines, A.P., 1981. Effect on blood lipids and haemostasis of a supplement of cod-liver oil, rich in eicosapentaenoic and docosahexaenoic acids, in healthy young men. Clin. Sci. (London) 61 (3), 317–324.
Sayanova, O., Napier, J.A., 2011. Transgenic oilseed crops as an alternative to fish oils. Prostagland. Leukot. Essent. Fatty Acid. 85 (5), 253–260.
Schuchardt, J.P., Hahn, A., 2013. Bioavailability of long-chain omega-3 fatty acids. Prostagland. Leukot. Essent. Fatty Acid. 89 (1), 1–8.
Scollan, N., et al., 2006. Innovations in beef production systems that enhance the nutritional and health value of beef lipids and their relationship with meat quality. Meat Sci. 74 (1), 17–33.
Ser, P.H., Watanabe, C., 2012. Fish advisories in the USA and Japan: risk communication and public awareness of a common idea with different backgrounds. Asia Pac. J. Clin. Nutr. 21 (4), 487–494.
Shimshack, J.P., Ward, M.B., 2010. Mercury advisories and household health trade-offs. J. Health Econ. 29 (5), 674–685.
Shimshack, J.P., Ward, M.B., Beatty, T.K.M., 2007. Mercury advisories: information, education, and fish consumption. J. Environ. Econ. Manage. 53 (2), 158–179.
Simopoulos, A.P., 1989. Summary of the NATO advanced research workshop on dietary omega 3 and omega 6 fatty acids: biological effects and nutritional essentiality. J. Nutr. 119 (4), 521–528.
Sioen, I.A., et al., 2006. Dietary intakes and food sources of fatty acids for Belgian women, focused on n-6 and n-3 polyunsaturated fatty acids. Lipids 41 (5), 415–422.
Sioen, L.A., et al., 2010. The influence of n-3 PUFA supplements and n-3 PUFA enriched foods on the n-3 LC PUFA intake of Flemish women. Lipids 45 (4), 313–320.
Skulas-Ray, A.C., et al., 2008. Omega-3 fatty acid concentrates in the treatment of moderate hypertriglyceridemia. Expert Opin. Pharmacother. 9 (7), 1237–1248.
Skulas-Ray, A.C., et al., 2011. Dose-response effects of omega-3 fatty acids on triglycerides, inflammation, and endothelial function in healthy persons with moderate hypertriglyceridemia. Am. J. Clin. Nutr. 93 (2), 243–252.
Skulas-Ray, A.C., et al., 2015. Red Blood Cell Docosapentaenoic Acid (DPA n-3) is inversely associated with triglycerides and C-reactive protein (CRP) in healthy adults and dose-dependently increases following n-3 fatty acid supplementation. Nutrients 7 (8), 5291.
Soto, D., Mena, G., 1999. Filter feeding by the freshwater mussel, *Diplodon chilensis*, as a biocontrol of salmon farming eutrophication. Aquaculture 171 (1-2), 65–81.
Spolaore, P., et al., 2006. Commercial applications of microalgae. J. Biosci. Bioeng. 101 (2), 87–96.
Sugano, M., Hirahara, F., 2000. Polyunsaturated fatty acids in the food chain in Japan. Am. J. Clin. Nutr. 71 (1 Suppl.), 189S–196S.
Sun, Q., et al., 2008. Blood concentrations of individual long-chain n-3 fatty acids and risk of nonfatal myocardial infarction. Am. J. Clin. Nutr. 88 (1), 216–223.
Surette, M.E., 2013. Dietary omega-3 PUFA and health: stearidonic acid-containing seed oils as effective and sustainable alternatives to traditional marine oils. Mol. Nutr. Food Res. 57 (5), 748–759.
Tacon, A., Feeding tomorrow's fish: keys for sustainability. Feeding Tomorrow's Fish. In: Cahiers Options Mediterraneennes, Tacon, A.G.J. and Basurco, B. (Eds.), 1997. 22: p. 11–33.
Tatarczyk, T., et al., 2007. Analysis of long-chain omega-3 fatty acid content in fish-oil supplements. Wien Klin Wochenschr 119 (13-14), 417–422.
Tavazzi, L., et al., 2008. Effect of n-3 polyunsaturated fatty acids in patients with chronic heart failure (the GISSI-HF trial): a randomised, double-blind, placebo-controlled trial. Lancet 372 (9645), 1223–1230.
Theophilus Olayiwola, B., et al., 2011. Differential effects of dietary lipids on growth performance, digestibility, fatty acid composition and histology of African catfish (*Heterobranchus longifilis*) fingerlings. Food Nutr. Sci. 2011.
Tou, J.C., Jaczynski, J., Chen, Y., 2007. Krill for human consumption: nutritional value and potential health benefits. Nutr. Rev. Washington 65 (2), 63.
Trivelpiece, W.Z., et al., 2011. Variability in krill biomass links harvesting and climate warming to penguin population changes in Antarctica. Proc. Natl. Acad Sci. USA 108 (18), 7625–7628.
Troell, M., et al., 1999. Ecological engineering in aquaculture: use of seaweeds for removing nutrients from intensive mariculture. J.Appl. Phycol. 11 (1), 89–97.
Truksa, M., et al., 2006. Metabolic engineering of plants to produce very long-chain polyunsaturated fatty acids. Transgenic Res. 15 (2), 131–137.
Turner, T.D., et al., 2015. Comparison of fatty acids in beef tissues from conventional, organic and natural feeding systems in western Canada. Can. J. Animal Sci. 95 (1), 49–58.
US Food and Drug Administration and Environmental Protection Agency, 2014. Fish: what pregnant women and parents should know.
US Food and Drug Administration and Environmental Protection Agency, 2004. Consumer advisory: What you need to know about mercury in fish and shellfish.
Ulven, S.M., et al., 2011. Metabolic effects of krill oil are essentially similar to those of fish oil but at lower dose of EPA and DHA, in healthy volunteers. Lipids 46 (1), 37–46.
Ursin, V.M., 2003. Modification of plant lipids for human health: development of functional land-based omega-3 fatty acids. J. Nutr. 133 (12), 4271–4274.
United States Department of Agriculture and United States Department of Health and Human Services (USDA, HSS), Dietary Guidelines for Americans, 2010. 2010, US Government Printing Office: Washington, DC.
Vannice, G., Rasmussen, H., 2014. Position of the academy of nutrition and dietetics: dietary fatty acids for healthy adults. J. Acad. Nutr. Diet 114 (1), 136–153.

Verbeke, W., et al., 2005. Consumer perception versus scientific evidence about health benefits and safety risks from fish consumption. Public Health Nutr. 8 (4), 422–429.

von Schacky, C., Weber, P.C., 1985. Metabolism and effects on platelet function of the purified eicosapentaenoic and docosahexaenoic acids in humans. J. Clin. Invest. 76 (6), 2446–2450.

Wachira, A.M., et al., 2002. Effects of dietary fat source and breed on the carcass composition, n-3 polyunsaturated fatty acid and conjugated linoleic acid content of sheep meat and adipose tissue. Br. J. Nutr. 88 (6), 697–709.

Walker, C.G., Jebb, S.A., Calder, P.C., 2013. Stearidonic acid as a supplemental source of omega-3 polyunsaturated fatty acids to enhance status for improved human health. Nutrition 29 (2), 363–369.

Ward, O.P., Singh, A., 2005. Omega-3/6 fatty acids: alternative sources of production. Process Biochem. 40 (12), 3627–3652.

Weaver, K.L., et al., 2008. The content of favorable and unfavorable polyunsaturated fatty acids found in commonly eaten fish. J. Am. Diet Assoc. 108 (7), 1178–1185.

Wei, M.Y., Jacobson, T.A., 2011. Effects of eicosapentaenoic acid versus docosahexaenoic acid on serum lipids: a systematic review and meta-analysis. Curr. Atheroscler. Rep. 13 (6), 474–483.

Whelan, J., 2009. Dietary stearidonic acid is a long chain (n-3) polyunsaturated fatty acid with potential health benefits. J. Nutr. 139 (1), 5–10.

Whelan, J., Rust, C., 2006. Innovative dietary sources of n-3 fatty acids. Ann. Rev. Nutr. 26, 75–103.

Whelan, J., Gouffon, J., Zhao, Y., 2012. Effects of dietary stearidonic acid on biomarkers of lipid metabolism. J. Nutr. 142 (3), 630S–634S.

Yokoyama, M., et al., 2007. Effects of eicosapentaenoic acid on major coronary events in hypercholesterolaemic patients (JELIS): a randomised open-label, blinded endpoint analysis. Lancet 369 (9567), 1090–1098.

Zlatanos, S., Laskaridis, K., 2007. Seasonal variation in the fatty acid composition of three Mediterranean fish–sardine (*Sardina pilchardus*), anchovy (*Engraulis encrasicholus*) and picarel (*Spicara smaris*). Food Chem. 103 (3), 725–728.

CHAPTER

4

Pregnant Women and Consumption of Fish: Where are We?

*M.A. Harris**, *C.J. Lammi-Keefe***

*Department of Food Science and Human Nutrition, College of Health and Human Sciences, Colorado State University, Fort Collins, Colorado, United States; **School of Nutrition and Food Sciences, Louisiana State University, Baton Rouge, Louisiana; Pennington Biomedical Research Center, Baton Rouge, Louisiana, United States

THE FISH PARADOX UNRAVELED: PREGNANT WOMEN SHOULD EAT MORE FISH FOR OPTIMAL BRAIN DEVELOPMENT IN THEIR CHILDREN

Scientific uncertainty, which once surrounded the consumption of fish and seafood by pregnant and breastfeeding women has been resolved. Numerous large epidemiologic studies have demonstrated that maternal DHA intake, attributable to seafood consumption, is associated with improved cognitive development. Long-term prospective studies in Great Britain (Daniels et al., 2004; Hibbeln et al., 2007; Leino et al., 2013), Europe (Zeilmaker et al., 2013), and the Republic of the Seychelles (Strain et al., 2008; Strain et al., 2012; Strain et al., 2015; Stokes-Riner et al., 2011; Davidson et al., 2011; Table 4.1) have demonstrated that women who eat greater than 12 ounces of fish per week give birth to babies with better cognitive performance. Similar results have been shown in studies conducted by researchers in the United States (Oken et al., 2008b) and Denmark (Oken et al., 2008b; Oken and Ballinger, 2008) which correlate fish consumption during pregnancy with cognitive development. Omega-3 intake from marine sources improved cognitive function in Inuit children whose seafood is known to contain high levels of methyl mercury (Jacobson et al., 2008). Since methyl mercury is a known neurotoxin and several studies suggested subtle adverse effects of methyl mercury exposure from seafood (Davidson et al., 2008; Jedrychowski et al., 2007; Freire et al., 2010), concern has been expressed that seafood consumption may impair neurocognitive development. However, the association of mercury in seafood and cognitive development is not as closely related as once thought. High intake of methyl mercury from seafood has not been shown to have adverse effects in other studies (Davidson et al., 1998; Myers et al., 2003). Seafood intake is overwhelmingly considered to be safe and beneficial for pregnant and breastfeeding women, at least in commercially caught fish at recommended levels of intake. Seemingly paradoxical is the observation that cognitive ability improves as both fish consumption and maternal mercury levels increase (Oken et al., 2008b). An explanation for this paradox is the protective effect of nutrients in fish; fish content of selenium exerts an apparent protective role against the neurotoxicity of methylmercury (Kahn & Wang, 2009) and omega-3 docosahexaenoic acid (DHA) (Boucher et al., 2011) is an essential nutrient for brain development. Seafood is the richest dietary source of omega-3 DHA. The FDA recently released the results of a quantitative assessment of the net effects of commercial seafood consumption on cognitive development (FDA, 2014). Thirty years of experience in the Seychelles (Strain et al., 2015) has confirmed the previous evidence that women consuming more than 12 ounces of fish per week give birth to children with the best cognitive performance.

OMEGA-3 DHA AND NEUROCOGNITIVE DEVELOPMENT

Omega-3 (n–3) DHA is a 22 carbon, 6 double bond n–3 fatty acid derived from the plant based linolenic acid (18 C:3 n–3, ALA) by a series of desaturation and elongation steps.

Large amounts of DHA are accreted in the developing fetal brain and retina during the last trimester of pregnancy and in the earliest months following birth (Innis, 1993). Research in animals and humans suggests that low maternal

Fish and Fish Oil in Health and Disease Prevention. http://dx.doi.org/10.1016/B978-0-12-802844-5.00004-X

TABLE 4.1 Epidemiological Studies of Fish Consumption During Pregnancy and Neurocognitive Development in Infants

Author and year	Population	Number of subjects	Measurement	Age at measurement	Effect of DHA supplementation
Daniels et al. (2004)	British ALSPAC	7421	MacArthur Communicative Development Inventory Denver Development Screening Test	15 months 18 months	Higher mean developmental scores for both the MacArthur Development Inventory and the Denver Development Screening Test (eg: MacArthur comprehension score for infants of fish consumers was 72 versus 68 for infants of nonconsumers)
Hibbeln et al. (2007)	BritishALSPAC	11875	IQ by Weschler Intelligence Scale for Children (n = 5449)	8 years	Maternal seafood intake in pregnancy < 340g/week associated with children in lower quartile for IQ; suboptimum outcomes for prosocial behavior, fine motor, communication, social development scores
Oken et al. (2008b)	United States	341	Peabody Picture Vocabulary Test (PPVT) Wide-Range Assessment of Visual Motor Abilities (WRAVMA)	3 years	Higher fish intake associated with better child cognitive test performance; higher mercury with poorer test scores effect; estimates for fish intake > 2 servings/week versus never: 2,2 (−2.6, 7.0) for PPVT; 6.4 (2.0, 10.8) for WRAVMA; for mercury in top decile, −4.5 (−8.5, −0.4) for PPVT and −4.6 (−8.3, −0.9) for WRAVMA
Oken et al. (2008a)	Danish	35,557	Yes–no queries about development[a]	6 months	Higher maternal fish intake and duration of breastfeeding associated with higher developmental scores for highest versus lowest quintile of fish intake
Oken et al., 2008a	Danish	25,446	Questionnaire about whether child could climb stairs, remove his/her socks and shoes, drink for cup, self-occupy for 15 min without adult participation, fetch an object when requested, write/draw, orient book correctly, use word-like sounds, put two words together; could child sit unsupported and walk unassisted	18.0–20.9 months	Higher maternal fish intake and duration of breastfeeding associated with higher developmental scores for highest versus lowest quintile of fish intake.
Jacobson et al. (2008)	Arctic Quebec	109	Assessment of relationship of DHA, polychlorinated biphenyls, mercury, and lead in cord plasma, maternal plasma, breastmilk. 6 and 11 months: infant growth, visual acuity (Teller Visual Acuity Card Test), cognitive, and motor function assessed with Fagan Test of Infant Intelligence (FTII). 11 months added mental and psychomotor indices of Bayley Scales of Infant Development, 2nd edition (BSID-II)	Inuit infants 6 and 11 months	Strong correlation between maternal and cord plasma phospholipid DHA. Higher cord DHA concentration associated with more optimal visual acuity, cognition, and motor development.
Leino et al. (2013)	Finland	3827	Quantitative benefit-risk assessment of child total IQ effects; assessed consumption data	Pregnant women	Beneficial child IQ effect of consumption of fatty fish during pregnancy; benefits outweigh risks
Zeilmaker et al. (2013)	Europe		Physiologically Based PharmacoKinetic modelling applied to calculate effect of prenatal methylmercury exposure and DHA on developing brain and children's IQ score	Pregnant women	Health benefits for children's IQ can be attained by focusing during pregnancy on fish species with high DHA content and low methylmercury content (avoiding the large predator fish)

Davidson et al. (1998)	Republic of Seychelles	711	Prenatal and postnatal methylmercury exposure Neurodevelopmental tests: McCarthy Scales of Children's Abilities; Preschool language Scale; Woodcock–Johnson Applied Problems and Letter and Word Recognition Tests of Achievement; Bender Gestalt Test; Child Behavior Checklist	Mother-child pairs Children: 66 months	Development of children to 66 months of age was not affected by high ocean fish diet of mothers during pregnancy
Myers et al. (2003)	Republic of Seychelles	779	Maternal prenatal methylmercury exposure Children at 9 years of age: neurocognitive (Wechsler intelligence test scale for children III full-scale IQ); language (Woodcock–Johnson test for achievement, letter-word recognition, and applied problems subtests and California verbal learning test); memory (visual memory subtest of wide-range assessment of memory & learning); motor and perceptual-motor (finger tapping, trailmaking, grooved pegboard, Bruininks–Oserestky test of motor proficiency); behavioral functions; sustained attention (Connor's continuous performance test)	Mother–infant pairs Children: 9 years	No adverse effects on child development
Davidson et al., 2008	Republic of Seychelles	300	Maternal prenatal and pregnancy methylmercury exposure Children: Bayley Scales of Infant Development-II at 9 and 30 months of age; measures of cognition & memory at 5, 9, and 25 months	Mother–child pairs children, BSID-II: 9 and 30 months Secondary measures: 5, 9, and 25 months.	Adverse association between methylmercury, maternal nutrition, and mean Psychomotor Development Index (PDI) score at 30 months of age, but no association in secondary analyses with PDI score and nutrition alone.
Strain et al. (2011)	Republic of Seychelles	229	Maternal serum ω-3 and ω-6 LCPUFA and associations with child development	Children children: BSID-II: 9 and 30 months	Psychomotor development index (PDI) positively associated with ω-3 LCPUFA and negatively associated with ω-6:ω-3 PUFA; adverse association of prenatal methylmercury and 30-month PDI.
Strain et al. (2012)	Republic of Seychelles	225	Serum ω-3 and ω-6 PUFA total lipids at 28 weeks pregnancy and delivery and maternal hair mercury at delivery and Preschool Language Scales: Preschool Language Scale–Revised edition; Woodcock–Johnson Scholastic Achievement Test, 2nd edition; Child Behavior Checklist; Kaufman Brief Intelligence Test	Mother–child pairs Children: 5 years	No adverse associations between mercury exposure and infant developmental outcomes; child Preschool Language Scale scores improved with increasing maternal serum DHA and decreased with increasing arachidonic acid
Strain et al. (2015)	Republic of Seychelles	1265	Maternal nonfasting serum total PUFAs; maternal hair methylmercury at delivery; Bayley Scales of Infant Development, MacArthur Bates Communicative, Development Inventories, Infant Behavior Questionnaire-Revised	Mother–child pairs Children: 20 months	No adverse associations between prenatal mercury exposure and child neurodevelopmental outcomes at age 20 months. Evidence of protective effect of maternal ω-3 polyunsaturated fatty acids for the Psychomotor Developmental Index
Stokes-Riner et al. (2011)	Republic of Seychelles	229	Maternal hair mercury; maternal blood at 28 weeks of pregnancy and at birth. Infant Bayley Scales of Infant Development-II Psychomotor Developmental Index at 9 and 30 months	Mother–child pairs children: 9 and 30 months	Higher maternal methylmercury was associated with lower child PDI scores and higher maternal ω-3 levels were associated with improved PDI scores.

(Continued)

TABLE 4.1 Epidemiological Studies of Fish Consumption During Pregnancy and Neurocognitive Development in Infants (*cont.*)

Author and year	Population	Number of subjects	Measurement	Age at measurement	Effect of DHA supplementation
Davidson et al. (2011)	Republic of Seychelles	600 371–462 for ful data sets	Behavior questionnaire (specific for the culture, including items from World Health Organization global school-based student health survey and US Centers for Disease Control and Prevention Youth Risk Behavior Survey from the Centers for Disease Control and Prevention 2003, Prevention); neurocognitive and behavioral testing; California Verbal Learning Test, subsets of Woodcock-Johnson Test of Scholastic Achievement-II; subsets of the Cambridge Neuropsychological Test Automated Battery; Wisconsin Card Sorting Test	Adolescents of main Cohort of Seychelles Child Development Study Adolescents: 17 years	No pattern of relationship between prenatal methylmercury and neurocognitive and behavioral testing of adolescents. Seafood (ω-3 fatty acids, other nutrients in fish?) appears to be protective during pregnancy and is important to health and development of children, with benefits extending into teen years.
Freire et al. (2010)	Granada, Spain	72	McCarthy Scales of Children's Abilities (motor and cognitive abilities)	Preschoolers (males, mean age, 51 months; range: 48–52 months)	Hair mercury of children was associated with decreases in general cognitive, memory, and verbal scores–cognitive delay. While environmental sources of mercury have been identified, consumption of oily fish was associated with total mercury in children's hair.
Jedrychowski et al., 2007	Poland	233	Usual dietary intakes by food frequency questionnaire at enrollment to study and by repeated 24-hour dietary recall 2nd trimester coupled with questionnaire about frequency of consumption of specific fish.	Mother–infant dyads (infants 1 year old, M and F, born 33–42 weeks of gestation, 91% born > 38 weeks)	Infant blood mercury level (geometric mean) was higher in infants with delayed neurocognitive and psychomotor performance and risk for delayed performance was greater for infants born to mothers with higher mercury levels.

[a] *A 13 item questionnaire about whether child could: hold up head, sit with straight back, roll back to front, sit unsupported, etc.*

DHA intake during pregnancy may result in suboptimal fetal DHA accretion. The effect of maternal DHA intake during pregnancy on brain development has been recently reviewed (Klemens et al., 2012; Gould et al., 2013; Lo et al., 2012). Further, maternal transfer of DHA across the placenta and fetal essential fatty acid status has been correlated with maternal levels of circulating DHA and DHA dietary intake (Innis, 2005; Al et al., 1995). Both maternal and fetal fatty acid status have been positively associated with various measures of infant cognitive development and central nervous system (CNS) maturity (Bouwstra et al., 2006; Colombo et al., 2004; Bakker et al., 2003), including sleep-state patterns in the newborn (Cheruku et al., 2002).

REQUIREMENTS FOR DHA DURING PREGNANCY TO SUPPORT CNS DEVELOPMENT

The brain and CNS have high concentrations of DHA and these affect a variety of nervous system functions including the uptake of ions (sodium, potassium, and calcium) which are involved in transmission of nervous impulses, cell surface receptor modification which affects nerve cell response to neurotransmitters and even gene expression (Fernstrom, 1999). DHA incorporation into the phospholipid membrane may alter these functions directly by altering membrane fluidity which alters receptor and ion channel conformation, or indirectly, by giving rise to "second messengers" which may affect nerve cell functions, such as excitation or nutrient exchange (Makrides et al., 1994).

The development of the visual pathway involves formation of a neural network to support the complex chain of events, or "visual cascade," which begins when light strikes the photoreceptors in the retina of the eye which in turn generates electrical signals that are sent to the bipolar and ganglion cells of the CNS, transmitting the signal along the optic nerve to the visual cortex. Retinal content of DHA increases during development and the retinal photoreceptor membranes contain the highest content of DHA in the body. Low retina DHA has been associated with decreased amplitude of the electroretinogram (ERG) signal in rats (Benolken et al., 1973). Although it is not possible to selectively separate visual function in the retina from the entire visual cascade, measurement of visual acuity has been used as a measure of the total "visual cascade" and brain cortical function in a number of studies (Dziechciarz et al., 2010; Helland et al., 2001; Malcolm et al., 2003; Judge et al., 2007a,b; Innis and Friesen, 2008; Smithers et al., 2011; Stein et al., 2012).

DHA to support these important developmental and functional roles of the CNS may be obtained from diet or converted from the 18 carbon essential n-3 fatty acid, α-linolenic acid (Fig. 4.1). However, fatty acid desaturase activity in the fetal and neonatal liver and in pregnant women is low (Szitany et al., 1999). Consequently, conversion of α-linolenic to DHA is limited and supplementation of pregnant women with ALA does not increase maternal nor neonatal circulating DHA (de Groot et al., 2004). Therefore, a source of preformed DHA is considered necessary to promote optimal brain and CNS development.

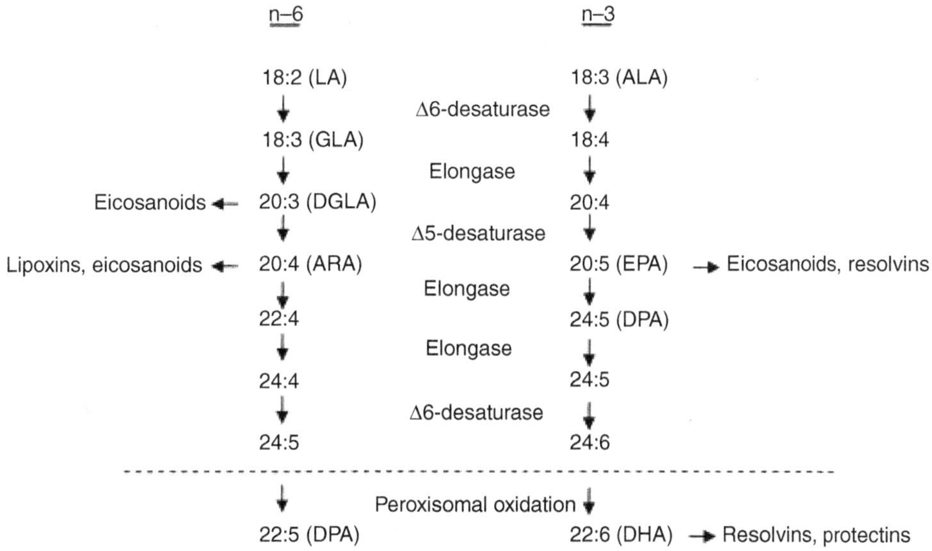

FIGURE 4.1 FAM: Fatty Acid Metabolism; LA: linoleic acid; GLA: gamma linoleic acid; DGLA: dihomogamma linolenic acid; DPA: docosapentaenoic acid; ARA: arachidonic acid; ALA: α-linolenic acid; EPA: eicosapentaenoic acid

DHA is thus an essential structural and functional component of brain and retinal tissue. Fetal brain accretion rates of DHA have been reported to be 14.5 mg per week in the 3rd trimester of pregnancy and continue at a rapid rate during the first 6 months of life (Martinez, 1992). A relationship between gestational age and the fatty acid composition of cerebral cortex and erythrocytes has been demonstrated in human subjects (Carver et al., 2001). Fifty-five percent of brain weight is lipid and DHA comprises 10–20% of total fatty acids (McNamara & Carlson, 2006), a large proportion of which is sequestered in the neuritis and developing synaptosomes during development. Decreased neuronal size and a reduced number of synaptic connections have been demonstrated in rat neurite cells incubated in DHA poor media (Calderon & Kim, 2004). The retina also accumulates DHA during gestation, and DHA deficiency during pregnancy has been shown to decrease photoreceptor DHA and visual acuity in rhesus monkeys (Neuringer et al., 1986). Defects in photoreceptor DHA content and function may not be completely reversible after birth (Anderson et al., 2005).

The role of DHA in visual development was used as the basis of the consensus recommendation that pregnant and breastfeeding women consume 200 mg DHA per day (Koletzko et al., 2007). However, human clinical trials in which pregnant women or infants perinatally have been supplemented with DHA have yielded inconsistent results (Makrides, 2013; Cohen et al., 2005). The greatest neurocognitive impacts have been demonstrated in infants tested up to 12 months of age and in preterm infants (Makrides, 2013) who were not sustained in utero for the entire third trimester of gestation and who therefore had suboptimal accretion of DHA during the entire critical period of brain development in the last trimester of pregnancy. The magnitude of the effect of postnatal DHA supplementation for the term infant is generally modest. A recent quantitative analysis predicted a 0.13 point improvement in a breastfed child's IQ for each 100 mg/day increase in maternal intake of DHA (Cohen et al., 2005).

Newer approaches to evaluate the effect of DHA during development have revolved around supplementation of women during the latter half of pregnancy through birth or through the first few months of breastfeeding. Fifteen RCTs of the effect of maternal DHA supplementation during pregnancy in which data were analyzed by treatment group have been published and are summarized in Tables 4.2 and 4.3.

Four of the RCTs (Helland et al., 2003; Tofail et al., 2006; Judge et al., 2007b; Helland et al., 2008) demonstrated positive effects by treatment on at least one outcome of cognitive development at one or more of the time points

TABLE 4.2 Effect of Effect of Maternal Supplementation with DHA in Pregnancy on Infant Sensory Outcomes

Author and year	Treatment	Completed Study	Timing	GA/ Age at measurement	Effect of DHA Supplementation
Helland et al. (2001)	1.18 g DHA and 0.8 g EPA as CLO Oil versus CO control	EEG CLO = 175 OO = 166	17–19th week of gestation through 3 months postpartum	2 days, 27 and 39 weeks	No effect EEG by treatment. Positive association cord plasma DHA in infants and number with mature EEG (n = 70) compared to immature EEG (n = 51) on day 2
Malcolm et al. (2003)	100 mg DHA as FO versus OA control	FO = 30 OA =26	15th week of gestation until delivery	FT/first week of life	Scotopic blue intensity ERG did not differ by supplement group; positive association with infant cord blood DHA
Judge et al. (2007a)	200 mg DHA/day as cereal-based bars control bars	DHA = 16 CON = 15	24th week of gestation until delivery	FT/4 months, 6 months	Improvement in behavioral (Teller card) visual acuity at 4 months, but no difference at 6 months
Innis and Friesen (2008)	400 mg DHA as FO versus CO/SO	FO = 67 CO/SO = 68	16th week of gestation until delivery	2 months	No effect on Teller card visual acuity
Smithers et al. (2011)	800 mg DHA as FO versus vegetable oil control Stratified to high or low post-natal feeding	FO = 91 CON= 94	18th–21st week gestation until delivery	4 months	No effect on VEP acuity nor VEP latency
Stein et al. (2012)	400 mg DHA as algal oil or CO/SO control	DHA = 679 CON = 817	18th–22nd week of gestation until delivery	FT/3 and 6 months	No effect on brainstem auditory evoked potentials

GA, gestational age at delivery; *FT*, full term (> 37 weeks); *PT*, preterm (< 37 week); *FO*, fish oil; *MTHFA*, 5-methyl tetrahydrofolic acid; *VEP*, visually evoked potential; *SO*, soybean oil; *OA*, oleic acid; *CO*, corn oil; *OO*, olive oil; *CLO*, cod liver oil; *K-ABC*, Kaufman Mental Assessment Battery for Children; and EEG, electroretinogram.

TABLE 4.3 Effect of Maternal Supplementation with DHA in Pregnancy on Infant Cognitive and Motor Outcomes

Author and year	Treatment	Completed Study	Timing	GA/ Age at measurement	Effect of DHA Supplementation
Helland et al. (2001)	1.18 g DHA and 0.8 g EPA as CLO Oil versus CO control	Fagan at 27th week CLO = 144, CO = 118, Fagan at 39 weeks CLO = 130 and CO = 115	17–19 weeks gestation through 3 months post partum	2 days, 27 and 39 weeks	No effect on Fagan test of novelty preference
Helland et al. (2003)	1.18 g DHA and 0.8 g EPA as CLO Oil versus CO control	CLO = 41 and CO = 45	17–19 weeks gestation through 3 months post partum	4 years	Improved K-ABC mental processing by treatment. Positive association with maternal DHA and EPA intake
Tofail et al. (2006)	1.2 g DHA + 1.8 g EPA as FO versus SO control	*N* = 249	25th week of gestation until delivery	FT/10 months	No difference in Bayley's MDI or PDI scales or behavioral outcomes by tx; positive association with DHA
Judge et al. (2007b)	200 mg DHA/day as cereal-based bars versus CO control bars	DHA = 14 CO = 16	24th week of gestation until delivery	FT/9 months	Improvement problem solving, no effect on recognition memory
Helland et al. (2008)	1.18 g DHA and 0.8 g EPA as CLO Oil versus CO control	CLO = 82 CO = 61	17–19 week gestation through 3 months post partum	7 years	No effect on K-ABC by treatment. Positive association of DHA status with improved sequential processing
Dunstan et al. (2008)	2.2 g DHA + 1.1 g EPA as FO versus OO control	FO = 33 and OO = 39	20th week of gestation until delivery	2.5 years	Improvement hand: eye coordination on Griffiths Mental Development Scales
Makrides et al. (2010)	800 mg DHA and 100 mg EPA versus sunflower oil control	FO = 351 CON = 375	<21 weeks of gestation until delivery	PT and FT/18 months	No effect on Bayley's language or cognitive scores
Van Goor et al. (2010)	200 mg DHA +/− 220 mg AA versus SO control	DHA = 22 DHA/AA = 41 CON = 36	14–20 weeks of gestation until 12th week post partum	FT/2 weeks, 12 weeks	Lower general movement quality with DHA alone compared to DHA + AA or control
Campoy et al. (2011)	500 mg DHA/150 mg EPA as FO +/− 400 ug MTHFA versus placebo	FO = 69 FO/MTHFA = 64 MTHFA = 65 Placebo = 80	22nd week of gestation until delivery After birth BF or formula matched to FO tx	FT/6.5 years	No effect on K-ABC

GA, gestational age at delivery; *FT*, full term (>37 week); *PT*, preterm (<37 week); *FO*, fish oil; *MTHFA*, 5-methyl tetrahydrofolic acid; *VEP*, visually evoked potential; *SO*, soybean oil; *OA*, oleic acid; *CO*, corn oil; *OO*, olive oil; *CLO*, cod liver oil; *K-ABC*, Kaufman Mental Assessment Battery for Children; and *EEG*, electroretinogram.

measured. The greatest number of studies (9 of the 15) (Helland et al., 2001; Malcolm et al., 2003; Innis and Friesen, 2008; Smithers et al., 2011; Helland et al., 2003; Helland et al., 2008; Makrides et al., 2010; Van Goor et al., 2010; Campoy et al., 2011) failed to demonstrate a positive effect of fish oil or DHA by treatment. Four of these (Helland et al., 2001; Malcolm et al., 2003; Helland et al., 2003; Helland et al., 2008) showed a positive association with DHA status. One study (Van Goor et al., 2010) showed a slightly negative effect of DHA supplementation without arachidonic acid (AA). Only one of the infant sensory studies showed an effect of prenatal DHA supplementation (Judge et al., 2007a,b). Methodological differences may account for differing results. Most of the visual studies measured the VEP which measures cortical response directly and with less variability than the Teller Visual Acuity Card Test. However, it should be considered that behavioral assessments may provide a better measure of what the infant actually perceives (Neuringer, 2000).

Results of prenatal supplementation trials neither support nor refute the effects of DHA upon neurocognitive development. There are a number of possible explanations for differences in the effect of prenatal DHA exposure on cognition. DHA status may play a role since maternal status has clearly been shown to affect infant status as determined by cord blood DHA. In order for supplementation to be effective, it must impact on maternal and neonatal DHA status. Studies of the effect of maternal DHA status during pregnancy and/or improved neonatal DHA status on infant cognitive development are generally lacking. A correlational study suggests that maternal DHA levels during pregnancy correlate with improved cognitive development in infants (Colombo et al., 2004). In this study, Columbo and Carlson examined DHA levels of mothers at birth (31 supplemented with 165 mg DHA/day during pregnancy and 38 unsupplemented) and looked at the duration and attention span of infants during the first 18 months of life. Infants whose mothers had the highest DHA had the shortest look duration at 4 and 6 months of age (associated with more rapid acquisition of signal at this age) but this advantage disappeared by 8 months. Subsequently, infants born to mothers who had the highest DHA levels demonstrated the most mature attention span and were less easily distracted at 12–18 months of age than infants born to mothers with lower DHA levels (Colombo et al., 2004). In a pilot study of eight infants, aged 4–6 months, born to mothers supplemented with 0, 300, or 600 mg DHA during the second half of pregnancy, Harris and Reece found cord RBC % total DHA to be positively correlated with Bayley's MDI Scales of Infant Development ($p = 0.05$) (Fig. 4.2).

Higher maternal DHA status at delivery has been positively associated with newborns' sleep patterns (more time in a wakeful state, decreased active:quiet sleep ratio, and less transitioning between sleep and wakefulness) characteristic of mature neurological maturity (Cheruku et al., 2002). It is interesting that over two decades ago early infant sleep patterns were associated with improved infant mental and motor development at 6 months of age (Freudigman and Thoman, 1993). More recently, maternal DHA status at birth was linked to infant sleep patterns (Cheruku et al., 2002; Lammi-Keefe et al., 2003) and this finding provided the basis for further investigation of maternal DHA status as a determinant of infant sleep, with the idea that infant sleep was determined in part by maturity of the central nervous system. A recent study has reported on the impact of an intervention with DHA during pregnancy on infant sleep patterns (Judge et al., 2012). In this study maternal consumption of a DHA-containing functional food beginning at 24 weeks of pregnancy until birth of the infants benefitted infant sleep patterning in the first 24 h after birth, with fewer arousals in quiet sleep on days 1 and 2, following birth. The significance of these studies (Cheruku et al., 2002; Lammi-Keefe et al., 2003; Judge et al., 2012) is that DHA status during

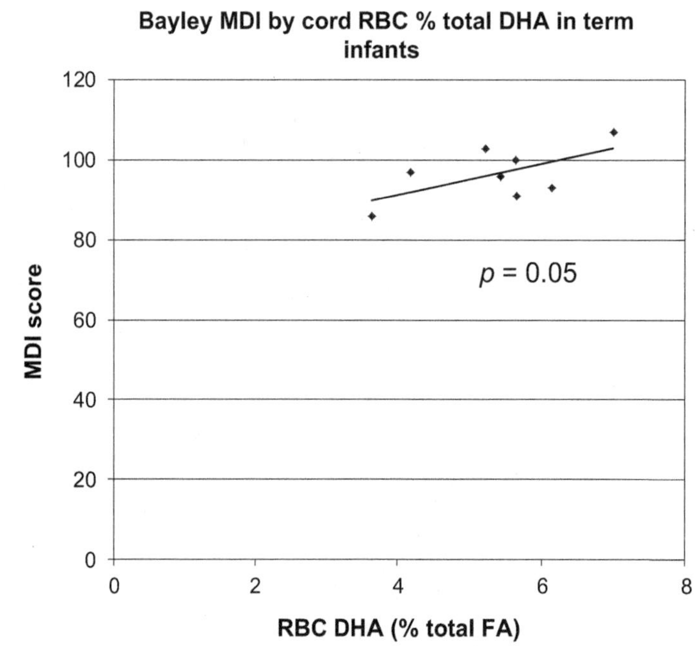

FIGURE 4.2 Harris M.A., Reece M.S. unpublished follow-up to "Omega3 for Baby and Me" trial

pregnancy can provide an advantage to the newborn that can be demonstrated in the immediate hours following birth. Furthermore, based on the earlier report of Freudigman and Thoman (1993) the earliest infant neurological state has significance for development out to at least 6 months of life. These studies suggest that in assessing study outcomes for DHA effect, the potential benefits of DHA supplementation during pregnancy and pregnancy and lactation on infant cognitive development may be more strongly related to infant DHA status than maternal 'supplementation group'.

Genetic differences in the ability to elongate and desaturate dietary sources of Omega-3 fatty acids to DHA likely play a role in individual response to supplementation. A number of single nucleotide polymorphisms in the delta-4 and -5 desaturase have been associated with maternal blood phospholipid and breastmilk DHA levels (Glaser et al., 2011).

In evaluating the potential for DHA's ability to affect neurological development, differences in measurements used to assess cognitive/developmental performance and age at measurement should be considered. Helland and coworkers demonstrated differences in cognitive development at age 4 (Helland et al., 2003) but not in early postnatal life (Helland et al., 2001); furthermore, effects in older children could only be demonstrated in relation to DHA status at 7 years of age (Helland et al., 2008). Sustained effects may require DHA throughout the period of rapid brain development in the first six to twelve months of post-natal life. Different measures of neurocognitive development (eg, visual processing, intelligence, motor and verbal performance) may represent domains which are more or less greatly impacted by DHA at various and different developmental periods. Additionally, a ceiling effect may exist and DHA may not have an effect in women already consuming an adequate amount of DHA in the diet.

Gender differences may explain in part cognitive response to Omega-3 DHA supplementation. Glaser and coworkers (Glaser et al., 2011) examined 4154 American children aged 6–16 years in the Third National Health and Nutrition Examination Survey (NHANES III), controlling a variety of confounders, and discovered a positive relationship between total Omega-3 fatty acid intake of 1 g or greater and cognitive test scores in both males (0.19 point increase) and females (0.38 point increase). However, in female children, the positive effects were twice as strong as in males ($p = 0.001$), suggesting female children may benefit more cognitively from increased DHA intakes (Lassek & Gaulin, 2011). In the DINO trial of early preterm infants, higher DHA supplementation, via DHA supplemented mothers breast milk or DHA supplemented formula, significantly improved BSID MDI scores ($p = 0.03$) and reduced the risk of mild [developmental quotient (DQ) < 85; $p = 0.01$] and severe (DQ < 70; $p = 0.02$) cognitive delay for girls at 18 months of age, while no effect was noted for boys (Smithers et al., 2008).

Recommended Intakes

The large numbers of individuals who have been studied in the prenatal supplementation trials demonstrate the safety of DHA supplementation during pregnancy (at least up to 800 mg/day in the largest studies). Currently there is no US DRI for DHA during pregnancy, lactation, or infancy although the United States Dietary Guidelines for Americans recommend 8–12 ounces of seafood per week for pregnant and lactating women (Department of Agriculture, 2015). Diets of many women of childbearing ages in Western countries are low in DHA (Department of Agriculture, 2012) and do not meet consensus recommendations (Koletzko et al., 2007). Data from the United States suggests that maternal DHA intakes average 60–80 mg/day (Judge et al., 2007a,b; Chen et al., 2010). Similar DHA intakes averaging 100 mg/day have been reported among pregnant women in Canada (Friesen and Innis, 2010). A study in the largely Mexican American population in western United States suggests that DHA intake may vary by ethnicity; mean intake in Hispanic whites were 140 mg/day compared to non-Hispanic whites which were 69 mg/day, in the range of other US studies (Harris et al., 2015). Similar DHA intakes averaging 100 mg/day have been reported among pregnant women in Canada (Jia et al., 2015). More recently evidence from Alberta, Canada suggests that intakes may have increased in women to an average of 122 mg DHA per day from food and an additional 80 mg/day from supplements (Oken et al., 2003). Table 4.4 provides selected sources of the long chain Omega-3 fatty acids. Health recommendations to decrease exposure to methyl mercury from the United State Department of Agriculture and Food and Drug Administration (http://www.usda.com), Health Canada and the Food Standards, Australia; FSANZ advice on mercury in fish (http://www.foodstandards.gov.newsroom/mediareleases/mediar) may further reduce intake.

There is clearly a need to educate both the public and health care providers on the importance of DHA to health throughout the life cycle.

TABLE 4.4 Selected Food Sources of Long Chain Omega-3 Fatty Acids

Food	Serving size	EPA (mg)	DHA (mg)
Herring, Atlantic (kippered)	3 oz	773	1002
Herring, Pacific	3 oz	1055	750
Salmon, Atlantic, (pink) cooked	3 oz	456	638
Salmon, Pacific (coho, wild cooked)	3 oz	340	560
Salmon, Pacific (canned)	3 oz	284	682
Tuna, Albacore (canned in water)	3 oz	535	198
Tuna, light (canned in water)	3 oz	40	189
Trout (rainbow, wild)	3 oz	398	442
Crab (King)	3 oz	250	100
Crab (Dungeness)	3 oz	239	96
Mackerel canned	3 oz	123	226
Cod, (Atlantic)	3 oz	131	—
Cod, (Pacific)	3 oz	87	146
Catfish (wild)	3 oz	85	116
Eggs (ordinary)	1 large	—	18
DHA enriched eggs	1 large	EPA + DHA combined	32*–160
DHA enriched milk	1 cup	—	32
DHA enriched peanut butter	2 TBSP	EPA + DHA combined	32*
DHA fortified orange juice	$\frac{1}{2}$ cup	EPA + DHA combined	50*

Source: USDA Nutrient Analysis (DB-SR16-1) and manufacturers data. All values are cooked, dry or as served.

References

Al, M.S., van Howelingen, A.C., Kester, A.D., Hasaart, T.H., deJong, A.E., Hornstra, G., 1995. Maternal essential fatty acid patterns during normal pregnant and their relationship to the neonatal essential fatty acid status. Br. J. Nutr. 74 (1), 55–68.

Anderson, G.J., Neuringer, M., Lin, D.S., Connor, W.E., Bakker, E.C., Hornstra, G., 2005. Can perinatal n-3 fatty acids deficiency be completely reversed after birth? Effects of retinal and brain biochemistry and visual function in rhesus monkeys. Pediatr. Res. 58 (5), 865–872.

Bakker, E.C., Ghys, A.J., Kester, A.D., Vles, J.S., Dubas, J.S., Blanco, C.E., Hornstra, G., 2003. Long-chain polyunsaturated fatty acids at birth and cognitive function at 7 y of age. Eur. J. Clin. Nutr. 57, 89–95.

Benolken, R.M., Anderson, R.E., Wheeler, T.G., 1973. Membrane fatty acids associated with the electrical response in visual excitation. Science 182, 1253–1254.

Boucher, O., Burden, M.J., Muckle, G., Saint-Amour, D., Ayotte, P., Dewailly, E., Jacobson, J.L., 2011. Neurophysiologic and neurobehavioral evidence of beneficial effects of prenatal omega-3 fatty acids intake on memory function at school age. Am. J. Clin. Nutr. 93 (5), 1025–1037.

Bouwstra, H., Dijck-Brouwer, D.A., Decsi, T., Boehm, E.R., Muskiet, F.A.J., Haddrs-Algra, M., 2006. Relationship between umbilical cord essential fatty acid content and quality of general movements of healthy term infants at 3 months. Pediatr. Res. 59 (5), 717–722.

Calderon, F., Kim, H.-Y., 2004. Docosahexaenoic acid promotes neurite growth in hippocampal neurons. J. Neurochem. 90 (4), 979–988.

Campoy, C., Escolano-Margarit, M.V., Ramos, R., Parilla-Roure, M., Csábi, G., Beyer, J., Koletzko, B., 2011. Effects of prenatal fish-oil and 5-methyltertrhydrofolate supplementation on cognitive development of children at 6.5 y of age. Am. J. Clin. Nutr. 94 (6 Suppl.), 1880S–1888S.

Carver, J.D., Benford, V.J., Han, B., Cantor, A.B., 2001. The relationship between age and the fatty acid composition of cerebral cortex and erythrocytes in human subjects. Brain Res. Bull. 56 (2), 79–85.

Chen, X., Scholl, T.O., Leskiw, M., Savaille, J., Stein, T.P., 2010. Differences in maternal circulating fatty acid composition and dietary fat intake in women with gestational diabetes mellitus or milk gestational hyperglycemia. Diab. Care 33 (9), 2049–2054.

Cheruku, S.R., Montgomery-Downs, H.E., Farkas, S.L., Thoman, E.B., Lammi-Keefe, C.J., 2002. Higher maternal plasma docosahexaenoic acid during pregnancy is associated with a more mature infant sleep-state patterning. Am. J. Clin. Nutr. 76 (3), 608–613.

Cohen, J.T., Bellinger, D.C., Connor, W.E., Shaywitz, B.A., 2005. A quantitative analysis of prenatal intake of n-3 polyunsaturated fatty acids on cognitive development. Am. J. Preventive Med. 29 (4), e12366–366.

Colombo, J., Kannass, K.N., Shaddy, D.J., Kundurthi, S., Maikronz, J.M., Anderson, C.J., Carlson, S., 2004. Maternal DHA and the development of attention in infancy and toddlerhood. Child Dev. 75 (4), 1254–1267.

Daniels, J.L., Longnecker, M.P., Rowland, A.S., Golding, J., 2004. ALSPAC Study Team University of Bristol Institute of Child Health. Fish intake during pregnancy and early cognitive development of offspring. Epidemiology 15 (4), 394–402.

Davidson, P.W., Cory-Slechta, D.A., Thurston, S.W., Huang, L.S., Shamlaye, C.F., Gunzler, D., Myers, G.J., 2011. Fish consumption and prenatal methylmercury exposure: cognitive and behavioral outcomes in the main cohort at 17 years from the Seychelles child development study. NeuroToxicology 32 (6), 711–717.
Davidson, P.W., Myers, G.J., Cox, C., Axtell, C., Shamlaye, C., Sloane-Reeves, J., Cernichiari, E., Needham, L., Choi, A., Wang, Y., Maths, B., Clarkson, T.W., 1998. Effects of prenatal and postnatal methylmercury exposure from fish consumption on neurodevelopment: outcomes at 66 months of age in the Seychelles Child Development Study. J. Am. Med. Assoc. 280 (8), 701–707.
Davidson, P.W., Strain, J.J., Myers, G.J., Thurston, S.W., Bonham, M.P., Shamlaye, C.F., Clarkson, T.W., 2008. Neurodevelopmental effects of maternal nutritional status and exposure to methylmercury from eating fish during pregnancy. NeuroToxicology 29 (5), 767–775.
de Groot, R.H., Hornstra, G., van Howelingen, A.C., Roumen, F., 2004. The effect of alpha-linolenic acid supplementation during pregnancy on maternal and neonatal polyunsaturated fatty acid status and pregnancy outcomes. Am. J. Clin. Nutr. 79 (2), 251–260.
Dunstan, J.A., Simmer, K., Dixon, G.M., Prescott, S.L., 2008. Cognitive assessment of children at age 2 ½ years after maternal fish oil supplementation in pregnancy: a randomized controlled trial. Archiv. Dis. Childhood Fetal Neonat. Ed. 93 (1), F45–F50.
Dziechciarz, P., Horvath, A., Szajewska, H., 2010. Effects of n-3 long chain polyunsaturated fatty acid supplementation during pregnancy and/or lactation on neurodevelopment and visual function in children: a systematic review of randomized controlled trials. J. Am. Coll. Nutr. 29 (5), 443–454.
Fernstrom, J.D., 1999. Effects of dietary polyunsaturated fatty acids on neuronal function. Lipids 34 (2), 161–169.
Freire, C., Ramos, R., Lopez-Espinosa, M.-J., Díez, S., Vioque, J., Ballester, F., Fernández, M.-F., 2010. Hair mercury levels, fish consumption, and cognitive development in preschool children from Granada Spain. Environ. Res. 110 (1), 96–104.
Freudigman, K., Thoman, E., 1993. Infant sleep during the first postnatal day and opportunity for assessment of vulnerability. Pediatrics 92, 373–379.
Friesen, R.W., Innis, S.M., 2010. Linoleic acid is associated with lower long-chain n–6 and n–3 fatty acids in red blood cell lipids of Canadian pregnant women. Am. J. Clin. Nutr. 91 (1), 23–31.
Glaser, C., Lattka, E., Rzehak, P., Steer, C., Koletzko, B., 2011. Genetic variation in polyunsaturated fatty acid metabolism and its potential relevance for human development and health. Maternal Child Nutr. 7, 27–40.
Gould, J.F., Smithers, L.G., Makrides, M., 2013. The effect of maternal omega-3 (n-3) LCPUFA supplementation during pregnancy on early childhood cognitive and visual development: a systematic review and meta-analysis of randomized controlled trials. Am. J. Clin. Nutr. 97 (3), 531–544.
Harris, M.A., Reece, M.S., McGregor, J.A., Wilson, J.W., Burke, S., Wheeler, M., Anderson, J.E., Auld, G.W., Allen, K.G.D.T., 2015. The effect of omega-3 docosahexaenoic acid (DHA) supplementation on gestational length:randomized trial of supplementation compared to nutrition education for increasing n-3 intake. Biomed. Res. Int. www.hindawi.con/journlas/bmri/aa/123078
Helland, I.B., Smith, L., Blomen, B., Saarem, K., Saugstad, O.D., Drevon, C.A., 2008. Effect of supplementing pregnant and lactating mothers with n-3 and n-6 very-long-chain fatty acids on children's IQ and body mass index at 7 years of age. Pediatrics 122 (2), e472–e479.
Helland, I.B., Smith, L., Saaren, K., Saugstad, O.D., Drevon, C.A., 2003. Maternal supplementation with very long chain n-3 fatty acids during pregnancy and lactation augments children's IQ at 4 years of age. Pediatrics 111 (1), e39–e44.
Helland, I.B., Saugstad, O.D., Smith, L., Saarem, K., Solvoll, K., Ganes, T., Drevon, C.A., 2001. Similar effects on infants of n-3 and n-6 fatty acids supplementation to pregnant and lactating women. Pediatrics 108 (5), e82.
Hibbeln, J.R., Davis, J.M., Steer, C., Emmett, P., Rogers, L., Williams, C., Golding, J., 2007. Maternal seafood consumption in pregnancy and neurodevelopmental outcomes in childhood (ALSPAC study): an observational cohort study. Lancet 369 (9561), 578–585.
Innis, S.M., 1993. The 1993 Borden Award Lecture Fatty acid requirements of the newborn. Can. J. Physiol. Pharmacol. 72, 1483–1492.
Innis, S.M., 2005. Essential fatty acids transfer and fetal development. Placenta 26 (Suppl. A), 26.
Innis, S.M., Friesen, R.W., 2008. Essential n-3 fatty acids in pregnant women and early visual acuity maturation in term infants. Am. J. Clin. Nutr. 87 (3), 548–557.
Jacobson, J.L., Jacobsen, S.W., Muckle, G., Kaplan-Estrin, M., Ayotte, P., Dewailly, E., 2008. Beneficial effects of a polyunsaturated fatty acid on infant development: evidence from the Inuit of artic Quebec. J. Pediatr. 152 (3), 356–364.
Jedrychowski, W., Perera, F., Jankowski, J., Rauh, V., Flak, E., Caldwell, K.L., Lisowska-Miszczyk, I., 2007. Fish consumption in pregnancy, cord mercury level and cognitive and psychomotor development of infants followed over the first three years of life: krakow epidemiologic study. Environ. Int. 33 (8), 1057–1062.
Jia, M., Pakseresht, M., Wattar, N., Wildgrove, J., Sontag, S., Andrews, M., Subhan, F.B., McCargar, L., Field, C.J., 2015. The APrON Study Team Women who take n-3 long chain polyunsaturated fatty acid supplements during pregnancy and lactation meet the recommended intake. Appl. Physiol. Nutr. Metab. 40 (5), 1–8.
Judge, M.P., Cong, X., Harel, O., Courville, A.P., Lammi-Keefe, C.J., 2012. Maternal consumption of a DHA-containing functional food benefits infant sleep patterning: an early neurodevelopmental measure. Early Human Dev. 88, 531–537.
Judge, M.P., Harel, O., Lammi-Keefe, C.J., 2007a. A docosahexaenoic acid-functional food during pregnancy benefits infant visual acuity at four but not six months of age. Lipids 42 (2), 117–122.
Judge, M.P., Harel, O., Lammi-Keefe, C.J., 2007b. Maternal consumption of a docosahexaenoic acid-containing functional food during pregnancy: benefit for infant performance on problem-solving but not on recognition memory tasks at 9 mo. Am. J. Clin. Nutr. 85 (6), 1572–1577.
Kahn, M.A.K., Wang, F., 2009. Mercury-selenium compounds and their toxicological significance: toward a molecular understanding of the mercury-selenium antagonism. Environ. Toxicol. Chem. 28 (8), 1567–1577.
Klemens, C.M., Salari, K., Mozurkewich, E.L., 2012. Assessing omega-3 fatty acid supplementation during pregnancy and lactation to optimize maternal mental health and childhood cognitive development. Clin. Lipidol. 7 (1), 93–109.
Koletzko, B., Cetin, I., Brenna, J.T., Perinatal Lipid Intake Working Group, 2007. Dietary fat intakes for pregnant and lactating women. Br. J. Nutr. 98 (05), 873–877.
Lammi-Keefe, C.J., Thoman, E.B., Cheruku, S.R., Montgomery-Downs, H.E., Farkas, S.L., Loosemore, E.D., DeMare, C.I., Keplinger, M.R., Mutungi, G., Judge, M.P., and Ibarorola, B., 2003. Sleep patterns of infants immediately after birth reflect DHA status and CNS maturity. In: Proc. Int. Cong. Essen. Fatty Acid. and Eicosanoid. Huang, Y-S, Lin, S-J, and Huang, P-C, Eds. AOCS Press, 105–111.
Lassek, W.D., Gaulin, S.J., 2011. Sex differences in the relationship of dietary fatty acids to cognitive measures in American children. Frontier. Evolut. Neurosci. 3, 5.

Leino, O., Karjalainen, A.K., Tuomisto, J.T., 2013. Effects of docosahexaenoic acid and methylmercury on child's brain development due to consumption of fish by Finnish mother during pregnancy: a probabilistic modeling approach. Food Chem. Toxicol. 54, 50–58.

Lo, A., Sienna, J., Mamak, E., Djokanovic, N., Westall, C., Koren, G., 2012. The effects of maternal supplementation of polyunsaturated fatty acids on visual, neurobehavioral and developmental outcomes of the child: a systematic review of the randomized trials. Obstetr. Gynecol. Int. 2015 (9).

McNamara, R.K., Carlson, S.E., 2006. Role of omega-3 fatty acids in brain development and function: potential implications for the pathogenesis and prevention of psychopathology. Prostagland. Leukotr. Essen. Fatty Acid. 75 (4–5), 329–349.

Makrides, M., 2013. DHA supplementation during the perinatal period and neurodevelopment: do some babies benefit more than others? Prostagland. Leukotr. Essen. Fatty Acid. 88 (1), 87–90.

Makrides, M., Neumann, M.A., Byard, R.W., Simmer, K., Gibson, R.A., 1994. Fatty acid composition of brain, retina, and erythrocytes in breast- and formula-fed infants. Am. J. Clin. Nutr. 60 (2), 189–194.

Makrides, M, Smithers, L.G., and Gibson, R., 2010. Role of long-chain polyunsaturated fatty acids neurological development and growth. Nestle Nutr. Workshop Ser. Pediatr. Prog., 65, 123–136.

Malcolm, C.A., Hamilton, R., McCulloch, D.L., Montgomery, C., Weaver, L.T., 2003. Scotopic electroretinogram in term infants born of mothers supplemented with docosahexaenoic acid during pregnancy. Investigative Ophthalmol. Vis. Sci. 44 (8), 3685–3691.

Martinez, M., 1992. Tissue levels of polyunsaturated fatty acids during early human development. J. Pediatr. 120, S129–S138, (4 Part 2).

Myers, G.J., Davidson, P.W., Cox, C., Shamlaye, C.F., Palumbo, D., Cernichiari, E., Clarkson, T.W., 2003. Prenatal methylmercury exposure from ocean fish consumption in the Seychelles Child Development Study. The Lancet 361 (9370), 1686–1692.

Neuringer, M., 2000. Infant vision and retinal function in studies of long-chain polyunsaturated fatty acids: methods, results and implications. Am. J. Clin. Nutr. 71 (1), 256S–267S.

Neuringer, M., Connor, W. E., Barstad, L., Luck, S., 1986. Biochemical and functional effects of prenatal and post-natal n-3 fatty acid deficiency on retina and brain in rhesus monkeys. Proc. Nat. Acad. Sci., 83 (11), 4021–4025.

Oken, E., Ballinger, D.C., 2008. Fish consumption, methtylmercury and child neurodevelopment. Curr. Opin. Pediatr. 20 (2), 178–183.

Oken, E., Kleinman, K.P., Berland, W.E., Simon, S.R., Rich-Edwards, J.W., Gillman, M.W., 2003. Decline in fish consumption among pregnant women after a national mercury advisory. Obstetr. Gynecol. 102 (2), 346–351.

Oken, E., Østerdal, M.L., Gillman, M.W., Knudsen, K.K., Halldorsson, T.I., StrØm, M., Olsen, S.F., 2008a. Associations of maternal fish intake during pregnancy and breastfeeding duration with attainment of developmental milestones in early childhood: a study from the Danish National Birth Cohort. Am. J. Clin. Nutr. 88 (3), 789–796.

Oken, E., Radesky, J.S., Wright, R.O., Bellinger, D.C., Amarasiriwardena, C.J., Kleinman, K.P., Gillman, M.W., 2008b. Maternal fish intake during pregnancy, blood mercury levels and child cognition at age 3 years in a U S. cohort. Am. J. Epidemiol. 167 (10), 1171–1181.

Smithers, L.G., Gibson, R.A., Makrides, M., 2011. Maternal supplementation with docosahexaenoic acid during pregnancy does not affect early visual development in the infant: a randomized controlled trial. Am. J. Clin. Nutr. 93 (6), 1293–1299.

Smithers, L.G., Gibson, R.A., McPhee, A., Makrides, M., 2008. Effect of two doses of docosahexaenoic acid (DHA) in the diet of preterm infants on infant fatty acid status: results from the DINO trial. Prostaglandins Leukot. Essent. Fatty Acids 79 (3–5), 141–146.

Stein, A.D., Wang, M., Rivera, J.A., Martorell, R., Ramakrishnan, U., 2012. Auditory- and visual-evoked potentials in Mexican infants are not affected by maternal supplementation with 400 mg/d docosahexaenoic acid in the second half of pregnancy. J. Nutr. 142 (8), 1577–1581.

Stokes-Riner, A.D., Thurston, S.W., Myers, G.J., Duffy, E.M., Wallace, J., Bonham, M., Davidson, P.W., 2011. A longitudinal analysis of prenatal exposure to methylmercury and fatty acids in the Seychelles. Neurotoxicol. Teratol. 33 (2), 325–328.

Strain, J.J., Davidson, P.W., Bonham, M.P., Duffy, E.M., Stokes-Reiner, A., Thurston, S.W., Wallace, J.M.W., Robson, P.J., Shamlaye, C.F., Georger, L.A., Sloane-Reeves, J., Chemichiari, E., Canfield, R.L., Cox, C., Huang, L.S., Janciuras, J., Myers, G.J., Clarkson, T.W., 2008. Associations of maternal long chain polyunsaturated fatty acids, methyl mercury, and infant development in the Seychelles Child Development Nutrition Study. Neurotoxicology 29 (5), 776–782.

Strain, J.J., Davidson, P.W., Bonham, M.P., Duffy, E.M., Stokes-Riner, A., Thurston, S.W., Wallace, J.M., Robson, P.J., Shamlaye, C.F., Georger, L.A., Sloane-Reeves, J., Cernichiari, E., Canfield, R.L., Cox, C., Huang, L.S., Janciuras, J., Myers, G.J., Clarkson, T.W., 2011. Currigendum to "Associations of maternal long-chain polyunsaturated fatty acids, methyl mercury, and infant development in the Seychelles Child Development Nutrition Study. Neurotoxicology 29 (5) (2008) 776–782." Neurotoxicology 32, 990.

Strain, J.J., Davidson, P.W., Thurston, S.W., Harrington, D., Mulhern, M.S., McAfee, A.J., Myers, G.J., 2012. Maternal PUFA status but not prenatal methylmercury exposure is associated with children's language functions at age five years in the Seychelles. J. Nutr. 142, 1943–1948.

Strain, J.J., Yeates, A.J., van Wijngaarden, E., Thurston, S.W., Mulhern, M.S., McSorley, E.M., Davidson, P.W., 2015. Prenatal exposure to methyl mercury from fish consumption and polyunsaturated fatty acids: association with child development at 20 mo of age in an observational study in the Republic of the Seychelles. Am. J. Clin. Nutr. 114, 100503.

Szitany, P., Koletzko, B., Mydilova, A., Demmelmair, H., 1999. Metabolism of 13C-labelled linoleic acid in newborn infants during the first week of life. Pediatr. Res. 45 (S5), 669–673.

Tofail, F., Kabir, I., Hamadani, J.D., Chowdhury, F., Yesmin, S., Mehreen, F., Huda, S.N., 2006. Supplementation of fish-oil and soy-oil during pregnancy and psychomotor development in infants. J. Health Popul. Nutr. 24 (1), 48–56.

United States Department of Agriculture, 2015–2020. Dietary Guidelines for Americans. http://health.gov/dietaryguidelines/2015/

United States Department of Agriculture, Agricultural Research Service, 2012. What We Eat In America, NHANES 2007–2008. http://www.ars.usda.gov/Services/docs.htm?docid=18349

US Food and Drug Administration (FDA), 2014. Qualitative Assessment of the New Effects on Neurocognitive Development from Eating Commercial Fish. http://www.fda.gov/downloads/Food/FoodborneIllnessContaminants/Metals/UCM396785.pdf

Van Goor, S.A., Dijck-Brouwer, D.A., Doornbos, B., Erwich, J.J.H.M., Schaafsma, A., Muskiet, F.A.J., Hadders-Algra, M., 2010. Supplementation with DHA but not DHA with arachidonic acid during pregnancy and lactation influences general movement quality in 12-week old term infants. Br. J. Nutr. 103 (02), 235–242.

Zeilmaker, M.J., Hoekstra, J., van Eijkeren, J.C., de Jong, N., Hart, A., Kennedy, M., Owen, H., Gunnlaugsdottir, H., 2013. Fish consumption during child bearing age: a quantitative risk-benefit analysis on neurodevelopment. Food Chem. Toxicol. 54, 30–34.

CHAPTER

5

Bioavailability of Lipids in Fish and Fish Oils

C. Genot*, A. Meynier*, N. Bernoud-Hubac**, M-C. Michalski**

*Biopolymères Interactions Assemblages, INRA, Nantes, France; **CarMeN Laboratory, INRA UMR1397, INSERM U1060, Université de Lyon, INSA-Lyon, Villeurbanne, France

INTRODUCTION: WHAT IS BIOAVAILABILITY?

Over the past 50 years, the health benefits of fish and fish lipid consumption have been proven and, amongst the active molecules, n–3 long chain fatty acids (n–3 LC-PUFA) have been put forward. Consequently, the most recent reviews on that topic do not concern solely fish lipids, but rather consider n–3 LC-PUFA as a whole including their different common dietary sources such as fish, fish oil, and other sources such as algae or krill. Currently, seafood is the primary dietary source of eicosapentaenoic acid (EPA; 20:5n–3) and docosahexaenoic acid (DHA; 22:6n–3). However, global fish stocks are declining and are not expected to meet future nutritional needs. Moreover, specific patients such as those with cardiovascular disease risk may benefit from higher intakes (Marangoni and Poli, 2013). As the intake of n–3 LC-PUFA was insufficient for several populations (Jacobsen et al., 2013) in relation to nutritional recommendations (EFSA, 2010), alternative solutions to fish consumption have been proposed to the consumers either as enriched foods or supplements, including specifically structured lipids (SLs) with high purity (Guo et al., 2005).

The daily intake of n–3 LC-PUFA such as EPA or DHA is in fact not equivalent to the amount that will be released in the gut from the ingested food (bioaccessibility) nor to the amount that reaches the systemic circulation (pharmacology definition of bioavailability) or its site of physiological activity (Schuchardt and Hahn, 2013). Recently, a huge number of studies have been published evaluating the potential effects of dietary n–3 LC-PUFA. However, and quite surprisingly, little scientific attention has been paid to the actual bioaccessibility and/or bioavailability of n–3 LC-PUFA in various foods and dietary supplements (Ghasemifard et al., 2014). It seems however that this information should help to better understand the observed health effects and the discrepancies observed between the different studies.

The aims of this chapter are to (1) summarize the lipid composition and specificity in fish and fish oils, (2) define their molecular and supramolecular carrier forms in different food products and supplements, (3) discuss their fate during digestion which partly determines their bioaccessibility, (4) review their health or metabolic impact as related to the supplied form. Finally, further thoughts are provided to better address this topic from the formulation, food or supplement processing viewpoint. Reviews are provided of specific metabolic studies evaluating fish oil bioavailability.

FROM FISH LIPIDS TO FISH FOODS AND OTHER FISH OIL DELIVERY SYSTEMS

Composition Specificities of Lipids in Fish and Fish Lipids

According to the CALIPSO survey, the lipid content of fish consumed in France varies between 20 g/100 g for eel, 13 g/100 g for salmon to less than 0.5 g/100 g for several lean fish (Sirot et al., 2008). This range of lipid content

Fish and Fish Oil in Health and Disease Prevention. http://dx.doi.org/10.1016/B978-0-12-802844-5.00005-1

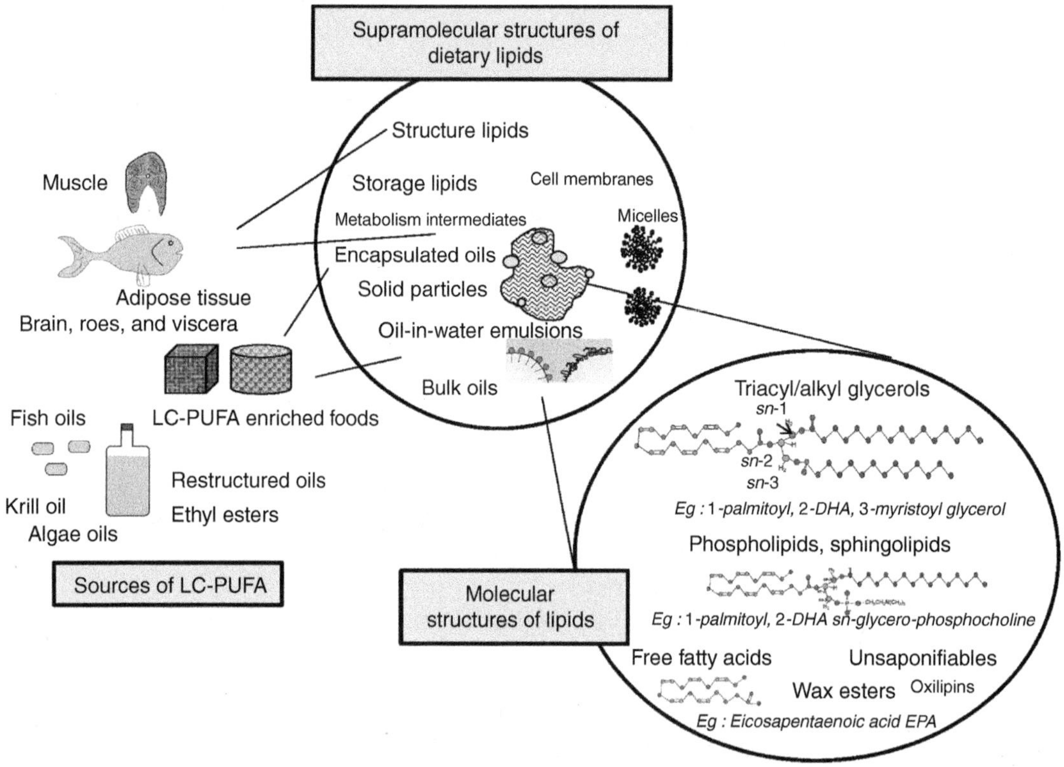

FIGURE 5.1 Molecular and supramolecular lipid structures in the wide sources of n-3 LC-PUFA.

reflects the range generally found in edible parts of fish, especially in muscle (Ackman, 2005). Nutritionally interesting lipids can also be found in other organs and fish by-products (Falch et al., 2006). In addition to interspecies and organ variations, fish lipid content is subject to large seasonal and physiological variations, including the effects of growing conditions (Ackman, 2005).

In fish lipids, as in all natural lipid sources, fatty acids (FA) are recognized as the prominent nutritional compounds. However, FA are building blocks of storage (triacylglycerols; TAGs) and membrane lipids (phospholipids = PL, sphingolipids, etc.) through ester or ether (alkyl glycerides, plasmalogens or diacylglyceryl ethers) bonds to glycerol, sphingosine or cholesterol (Fig. 5.1). They can also be part of wax esters, present in appreciable amounts in certain fish muscles and organs (de Koning, 2005; Scano et al., 2008), although the hydrolysis of wax esters in the human digestive tract and the bioavailability of theses FA is questionable. Nonesterified fatty acids (NEFA), or free fatty acids (FFAs), are only minor components present generally at low levels (<1–2%) in native lipids while they may range up to 5% or even 10% in fish oils due to *postmortem* hydrolysis (Ackman, 2005). High amounts of NEFA are generally considered as deleterious for product quality, even if they do not present any nutritional or toxicological issue. Indeed, easy calculation evidence shows that that 1 g of lipid in the form of pure TAGs provides a maximum of 960 mg FA with the ratio being smaller for fish and vegetable oils (750–930 mg/g), due in part, to the presence of unsaponifiable material. The FA quantity per gram of total material is even smaller for lecithins and pure PL (490–270 mg/g; Kabri et al., 2013).

Fish Lipids Carry a Large Range of Fatty Chains, Including Omega-3 FA

Fish are renowned as the main source of the long-chain highly unsaturated omega-3 fatty acids (LC n–3 PUFAs or HUFA), EPA, docosapentaenoic (DPA; 22:5n–3) and DHA acids in the human diet (Jacobsen et al., 2013). They also contain 18:3n–3 (linolenic acid) and 18:4n–3 in lesser concentrations. However, the n–3 FA composition of fish depends on fish species, diet, age, and growing conditions. In general, colder temperatures lead to an increase in unsaturation in lipids, thus maintaining membrane fluidity (Miller et al., 2008). Typically, a serving of lean fish (ie, cod) could provide 0.2–0.3 g LC n–3 PUFAs while 1.5–3.0 g could be provided by a serving of oily fish (ie, salmon or mackerel; Jacobsen et al., 2013). These beneficial FAs are present in the different organs of the animals at various levels, depending on the organ and the metabolic characteristics of the species. Fish by-products such as roe, liver (cod), and salmon or tuna head are thus considered important sources for the production of oils or lecithins rich in LC n–3 PUFA (Falch et al., 2006; Shirai et al., 2006). Besides the fish sources, LC n–3 PUFA are more generally obtained from other marine sources, including marine mammals, krill oils, algae, and from oleaginous microorganisms (Breivik, 2007; Jacobsen et al., 2013).

FAs from the omega-6 (n–6) series, namely linoleic (18:2 n–6) and arachidonic acids (20:4 n–6), are also found in low amounts in sea-dwelling fish (0.4–14.2%, usually less than 1% in wild fish) while fresh water fish contains 2.4–21.9% n–6 PUFA (Lei et al., 2012). Besides PUFA, fish contains saturated fatty acids (SFA), mainly C14, C16, C18 which provides 9–50% of total FA, and monounsaturated fatty acids (MUFA: C16:1 n–7, C18:1 n–9, C20:1, C22:1; Jacobsen et al., 2013). In total, if about 16 FAs are commonly mentioned in composition tables, 12 account for about 90% of total FAs found in fish. More than 48 different FAs can be detected in the lipid extracts of fish including odd-carbon FA, branched and conjugated FA. For instance, in freshwater fish, conjugated FA, including 9c11t-18:2 (up to 1% of total FA), branched FAs (TAG: 1.7–5.9%; PL: 1.6–3%) and saturated and unsaturated odd-carbon fatty acids (TAG: 5.9–14.74%; PL : 3.2% in PC to 7.9% in PE; Lei et al., 2012). In the presence of wax esters, saturated and unsaturated (C14–C22) fatty alcohols can be also found.

For nutritional and other applications, after extraction, fish oils are generally refined (successive steps including degumming, neutralization, washing, drying, bleaching, filtration, and deodorization). They can be also subject to fractionation techniques and/or enzymatic processing to obtain material with the targeted characteristics (Breivik, 2007).

In Fish, the FA Carrier Molecules are very Diverse: TAG Versus PL and Position of FA Within

Lipid Classes and Molecular Species

TAGs are generally the main constituents of fish oils. They are composed of numerous molecular species characterized by a defined combination of three FAs, similar or different, esterified to the glycerol backbone (Fig. 5.1). Thus, in menhaden oil, 253 TAGs were identified and quantified containing 0 (trisaturated TAG) to 18 unsaturations (tri-DHA), the TAGs found in the highest amounts being DHA/palmitic (P)/P (4.4 wt%) and EPA/P/P (4 wt%) (Beccaria et al., 2015). This presence of saturated and unsaturated TAGs explains the thermal properties of fish oils and provides a clue for the fractionation of fish oils and allows oils to be enriched in the beneficial FA (Breivik, 2007).

PLs present as membrane lipids in fish organs are generally present at low percentages in crude and refined fish oil. They concentrate in fish lecithins and extracts prepared from specific organs such as head PLs. They also represent 30–65% of krill oil. Fish PLs tend to have high proportions of DHA and less EPA compared to TAGs (more EPA than DHA). The major PL in marine sources is phosphatidyl choline (PC), whereas phosphatidyl ethanolamine (PE) is the second most abundant. Phosphatidylinositol (PI), phosphatidylserine (PS), lysophosphatidylcholine (lyso-PC), and sphingomyelin are found in smaller amounts. Each PL class is composed of different molecular species defined by nature of the fatty chains. In the muscle of Atlantic salmon, the predominant molecular species are for PC 16:0/18:1; 16:0/20:5, and 16:0/22:6 followed by 16:0/22:5 and for PE: 16:0/22:6, 18:0/20:5, and 18:0/22:6 (Miller et al., 2006).

Regiospecificity of FA in TAGs and PLs

The location of fatty chains at position sn–1/3 of sn–2 of glycerol in TAGs and PLs (Fig. 5.1) is of nutritional importance because the lipid molecules must be hydrolyzed to produce the absorbable 2-monoacylglycerides (2-MAG) and NEFA. Early studies evidenced that in fish TAGs and PLs, LC n–3 PUFA tend to be located at the sn–2 position of glycerol backbone, contrary to marine mammals (Aursand et al., 1995; Brockerhoff and Ackman, 1967). The regiospecificity of 46 TAGs was characterized in tuna oil; among them 5 TAGs contained 3 HUFAs (Baiocchi et al., 2015). For combinations of DHA or EPA with two palmitic acids in TAG molecular species, DHA or EPA were mainly at the sn–2 position in fish. Conversely, they concentrated at the sn–1 position in marine mammals (Gotoh et al., 2011). The binding position tendency of HUFA in TAG positional isomers consisting of two HUFAs and one palmitic acid was the same as that for combinations of one HUFA and two palmitic acids. In a more recent study DHA was found preferentially located at the sn–2 position, while EPA was observed at near equal levels in all positions (Cubero Herrera et al., 2013). Differences between species can be underlined however. For instance, salmon oil contained a greater percentage of PUFA 18:3 (n–3), 20:4 (n–3), 20:5 (n–3), 22:5 (n–3), and 22:6 (n–3) at the sn–2 position of the TAG as compared to menhaden oil, in which PUFA of were randomly distributed (Nwosu and Boyd, 1997). In fillets of Atlantic salmon, ~50% of EPA and ~80% of DHA were located in the sn–2 position of TAGs (Ruiz-Lopez et al., 2015). In PLs, about 90% of DHA was located in the PC sn–2 position, independently of the diet. For EPA, ~80% was located in the PC sn–2 position but fish fed a vegetable-rich diet carrying a low level of EPA + DHA had more EPA in the sn–2 position (83%) than when the diet provided more EPA + DHA (77% EPA in sn–2 position; Ruiz-Lopez et al., 2015).

In freshwater fish, C16, EPA, and DHA were preferentially located at the sn–2 position of TAGs, while both SFA and MUFA occupied the sn–1 position of PL (Lei et al., 2012).

Unsaponifiable Fraction, Contaminants, and Neoformed Compounds

Besides the glyceride species and other FA carrying molecules, fish products contain an unsaponifiable fraction that represents a high proportion in lipids of certain fish and organs. For instance, the unsaponifiable fraction represents 50–80% of the liver of deep sea sharks. It is mainly composed of squalene, a highly unsaturated triterpene ($C_{30}H_{50}$), widespread in the animal kingdom where it is an intermediate for the biosynthesis of phytosterol or cholesterol (Popa et al., 2014; Spanova and Daum, 2011). Cholesterol and vitamin E (tocopherols), D3 and A, and carotenoids are also found in lipids of fish. Some of these compounds (eg, tocopherols, squalene, and carotenoids) exhibit antioxidant activity and therefore provide HUFAs protection against oxidative attacks during food processing and during digestion (Jacobsen et al., 2013) which limits quantitative losses of the beneficial FA and guarantees the actual amounts available for absorption.

Fish food products and fish lipids also contain compounds issued from in vivo oxidative metabolism (oxilipins produced by enzymatic and nonenzymatic pathways) or from *postmortem* oxidative processes (lipid oxidation products: hydroperoxydes, epoxides, biologically active aldehydes such as malondialdehyde, 4-hydroxynonenal, and 4-hydroxyhexenal, etc.) and neoformed compounds generated during fish processing (storage, drying, cooking, etc.) or during oil and lecithins extraction and processing, including storage (Awada et al., 2012; Hsieh and Kinsella, 1989; Lu et al., 2012; Viau et al., 2015). Of note, a strategy to prevent oxidation is to incorporate DHA into a lipid molecule. Indeed, it has been demonstrated that DHA esterified in PLs is less easily oxidizable than in the other forms of either FFA, EEs, or even TAGs (Lyberg et al., 2005; Song et al., 1997). Fish lipids may also contain hydrophobic contaminants, concentrated in the lipid fraction of living species. These contaminants include persistent organic pollutants (POPs), such as, polychlorinated biphenyl (PCB), polybrominated diphenylether (PBDE), organochlorine pesticides, polycyclic aromatic hydrocarbons, dioxin, and heavy metals. The presence of these compounds should be controlled, and recommendations have been made by international safety agencies (EFSA, 2005; Usydus et al., 2008).

Fish Lipid Supramolecular Structures in Fish, Foods, and Delivery Systems

Lipids are not only characterized by their molecular structure, but also by the arrangement of their molecules in a given environment. The main external parameters that drive the molecular arrangement of lipid molecules are temperature and interaction with water. However, for similar compositions of the media, very different structures can be obtained at the colloid and mesoscale levels depending on how the system was obtained. Basically, one can distinguish the structures of lipids found in the native biological material (cell membranes, storage organelles, and tissues) and from those obtained after processing, especially when extraction, fractionation, formulation steps have been applied (Fig. 5.1). For fish oils various delivery systems structured at the micro- and nanoscales (submicro and nanoemulsions, solid particles, etc.) have been developed (Jacobsen et al., 2013; McClements, 2010; Michalski et al., 2013). The objectives are to protect the oxidation sensitive molecules (HUFAs), to avoid offodors and to control the in vivo delivery.

TAGs are highly hydrophobic, whereas PLs are amphiphilic due to their polar head groups. Hence, the physical–chemical properties of these two groups of lipid structures are different. Only PLs are able to directly interact with water through hydration of their polar heads to form micelles, liposomes, or other structured assemblies in the presence of water. The thermal behavior of lipids is determined by the distribution of chain length and unsaturation of the molecular species. As both unsaturated and highly unsaturated species are present in fish lipids, they exhibit a large range of melting and crystallization temperatures. However, at ambient and/or body temperature, fish lipids are at liquid state. This means that bulk TAGs are in a fluid, nonordered state while polar lipids in contact with water are in liquid–crystalline state. For instance, in cell membranes the lipids are organized in fluid lamellar phases in which the fatty chains face to form lipid bilayers incorporating cholesterol and membrane proteins. To obtain stable dispersions of TAGs in water (oil-in-water emulsions), the presence of surface active compounds (emulsifiers) is compulsory (Jacobsen et al., 2013). In n–3 LC PUFA enriched-foods, the fish oil is often dispersed in the other matrix constituents, forming an emulsified system. This emulsion can either be formed when all food ingredients are mixed together or prepared separately to be used as well during the process. The size of the oil droplets and the nature of the compounds that stabilize the droplets are highly variable, which can impact the bioavailability of the nutrients. Droplets can range from about 50 nm to several micrometers. At a constant oil phase fraction, the smaller the droplets, the larger the interfacial area; for instance, a decrease by 10× of the diameter of the droplets multiplies the droplet number and the interfacial area by 1000. The interface layer can be composed of very different emulsifying molecules (small size surfactants such as polar lipids, proteins, etc.), possibly forming multilayers capable of resisting digestive enzymes and delaying nutrient delivery. Microencapsulation technology using protein or carbohydrate coatings is also used to protect foods enriched in fish oils and various other food products (bread and baked foods, infant food, yogurts, cheeses, meat products, etc.), without impacting their taste and shelf-life.

Notably, structured lipids (SLs) or custom-made lipids can supply functional FA such as LC n–3 PUFA because of their specific positioning in the glycerol structure. The term SLs indeed refers to lipids which are restructured, in order to chemically or enzymatically modify the composition and/or position of their FA, in contrast to natural oils and fats (Babayan, 1987). As natural fish lipids, SLs self-organize as explained above according to their physicochemical properties and medium composition.

DIGESTION AND BIOACCESSIBILITY OF FISH LIPIDS

Dietary lipids accounted from one third up to 40% of our daily energy intake, among which 90% are made up of TAGs. From mouth to intestine, lipids are subjected to physical and chemical transformations that finally produce absorbable species, namely nonesterified or free fatty acids (NEFA, FFA) and 2-MAGs. These entities are released from the lipid molecular structures by various lipases and incorporated during the intestinal step to mixed micelles that are easily absorbed by the intestinal epithelial cells. The fraction of FA released from the food and incorporated into transport structure such as mixed micelles or vesicles is referred as the bioaccessible fraction. A huge amount of literature has detailed the actual knowledge on lipid digestion. The following reviews and the references therein show the main elements that modulate digestion, bioaccessibility, and bioavailability of lipids (Armand, 2007; Lairon, 2009; Thomas et al., 2012). Provided that the most sensitive FAs (namely LC-PUFA) have been protected against oxidative attack during the whole process, and excluding specific pathological situations, the total amount of bioaccessible FA fits well with the total ingested amounts of FA, whatever the lipids, the FA, and the ingested material. Differences do however reside in the FA release kinetics, and thus in postprandial bioaccessibility affecting prandial/postprandial lipemia. Indeed, a large set of parameters such as the molecular and supramolecular organization of the lipids and individual physiologies are implied in these kinetic variations.

What Occurs to Fish Lipids After Ingestion?

Food and lipid digestion starts in the mouth. Here, the mechanical effects of mastication and dilution by saliva are associated to several enzymatic reactions. The temperature also progressively approaches the body temperature. Mastication first generates breakage of solid and cellular foods into small pieces that can be swallowed; the original millimeter to micrometer structures are more or less broken and mixed together. Saliva secretion, mainly from parotid gland, is stimulated by chewing. Food and saliva are put into contact in the shear conditions induced by mastication. Thus, in the mouth, due to dilution effect of the saliva, the pH and ionic strength of the aqueous environment of biomolecules changes. Bulk fat is dispersed into large globules partly stabilized by food and saliva surface-active molecules. The lipid contact surface, available for the next steps of digestion, consequently increases. Lipolysis in the oral cavity due to lipases present in the saliva or carried in the foods, could produce enough FFA to be involved in the orosensory detection of fat (Kawai and Fushiki, 2003) and initiate fat digestion (Valdez and Fox, 1991). Fat or fatty acid receptors present in the mouth would be also activated and signal further down the gastrointestinal tract (GIT), the presence of fat. This message leads to physiological and hormonal conditioning of the GIT, and makes it ready for fat digestion. Nevertheless, the consequences of these in-mouth modifications of lipid structures on their later fate in the GIT are not actually known. Regarding the oxidative fate of the lipids during digestion, which can be critical for LC n–3 PUFA, the saliva contains a large array of molecules with potential antioxidant or prooxidant activities. This leads to very large range of individual balances for antioxidant/prooxidant activity of the saliva when the bolus reaches the stomach, depending on physiological factors. At this step, the bolus in the stomach is composed of a mixture of the chewed foods ingested during the entire meal diluted by the saliva.

The stomach can be considered as is a bioreactor in which lipolysis is initiated, but capable of favoring lipid oxidation. The bolus is mixed with the gastric juice (pH 1–3). After an increase related to the buffering ability of the ingested food (up to 7), its pH progressively decreases to pH around 2. This physicochemical action is combined with the mechanical action due to stomach peristaltic movements, active protein and carbohydrate hydrolysis by pepsin and amylases (already present in the saliva) and partial hydrolysis of TAGs by the gastric lipase. Gastric lipolysis accounts for 5–40% of ingested triacylglycerols. Generated surfactants (FFA, diglycerides, amphiphilic peptides) participate to further structural reorganizations of the lipids. The remaining bulk fat is coarsely emulsified whereas, depending on their interface composition and structure, small droplets can partially coalesce under the joint actions of flocculation induced by mucin, protein hydrolysis and acid pH (Armand, 2007; Lairon, 2009).

The increase of lipid–gastric medium exchange surface, the acidic conditions, the presence of oxygen and pro-oxidant (ie, dietary iron and heme proteins: hemoglobin and myoglobin from meat products) favor lipid oxidation. The rate of the reaction also depends on initial lipid structures (nature of the interfacial membranes surrounding the lipid droplets; encapsulation in stomach-digestion resistant structures) and the presence of dietary antioxidants (tocopherols, phenolic compounds, and melanoidins Kanner and Lapidot, 2001).

The final release and absorption of FFA, MAG, and oxidized species takes place in the duodenum. The partially hydrolyzed and emulsified lipids are delivered into the small intestine where they are mixed with pancreatico-biliary and intestinal juices. These juices contain bile salts, phospholipids, pancreatic lipase, colipase, proteases, ion minerals, and bicarbonate among others. It results in alkalization of the chyme and additional modifications of the lipid interface and lipid structures. Lipolysis, proteolysis, and amylolysis are completed. Pancreatic lipase selectively hydrolyses DPA over EPA and DHA due to location of the first double bonds in the fatty acid rather than regioselectivity (Akanbi et al., 2014). Mixed micelles and vesicles are formed allowing the absorption of FA and monoglycerides. Unlike the prooxidant gastric environment, the intestinal environment is neutral or slightly basic, of reducing nature and is assumed to be anaerobic. Nevertheless, oxygen pressure approaching air-saturation was measured in the upper parts of duodenum and jejunum in the pork (He et al., 1999), and a gradient of oxygen concentration from stomach to the colon, with nonzero concentration in the duodenal part of GIT was found in the mice (Hillman et al., 1993). Pancreatico-biliary juice contains free radical scavengers and compounds capable to induce the decomposition of the primary products of lipid oxidation (Terao et al., 1995) or to reduce hydroperoxides (Aw, 2005). Gastrointestinal glutathione peroxidase has been proposed as a barrier against the absorption of dietary hydroperoxides (Wingler et al., 2000).

Bioaccessibility of n–3 PUFA, Molecular, and Supramolecular Structure

Despite the huge amount of literature on n–3 lipids, on the one hand, and on in vitro digestion of lipids on the other hand, few data were concerned with the impact of molecular or supramolecular structures of n–3 lipids on their bioaccessibility. The FA release during in vitro digestion was found to be similar from salmon oil and muscle (Aarak et al., 2014), suggesting a minor impact of food matrix. The same research group investigated the impact of meal composition on the FA release from salmon muscle. They reported that barley addition led to a decrease of the overall release of FA, whereas in presence of broccoli, the lipolysis was initially inhibited and increased from 80 min to 140 min, when digestion of salmon muscle leveled off (Aarak et al., 2013). When incorporated in a plain yogurt, the bioaccessibility of EPA was higher from PL than from MAG or TAG sources (Domoto et al., 2013) as revealed by a dynamic in vitro system.

The role of supramolecular organization of lipids on their digestion was recently highlighted (Marze, 2013; McClements et al., 2009; Michalski et al., 2013) but few studies to date quantified its impact on the individual bioaccessibility of individual FA. Because bioavailability is related to the fate of lipids after absorption and several metabolic transformations, a deeper knowledge of the individual bioaccessibility of each FA as related to the initial molecular and supramolecular structure of their carrier in ingested foods could be helpful to understand the results on bioavailability, which must contain reliable information on the composition and structure of ingested lipids (Fig. 5.2).

BIOAVAILABILITY OF FISH LIPIDS ACCORDING TO DIFFERENT MOLECULAR AND SUPRAMOLECULAR STRUCTURES AND THE FOOD PRODUCT

Bioavailability of n–3 LC-PUFA can be Modified by the Molecular Form of Lipids

The bioavailability of n–3 LC PUFA can be affected by their chemical form. As reviewed above, LC n–3 PUFA are commonly found in TAGs, FFA, EEs form or in phospholipids (PLs). Similar incorporation rates in plasma lipids of EPA and DHA were reported in humans after 14 days of supplementation with EEs or TAGs (Krokan et al., 1993). This is consistent with other data (Nordoy et al., 1991), despite a lower hydrolysis rate by pancreatic lipases for EEs than for TAGs (Krokan et al., 1993). Conversely, the incorporation in plasma of EPA and DHA in humans, after a single bolus, was also lower after EEs than TAG intake (Lawson and Hughes, 1988). In contrast to acute studies,

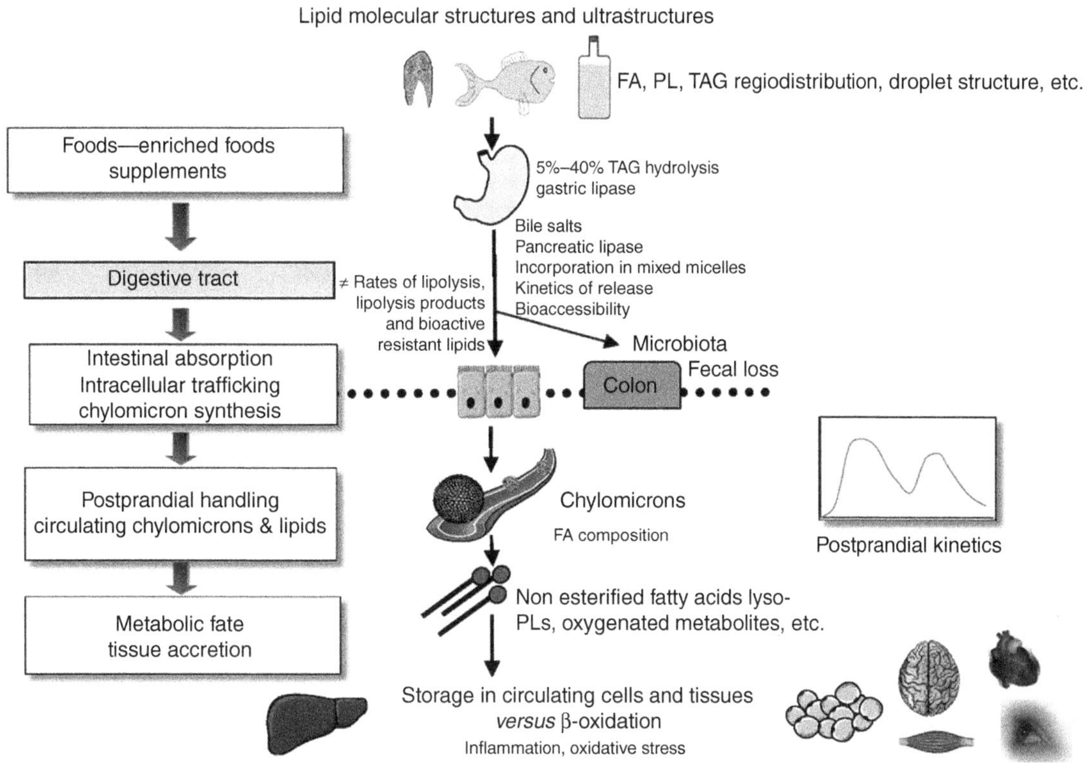

FIGURE 5.2 Fate of fish lipids after ingestion: from gut-driven bioaccessibility to bioavailability and metabolic fate and impact.

in a 6-month-supplementation study in humans with identical doses of EPA + DHA, TAG carrier led to a faster and higher increase in the omega-3 index than EE carrier (Neubronner et al., 2011).

The highest bioavailability was obtained with FFA, conversely to data obtained in rats with marine free FA (De Schrijver et al., 1991). Conflicting results were obtained in rodents. In rats, EEs were more efficient to increase the amount of EPA in plasma PL and cholesterol esters in the rat, than TAGs or PLs (Hamazaki et al., 1987). In mice, DHA-PLs and DHA-TAGs were more efficient than DHA as FFAs or EEs in increasing the n-3 PUFA concentration in mouse organs after 1 week of supplementation in a low- or high-fat diet (Ding et al., 2013). Importantly, the kinetics of EPA and DHA absorption, rather than the total amount of FA in plasma several hours after consumption, were influenced by the carrier form (Ikeda et al., 1993; Ikeda et al., 1995), suggesting that, for a given molecular form, the type of FA can impact its bioavailability: DPA and EPA, provided as FFA, are metabolized differently in rodents and humans (Fard et al., 2014; Sinclair et al., 2013). Both in animals and humans, dietary 1,3-DAG have been shown to present a hypotriglyceridemic effect and also to reduce postprandial lipemia compared with TAGs with a similar FA composition (Hara et al., 1993; Maki et al., 2009; Saito et al., 2006; Taguchi et al., 2000). However, DAG-DHA and TAG-DHA would have similar effects on lowering triglyceridemia in the rat (Tamai et al., 2007); whether further incorporation of DHA in plasma lipids and tissues would be different remains to be elucidated.

PLs Versus TGs and PL-Containing Oils

LC n–3 PUFA in PLs Versus TAGs

In the rat, feeding liposomes of marine PLs compared to TAG oil leads to a more efficient incorporation of n–3 FA in plasma and liver lipids (Cansell et al., 2006; Cansell et al., 2003), but to a similar hypotriglyceridemic effect after 2 weeks of feeding (Cansell et al., 2006). Dietary PLs also induced a higher expression and activity of CPT-I in the liver, and an upregulation of intracellular proteins involved in free FA uptake and lipid synthesis, which could probably lead to a greater β-oxidation of EPA (Cansell et al., 2009). However, in such studies, the relative impact of the carrier molecules (PLs versus TAGs) and of the dispersion state of these molecules (liposomes versus oil) cannot be delinked. Regarding wider metabolic impact, the supplementation of PLs containing LC n–3 PUFAs as PLs in a high fat diet in mice had a major effect on decreasing adipocyte size that was not observed using TAGs (Awada et al., 2013), possibly due to an improved modulation of the endocannabinoid system activity in the white adipose tissue (Rossmeisl et al., 2012). A preferential uptake of DHA by human erythrocytes was reported when DHA was provided as phosphatidylcholine (PC)-DHA compared to TAG-DHA (Lemaitre-Delaunay et al., 1999). Additionally, a preferential brain incorporation of 2-DHA-LysoPC over free DHA was observed in the young rat (Thies et al., 1994), and a preference for 2-DHA-LysoPC to cross a re-constituted blood brain barrier compared to free DHA (Bernoud et al., 1999). Altogether, these results may partly explain differences observed between PL-rich krill oil and TAG-rich fish oil in clinical trials in humans (Bunea et al., 2004; Kidd, 2007; Tou et al., 2007).

Natural Sources of LC n–3 PUFA in PLs: Krill and Egg

Numerous studies showed that supplementation with EPA and DHA in PLs from krill oil, exerts stronger biological effects compared with EPA and DHA in TAGs from fish oil at similar n–3 PUFA doses. Moreover, in mice transgenic for TNF-α with similar doses of n–3 PUFAs from krill oil, appear to exert a greater potential to promote lipid catabolism than fish oil, although no differences in the levels of inflammatory markers could be observed (Vigerust et al., 2013). Fish and krill oils act with different efficiency and also partially via different mechanisms: krill oil specifically decreased the expression of genes involved in the early steps of isoprenoid/cholesterol and lipid synthesis while fish oil mainly increased the expression of several genes involved in fatty acid metabolism (Tillander et al., 2014). Other reviews report clinical trials showing superior effects of krill oil versus fish oil in increasing plasma LC n–3 PUFA. (Burri, 2011). Of note, this effect was maintained even with constant intake of n–6 PUFA among products, showing the impact of the structure of the molecular carrier rather than the FA profile of krill oil (Ramprasath et al., 2014). Importantly, however in a clinical prevention context, concentrated fish oil providing fourfold higher EPA + DHA than krill oil, and twofold higher than salmon oil and was found to exert the most beneficial effects in terms of increasing plasma n–3 PUFA and reducing several cardio-metabolic risk factors (Laidlaw et al., 2014). Another natural PL source can be oil from the micro-algae *Nannochloropsis oculata*, which contains a significant amount of EPA in PLs and glycolipids and no DHA (Kagan et al., 2013). During a postprandial test in humans, the incremental AUC for EPA was greater with algal oil than with krill oil, while no difference was observed for the iAUC of DHA (Kagan et al., 2013). Complementary studies in rodents showed similar tissue uptake of LC n–3 PUFA from both oils, despite the fact that the algal oil contained less EPA: an impact of glycolipids on digestibility was suggested (Kagan et al., 2015). Herring roe was another product rich in PLs containing EPA and DHA and reported to improve the incorporation of n–3 PUFA in the plasma of healthy adults (Bjorndal et al., 2014). Interestingly, opposite results were obtained in piglets fed DHA for 16 days as TAGs from unicellular algae oil, which induced higher total DHA concentration in plasma than DHA provided as egg PL, despite similar FA profiles; again suggesting the importance of the molecular carrier (TAG or PL; Mathews et al., 2002). Both in the rat and in elderly humans, dietary supplementation with DHA-rich egg PL induced increased DHA and ARA accretion in plasma and erythrocyte membranes (certainly due to the fact that egg PLs contain ~4% ARA for ~7.6% DHA); in contrast, a depletion in ARA was observed for supplementation with DHA in TAGs of fish oil (Gerbi et al., 2004; Payet et al., 2004).

Structured TAG and Oils with Different TAG Structures

Structured TAG Molecules Containing LC n–3 PUFA

Regarding the synthesis of SLs in the form of TAG with specific FAs at each position of the glycerol backbone as nutritional and health supplements, World Health Organization recommends Oil Technologists and Nutritionists an ideal oil which would have the SFA/MUFA/PUFA ratio of 1/1/1 (Trivedi and Singh, 2005). A new type of SLs in food industries has been developed called medium and long-chain TAGs (MLCTs), combining LC-FA of physiological interest such as DHA together with medium-chain FA that provide an efficient energy source. Usually, synthetic TAGs have LC-PUFAs located at the internal position with MCFAs at the external positions. A structured oil containing mostly PUFA on *sn*–2 and 10:0 on sn–1,3 position resulted in a significantly higher lymphatic transport of EPA and DHA during postprandial kinetics compared with a randomized oil (Christensen et al., 1995). However, cumulative amounts after 24 h were not significantly different (Christensen et al., 1995). In another study, lymphatic absorption of PUFA was similar using two types of structured TAGs with similar compositions (40% of 10:0 and 40% of PUFA) but with PUFA located mainly on sn–2 (MLM) or on sn–1,3 (LML) (Porsgaard et al., 2005). In turn, native fish oil that contained less PUFA (28%) resulted in higher PUFA absorption than the SLs in the first 8 h of digestion; longer overall absorption being similar among the three lipid sources (Porsgaard et al., 2005). In humans, a significant reduction of total plasma TAGs, was observed after a dietary test intake containing 72% medium-chain FAs and 22% n–3 LC-PUFAs. This is likely due to increased β-oxidation with synergistic effects of MCFAs and LC-PUFAs (Beermann et al., 2003). Displacing PUFAs from the critical sn–2 position by substitution with SFAs is hypothesized to cause lipid and lipoprotein abnormalities (Karupaiah and

Sundram, 2007). The authors stated that it is still too early to conclude on the behaviour of unusual positional distribution of FAs in TAGs species originating from oils.

Marine Mammal Oils with Different Positions of LC n–3 PUFA on TAG

Conversely to fish oil, oils from marine mammals such as whales or seals are composed of TAG with PUFA located mainly on sn–1,3 positions (Ackman, 1988). In vitro studies showed that DHA and EPA from whale oil are less easily released by pancreatic lipases than other FA such as 16:0 and 18:1 (Bottino et al., 1967). Because DPA (22:5 n–3) on external positions did not present such a resistance to lipolysis, this suggests that the latter phenomenon could be due to steric constraints due to the double bond located close to the carboxyl group independently from FA location on TAG, (Bottino et al., 1967; Yang et al., 1990). After an intragastric administration of fish oil or seal oil in rats, postprandial kinetics of EPA and DHA in the lymph showed that n–3 PUFA were better absorbed from fish oil during the first hours of digestion (Christensen et al., 1994). However, this effect did not remain significant regarding total assimilation after 24 h, showing a difference between acute and longer term effects of TAG structure. After seal oil administration compared with fish oil, a significantly higher load of n–3 PUFA was esterified in the sn–1,3 positions of chylomicron TAG (Christensen and Hoy, 1996). In chronic designs, feeding rats with seal oil, in which EPA or DHA is located at the sn-1,3-positions of TAGs, more effectively reduced plasma and liver TAG levels through suppression of FA synthesis than fish oil in which EPA and DHA are located at the sn–2 position (Yoshida et al., 1996). Studies in humans should be done as the issue merits further investigation.

Bioavailability of Fish LC-PUFA May Depend on the Supramolecular Organization of Lipids

Fish Lipids in Fish Muscle

Regarding fish products, numerous clinical and epidemiological studies report that the consumption of fat-rich fish or capsules of fish oil rich in LC n–3 PUFA exerts a protective effect against the cardiovascular diseases. However, while a low intake of fat-rich fish is sufficient to observe beneficial cardiovascular effects (Guichardant et al., 2004; He et al., 2002), the doses provided by the dietary complements are generally much higher than those brought by the diet (Bucher et al., 2002). Moreover, n–3 PUFA were reported to be better incorporated in plasma lipids when consumed from salmon than from cod liver oil, despite the threefold higher content of EPA + DHA in cod liver oil compared with salmon meat (Elvevoll et al., 2006). Interestingly, such effects on plasma lipids and lipoproteins were also observed in hyperlipidemic subjects after the consumption of fish rather than fish oil (Cobiac et al., 1991). Some authors suggested that the better absorption of n–3 PUFA would result from the dispersed state of TAG in fish (Elvevoll et al., 2006), that is an impact of their supramolecular structure as lipid droplets. However, an effect of the entire structure of this specific food matrix is also possible. In this respect, recent in vitro digestion studies showed that greater proportion of microencapsulated tuna oil was hydrolyzed (~75%) when it was brought in a liquid matrix (orange juice or yogurt) than in a solid matrix (cereal bar; ~62%) (Shen et al., 2011). A further study in ileostomized patients showed that the food matrix in which the microencapsulated oil was delivered may alter the transit kinetics of the n–3 PUFA through the small intestine, with a slower transit time with the cereal bar matrix despite similar total intestinal absorption (Sanguansri et al., 2013). The differences between the regular consumption of fish and the consumption of dietary complements as sources of n–3 PUFA were discussed in a review (He, 2009).

Fish Oil Emulsions and Microcapsules

Fish oil can be provided either in free form in capsules or as emulsion droplets to be used in an enriched drink or food. Regular oil-in-water emulsions are the most commonly used to encapsulate lipophilic molecules such as n–3 PUFA. In humans, ingestion of an emulsified oil results in higher levels of plasma TAGs (postprandial area under the curve over 9 h) and of EPA and DHA in plasma lipids, compared to the same oil ingested in the nonemulsified state (Garaiova et al., 2007). In humans the absorption of n–3 PUFA, evaluated from the FA composition of plasma PLs for 48 h after ingestion, was enhanced after the ingestion of a single dose of emulsified fish oil, as compared with nonemulsified oil provided by a capsule (Raatz et al., 2009). The proposed mechanism was that emulsification favored the action of digestive lipases by simplifying the emulsification that occurs in the stomach, as previously reported (Borel et al., 1994). Interestingly in humans, the hydrolysis of TAGs by gastric and pancreatic lipases was found to be more efficient with emulsion droplets of small size (0.7 μm) than with larger droplet (10 μm), in emulsions containing, among others, fish oil, olive oil, and soybean lecithin (Armand et al., 1999). Moreover in rats, a nanoemulsion of fish oil was found to result in a greater intestinal lipid absorption than a regular emulsion of the same oil (Dey et al., 2012). In rats, a microemulsion of fish oil formulated with phospholipids significantly enhanced DHA levels in the serum, liver, heart, and brain tissues (Sugasini and Lokesh, 2013). Of note, the composition of the fish oil emulsion such as the choice of the emulsifier can also have an impact of PUFA oxidation in digestive media (Kenmogne-Domguia et al., 2014). Altogether, both the dispersion state as droplets and the direct impact of the emulsifier itself can impact the bioavailability of LC n–3 PUFA-rich oils. In contrast, microencapsulation of fish oil was reported to slow down its intestinal transit in rats (Augustin et al., 2011), probably due to the composition of the microcapsule interface. In humans, increases in plasma and erythrocyte n–3 FA values were similar regardless of providing fish oil as a capsule with a glass of milk or in microencapsulated form in a milk matrix, with both achieving an omega-3 index in plasma of ~6% after 4 weeks (Sanguansri et al., 2015). Interestingly, it was recently demonstrated, both in normal weight and in healthy obese humans, that the enhancement of milk FA absorption by emulsification also resulted in enhanced beta-oxidation of exogenous FA (Vors et al., 2013). Therefore, whether fish oil emulsification would result in a greater beta-oxidation LC n–3 PUFA would deserve to be elucidated in order to enhance their bioavailability in terms of metabolic targets and functions in plasma and in different tissues.

CONCLUSION AND FUTURE PROSPECTS

Despite the abundant literature on the n–3 LC-PUFA and their health effects, it remains difficult to propose a rational approach to propose dietary strategies to improve health. To overcome this gap, it seems that a dual approach should be preferred, involving both the type and properties of food products or supplements and the metabolic requirements according to the age and metabolic status. Altogether, as recently reviewed in details, there is a need to systematically investigate the bioavailability of omega-3 FA formulations, which might be a key to designing more effective studies in the future, with an aim to lead to more efficient recommendations for dietary intakes (Ghasemifard et al., 2014; Schuchardt and Hahn, 2013).

To date, some crucial information such as the exact nature of the lipids added to the diet, the nature and amount of individual FA, and associated antioxidants is often missing in the presentation of the experimental design of metabolic studies. Moreover, studies have shown that the consumption of oxidation products of PUFA could modulate their metabolic effects; it would be desirable to assess the level of oxidation of ingested lipids in the nutritional studies. Similarly, the food formulation and processing are too often insufficiently described. If the role of supramolecular organization of lipid on their digestion has been frequently evoked, rare quantitative data described the kinetics of individual n–3 LC PUFA bioaccessibility (release in the gut) as a function of their initial molecular and/or supramolecular organization. Such data could be used to screen various lipid formulations according their kinetics of release after digestion. Future studies in humans should include designs with well controlled amounts of n–3 LC PUFA in each molecular form, with adequate description of their physico-chemical characteristics according to the carrier form, and studying metabolic fate exhaustively, including fecal loss.

Importantly, there is a growing demand by the food and pharmaceutical industry that has stimulated an extensive search for synthetic methods to produce specific PLs with new combination of FAs, notably to enrich certain PL species with EPA and DHA. New structured molecules seem to be promising. A synthesis of a particular structured PC containing an acetyl group at the sn–1 position to mimic 2-DHA-LysoPC, and prevent the acyl migration thus ensuring structure stability, has been designed (Polette et al., 1999). This new structured PC, named AceDoPC, has been recently shown to be a specific carrier of DHA to the brain (Hachem et al., 2015); applications as oral supplementation now deserves further investigation.

To improve the efficiency of the delivery systems of n–3 LC PUFA, questions of the targeted population and metabolic impact should be clearly addressed. In this context, the optimal delivery system would probably be different to increase the proportion of DHA in the retina or to lower the circulating TAG. Similar considerations can be made for the general population (healthy adults) or for targeted ones (eg, newborn, infant, elderly, metabolic disorders).

References

Aarak, K.E., Kirkhus, B., Johansen, S., Vegarud, G.E., Borge, G.I.A., 2014. Effect of broccoli phytochemical extract on release of fatty acids from salmon muscle and salmon oil during in vitro digestion. Food Funct. 5, 2331–2337.

Aarak, K.E., Rigby, N.M., Kirkhus, B., Salt, L.J., Sahlstrom, S., Bengtsson, G.B., Vegarud, G.E., Mackie, A.R., 2013. The impact of meal composition on the release of fatty acids from salmon during in vitro gastrointestinal digestion. Food Funct. 4, 1819–1826.

Ackman, R.G., 1988. Some possible effects on lipid biochemistry of differences in the distribution on glycerol of long-chain n-3 fatty acids in the fats of marine fish and marine mammals. Atherosclerosis 70, 171–173.

Ackman, R.G., 2005. Fish oils. In: Bailey's industrial oil and fat products, sixth ed. John Wiley and Sons, Inc. 279–317.

Akanbi, T.O., Sinclair, A.J., Barrow, C.J., 2014. Pancreatic lipase selectively hydrolyses dpa over epa and dha due to location of double bonds in the fatty acid rather than regioselectivity. Food Chem. 160, 61–66.

Armand, M., 2007. Lipases and lipolysis in the human digestive tract: Where do we stand ? Curr. Opin. Clin. Nutr. Metab. Care 10, 156–164.

Armand, M., Pasquier, B., Andre, M., Borel, P., Senft, M., Peyrot, J., Salducci, J., Portugal, H., Jaussan, V., Lairon, D., 1999. Digestion and absorption of 2 fat emulsions with different droplet sizes in the human digestive tract. Am. J. Clin. Nutr. 70, 1096–1106.

Augustin, M.A., Patten, G., De Luca, A., Abeywardena, M., Lockett, T., Head, R., Sanguansri, L., 2011. Intestinal passage of microencapsulated fish oil in rats following oral administration. Food Funct. 2, 684–696.

Aursand, M., Jorgensen, L., Grasdalen, H., 1995. Positional distribution of omega-3 fatty acids in marine lipid triacylglycerols by high-resolution c-14 nuclear magnetic resonance spectroscopy. J. Am. Oil Chem. Soc. 72, 293–297.

Aw, T.Y., 2005. Intestinal glutathione: determinant of mucosal peroxide transport, metabolism, and oxidative susceptibility. Toxicol. Appl. Pharmacol. 204, 320–328.

Awada, M., Meynier, A., Soulage, C.O., Hadji, L., Geloen, A., Viau, M., Ribourg, L., Benoit, B., Debard, C., Guichardant, M., Lagarde, M., Genot, C., Michalski, M.C., 2013. N-3 pufa added to high-fat diets affect differently adiposity and inflammation when carried by phospholipids or triacylglycerols in mice. Nutr. Metab. (London) 10, 23.

Awada, M., Soulage, C.O., Meynier, A., Debard, C., Plaisancie, P., Benoit, B., Picard, G., Loizon, E., Chauvin, M.A., Estienne, M., Peretti, N., Guichardant, M., Lagarde, M., Genot, C., Michalski, M.C., 2012. Dietary oxidized n-3 pufa induce oxidative stress and inflammation: role of intestinal absorption of 4-hhe and reactivity in intestinal cells. J. Lipid Res. 53, 2069–2080.

Babayan, V.K., 1987. Medium chain triglycerides and structured lipids. Lipids 22, 417–420.

Baiocchi, C., Medana, C., Dal Bello, F., Giancotti, V., Aigotti, R., Gastaldi, D., 2015. Analysis of regioisomers of polyunsaturated triacylglycerols in marine matrices by hplc/hrms. Food Chem. 166, 551–560.

Beccaria, M., Costa, R., Sullini, G., Grasso, E., Cacciola, F., Dugo, P., Mondello, L., 2015. Determination of the triacylglycerol fraction in fish oil by comprehensive liquid chromatography techniques with the support of gas chromatography and mass spectrometry data. Anal. Bioanal. Chem. 407, 5211–5225.

Beermann, C., Jelinek, J., Reinecker, T., Hauenschild, A., Boehm, G., Klor, H.U., 2003. Short term effects of dietary medium-chain fatty acids and n-3 long-chain polyunsaturated fatty acids on the fat metabolism of healthy volunteers. Lipids Health Dis. 2, 10.

Bernoud, N., Fenart, L., Moliere, P., Dehouck, M.P., Lagarde, M., Cecchelli, R., Lecerf, J., 1999. Preferential transfer of 2-docosahexaenoyl-1-lysophosphatidylcholine through an in vitro blood-brain barrier over unesterified docosahexaenoic acid. J. Neurochem. 72, 338–345.

Bjorndal, B., Strand, E., Gjerde, J., Bohov, P., Svardal, A., Diehl, B.W.K., Innis, S.M., Berger, A., Berge, R.K., 2014. Phospholipids from herring roe improve plasma lipids and glucose tolerance in healthy, young adults. Lipids Health Dis. 13.

Borel, P., Armand, M., Ythier, P., Dutot, G., Melin, C., Senft, M., Lafont, H., Lairon, D., 1994. Hydrolysis of emulsions with different triglycerides and droplet sizes by gastric lipase in vitro effect on pancreatic lipase activity. J. Nutr. Biochem. 5, 124–133.

Bottino, N.R., Vandenburg, G.A., Reiser, R., 1967. Resistance of certain long-chain polyunsaturated fatty acids of marine oils to pancreatic lipase hydrolysis. Lipids 2, 489–493.

Breivik, H., 2007. Long-chain omega-3 speciality oils. The Oily Press (PJ Barnes & Associates), Bridgewater, pp. 314.

Brockerhoff, H., Ackman, R.G., 1967. Positional distribution of isomers of monoenoic fatty acids in animal glycerolipids. J. Lipid Res. 8, 661–666.

Bucher, H.C., Hengstler, P., Schindler, C., Meier, G., 2002. N-3 polyunsaturated fatty acids in coronary heart disease: a meta-analysis of randomized controlled trials. Am. J. Med. 112, 298–304.

Bunea, R., El Farrah, K., Deutsch, L., 2004. Evaluation of the effects of neptune krill oil on the clinical course of hyperlipidemia. Altern. Med. Rev. 9, 420–428.

Burri, L., 2011. The power of omega-3 phospholipids omega-3 fatty acids from superba (tm) krill oil show increased bioavailability compared to triglyceride omega-3s. Agro Food Industry Hi-Tech. 22, 10.

Cansell, M., Moussaoui, N., Petit, A.P., Denizot, A., Combe, N., 2006. Feeding rats with liposomes or fish oil differently affects their lipid metabolism. Eur. J. Lipid Sci. Technol. 108, 459–467.

Cansell, M., Nacka, F., Combe, N., 2003. Marine lipid-based liposomes increase in vivo fa bioavailability. Lipids 38, 551–559.

Cansell, M.S., Battin, A., Degrace, P., Gresti, J., Clouet, P., Combe, N., 2009. Early dissimilar fates of liver eicosapentaenoic acid in rats fed liposomes or fish oil and gene expression related to lipid metabolism. Lipids 44, 237–247.

Christensen, M.S., Hoy, C.E., 1996. Effects of dietary triacylglycerol structure on triacylglycerols of resultant chylomicrons from fish oil- and seal oil-fed rats. Lipids 31, 341–344.

Christensen, M.S., Hoy, C.E., Becker, C.C., Redgrave, T.G., 1995. Intestinal absorption and lymphatic transport of eicosapentaenoic (epa), docosahexaenoic (dha), and decanoic acids: dependence on intramolecular triacylglycerol structure. Am. J. Clin. Nutr. 61, 56–61.

Christensen, M.S., Hoy, C.E., Redgrave, T.G., 1994. Lymphatic absorption of n-3 polyunsaturated fatty acids from marine oils with different intramolecular fatty acid distributions. Biochem. Biophys. Acta 1215, 198–204.

Cobiac, L., Clifton, P.M., Abbey, M., Belling, G.B., Nestel, P.J., 1991. Lipid, lipoprotein, and hemostatic effects of fish vs fish-oil n-3 fatty acids in mildly hyperlipidemic males. Am. J. Clin. Nutr. 53, 1210–1216.

Cubero Herrera, L., Ramaley, L., Potvin, M.A., Melanson, J.E., 2013. A method for determining regioisomer abundances of polyunsaturated triacylglycerols in omega-3 enriched fish oils using reversed-phase liquid chromatography and triple-stage mass spectrometry. Food Chem. 139, 655–662.

de Koning, A.J., 2005. Phospholipids of marine origin: the orange roughy (*Hoplostethus atlanticus*). South African J. Sci. 101, 414–416.

De Schrijver, R., Vermeulen, D., Backx, S., 1991. Digestion and absorption of free and esterified fish oil fatty acids in rats. Lipids 26, 400–404.

Dey, T.K., Ghosh, S., Ghosh, M., Koley, H., Dhar, P., 2012. Comparative study of gastrointestinal absorption of epa & dha rich fish oil from nano and conventional emulsion formulation in rats. Food Res. Int. 49, 72–79.

Ding, N., Xue, Y., Tang, X., Sun, Z.-M., Yanagita, T., Xue, C.-H., Wang, Y.-M., 2013. Short-term effects of different fish oil formulations on tissue absorption of docosahexaenoic acid in mice fed high- and low-fat diets. J. Oleo Sci. 62, 883–891.

Domoto, N., Koenen, M.E., Havenaar, R., Mikajiri, A., Chu, B.-S., 2013. The bioaccessibility of eicosapentaenoic acid was higher from phospholipid food products than from mono- and triacylglycerol food products in a dynamic gastrointestinal model. Food Sci. Nutr. 1, 409–415.

EFSA, 2005. Opinion of the scientific panel on contaminants in the food chain [contam] related to the safety assessment of wild and farmed fish. EFSA J.

EFSA, 2010. Scientific opinion on dietary reference values for fats, including saturated fatty acids, polyunsaturated fatty acids, monounsaturated fatty acids, trans fatty acids, and cholesterol[1]. Efsa panel on dietetic products, nutrition, and allergies (nda)[2], EFSA J., vol. 8, pp.1461.

Elvevoll, E.O., Barstad, H., Breimo, E.S., Brox, J., Eilertsen, K.E., Lund, T., Olsen, J.O., Osterud, B., 2006. Enhanced incorporation of n-3 fatty acids from fish compared with fish oils. Lipids 41, 1109–1114.

Falch, E., Rustad, T., Aursand, M., 2006. By-products from gadiform species as raw material for production of marine lipids as ingredients in food or feed. Proc. Biochem. 41, 666–674.

Fard, S.G., Linderborg, K.M., Turchini, G.M., Sinclair, A.J., 2014. Comparison of the bioavailability of docosapentaenoic acid (dpa 22 5n-3) and eicosapentaenoic acid (epa 20 5n-3) in the rat. Prostagland. Leukotrien. Essen. Fatty Acid. 90, 23–26.

Garaiova, I., Guschina, I.A., Plummer, S.F., Tang, J., Wang, D., Plummer, N.T., 2007. A randomised cross-over trial in healthy adults indicating improved absorption of omega-3 fatty acids by pre-emulsification. Nutr. J. 6.

Gerbi, A., Bernard, M., Gleize, B., Coste, T.C., Maixent, J.M., Lan, C., Paganelli, F., Pieroni, G., 2004. Dose dependent accretion of docosahexaenoic acid (dha) in cardiac membranes of rats fed egg yolk powder enriched in dha. Cell. Mol. Biol. 50, 855–860.

Ghasemifard, S., Turchini, G.M., Sinclair, A.J., 2014. Omega-3 long chain fatty acid "bioavailability": a review of evidence and methodological considerations. Prog. Lipid Res. 56, 92–108.

Gotoh, N., Matsumoto, Y., Nagai, T., Mizobe, H., Otake, I., Ichioka, K., Kuroda, I., Watanabe, H., Noguchi, N., Wada, S., 2011. Actual ratios of triacylglycerol positional isomers consisting of saturated and highly unsaturated fatty acids in fishes and marine mammals. Food Chem. 127, 467–472.

Guichardant, M., Chantegrel, B., Deshayes, C., Doutheau, A., Molière, P., Lagarde, M., 2004. Specific markers of lipid peroxidation issued from n-3 and n-6 fatty acids. Biochem. Soc. Trans. 32, 139–140.

Guo, Z., Vikbjerg, A.F., Xu, X., 2005. Enzymatic modification of phospholipids for functional applications and human nutrition. Biotechnol. Adv. 23, 203–259.

Hachem, M., Geloen, A., Van, A.L., Foumaux, B., Fenart, L., Gosselet, F., Da Silva, P., Breton, G., Lagarde, M., Picq, M., Bernoud-Hubac, N., 2015. Efficient docosahexaenoic acid uptake by the brain from a structured phospholipid. Mol. Neurobiol.

Hamazaki, T., Urakaze, M., Makuta, M., Ozawa, A., Soda, Y., Tatsumi, H., Yano, S., Kumagai, A., 1987. Intake of different eicosapentaenoic acid-containing lipids and fatty acid pattern of plasma lipids in the rats. Lipids 22, 994–998.

Hara, K., Onizawa, K., Honda, H., Otsuji, K., Ide, T., Murata, M., 1993. Dietary diacylglycerol-dependent reduction in serum triacylglycerol concentration in rats. Ann. Nutr. Metab. 37, 185–191.

He, G.L., Shankar, R.A., Chzhan, M., Samouilov, A., Kuppusamy, P., Zweier, J.L., 1999. Noninvasive measurement of anatomic structure and intraluminal oxygenation in the gastrointestinal tract of living mice with spatial and spectral epr imaging. Proc. Nat. Acad. Sci. USA. 96, 4596-4591.

He, K., 2009. Fish, long-chain omega-3 polyunsaturated fatty acids and prevention of cardiovascular disease—eat fish or take fish oil supplement? Prog. Cardiovasc. Dis. 52, 95–114.

He, K., Rimm, E.B., Merchant, A., Rosner, B.A., Stampfer, M.J., Willett, W.C., Ascherio, A., 2002. Fish consumption and risk of stroke in men. Jama. 288, 3130–3136.

Hillman, K., Whyte, A.L., Stewart, C.S., 1993. Dissolved oxygen in the porcine gastrointestinal tract. Letters Appl. Microbiol. 16, 299–302.

Hsieh, R.J., Kinsella, J.E., 1989. Oxidation of polyunsaturated fatty acids: mechanisms, products, and inhibition with emphasis on fish. Adv. Food Nutr. Res. 33, 233–241.

Ikeda, I., Imasato, Y., Nagao, H., Sasaki, E., Sugano, M., Imaizumi, K., Yazawa, K., 1993. Lymphatic transport of eicosapentaenoic and docosahexaenoic acids as triglyceride, ethyl ester and free acid, and their effect on cholesterol transport in rats. Life Sci. 52, 1371–1379.

Ikeda, I., Sasaki, E., Yasunami, H., Nomiyama, S., Nakayama, M., Sugano, M., Imaizumi, K., Yazawa, K., 1995. Digestion and lymphatic transport of eicosapentaenoic and docosahexaenoic acids given in the form of triacylglycerol, free acid and ethyl ester in rats. Biochem. Biophys. Acta 1259, 297–304.

Jacobsen, C., Skall Nielsen, Frisenfeldt Horn, A., Moltke Sorensen, A.D. (Eds.), 2013. Food Enrichment with Omega-3 Fatty Acids. Woolhead Publishing Limited, Cambridge.

Kabri, T.H., Meynier, A., Bontemps, D., Gaillard, C., Foucat, L., Linder, M., Genot, C., 2013. Formulation of sub-micron emulsions containing docosahexaenoic acid esterified in triacylglycerols or phospholipids. Eur. J. Lipid Sci. Technol. 115, 1294–1308.

Kagan, M.L., Levy, A., Leikin-Frenkel, A., 2015. Comparative study of tissue deposition of omega-3 fatty acids from polar-lipid rich oil of the microalgae nannochloropsis oculata with krill oil in rats. Food Func. 6, 186–192.

Kagan, M.L., West, A.L., Zante, C., Calder, P.C., 2013. Acute appearance of fatty acids in human plasma - a comparative study between polar-lipid rich oil from the microalgae nannochloropsis oculata and krill oil in healthy young males. Lipids in Health and Disease 12.

Kanner, J., Lapidot, T., 2001. The stomach as a bioreactor: dietary lipid peroxidation in the gastric fluid and the effects of plant-derived antioxidants. Free Radical Biol. Med. 31, 1388–1395.

Karupaiah, T., Sundram, K., 2007. Effects of stereospecific positioning of fatty acids in triacylglycerol structures in native and randomized fats: A review of their nutritional implications. Nutr. Metabol. 4, 16.

Kawai, T., Fushiki, T., 2003. Importance of lipolysis in oral cavity for orosensory detection of fat. Am. J. Physiol. Regul. Integr. Compar. Physiol. 285, R447–R454.

Kenmogne-Domguia, H.B., Moisan, S., Viau, M., Genot, C., Meynier, A., 2014. The initial characteristics of marine oil emulsions and the composition of the media inflect lipid oxidation during in vitro gastrointestinal digestion. Food Chem. 152, 146–154.

Kidd, P.M., 2007. Omega-3 dha and epa for cognition, behavior, and mood: clinical findings and structural-functional synergies with cell membrane phospholipids. Altern. Med. Rev. 12, 207–227.

Krokan, H.E., Bjerve, K.S., Mork, E., 1993. The enteral bioavailability of eicosapentaenoic acid and docosahexaenoic acid is as good from ethyl esters as from glyceryl esters in spite of lower hydrolytic rates by pancreatic lipase in vitro. Biochem. Biophys. Acta. 1168, 59–67.

Laidlaw, M., Cockerline, C.A., Rowe, W.J. 2014. A randomized clinical trial to determine the efficacy of manufacturers' recommended doses of omega-3 fatty acids from different sources in facilitating cardiovascular disease risk reduction. Lipids in Health and Disease 13.

Lairon, D., 2009. Digestion and absorption of lipids. In: McClements, D.J., Decker, E.A. (Eds.), Designing Functional Foods. Measuring and Controlling Food Structure Breakdown and Nutrient Absoprtion. Woodhead Publishing Oxford, pp. 68–93.

Lawson, L.D., Hughes, B.G., 1988. Human absorption of fish oil fatty acids as triacylglycerols, free acids, or ethyl esters. Biochem. Biophys. Res. Commun. 152, 328–335.

Lei, L., Li, J., Li, G.Y., Hu, J.N., Tang, L., Liu, R., Fan, Y.W., Deng, Z.Y., 2012. Stereospecific analysis of triacylglycerol and phospholipid fractions of five wild freshwater fish from poyang lake. J. Agri. Food Chem. 60, 1857–1864.

Lemaitre-Delaunay, D., Pachiaudi, C., Laville, M., Pousin, J., Armstrong, M., Lagarde, M., 1999. Blood compartmental metabolism of docosahexaenoic acid (dha) in humans after ingestion of a single dose of [(13)c]dha in phosphatidylcholine. J. Lipid Res. 40, 1867–1874.

Lu, F.S.H., Nielsen, N.S., Baron, C.P., Jacobsen, C., 2012. Oxidative degradation and non-enzymatic browning due to the interaction between oxidised lipids and primary amine groups in different marine pl emulsions. Food Chem. 135, 2887–2896.

Lyberg, A.M., Fasoli, E., Adlercreutz, P., 2005. Monitoring the oxidation of docosahexaenoic acid in lipids. Lipids 40, 969–979.

Maki, K.C., Mustad, V., Dicklin, M.R., Geohas, J., 2009. Postprandial metabolism with 1,3-diacylglycerol oil versus equivalent intakes of long-chain and medium-chain triacylglycerol oils. Nutrition 25, 627–633.

Marangoni, F., Poli, A., 2013. N-3 fatty acids: functional differences between food intake, oral supplementation and drug treatments. Int. J. Cardiol. 170, S12–S15.

Marze, S., 2013. Bioaccessibility of nutrients and micronutrients from dispersed food systems: impact of the multiscale bulk and interfacial structures. Critical Rev. Food Sci. Nutr. 53, 76–108.

Mathews, S.A., Oliver, W.T., Phillips, O.T., Odle, J., Diersen-Schade, D.A., Harrell, R.J., 2002. Comparison of triglycerides and phospholipids as supplemental sources of dietary long-chain polyunsaturated fatty acids in piglets. J. Nutr. 132, 3081–3089.

McClements, D.J., 2010. Emulsion design to improve the delivery of functional lipophilic components. Ann. Rev. Food Sci. Technol. 1 (1), 241–269.

McClements, D.J., Decker, E.A., Park, Y., 2009. Controlling lipid bioavailability through physicochemical and structural approaches. Critic. Rev. Food Sci. Nutr. 49, 48–67.

Michalski, M.C., Genot, C., Gayet, C., Lopez, C., Fine, F., Joffre, F., Vendeuvre, J.L., Bouvier, J., Chardigny, J.M., Raynal-Ljutovac, K., 2013. Multiscale structures of lipids in foods as parameters affecting fatty acid bioavailability and lipid metabolism. Prog. Lipid Res. 52, 354–373.

Miller, M.R., Nichols, P.D., Barnes, J., Davies, N.W., Peacock, E.J., Carter, C.G., 2006. Regiospecificity profiles of storage and membrane lipids from the gill and muscle tissue of atlantic salmon (salmo salar l) grown at elevated temperature. Lipids 41, 865–876.

Miller, M.R., Nichols, P.D., Carter, C.G., 2008. N-3 oil sources for use in aquaculture - alternatives to the unsustainable harvest of wild fish. Nutr. Res. Rev. 21, 85–96.

Neubronner, J., Schuchardt, J.P., Kressel, G., Merkel, M., von Schacky, C., Hahn, A., 2011. Enhanced increase of omega-3 index in response to long-term n-3 fatty acid supplementation from triacylglycerides versus ethyl esters. Eur. J. Clin. Nutr. 65, 247–254.

Nordoy, A., Barstad, L., Connor, W.E., Hatcher, L., 1991. Absorption of the n-3 eicosapentaenoic and docosahexaenoic acids as ethyl esters and triglycerides by humans. Am. J. Clin. Nutr. 53, 1185–1190.

Nwosu, C.V., Boyd, L.C., 1997. Positional distribution of fatty acids on triacylglycerols of menhaden (brevoortia tyrannis) and salmon (salmo salar) oils. J. Food Lipid. 4, 65–74.

Payet, M., Esmail, M.H., Polichetti, E., Le Brun, G., Adjemout, L., Donnarel, G., Portugal, H., Pieroni, G., 2004. Docosahexaenoic acid-enriched egg consumption induces accretion of arachidonic acid in erythrocytes of elderly patients. Br. J. Nutr. 91, 789–796.

Polette, A., Deshayes, C., Chantegrel, B., Croset, M., Armstrong, J.M., Lagarde, M., 1999. Synthesis of acetyl,docosahexaenoyl-glycerophosphocholine and its characterization using nuclear magnetic resonance. Lipids 34, 1333–1337.

Popa, I., Babeanu, N.E., Nita, S., Popa, O., 2014. Squalene - natural resources and applications. Farmacia 62, 840–862.

Porsgaard, T., Xu, X., Gottsche, J., Mu, H., 2005. Differences in the intramolecular structure of structured oils do not affect pancreatic lipase activity in vitro or the absorption by rats of (n-3) fatty acids. J. Nutr. 135, 1705–1711.

Raatz, S.K., Redmon, J.B., Wimmergren, N., Donadio, J.V., Bibus, D.M., 2009. Enhanced absorption of n-3 fatty acids from emulsified compared with encapsulated fish oil. J. Am. Diet Assoc. 109, 1076–1081.

Ramprasath, V.R., Eyal, I., Zchut, S., Jones, P.J.H., 2014. Response to commentary on a trial comparing krill oil versus fish oil. Lipids in Health and Disease 13.

Rossmeisl, M., Jilkova, Z.M., Kuda, O., Jelenik, T., Medrikova, D., Stankova, B., Kristinsson, B., Haraldsson, G.G., Svensen, H., Stoknes, I., Sjovall, P., Magnusson, Y., Balvers, M.G.J., Verhoeckx, K.C.M., Tvrzicka, E., Bryhn, M., Kopecky, J., 2012. Metabolic effects of n-3 pufa as phospholipids are superior to triglycerides in mice fed a high-fat diet: Possible role of endocannabinoids. Plos One 7.

Ruiz-Lopez, N., Stubhaug, I., Ipharraguerre, I., Rimbach, G., Menoyo, D., 2015. Positional distribution of fatty acids in triacylglycerols and phospholipids from fillets of atlantic salmon (*Salmo salar*) fed vegetable and fish oil blends. Marine Drug. 13, 4255–4269.

Saito, S., Tomonobu, K., Hase, T., Tokimitsu, I., 2006. Effects of diacylglycerol on postprandial energy expenditure and respiratory quotient in healthy subjects. Nutrition 22, 30–35.

Sanguansri, L., Augustin, M.A., Lockett, T.J., Abeywardena, M.Y., Royle, P.J., Mano, M.T., Patten, G.S., 2015. Bioequivalence of n-3 fatty acids from microencapsulated fish oil formulations in human subjects. Br. J. Nutr. 113, 822–831.

Sanguansri, L., Shen, Z., Weerakkody, R., Barnes, M., Lockett, T., Augustin, M.A., 2013. Omega-3 fatty acids in ileal effluent after consuming different foods containing microencapsulated fish oil powder - an ileostomy study. Food Func. 4, 74–82.

Scano, P., Rosa, A., Marincola, F.C., Locci, E., Melis, M.P., Dessi, M.A., Lai, A., 2008. C-13 nmr, gc and hplc characterization of lipid components of the salted and dried mullet (*Mugil cephalus*) roe "bottarga". Chem. Phys. Lipids 151, 69–76.

Schuchardt, J.P., Hahn, A., 2013. Bioavailability of long-chain omega-3 fatty acids. Prostagland. Leukotr. Essen. Fatty Acid 89, 1–8.

Shen, Z., Apriani, C., Weerakkody, R., Sanguansri, L., Augustin, M.A., 2011. Food matrix effects on in vitro digestion of microencapsulated tuna oil powder. J. Agri. Food Chem. 59, 8442–8449.

Shirai, N., Higuchi, T., Suzuki, H., 2006. Analysis of lipid classes and the fatty acid composition of the salted fish roe food products, ikura, tarako, tobiko and kazunoko. Food Chem. 94, 61–67.

Sinclair, A., Linderborg, K., Cameron-Smith, D., 2013. Postprandial metabolism of docosapentaenoic acid (DPA, 22 5n-3) and eicosapentaenoic acid (EPA 20 5n-3) in humans. Ann. Nutr. Metabol. 63, 59–159.

Sirot, V., Oseredczuk, M., Bemrah-Aouachria, N., Volatier, J.L., Leblanc, J.C., 2008. Lipid and fatty acid composition of fish and seafood consumed in france: Calipso study. J. Food Comp. Anal. 21, 8–16.

Song, J.H., Inoue, Y., Miyazawa, T., 1997. Oxidative stability of docosahexaenoic acid-containing oils in the form of phospholipids, triacylglycerols, and ethyl esters. Biosci. Biotechnol. Biochem. 61, 2085–2088.

Spanova, M., Daum, G., 2011. Squalene - biochemistry, molecular biology, process biotechnology, and applications. Eur. J. Lipid Sci. Technol. 113, 1299–1320.

Sugasini, D., Lokesh, B.R., 2013. Enhanced incorporation of docosahexaenoic acid in serum, heart, and brain of rats given microemulsions of fish oil. Mol. Cell. Biochem. 382, 203–216.

Taguchi, H., Watanabe, H., Onizawa, K., Nagao, T., Gotoh, N., Yasukawa, T., Tsushima, R., Shimasaki, H., Itakura, H., 2000. Double-blind controlled study on the effects of dietary diacylglycerol on postprandial serum and chylomicron triacylglycerol responses in healthy humans. J. Am. Coll. Nutr. 19, 789–796.

Tamai, T., Murota, I., Maruyama, K., Baba, T., Toyama, T., Watanabe, N., Kudo, N., Kawashima, Y., 2007. Effects of supplemented diacylglycerol rich in docosahexaenoic acid on serum triacylglycerol in a diet-induced hyperlipidemic model of rats are essentially equivalent to those of triacylglycerol rich in docosahexaenoic acid. Biol. Pharm. Bull. 30, 2381–2388.

Terao, J., Ingemansson, T., Ioku, K., Yuki, H., Ito, Y., 1995. Effects of rat bile-panceratic juice on fe2+ induced peroxidation of phospholipids. Biosci. Biotechnol. Biochem. 59, 55–58.

Thies, F., Pillon, C., Moliere, P., Lagarde, M., Lecerf, J., 1994. Preferential incorporation of sn-2 lysopc dha over unesterified dha in the young rat brain. Am. J. Physiol. 267, R1273–1279.

Thomas, N., Holm, R., Rades, T., Mullertz, A., 2012. Characterising lipid lipolysis and its implication in lipid-based formulation development. Aaps. J. 14, 860–871.

Tillander, V., Bjorndal, B., Burri, L., Bohov, P., Skorve, J., Berge, R.K., Alexson, S.E.H., 2014. Fish oil and krill oil supplementations differentially regulate lipid catabolic and synthetic pathways in mice. Nutr. Metabol. 11.

Tou, J.C., Jaczynski, J., Chen, Y.C., 2007. Krill for human consumption: nutritional value and potential health benefits. Nutr. Rev. 65, 63–77.

Trivedi, R., Singh, R.P., 2005. Modification of oils and fats to produce structured lipids. J. Oleo Sci. 54, 423–430.

Usydus, Z., Szlinder-Richert, J., Polak-Juszczak, L., Kanderska, J., Adamczyk, M., Malesa-Ciecwierz, M., Ruczynska, W., 2008. Food of marine origin: between benefits and potential risks part 1. Canned fish on the polish market. Food Chem. 111, 556–563.

Valdez, I.H., Fox, P.C., 1991. Interactions of the salivary and gastrointestinal systems 1. The role of saliva in digestion. Digestive Dis. 9, 125–132.

Viau, M., Genot, C., Ribourg, L., Meynier, A., 2015. Amounts of the reactive aldehydes, malonaldehyde, 4-hydroxy-2-hexenal and 4-hydroxy-2-nonenal in fresh and oxidized edible oils do not necessary reflect their peroxide and anisidine values. Eur. J. Lipid Sci. Technol.

Vigerust, N.F., Bjorndal, B., Bohov, P., Brattelid, T., Svardal, A., Berge, R.K., 2013. Krill oil versus fish oil in modulation of inflammation and lipid metabolism in mice transgenic for tnf-alpha. Eur. J. Nutr. 52, 1315–1325.

Vors, C., Pineau, G., Gabert, L., Drai, J., Louche-Pelissier, C., Defoort, C., Lairon, D., Désage, M., Danthine, S., Lambert-Porcheron, S., Vidal, H., Laville, M., Michalski, M.C., 2013. Modulating absorption and postprandial handling of dietary fatty acids by structuring fat in the meal: a randomized cross-over clinical trial. Am. J. Clin. Nutr. 97, 23–26.

Wingler, K., Muller, C., Schmehl, K., Florian, S., Brigelius-Floché, R., 2000. Gastrointestinal glutathion peroxidase prevents transport of lipid hydroperoxides in caco-2 cells. Gastroenterology 119, 420–430.

Yang, L.Y., Kuksis, A., Myher, J.J., 1990. Lipolysis of menhaden oil triacylglycerols and the corresponding fatty acid alkyl esters by pancreatic lipase in vitro: a reexamination. J. Lipid Res. 31, 137–147.

Yoshida, H., Kumamaru, J., Mawatari, M., Ikeda, I., Imaizumi, K., Tsuji, H., Seto, A., 1996. Lymphatic absorption of seal and fish oils and their effect on lipid metabolism and eicosanoid production in rats. Biosci. Biotechnol. Biochem. 60, 1293–1298.

CHAPTER

6

Fish Oils in Human Nutrition: History and Current Status

H.B. Rice, A. Ismail

Global Organization for EPA and DHA Omega-3s (GOED), Salt Lake City, Utah, United States

INTRODUCTION

The fish oil industry can be traced back to the 1770s when the first cod liver oils were marketed in the United Kingdom. The following excerpt describes the putative benefits from that time (Waring, 1886).

> *Cod-liver Oil has for a long period been esteemed in Germany and Holland in the treatment of scrofulous and rheumatic diseases. It was introduced into England by Dr. Percival, in 1771, as a remedy for chronic rheumatism, and was employed in the Manchester Infirmary some time after this period. It however fell into disuse, till Schenk published an account of sixteen cases of chronic rheumatism successfully treated by it. It was not, however, till 1841 that its value was fully ascertained by British practitioners, when Dr. J.H. Bennett published an essay on its properties; since that date it has been fully recognized as a remedy of great power and usefulness in tubercular disease; so much so, that in one year (1853) not less than six hundred gallons were administered in one institution-the London Hospital for Consumption and Diseases of the Chest.*

Today, the primary reason people take fish oil is for its cardiovascular benefits. In the 1970s, Danish physicians Jorn Dyerberg and Hans Olaf Bang provided the first evidence that the fatty acids in fish have beneficial effects on coronary heart disease (Bang et al., 1976; Dyerberg et al., 1978). Their hypothesis-generating observations stimulated high quality preclinical and clinical research resulting in significant scientific substantiation for the benefits of the long-chain omega-3 fatty acids, eicosapentaenoic acid (EPA), and docosahexaenoic acid (DHA).

In addition to its cardiovascular benefits, fish oil, rich in EPA and DHA, is sought after for health benefits associated with the brain and eyes, as well as general inflammation and multiple inflammatory conditions. Pregnant and lactating women also take fish oil to benefit their unborn fetuses and babies, respectively.

Sources of EPA and DHA oils have been marketed for centuries, primarily in the form of cod liver oil, but only since the 1980s has the market evolved into what it is today: an industry that has diversified the sources of oils it uses, has grown at double-digit rates for more than 30 years, and counts hundreds of millions of consumers in its user base. In 2012, it was estimated that consumers spent more than $26 billion on products containing EPA and DHA oils worldwide (Packaged Facts, 2012), in applications ranging from dietary supplements to fortified foods.

MARKET

The specific applications in which consumers choose to spend their money on EPA and DHA products is quite diverse, but there are significant differences in how these products are formulated and many applications only have minor inclusions of EPA and DHA. The Global Organization for EPA and DHA (GOED) conducts an annual market research project that illustrates this. In 2013, 79% of the 89,000 tons of EPA and DHA oils consumed were purchased as dietary supplements (GOED, 2014), but no single segment represented more than 40% of the money consumers spent. Infant formulas were the largest segment in terms of consumer spending at slightly over $10 billion, but supplements only came in at $3.2 billion, less than 12% of the total consumer spending despite accounting for the largest volume.

Fish and Fish Oil in Health and Disease Prevention. http://dx.doi.org/10.1016/B978-0-12-802844-5.00006-3

The market is almost entirely supplied by fish oils by volume, which accounted for more than 86,000 tons of supply in 2013. However, other sources, like krill and algae, have created significant value from low volumes. These nonfish sources of EPA and DHA oil accounted for 18% of the value of omega-3 ingredients sold in 2013, but only 3% of the volume (GOED, 2014).

Globally, the primary markets are in developed countries, with the United States, Europe, Japan, Australia, and Canada accounting for 74% of the consumption of EPA and DHA oils but only 17% of the world population (GOED, 2014). Most of these markets are slowing though, and the market's attention is shifting quickly to Asia where high growth is still forecasted for many years to come.

Dietary Supplements

The dietary supplement market is the oldest and largest consumer segment in terms of volume consumption. It is a market that is largely broken into two segments: Natural fish oils and concentrated fish oils that deliver higher amounts of EPA and DHA per unit of volume. The traditional lifecycle of the consumer in most regions of the world has been to enter the market consuming a natural fish oil supplement, after which a portion of consumers will "upgrade" to higher value concentrates to either increase their EPA and DHA consumption or get the same dosage in a smaller serving size. Some consumers leave the market as well, usually citing sensory issues as the main cause. The krill oil industry has been successful at rerecruiting many of these consumers, with one survey showing that nearly half of krill consumers had previously left the category (Discovery Research Group, 2012).

The United States is the largest market for omega-3 supplements at 33% of global demand (GOED, 2014). While omega-3s are generally recognized for their cardiovascular benefits, with nearly 80% of consumers identifying that they are beneficial for heart health, only 42% of American omega-3 supplement users are concerned about their heart. This is a key driver for the market, but 73% of omega-3 consumers are trying to actively manage their overall wellness and 34% are concerned about their cognitive health (GOED, 2015a). These figures indicate that consumers are not assigning a singular benefit to omega-3s, but instead view them as important nutrients for contribution to their overall health. These results are similar to other regions as well, but there are some countries where market growth has been driven by specific key health factors. In Australia, for example, most omega-3 consumers attribute joint health benefits to omega-3 supplements, while in China and parts of Asia, DHA's brain development benefits are most well-known.

Pharmaceuticals

The pharmaceutical market is the newest development for omega-3s, but it is growing rapidly and has great potential. There are currently four approved pharmaceuticals in the world utilizing EPA and/or DHA in very high concentrations (85–97%), and all of which are derived from fish oils. Most of the pharmaceuticals that are approved today target hypertriglyceridemia or problems associated with hyperlipidemia, aspects of cardiovascular health. Globally, consumers are spending more than $2 billion on these products, but the United States market alone accounts for nearly $1.2 billion of the global sales (Packaged Facts, 2012).

For these existing products, the market is changing very rapidly. The first two products, Omacor® from Pronova BioPharma ASA and Epadel from Mochida Pharmaceutical Co., LTD now face competition from generic versions of the drugs. However, the market does not behave like other traditional generic pharmaceuticals that are priced 90% below their branded counterparts. Instead, these fish oil concentrates have very high production costs and the generic manufacturers do not actually own the production, and in fact often own the highest cost technologies due to their only recent entrance in the market. This means that the generics are only priced 20–30% lower than the branded alternatives. In addition to the generics, OTC versions of Epadel exist in Japan but have had only limited success because pharmacists still require patients to regularly visit doctors before they will sell them the product.

The market potential in the pharmaceutical market is still very significant because the pipeline of products still in research and development has both depth and breadth. While the four approved pharmaceuticals largely compete in the same arena, there are more than 50 new pharmaceuticals derived from EPA and DHA in development but they are targeting 32 different health conditions (GOED, 2015(b)). The typical pharmaceutical R&D pipeline always has a lot of products that never make it all the way to market, but many of these are already in Phase II or Phase III clinical trials and have surpassed the most difficult milestones.

Infant Formula

The infant formula market actually accounts for the greatest portion of consumer spending on omega-3 products, totaling more than $10.2 billion (Packaged Facts, 2012), but this is primarily due to the high cost of other ingredients in the formula. By volume, only 3% of omega-3 oils are consumed via infant formula, but the other components of formula notwithstanding, it is still a high value segment accounting for 13% of the value of omega-3 ingredients consumed (GOED, 2014). Regardless, there has been rapid growth in the incorporation of DHA into infant formulas around the world due to its importance in the developing neurological systems of infants. In most developed countries of the world, nearly every formula sold contains DHA. In the developing world, penetration into formulas is difficult to determine, but there is still ample room for growth as most infant formula companies sell value-priced lines of formula that do not contain DHA.

The market for DHA in infant formulas is supplied primarily by two sources, algal and tuna oils, because both have higher content of DHA than EPA, a key requirement for those markets. Algal oils supply 31% of the market, but are much higher value and account for 58% of the value of DHA oils going into infant formulas (GOED, 2014). The primary reason for this disparity is that tuna oils typically contain 24–26% DHA while the algal oils available in the market contain 40–45% DHA.

Regardless, algal oils have been successful in the North American market where they retain significant intellectual property via use of patents, retaining a 96% share of the market. Tuna oils, on the other hand, have been successful particularly in developing markets where cheaper alternatives are attractive to keep costs lower for consumers and developed countries where patents have expired related to algal DHA.

Growth in infant formulas has largely followed population growth trends in the developed world, but in developing countries it is following the growth in the size of the middle class. However, economic growth appears to be slowing in major developing markets like China and the rest of Asia, which may mean there is a lower growth outlook for DHA ingredients in this sector in the short term, while long-term fundamentals still look strong.

Clinical Nutrition

The market for clinical nutrition products with omega-3s has aspects that are similar to both the dietary supplement and pharmaceutical markets. There are some products, like enteral and parenteral nutrition products that are used for therapeutic uses and require government approvals, while medical foods and similar products are used for nutritional management and do not require similar levels of approval. Together these products account for $1.4 billion in consumer spending (Packaged Facts, 2012) and 1,200 tons of consumption of EPA and DHA oils (GOED, 2014).

Overall it is a relatively small category, but there are significant expectations for growth if the parenteral and enteral nutrition products can gain regulatory approval in markets like the United States and China, where they are currently only in limited use. Europe is the leading market for these products today, with nearly 37% of the oils being consumed in these applications. By contrast, the United States market, which is a larger market for both pharmaceuticals and supplements, only has a 20% share of consumption of clinical nutrition products (GOED, 2014).

These products are generally supplied by natural refined fish oils or concentrates with 40–50% EPA and DHA today (GOED, 2014), but there is interest in using plant-based sources of EPA and DHA like algae. Despite the medical nature of this market, it does tend to be price sensitive, and the higher costs of producing algal oils today is still a barrier.

The prospects for omega-3 clinical nutrition products appear to be bullish, as the patients using these products tend to be critically ill and often have significant nutritional deficiencies or problems with nutrient metabolism, so the effect is often more pronounced. Most of the studies using EPA and DHA in these areas show results that are both clinically and statistically significant, but the greater challenge lies in obtaining regulatory approvals. For instance, in Europe it is standard protocol that critically ill premature infants receive EPA and DHA emulsions because they have been associated with very high survival rates, but in the United States, regulatory authorities require placebo-controlled studies before approving these products. This is difficult because doctors are unwilling to run studies with a placebo group when mortality reductions are clearly evident in the test group of infants. These issues can be managed, but it takes time and often a longer approval process than pharmaceuticals. Other health conditions that may drive this market going forward include surgery recovery and complication rates, cystic fibrosis, fatty liver disease, cancer cachexia, and HIV/AIDS care.

Functional Foods

The omega-3 functional food market grew very rapidly in the late 1990s and early 2000s and many ingredient companies began to divert significant resources into developing specialized forms of omega-3s that could adapt to food processing technologies. However, the market quickly matured and growth slowed as food marketers had a difficult time finding ways to position the benefits of EPA and DHA to the consumer. There were some foods, like yogurts targeting children, where food manufacturers discovered they could eliminate the more costly omega-3s and still provide other cheaper nutrients that were valuable for children that effectively had the same message for the consumer, a healthier alternative for your child. In other cases, food companies were putting an inherently healthy

EPA and DHA ingredient in an unhealthy food matrix and the consumers were just confused by the proposition, like in the case of chocolate puddings with DHA. However, despite these missteps, GOED is aware of at least a dozen food products fortified with EPA and DHA that have the equivalent of more than $100 million in retail sales in their respective markets, so success is possible with the right value proposition.

The functional food market accounted for $7.9 billion in global consumer spending, or 31% of all consumer spending on omega-3 products (Packaged Facts, 2012). By volume, however, it was a small category with only 4000 tons of omega-3 oils going into these applications, or 3% of total volume (GOED, 2014). Similar to infant formula, the ultimate retail price the consumer pays are primarily for other ingredients in the food matrix, rather than the omega-3s specifically. In fact, these products will often have between 32mg and 50mg of EPA and DHA per serving, which is small compared to the 300–1000 mg dosages you find in supplements. This can create a conflict between the food and supplement industries, but they have different philosophies. With foods, the primary nutrient delivery goal is to deliver the daily supply of a nutrient over multiple servings since you have more than one dietary occasion per day, so the dosages of EPA and DHA are generally based on daily intake recommendations. By contrast, supplements are trying to deliver the entire dosage in a single serving and the formulations are often based on recommendations from scientific groups or in response to competing products in the market.

The growth prospects are still positive for functional foods, but many industry observers feel that recommended intakes are required for these products to thrive, since new product development will be driven by the types of claims companies can make. Without a daily intake recommendation, for instance, a company would not have a threshold for being able to say they provide a "good source" of these nutrients. Most developed countries have recently adopted such intakes, so these industry observers are watching the food market in these countries with keen interest, but are generally waiting for the United States and Canada to adopt recommended intakes since they tend to lead global food development trends.

CLAIMS

EPA- and DHA-rich oils, like other foods and dietary/food supplements, are marketed with claims. Provided that they are scientifically substantiated, nutrition and health claims can help consumers make well-informed choices. Regardless of where a fish oil is sold, they must comply with the regulations applicable to that jurisdiction(s), including those for nutrition and health claims. What follows is information on claims from different geographies around the world. Compared to other geographies, significant details are provided concerning the United States. This is because the United States has not been as progressive and supportive of realizing the public health benefits of the long-chain omega-3s, EPA and DHA. For example, the United States does not recognize beneficial levels associated with EPA and DHA. This has resulted in a ban on the use of nutrient content claims associated with EPA and DHA. In addition, no FDA-approved health claim accurately reflects the current status of the science.

United States

In the United States, there are three broad categories of claims that are permissible in the labeling of dietary supplements and foods, including: structure/function claims, nutrient content claims, and health claims.

Structure/Function Claims

Structure/function claims may describe the role of a nutrient or dietary ingredient intended to affect the normal structure or function of the human body. These types of claims are not preapproved by the FDA, but the manufacturer is required to have substantiation that the claim is truthful and not misleading. Since these claims do not require preapproval, there are no specific claims to discuss; therefore, it is recommended that the reader seeks further guidance from the FDA website (www.fda.gov).

Nutrient Content Claims

The FDA received three notifications (Jan. 2004, Jan. 2005, and Dec. 2005) under the Food and Drug Administration Modernization Act (FDAMA) of 1997 (FDA, 1997) about nutrient content claims for alpha-linolenic acid (ALA), DHA, or EPA omega-3 fatty acids based on authoritative statements from the Institute of Medicine's (IOM) Dietary Reference Intake Report (Institute of Medicine, 2005). Because the notifications did not receive objection from the FDA, they were deemed authorized for use in food (including dietary supplements) labeling; however, on Nov. 27, 2007, the FDA published a Notice of Proposed Rulemaking that would prohibit the use of the nutrient content claims for EPA and DHA should a Final Rule be published (FDA, 2007). FDA proposed to conclude that the statements "do not identify a nutrient level, or reference value, for EPA and/or DHA that FDA could use to establish by regulation a label reference value for use in nutrition labeling." FDA also noted the IOM Final Report "does not establish a DRI (dietary reference intake) in any form for either EPA or DHA." Because the IOM Final Report does not identify a nutrient level to which the EPA and DHA claims refer, FDA notes the statements do not meet the FDAMA requirements.

On Apr. 28, 2014, the FDA issued its Final Rule (FDA, 2014) reiterating its position found in the Notice of Proposed Rulemaking. The effective date for the Final Rule is Jan. 1, 2016 which means that the previously notified nutrient content claims related to EPA and DHA can no longer be used after that date. The Final Rule reflects neither the well-substantiated benefits associated with EPA and DHA nor any FDA assessment of the science. Quite simply, the Final Rule is about statutory requirements.

The industry considers nutrient content claims for EPA and DHA to be critical in order to communicate the importance of these fatty acids. To this end, a DRI for EPA and DHA is needed. Once a DRI is established, the FDA can be petitioned to use EPA and DHA specific nutrient content claims based on the level set during the DRI review. In the absence of any objection, 120 days after submitting a petition to the FDA, the nutrient content claims can be used. The timeline for establishing a DRI for EPA and DHA is debatable.

On Sep. 3, 2009, GOED and eight other associations/organizations submitted a Citizen Petition to the IOM requesting it to convene an expert panel to update DRIs for EPA and DHA. The petition was not considered at that time. On Jul. 31, 2013, GOED nominated EPA and DHA for DRI review in response to a call for nominations from Canada and the United States. On Aug. 15, 2014, it was announced that EPA and DHA, along with three other nutrients, had been selected as top priority nutrients for DRI reviews. At the time of prioritization, it was decided that before a DRI review would be undertaken that a workshop was needed to discuss whether, and how, chronic disease outcomes can be incorporated into the process of setting DRI values. The workshop entitled "Options for Consideration of Chronic Disease Endpoints for Dietary Reference Intakes" took place on Mar. 10 and 11, 2015. Originally, it was anticipated that the workshop would conclude with a recommendation for whether or not chronic disease risk reduction could be used as an endpoint to establish DRIs. This was not the case. The purpose of the workshop was not to come to consensus, rather to inform the IOM about the issues associated with using chronic diseases as endpoints. While it is known that two to three manuscripts, based on the workshop discussions, will be submitted for publication as a means to inform the IOM, due to a lack of transparency in the overall process, it's not clear what will happen after that. The bottom line, however, is that it will be several years before the next DRI review is commenced.

Health Claims

In the United States, the following qualified health claim is permitted for use to market conventional foods and dietary supplements containing EPA and DHA: "Supportive but not conclusive research shows that consumption of EPA and DHA omega-3 fatty acids may reduce the risk of coronary heart disease. One serving of [Name of the food] provides [ ] gram of EPA and DHA omega-3 fatty acids. [See nutrition information for total fat, saturated fat, and cholesterol content.]" The claim's specific conditions of use can be found in either of the two letters of enforcement discretion (FDA, 2004a; FDA, 2004b) from the FDA.

Skip ahead almost 10 years to Nov. 2013 when GOED submitted a health claim petition for EPA and DHA and the reduction of blood pressure in the general population. The petition was based on a metaanalysis of 70 randomized clinical trials and concluded that provision of EPA + DHA reduces systolic blood pressure, while provision of $\geq$ 2 g reduces diastolic blood pressure (Miller et al., 2014). In Jul. 2014, the FDA informed GOED that, based on the Agency's preliminary review of the health claim petition, it was unlikely to meet the standard of significant scientific agreement (SSA). For this reason, GOED was given the option to agree to a qualified health claim (QHC) review. GOED agreed to the review change and so started the formal review process. A decision from the FDA was due May 2015, but the FDA requested a 90 day extension with a new decision date of Aug. 2015.

European Union

Nutrition Claims (European Commission, 2010)

The nutrition claims for 'source of omega-3 fatty acids' and 'high in omega-3 fatty acids' were adopted on Feb. 9, 2010 and entered into force on Mar. 1, 2010. According to the Commission,

> *Concerning the claims 'Source of omega-3 fatty acids' and 'High in omega-3 fatty acids', the conditions of use should distinguish between the two types [short- versus long-chain] of omega-3 fatty acids, which have different physiological roles and for which different levels of consumption are recommended. Furthermore, those conditions of use should establish a minimum quantity requested per 100 g and 100 kcal of product in order to ensure that only foods providing a significant amount of omega-3 fatty acids at their level of consumption can bear those claims.*

The nutrition claims for EPA and DHA are as follows:

- A claim that a food is a 'source of omega-3 fatty acids', and any claim likely to have the same meaning for the consumer may only be made where the product contains at least 40 mg of the sum of EPA and DHA per 100 g and per 100 kcal.
- A claim that a food is 'high in omega-3 fatty acids', and any claim likely to have the same meaning for the consumer may only be made where the product contains at least 80 mg of the sum of EPA and DHA per 100 g and per 100 kcal.

Health Claims (European Commission, 2006)

In the European Union (EU), the European Food Safety Authority (EFSA) has returned more positive opinions for the benefits of EPA and DHA than any other nutrient. Given the strict regulatory regime under which the evaluations have been conducted, this is testament to the well-established benefits associated with the long-chain omega-3s. In the EU, health claims are classified as either Article 13 (health claims other than those referring to the reduction of disease risk and to children's development and health) or Article 14 [reduction of disease risk claims (1)(a) and claims referring to children's development and health (1)(b)]. Thus far, nine health claims, including six Article 13(1) and three Article 14(1)(b) claims have been authorized for use.

Article 13(1)

Claim: DHA contributes to the maintenance of normal brain function (European Commission, 2012)
Conditions of use: The claim may be used only for food which contains at least 40 mg of DHA per 100 g and per 100 kcal. In order to bear the claim, information shall be given to the consumer that the beneficial effect is obtained with a daily intake of 250 mg of DHA.

Claim: DHA contributes to the maintenance of normal vision (European Commission, 2012)
Conditions of use: The claim may be used only for food which contains at least 40 mg of DHA per 100 g and per 100 kcal. In order to bear the claim, information shall be given to the consumer that the beneficial effect is obtained with a daily intake of 250 mg of DHA.

Claim: EPA and DHA contribute to the normal function of the heart (European Commission, 2012)
Conditions of use: The claim may be used only for food which is at least a source of EPA and DHA as referred to in the claim "Source of Omega-3 Fatty Acids". In order to bear the claim, information shall be given to the consumer that the beneficial effect is obtained with a daily intake of 250 mg of EPA and DHA.

Claim: DHA contributes to the maintenance of normal blood triglyceride levels (European Commission, 2013)
Conditions of use: The claim may be used only for food which provides a daily intake of 2 g of DHA and which contains DHA in combination with eicosapentaenoic acid (EPA). In order to bear the claim, information shall be given to the consumer that the beneficial effect is obtained with a daily intake of 2 g of DHA. When the claim is used on food supplements and/or fortified foods information shall also be given to consumers not to exceed a supplemental daily intake of 5 g of EPA and DHA combined. The claim shall not be used for foods targeting children.

Claim: DHA and EPA contribute to the maintenance of normal blood pressure (European Commission, 2013)
Conditions of use: The claim may be used only for food which provides a daily intake of 3 g of EPA and DHA. In order to bear the claim, information shall be given to the consumer that the beneficial effect is obtained with a daily intake of 3 g of EPA and DHA. When the claim is used on food supplements and/or fortified foods, information shall also be given to consumers not to exceed a supplemental daily intake of 5 g of EPA and DHA combined. The claim shall not be used for foods targeting children.

Claim: DHA contributes to the maintenance of normal blood triglyceride levels (European Commission, 2013)
Conditions of use: The claim may be used only for food which provides a daily intake of 2 g of EPA and DHA. In order to bear the claim, information shall be given to the consumer that the beneficial effect is obtained with a daily intake of 2 g of EPA and DHA. When the claim is used on food supplements and/or fortified foods, information shall also be given to consumers not to exceed a supplemental daily intake of 5 g of EPA and DHA combined. The claim shall not be used for foods targeting children.

Article 14(1)(b)

Claim: Docosahexaenoic acid (DHA) maternal intake contributes to the normal brain development of the fetus and breastfed infants (European Commission, 2011)

Conditions of Use: Information shall be given to pregnant and lactating women that the beneficial effect is obtained with a daily intake of 200 mg of DHA in addition to the recommended daily intake for omega-3 fatty acids for adults, that is: 250 mg DHA and EPA. The claim can be used only for food which provides a daily intake of at least 200 mg DHA.

Claim: Docosahexaenoic acid (DHA) intake contributes to the normal visual development of infants up to 12 months of age (European Commission, 2011)
Conditions of use: Information shall be given to the consumer that the beneficial effect is obtained with a daily intake of 100 mg of DHA. When the claim is used on follow-on formula, the food shall contain at least 0.3 % of the total fatty acids as DHA.

Claim: Docosahexaenoic acid (DHA) maternal intake contributes to the normal development of the eye of the fetus and breastfed infants (European Commission, 2011)
Conditions of Use: Information shall be given to pregnant and lactating women that the beneficial effect is obtained with a daily intake of 200 mg of DHA in addition to the recommended daily intake for omega-3 fatty acids for adults, that is: 250 mg DHA and eicosapentaenoic acid (EPA). The claim can be used only for food which provides a daily intake of at least 200 mg DHA.

Japan

In Japan, the Consumer Affairs Agency (CAA) has jurisdiction over the three categories of health claims for foods, including: Foods with Function Claims, Foods with Nutrient Function Claims (FNFC), and Foods for Specified Health Uses (FOSHU).

Foods with Function Claims

Foods with Function Claims is a new category of claims and foods in this category are permitted to make claims about the health benefit of the finished product or active ingredient if a notification with appropriate scientific substantiation (ie, clinical trial or systematic review) is submitted to the CAA at least 60 days prior to the product launch. Nutrients associated with Japanese DRIs are not permitted to use these types of claims; however, some constituents associated with nutrients with Japanese DRIs are permitted. For the fish oil industry, this means that a food whose active ingredient is omega-3 fatty acids cannot be a Food with Function Claims, but when the active ingredient is EPA or DHA, such food can be a Food with Function Claims. Foods with Function Claims cannot be used to market products to individuals with disease, children, or expectant mothers (including those who are planning to become pregnant).

Foods with Nutrient Function Claims (FNFC)

Beginning Apr. 1, 2014, n–3 fatty acids, but not EPA and DHA, were added to the FNFC system. FNFC refers to all food that is labeled with the nutrient function claims, and these foods may be freely manufactured and distributed without any permission from or notification to the national government, if it meets the established standards and specifications. The added claim is "n–3 fatty acids is a nutrient which helps maintain healthy skin" with a regulatory defined range of 0.6–2.0 g/day. The mandatory statements that must accompany this claim include: "Excess intake of this product neither cures your disease nor promotes your health. Please comply with the advisable daily intake" and "This food product differs from Foods for Specified Health Uses and has not been examined particularly by the Secretary General of Consumer Affairs Agency."

Foods for Specified Health Uses (FOSHU)

There is one claim associated with FOSHU and it is "As this product contains DHA or EPA, it has the action of lowering serum triglycerides. It is a food suited for the person who worries about serum triglycerides." The finished product must carry the following warning: "This product is not a preventive nor a curative medicine for hyperlipidemia. Persons under treatment should consult with a doctor." Since FOSHU approval is product-specific, this claim does not apply to every product.

Australia New Zealand

Nutrition Content Claims (Australia New Zealand, 2013)

For use with foods (not complementary medicines), there are three nutrition content claims associated with EPA and DHA.

- Contains omega-3 fatty acids
  - Condition of use: food contains ≥ 30 mg total EPA and DHA per serving
- Good source of omega-3 fatty acids
  - Condition of use: food contains ≥ 60 mg total EPA and DHA per serving
- Increased omega-3 fatty acids
  - Condition of use: food contains ≥ 25% more omega-3 fatty acids than in the same quantity of reference food

Health Claims (Australia New Zealand, 2013)

For use with foods (not complementary medicines), the following general level health claim can be used, "EPA and DHA (but not omega-3) contribute to heart health" provided the food contains a minimum of 50 mg EPA and DHA combined in a serving of food. Also, other than for fish or fish products with no added saturated fatty acids, the food must contain: ≤ 28% saturated fatty acids and trans fatty acids; or ≤ 5 g per 100 g saturated fatty acids and trans fatty acids.

Canada

Nutrient Content Claims (Canadian Food Inspection Agency, online(a))

The following nutrient content claims can be used on food: "source of", "contains" or "provides" omega-3 polyunsaturated fatty acids or "xg of omega-3 fatty acids (or DHA or EPA and DHA) per Y serving" provided there is ≥ 0.3 g of omega-3 polyunsaturated fatty acids per reference amount and serving of stated size or per 100 g, if the food is a prepackaged meal.

Health Claims

In Canada, there is one claim permitted for use on food products (nutrient function claim) and multiple claims permitted for Natural Health Products (NHPs). Note that in order to market natural health products in Canada, the applicable regulations require first obtaining the necessary product and site licenses. For more information, visit Health Canada's website at http://www.hc-sc.gc.ca/index-eng.php.

Food *(Canadian Food Inspection Agency, online(b))*

Nutrient function claim: "DHA, an omega-3 fatty acid, supports the normal physical development of the brain, eyes and nerves primarily in children under two year of age."

NHP-Cod Liver Oil *(http://webprod.hc-sc.gc.ca/nhpid-bdipsn/atReq.do?atid=cod.liver.oil&lang=eng)*

- For products providing 100–1360 mg eicosapentaenoic acid (EPA) + docosahexaenoic acid (DHA), per day:
  - "Source of omega-3 fatty acids for the maintenance of good health"
  - "Source of eicosapentaenoic acid (EPA) and docosahexaenoic acid (DHA) for the maintenance of good health"
- For products providing 100–1360 mg EPA + DHA including at least 100 mg DHA, per day:
  - "Helps support cognitive health and/or brain function"
- For products providing 150–1360 mg EPA + DHA including at least 150 mg DHA, per day:
  - "Helps support the development of the brain, eyes and nerves in children up to 12 years of age"

NHP-Fish Oil *(http://webprod.hc-sc.gc.ca/nhpid-bdipsn/monoReq.do?id=88&lang=eng)*

- For products providing 100– 3000 mg EPA + DHA, per day:
  - "Source of omega-3 fatty acids for the maintenance of good health."
  - "Source of eicosapentaenoic acid (EPA) and docosahexaenoic acid (DHA) for the maintenance of good health"
- For products providing 500–3000 mg EPA + DHA and containing a ratio of EPA:DHA between 0.5:1 and 2:1, per day:
  - "Helps maintain/support cardiovascular health"
- For products providing 1000– 3000 mg EPA + DHA and containing a ratio of EPA:DHA between 0.5:1 and 2:1, per day:
  - "Helps to reduce serum triglycerides/triacylglycerols"

- For products providing 2800–3000 mg EPA + DHA and containing a ratio of EPA:DHA between 0.5:1 and 2:1, per day:
  - "In conjunction with conventional therapy, helps to reduce the pain of rheumatoid arthritis in adults"
- For products providing 100–3000 mg EPA + DHA, including at least 100 mg DHA, per day:
  - "Helps support cognitive health and/or brain function"
- For products providing 150–2000 mg EPA + DHA, including at least 150 mg DHA, per day:
  - "Helps support the development of the brain, eyes and nerves in children up to 12 years of age"
- For products providing 1500–3000 mg EPA + DHA and containing a ratio of EPA:DHA between 1.75:1 and 2:1, including at least 1,000 mg EPA, per day:
  - "Helps to promote healthy mood balance"

NHP-Krill Oil ***(http://webprod.hc-sc.gc.ca/nhpid-bdipsn/monoReq.do?id=205&lang=eng)***

- "Source of omega-3 fatty acids for the maintenance of good health"
- "Source of eicosapentaenoic acid (EPA) and docosahexaenoic acid (DHA) for the maintenance of good health"

NHP-Seal Oil ***(http://webprod.hc-sc.gc.ca/nhpid-bdipsn/atReq.do?atid=seal.oil&lang=eng)***

- For products providing 100–3000 mg EPA + DHA + docosapentaenoic acid (DPA), per day:
  - "Source of omega-3 fatty acids for the maintenance of good health"
  - "Source of eicosapentaenoic acid (EPA), docosahexaenoic acid (DHA), and docosapentaenoic acid (DPA) for the maintenance of good health"
- For products providing 150–2000 mg EPA + DHA + DPA, including at least 150 mg DHA, per day:
  - "Helps to support the development of the brain, eyes and nerves in children up to 12 years of age"

CONCLUSION

EPA- and DHA-rich oils have been marketed for centuries. Globally, consumers spend billions of dollars each year to reap the health benefits of EPA- and DHA-rich oils. In addition to their cardiovascular benefits, these oils are sought after for health benefits associated with the brain and eyes, as well as general inflammation and multiple inflammatory conditions. Pregnant and lactating women also take fish oil to benefit their unborn fetuses and babies, respectively. The majority of these oils are sold in developed countries. The markets for these oils include: dietary supplements, pharmaceuticals, infant formula, clinical nutrition, and functional foods. Provided that they are scientifically substantiated, claims can help consumers make well-informed choices, but all claims must comply with the regulations applicable to the jurisdiction(s) where the oils are sold.

References

Australia New Zealand, 2013. Australia New Zealand Food Standards Code - Standard 1.2.7 - Nutrition, Health and Related Claims. Federal Register of Legislative Instruments F2013L00054. http://www.comlaw.gov.au/Series/F2013L00054

Bang, H.O., Dyerberg, J., Home, N., 1976. The composition of food consumed by Greenland Eskimos. Acta Med. Scand. 200, 69–73.

Canadian Food Inspection Agency, online(a). Acceptable Nutrient Function Claims. http://www.inspection.gc.ca/food/labelling/food-labelling-for-industry/health-claims/eng/1392834838383/1392834887794?chap=8#s16c8

Canadian Food Inspection Agency, online(b). Specific Nutrient Content Claims. http://www.inspection.gc.ca/food/labelling/food-labelling-for-industry/nutrient-content/specific-claim-requirements/eng/1389907770176/1389907817577?chap=7

Discovery Research Group, 2012. Research Report: Omega-3 Supplement Use Survey. Discovery Research Group, Salt Lake City.

Dyerberg, J., Bang, H.O., Stofferson, E., Moncada, S., Vane, J.R., 1978. Eicosapentaenoic acid and prevention of thrombosis and atherosclerosis. Lancet 2, 117–119.

European Commission, 2006. Regulation (EC) No 1924/2006 of the European Parliament and of the Council of 20 December 2006 on nutrition and health claims made on foods. http://eur-lex.europa.eu/LexUriServ/LexUriServ.do?uri=OJ:L:2007:012:0003:0018:EN:PDF

European Commission, 2010. Commission Regulation (EC) No 116/2010 of 9 February 2010 amending Regulation (EC) No 1924/2006 of the European Parliament and of the Council with regard to the list of nutrition claims. http://eur-lex.europa.eu/LexUriServ/LexUriServ.do?uri=OJ:L:2010:037:0016:0018:EN:PDF

European Commission, 2011. Commission Regulation (EU) No 440/2011 of 6 May 2011 on the authorisation and refusal of authorisation of certain health claims made on foods and referring to children's development and health. http://eur-lex.europa.eu/legal-content/EN/TXT/PDF/?uri=CELEX:32011R0440&from=EN

European Commission, 2012. Commission Regulation (EU) No 432/2012 of 16 May 2012 establishing a list of permitted health claims made on foods, other than those referring to the reduction of disease risk and to children's development and health. http://eur-lex.europa.eu/LexUriServ/LexUriServ.do?uri=OJ:L:2012:136:0001:0040:en:PDF

European Commission, 2013. Commission Regulation (EU) No 536/2013 of 11 June 2013 amending Regulation (EU) No 432/2012 establishing a list of permitted health claims made on foods other than those referring to the reduction of disease risk and to children's development and health. http://eur-lex.europa.eu/LexUriServ/LexUriServ.do?uri=OJ:L:2013:160:0004:0008:EN:PDF

GOED, 2014. EPA & DHA Ingredient Market Overview 2012–13. GOED, Salt Lake City.

GOED, 2015. Proprietary consumer surveys conducted in 12 countries 2013–15. GOED, Salt Lake City.

GOED, 2015. The Pharmaceutical Market for EPA and DHA Omega-3s. https://docs.google.com/presentation/d/1aqu-Z0gxi4oOXum7oFKqjNZ701UZdzmpu5G9b85WGqE/pub?start=false&loop=false&delayms=3000

Institute of Medicine, 2005. Dietary Reference Intakes for Energy, Carbohydrates, Fiber, Fat, Fatty Acids, Cholesterol, Protein, and Amino Acids. The National Academies Press, Washington, D.C. http://www.nal.usda.gov/fnic/DRI/DRI_Energy/energy_full_report.pdf

Miller, P.E., Van Elswyk, M., Alexander, D.D., 2014. Long-chain omega-3 fatty acids eicosapentaenoic acid and docosahexaenoic acid and blood pressure: a meta-analysis of randomized controlled trials. Am. J. Hypertens. 27, 885–896.

Packaged Facts, 2012. Global Market for EPA/DHA Omega-3 Products. Packaged Facts, Rockville.

United States FDA, 1997. Food and Drug Administration Modernization Act (FDAMA) of 1997. http://www.fda.gov/downloads/RegulatoryInformation/Legislation/FederalFoodDrugandCosmeticActFDCAct/SignificantAmendmentstotheFDCAct/FDAMA/FullTextofFDAMAlaw/UCM089145.pdf

United States FDA, 2004. Letter Responding to Health Claim Petition dated June 23, 2003 (Wellness petition): Omega-3 Fatty Acids and Reduced Risk of Coronary Heart Disease (Docket No. 2003Q-0401). http://www.fda.gov/Food/IngredientsPackagingLabeling/LabelingNutrition/ucm072936.htm

United States FDA, 2004. Letter Responding to Health Claim Petition dated Nov. 3, 2003 (Martek Petition): Omega-3 Fatty Acids and Reduced Risk of Coronary Heart Disease (Docket No. 2003Q-0401). http://www.fda.gov/Food/IngredientsPackagingLabeling/LabelingNutrition/ucm072932.htm

United States FDA, 2007. Food Labeling: Nutrient Content Claims; Alpha-Linolenic Acid, Eicosapentaenoic Acid, and Docosahexaenoic Acid Omega-3 Fatty Acids. Notice of Proposed Rulemaking. Federal Register 72, 66103-66118. http://www.fda.gov/OHRMS/DOCKETS/98fr/E7-22991.pdf

United States FDA, 2014. Food Labeling: Nutrient Content Claims; Alpha-Linolenic Acid, Eicosapentaenoic Acid, and Docosahexaenoic Acid Omega-3 Fatty Acids. Final Rule. Federal Register 79, 23262-23273. http://www.gpo.gov/fdsys/pkg/FR-2014-04-28/pdf/2014-09492.pdf

Waring, E.J., 1886. In: Blakiston, P. (Ed.), A Manual of Practical Therapeutics: Considered with Reference to Articles of the Materia Medica. Fourth ed. Son & Co., Philadelphia.

P A R T I I

FISH AND FISH OIL NUTRITION IN THE LIFE CYCLE

CHAPTER

7

Omega 3 Fatty Acids Counterbalance Actions of Omega-6 Fatty Acids

B. Lands

American Society for Nutrition, College Park, Maryland, United States

BALANCING OUR OPTIONS

Human health is not a simple, single thing. It is a balance among thousands of different processes involving gene-defined proteins responding to environmentally based stimuli. These responses form an intricate network of actions mediated and modulated by a balanced set of signals from nerves and bioactive molecules. However, year on year some of the physiological processes drift unintentionally from healthy physiology toward pathophysiology. Molecular mediators of those transitions are objective biomarkers to monitor the drift. While advanced age inevitably brings death, many troubling chronic disorders familiar to the aged need not be inevitable. Evidence indicates that eating sea foods, fish, and fish oil can diminish the risk for some progressive chronic disorders and delay the condition we call ageing. The way that this happens is a story worth reading.

The story of fish, fish oil, and human health involves foods and vitamins and hormones interacting in a balanced network that gives us a healthy life (Lands, 1986). Weaving in and out of the story and affecting the network are two different types of essential vitamin-like nutrients, omega-3 (n–3) and omega-6 (n–6) fatty acids. They provide useful biomarkers of health status, and they drive health conditions. Humans and all vertebrates need these two vital types of nutrient that plants continually make and provide. We eat them and convert them into potent hormone-like mediators that modulate and balance most of our physiological events.

Scientists know how seafood differs from many other foods as their nutrients affect health outcomes in important ways. When people learn more about how that happens, they are likely to reexamine their current choice of foods. This story tells how the balance of the n–3 and n–6 nutrients in foods has health outcomes that will likely prompt us every day to weigh and balance our options for the foods that we eat. Examining the consequences of nutrient balance on the resultant biomarkers in our tissues and on a predisposition for preventable health conditions is the goal of this review.

TWO TISSUE BIOMARKERS PREDICT HEALTH RISK DIFFERENTLY

Biomarkers are objective indicators of tissue conditions and their likely health outcomes. They are important for health risk assessment. Some have a specific narrow predictive ability, and some correlate with multiple unwanted health conditions. They can be called "risk factors" when they reliably predict a risk for what might happen to our health. Many factors and biomarkers predict some degree of risk. However, the most important biomarkers are intermediates in the chain of events that actually cause the clinical condition. Those intermediates are often valid surrogates for a person's clinical status. Lowering those surrogates can lower the risk for harm from the clinical condition.

One convenient biomarker for general health risk assessment (HRA) is the percent of n–6 in the highly unsaturated fatty acids (HUFA) of blood lipids (Bibus and Lands, 2015). Put simply, people with more n–6 than n–3 HUFA (ie, more than 50% n–6 in HUFA) have a greater risk for unwanted health conditions than those with less n–6 than

Fish and Fish Oil in Health and Disease Prevention. http://dx.doi.org/10.1016/B978-0-12-802844-5.00007-5

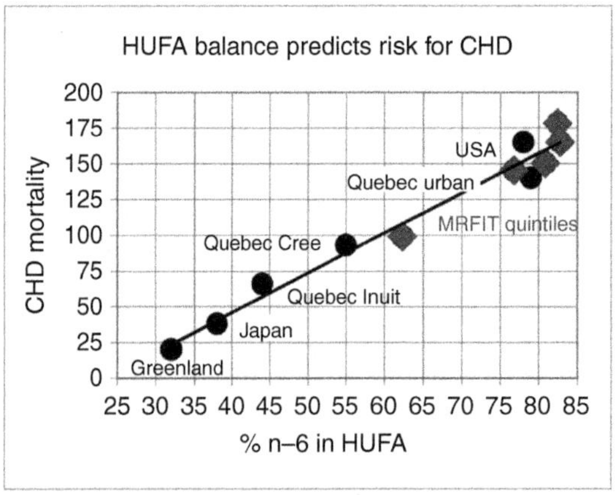

FIGURE 7.1 **HUFA balance predicts health risk.** Death rates from coronary heart disease (expressed per 100,000 population) are higher for people with higher %n–6 in HUFA. The five *diamonds* at the upper right are quintiles of the MRFIT control group. *Source: This figure was made from data in Lands (2003a).*

n–3 HUFA. The risk can be estimated by a simple finger-tip blood-spot analysis (Bibus and Lands, 2015). Fig. 7.1 shows that the HUFA balance has a wide range of values (25–85% n–6 in HUFA) among diverse groups of humans often regarded as healthy but living with very different risk for an unwanted health condition.

Considering Blood HUFA Balance

The linear relationship of heart attack deaths with %n–6 in HUFA in Fig. 7.1 shows progressively higher risk for people with progressively higher values with no obvious optimum point. Much is now known about how HUFA balance influences CHD mortality. An important first step in understanding was to recognize how closely the HRA measurement of HUFA balance associates with certain health conditions (Lands et al., 1992).

The Multiple Risk Factor Intervention Trial (MRFIT) was a large, multicenter clinical trial (Stamler et al., 2012) that considered a number of biomarkers related to cardiovascular disease (CVD). Results for 6,000 people in the untreated control group are shown as five quintiles (red diamonds) in the upper right side of Fig. 7.1. Most of the people in the trial had estimated HUFA balance values near 80% n–6 in HUFA (Lands, 2003a). However, the quintile with the lowest estimated value (near 60% n–6 in HUFA) had about one-half the deaths seen for people in the other quintiles. In a similar way, a large provincial CVD study in Canada showed that people in Cree communities of Quebec with average HRA values near 45% n–6 in HUFA (Dewailly et al., 2002) had about half the CVD mortality rate of people in urban Quebec who had average HRA values near 75% (Dewailly et al., 2001a).

An important aspect of the ethnic food habits for the diverse populations studied is the predominance of fish and fish oils in daily foods of people at the lower left of Fig. 7.1. People in Inuit communities of Quebec and Greenland had lower HRA values and lower incidence of CVD death (Dewailly et al., 2001b; Stark et al., 2002). Also, the average %n–6 in HUFA measured among Japanese people was below 50% (Kobayashi et al., 2001; Lands, 2003b), and the Japanese CVD mortality rate was much less than that for Americans. The strong correlation of the HRA value with CVD risk ($r^2 = 0.99$) in Fig. 7.1 is a stimulus to learn how to interpret and benefit from that relationship.

A striking example of high and low HUFA balance values associated with death occurred for prostate cancer (Marugame and Mizuno, 2005). Five different countries in 1970 had age-adjusted prostate cancer death rates (per 100,000) that were approximately 50 in Japan, 300 in Italy, and about 500 in the United States, United Kingdom, and France. At that time, the corresponding average HRA values of %n–6 in HUFA in those countries were about 35%, 60%, and 70–80%, respectively. While the death rates and the HRA values in the United States, United Kingdom, and France remained relatively unchanged during the next 30 years, average HRA values in Japan rose from 35 to 50%, and the death rate rose from 50 to 150. During that time in Italy, the average HRA value rose from 60 to 70% and the death rate rose from 300 to 500 per 100,000 population. Specific factors causing prevalent prostatic hyperplasia in older men worldwide to transition into fatal malignancy are not identified. Whatever causes higher prostate cancer death rates to associate with higher tissue percentage of n–6 in HUFA merits careful interpretation. Clues to enhanced tumor proliferation are briefly noted in the Section on *Inflammation has Many Outcomes*.

Most scientists caution the public that correlation alone must not be taken as proof that the HRA measurement is monitoring a cause of death. The correlation of the percentage of n–6 in HUFA with CVD first appeared with fragmentary data (Lands et al., 1992). By the time the strong correlation ($r^2 = 0.99$) became evident (Lands, 2003a), clinicians already had decades of experience using a different biomarker, blood cholesterol, to predict risk for CVD, and heart attacks. Many committees of biomedical experts have agreed that blood cholesterol was an important and useful predictor for risk of a heart attack.

Considering Blood Cholesterol Levels

Among Americans, higher levels of cholesterol associate with higher rates of CVD death. However, two very large expensive clinical trials attempted to lower the cholesterol and the risk of death without finding clear evidence that cholesterol has a causal role (reviewed by Lands, 2008). Before starting another large study, the United States National Institutes of Health convened a Consensus Conference of 14 experts to review the evidence in 1984. The experts unanimously declared cholesterol to be a cause of CVD (Consensus, 1985), and new studies with cholesterol-lowering drugs were initiated. Public health messages worldwide gave advice for people to monitor their plasma cholesterol level and to take steps to lower it if it was above 220 mg/100 mL. Plasma cholesterol had become regarded as a valid surrogate for the clinical condition of CVD without a clearly identified mechanism by which it actually mediated pathophysiology (Lands, 2015a).

An important aspect of blood cholesterol levels was noted by the Consensus Conference, but poorly implemented. The experts recognized that excess food energy elevated levels of cholesterol, and they urged removing that cause by *"use of diet as a primary mode of therapy"*. They noted that *"Drug therapy should be used only after a careful trial of diet modification using the most rigorous diet appropriate"* and *"Even when drugs seem appropriate, it is important to stress that maximal diet therapy should be continued."* What occurred after that was an explosive financial investment in developing, marketing and using cholesterol-lowering drugs while the nation experienced a steady rise in the prevalence of food energy imbalance and obesity. Advice to decrease the causal food energy imbalances was not effectively implemented.

After a large clinical trial, ENHANCE (Kastelein et al., 2008), lowered blood cholesterol levels without a corresponding lowering of cardiovascular events, doubts about the causal role of cholesterol in CVD began to appear in the public media (Carey, 2008; Couzin, 2008). Was cholesterol just an associated consequence of the acknowledged underlying cause, food energy imbalance, which elevates both cholesterol and the disease process? Questions about how the large, expensive drug-treatment study failed to lower unwanted clinical conditions created public confusion and concern. The key hypothesis in designing the intervention had been to regard the associated biomarker, cholesterol, as a causal mediator of pathophysiology and therefore a valid surrogate for the disease. If the cholesterol level were mediating the disease, then lowering cholesterol should lower the risk of disease. That did not occur with the ENHANCE Trial. Of course, if cholesterol were not the cause, lowering it would not necessarily lower the disease. Now people could consider the question: if the cholesterol biomarker was not mediating the risk of disease, what was?

In this regard, a large 25-year multinational clinical study (Verschuren et al., 1995) found that blood cholesterol levels predict risk for cardiovascular death only to the extent that people's HUFA balance has n–6 HUFA exceeding n–3 HUFA (ie, when percentage of n–6 in HUFA is greater than 50%). Fig. 7.2 shows that the blood cholesterol

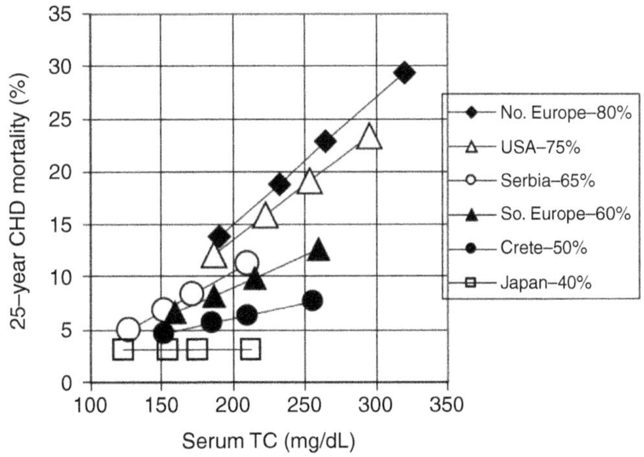

FIGURE 7.2 **HUFA balances alter the relationship of deaths to cholesterol levels.** Results from the 25-year follow-up for the Seven Countries Study (Verschuren et al., 1995) were discussed in an earlier review (Lands, 2008) which noted that "Food energy imbalances which elevate blood cholesterol may be fatal only to the degree that omega-6 (n–6) exceeds omega-3 (n–3) in tissue HUFA." Northern Europe and Southern Europe have abbreviations "No." and "So.," respectively. *Source: Reprinted from Lands, 2008, Figure 13.*

level is predictive for people in the USA and Northern Europe (with HRA values near 75–80%). However, it has no association with mortality for Japanese people who had average HRA biomarker levels near 40–50% n–6 in HUFA (Lands, 2003b). Extensive data from 173,539 subjects confirmed that Japanese death rates were not higher with higher blood cholesterol levels (Ogushi et al., 2009). In fact, death rates for Japanese with 240 mg cholesterol/100 mL were lower than those for Japanese with 160 mg cholesterol/100 mL.

Paradoxical results from Japan give a reminder that a wide range of blood cholesterol levels occur in humans regarded as healthy. Fig. 7.1 shows the observed death rate for the "generally healthy" USA population with a high average HRA value (indicating a high risk of harm) is only 200 per year for 100,000 people. The prediction of a high risk for harm in a group of people can alert them to take steps to avoid harm. However, designing effective interventions requires knowledge of explicit interactions that allow different proportions of HUFA to alter blood cholesterol's ability to be an effective HRA predictor. The Section on *HUFA Balance Affects Food Energy Toxicity* examines how the percentage of n–6 in HUFA biomarker can be a valid surrogate for the clinical condition among different ethnic groups when cholesterol is not. Another step forward in understanding that association came when we learned how a high or low status of the tissue HUFA biomarker is controlled by the balance of n–3 and n–6 nutrients present in different ethnic food habits.

TWO ESSENTIAL NUTRIENTS COMPETE FOR A PLACE IN LIFE

The two most abundant essential fatty acids in nature are linoleic (18:2n–6) and alpha-linolenic (18:3n—3) acids. These two 18-carbon polyunsaturated fatty acids (PUFA) are made by plant foliage and algae. Accompanying them in some cases are lesser amounts of two PUFA homologs, gamma-linolenic (18:3n–6) and stearidonic (18:4n–3) acids. Animals and humans cannot make the n–3 and n–6 essential fatty acids and must obtain them from foods (Burr and Burr, 1930; Lands, 2015c). After being eaten by animals, the n–3 and n–6 18-carbon PUFAs are further metabolized by an array of desaturating and elongating enzymes to form two closely-related families of 20- and 22-carbon highly unsaturated fatty acids (HUFA) shown in Fig. 7.3. Most of the enzymes that add more double bonds and extend the chain length of these very similar fatty acids do not discriminate appreciably between the n–3 and n–6 structures.

Indiscriminate actions with regard to the terminal double bond structure occur also with other lipid metabolizing enzymes that form and hydrolyze the acyl-CoA derivatives as well as the esters in triglycerides and phospholipids. The lack of discrimination by those enzymes causes the relative availability of competing acids to strongly influence the relative amounts of product accumulated in n–3 and n–6 HUFA. In this way, the balance of n–3 and n–6

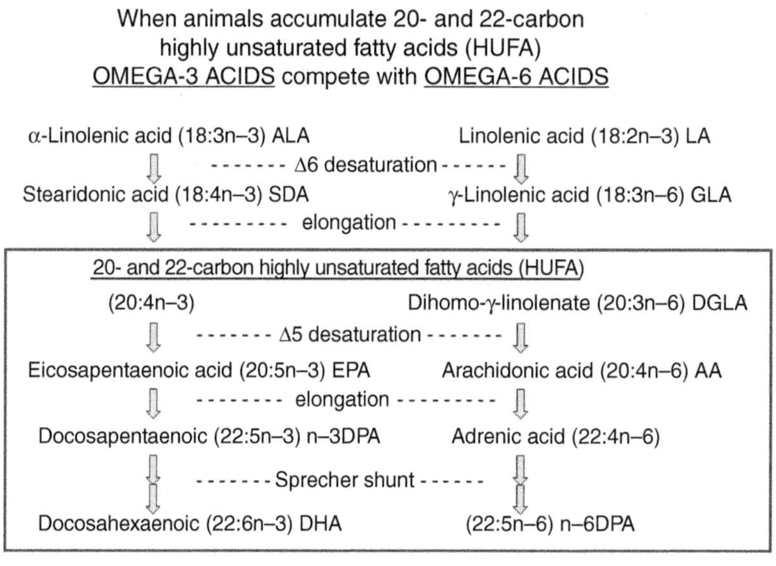

FIGURE 7.3 **The n-3 and n-6 PUFA compete while forming HUFA.** The four 18-carbon PUFA found in plants are converted in animals by multiple enzymatic steps to 20- and 22-carbon HUFA and stored in tissue lipids. *Source: Reprinted from Lands, 2015c, Figure 2.*

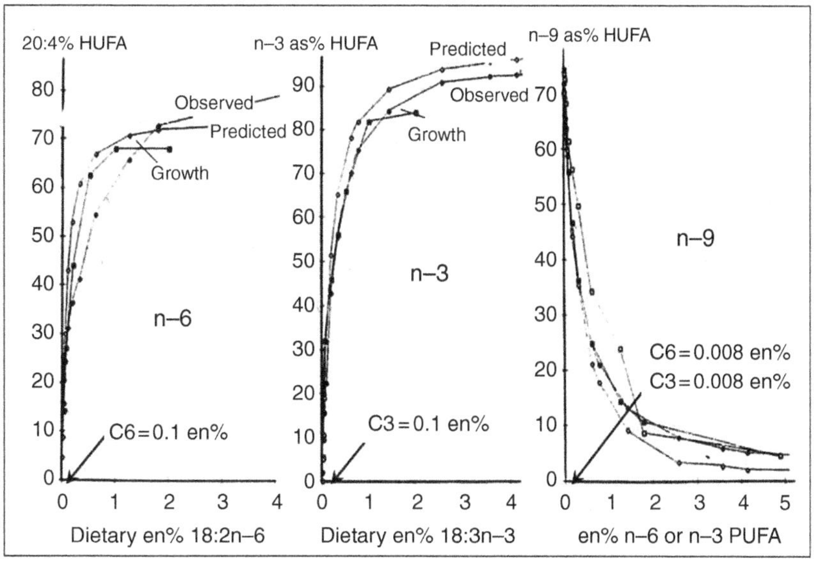

FIGURE 7.4 **Competitive hyperbolic dynamics in accumulating and displacing HUFA.**

nutrients in daily foods determines the balance of n–3 and n–6 HUFA maintained in tissues (Lands, 2014). That food-determined balance is the HRA value which predicts health outcomes as noted above.

Details of the dynamics of conversion and accumulation into tissue HUFA by competing dietary linoleic and alpha-linolenic acids were elegantly documented by Mohrhauer and Holman many years ago (Mohrhauer and Holman, 1963a, 1963b). The efficiency of these two acids in forming and accumulating n–3 and n–6 HUFA and in supporting growth of young animals was seen in a sensitive dose-response manner that had a midpoint dietary dose for both HUFA accumulation and growth near 0.1% of food energy (0.1 en%) (Fig. 7.4). Competition was evident for forming and accumulating the n–9 HUFA, 20:3n–9, from oleic acid already present in animal tissues. Fig. 7.4 shows efficient displacement of the n–9 HUFA from tissue lipids as the dietary supply of either n–3 or n–6 nutrient increased.

Oleic (18:1n–9), palmitic (16:0), and stearic (18:0) acids are major forms of energy storage in humans. They are made and accumulated from the key intermediate in food energy metabolism, acetyl-CoA. In the absence of dietary polyunsaturated acids which compete for the elongation and desaturation enzymes, the oleate made by animals accumulates in tissues as the n–9 HUFA, 20:3n–9. However, Fig. 7.4 shows that very small daily amounts of n–3 or n–6 nutrients (0.1 en%) are quite efficient in competitively lowering this accumulation as they form HUFA that displace the 20:3n–9. Dietary supplies of about 0.5 en% n–3 or n–6 nutrients which gave a level of accumulated HUFA greater than the n–9 HUFA were adequate to support growth of the young animals.

Quantitative Description of Diet-Tissue Dynamics

The accumulation of HUFA in animal tissues (Fig. 7.4) fits a simple hyperbolic pattern commonly seen for enzyme-catalyzed processes that involve saturable catalytic sites. Quantitative descriptions of how dietary abundance affects the accumulation of product in a competitive hyperbolic process fit a pattern familiar to all enzymologists.

$$\text{Rate} = \frac{V_{max}}{\left[1+K_s\left(1+\frac{I}{K_i}\right)/S\right]} \tag{7.1}$$

Where the maximum rate is V_{max}, substrate concentration is S, K_s is the substrate concentration giving half-maximal reaction rate, competitor concentration is I, and K_i is the competitor concentration giving half maximal inhibition.

The early diet-tissue results with laboratory animals (Mohrhauer and Holman, 1963a, 1963b) were confirmed and fitted to the predictive Eq. (7.1) in which constants for midpoint values of dietary supply were near 0.05 en% for both n–3 and n–6 nutrients (Lands et al., 1990). Surprisingly, the equation and constants developed for laboratory animals also fit closely with results from human volunteers eating standardized diets in a clinical study

(Lands et al., 1992). This result affirms the value of studying laboratory animals to understand basic aspects of lipid metabolism in humans.

Experimental results from rats allowed researchers to study in detail the essentiality of linoleic and alpha-linolenic acids for mammals. Importantly, animal studies determined accurately the small amounts of these essential nutrients needed to prevent the pathophysiology of deficiency. It is not ethical to create pathophysiology in humans to determine the borderline between deficiency and adequacy. However, limited results from a unique study of human infants (Hansen et al., 1963) fit closely with the more detailed data obtained from laboratory animals. With progressively lower dietary supply of dietary linoleic acid, the transition from healthy physiology to deficient pathophysiology for human babies was near 0.1 en%. That study was done decades ago and will never be done again.

Later observations of healthy infants in the United Kingdom, indicated that minimum requirements for linoleate must be below 0.5 en% (Cuthbertson, 1976). There is no longer a need to examine further the lower boundary between healthy physiology and pathophysiology. Most foods clearly provide more than enough essential n–6 nutrients. However, this review will later address the apparently narrow therapeutic window for n–6 linoleate (Lands, 2014) and the harmful impact of chronic daily intakes over 10 times the lowest effective amount.

Because of a growing interest in the 1980's about the impact of seafood on health (Lands, 1986), the empirical equation was expanded to include dietary n–3 and n–6 HUFA. The expanded equation (Lands et al., 1992) predicts the likely proportion of n–6 in HUFA (or n–3 in HUFA) by using the intake of four types of essential nutrients: n–3 and n–6 18-carbon PUFA plus n–3 and n–6 20- and 22-carbon HUFA. It allowed investigators in a small blinded clinical study to estimate accurately the number of fish oil capsules that individuals had been eating as daily dietary supplements. Overall, the expanded diet-tissue relationship (Eq. 7.2) fit results obtained with rats, mice, and humans. The equation successfully predicts the observed tissue HUFA balance reported from 34 different published studies of nearly 4,000 people in 92 groups from 11 different countries (Strandjord et al., submitted).

$$20:3+20:4\text{n}-6\,\text{in HUFA}=\frac{100}{1+\dfrac{HC_6}{\text{en}\%H6}\left(1+\dfrac{\text{en}\%H3}{HC_3}\right)}+\frac{100}{1+\dfrac{PC_6}{\text{en}\%P6}\left(1+\dfrac{\text{en}\%P3}{PC_3}+\dfrac{\text{en}\%H3}{HI_3}+\dfrac{\text{en}\%O}{C_0}+\dfrac{\text{en}\%P6}{K_S}\right)} \tag{7.2}$$

where, $HC_3=3.0; HC_6=0.70; PC_3=0.0555; PC_6=0.0441; HI_3=0.005; HI_6=0.040; C_0=5.0;$ and $K_S=0.175$.

When embedded into a simple spreadsheet calculator (Calculator, 2002), the equation combines the dietary intake of four fatty acids and estimates the likely HRA outcome in terms of %n–6 in HUFA to help clinical researchers design new dietary interventions. The calculator quickly shows competing impacts of n–3 and n–6 nutrients on the HUFA balance. While this approach aids designers of clinical trials, most food choices made by the public are based on individual familiar food items. People choose diverse food items and combine them in personal daily menu plans that fit their personal tastes. Something was needed to help individuals choose diverse food items to obtain and maintain a desired HUFA balance.

To estimate the likely outcome from a full daily menu of foods, Eq. (7.2) was combined with food data from the USDA Nutrient Database (USDA website) in an interactive, personalized menu planning software program. The program combined the amounts of eleven different n–3 and n–6 nutrients (expressed as en%) to estimate the likely HUFA balance resulting from the multiple food choices in a day's menu plan. The flexible adaptation of people's HUFA balance to the intake of various food combinations is illustrated by seven daily menu plans that combined familiar foods in combinations that give very different HRA values: 15%, 26%, 35%, 50%, 63%, 71%, and 91% (Lands, 2005).

Recognizing the Impact of Each Food Item

The impact of each individual food item on the HRA value is more easily evident when the contents of eleven competing n–3 and n–6 nutrients are converted into an Omega 3-6 Balance Score (Lands and Lamoreaux, 2012). The conversion uses the difference in the milligram per kilocalorie content (related to en%) to describe the essential fatty acid balance in an individual food item. The resulting Score is positive when n–3 exceed n–6 nutrients, and it is negative when n–6 exceed n–3 nutrients. As seen earlier with the competitive, hyperbolic equation, the HRA value of %n–6 in HUFA has a predictable relationship with the calorie-weighted average balance of n–3 and n–6 nutrients in foods eaten. Foods that have positive scores will increase the percentage of n–3 in HUFA, whereas foods with negative scores will decrease the %n–3 in HUFA (ie, increase the percentage of n6 in HUFA). Tissue HUFA balance values ranging from 20% to 80% n–6 in HUFA (Fig. 7.1) correspond to eating foods with average Omega 3-6 Balance Scores ranging from +3 to −7.

Individual food Scores vary from −100 to +200. Examples of Scores for familiar foods are: almonds, −22; avocado, −11; beef frankfurter, −3; cabbage, 0; carrots, −3; cashews, −13; caviar, +166; cauliflower, +3; cheddar cheese, −1; cheese pizza, −7; Cheerios, −4; chicken nuggets, −18; egg, −17; flax oil, +46; flaxmeal, +32; french fries, −10; green beans +1; ice cream, −1; kidney bean, 0; kippered herring, +70; mayonnaise, −36; milk, −1; oyster, +59; pepperoni, −7; potato, 0; potato salad, −21; pistachio, −23; rice, 0; salmon, +46; snack crackers, −18; tofu, −26; trout, +36; turkey, −8; turnip, +1; vegetable oils (canola, −10; corn, −59; olive, −10; grapeseed, −79; poppyseed, −71; soybean, −50); yogurt, 0.

The 100 most eaten foods in the USA (Haytowitz, 2012) have an unweighted average balance score of −6.2 (Lands and Lamoreaux, 2012), which corresponds to an HRA value near 75% n–6 in HUFA (between the 71% estimated for American nurses (Lands, 2015b; Table 1) and the 81% reported for American soldiers (Lin et al., 2014; Table 6). If ten foods with the most negative Scores were removed, the remaining 90 items would have an average Balance Score near −3.2, which corresponds to an HRA value near 61% n–6 in HUFA; a value typically seen with a traditional Mediterranean lifestyle and its lower risk for CVD. This aspect is likely the reason that a Mediterranean lifestyle became regarded as a healthy choice.

The percentage of n–6 in HUFA biomarker is an inescapable consequence of dietary habits, and it also strongly predicts unwanted health conditions like CVD that the National Heart Lung and Blood Institute plus the Centers for Disease Control regard as preventable (NHLBI, 2013). Knowing that CVD is preventable makes it paradoxical that more than two-thirds of Americans over 60 years of age currently have this disease (NHLBI, 2013). Some important information is missing in public dialogs to maintain this very high prevalence. Actions need to be taken to identify explicit ways in which the biomarker acts at the border between healthy physiology and pathophysiology so that appropriate steps can be taken to prevent further harm.

TWO FAMILIES OF EICOSANOIDS HAVE DIFFERENT IMPACTS

Knowing that the food-based biomarker percentage of n–6 in HUFA predicts chronic inflammatory and thrombotic aspects of CVD opens the question of how to use that knowledge. If the percentage of n–6 in HUFA is merely a related, predictive sign, lowering it may not lower the risk for disease in the way that lowering a valid surrogate would. However, the percentage of n–6 in HUFA develops from everyday food habits, and it mediates pathophysiology. Altering foods to lower it will likely lower the risk for CVD. Fifty years of biomedical evidence on HUFA-derived eicosanoids provide a basis for choosing effective preventive nutrition actions (Lands, 2015d).

Recognizing n–3 and n–6 Eicosanoids

The conversion of tissue HUFA into potent hormone-like mediators of physiology has a key role in human health (Lands, 1986, 2005). The conversion was first described simultaneously in 1964 by two different laboratories (van Dorp et al., 1964; Bergstrom et al., 1964). A highly stereospecific enzyme-catalyzed oxidation of the HUFA, arachidonate (20:4n–6), produced the cyclic oxidized n–6 derivative, prostaglandin E_2, which has potent biological actions. While the enzyme reacts with stereospecific control during the oxidation, it acts with other HUFA containing different numbers of double bonds to give prostaglandin E_1 from 20:3n–6 and prostaglandin E_3 from 20:5n–3 (Bergstroem et al., 1964). The different prostaglandins were quickly seen to have different potencies in affecting fatty acid mobilization from adipose tissue (Steinberg et al., 1964). Those different potencies are the beginning of understanding how HUFA balance affects human health.

What followed after that discovery was an explosive increase in biomedical research that discovered and interpreted many bioactive eicosanoid mediators formed from HUFA (Fig. 7.5). Eventually, three types of fatty acid oxidizing enzymes, cyclooxygenases, lipoxygenases, and cytochrome P450 oxidases, were recognized to generate three different families of bioactive lipid signaling agents: prostaglandins, leukotrienes, and epoxides (Lands, 2012). Other bioactive materials from n–3 HUFA (eg, resolvins, maresins, protectins; Spite et al., 2014) may counteract n–6-mediated disorders, emphasizing the benefit of a HUFA balance with more n–3 than n–6 HUFA. Each new mediator had one or more specific membrane-bound receptors that bound the eicosanoid and transmitted a signal into the cell and affected cell physiology. The enzymes and receptors became targets for designing new drugs that selectively altered the intensity of eicosanoid actions. The past few decades gave extensive evidence for eicosanoid actions at one or more diverse eicosanoid receptors which became recognized to occur on nearly every cell and tissue in the body.

Different Potencies in Eicosanoid Actions

As noted earlier, the enzymes converting dietary n–3 and n–6 18-carbon PUFA into the 20- and 22-carbon HUFA and accumulating them in tissue phospholipids are not appreciably influenced by different n–3 and n–6 structural

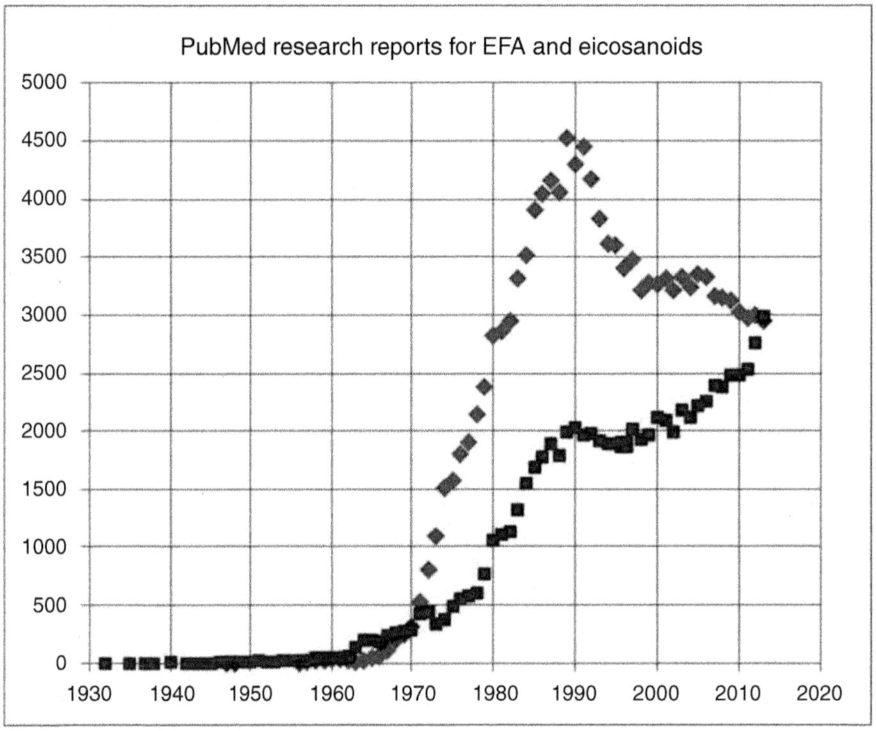

FIGURE 7.5 **Research reports for essential fatty acids and eicosanoids.** *Dark gray (red in the online version) squares* indicate annual reports retrieved by PubMed for the combined terms: essential fatty acids or linoleic or linolenic or arachidonic or eicosapentaenoic or docosahexaenoic. *Gray (blue in the online version) diamonds* indicate annual reports retrieved for the term: eicosanoids. *Source: Reprinted from Lands, 2015c, Figure 3.*

features. That allows the relative abundance in the diet to be the major factor controlling the HUFA balance accumulated in tissues. Relatively indiscriminate action also occurs with phospholipase release of HUFA from tissue phospholipids (Leslie, 2004), making the relative abundance of accumulated n–3 and n–6 tissue HUFA affect the relative amounts of substrate made available to the oxidizing enzymes that form potent eicosanoids (Fig. 7.6). In contrast to the phospholipase $cPLA_2$ lack of specificity, some of the enzymes that convert HUFA into bioactive mediators and some of the receptors that transduce mediator signals into physiological responses selectively discriminate between n–3 and n–6 structures (Wada et al., 2007). The biomedical community is still in the early stages of recognizing the extremely broad impact that HUFA balance has on physiological signals that result from release of HUFA from tissue membranes.

The cyclooxygenases, COX-1 and COX-2, form prostaglandin H more intensely with n-6 arachidonic acid (20:4n-6) than n-3 eicosapentaenoic acid (20:5n-3) (Wada et al., 2007). The PGD synthase and PGE synthase also form n-6 products more rapidly than n–3 products. Finally, all four EP receptors work several-fold more intensely with the n–6 PGE_2 than the n–3 PGE_3. These selectives mean that physiological processes amplified by prostaglandin derivatives are more intense when the tissue HUFA balance has more than 50%n–6 in HUFA compared to having less. Intense n–6 actions by prostaglandin receptors sometimes shift healthy physiology toward pathophysiology, enhancing chronic inflammatory processes during atherogenesis and thrombotic platelet aggregation in heart attacks (Lands, 2015d).

The 5-lipoxygenase that forms leukotriene A acts equally well with n–3 and n–6 substrates, but conversion of the n–6 LTA_4 to cysteinyl leukotrienes is much more intense than with the n–3 LTA_5 (Murphy et al., 1981; Soderstrom et al., 1992). As a result, broncho-pulmonary distress in asthma and chronic obstructive pulmonary disease (COPD) is greater when the percentage of n–6 in HUFA is high. A major driver of immune-inflammatory conditions comes from selective action of the high affinity BLT_1 receptor signaling that has a 100-fold greater intensity with n–6 LTB_4 compared to n–3 LTB_5 (Lee et al., 1988).

The bottom row of information in Fig. 7.6 shows relative responses of G-protein-coupled eicosanoid receptors elicited by n–3 ligands compared to n–6 ligands. When bound to their ligand, prostanoid receptors (DP; EP_2; EP_4; IP) signal into the cells via Gs-activated adenylylcyclase which increases cAMP-stimulated protein kinase A (PKA) actions. Alternatively, prostanoid EP_3 receptor signals into the cell via Gi, inhibiting adenylyl cyclase and lowering cAMP stimulation of PKA activity. The prostanoid receptors EP_1, EP_3, FP, and TP signal into the cell via Gq, activating

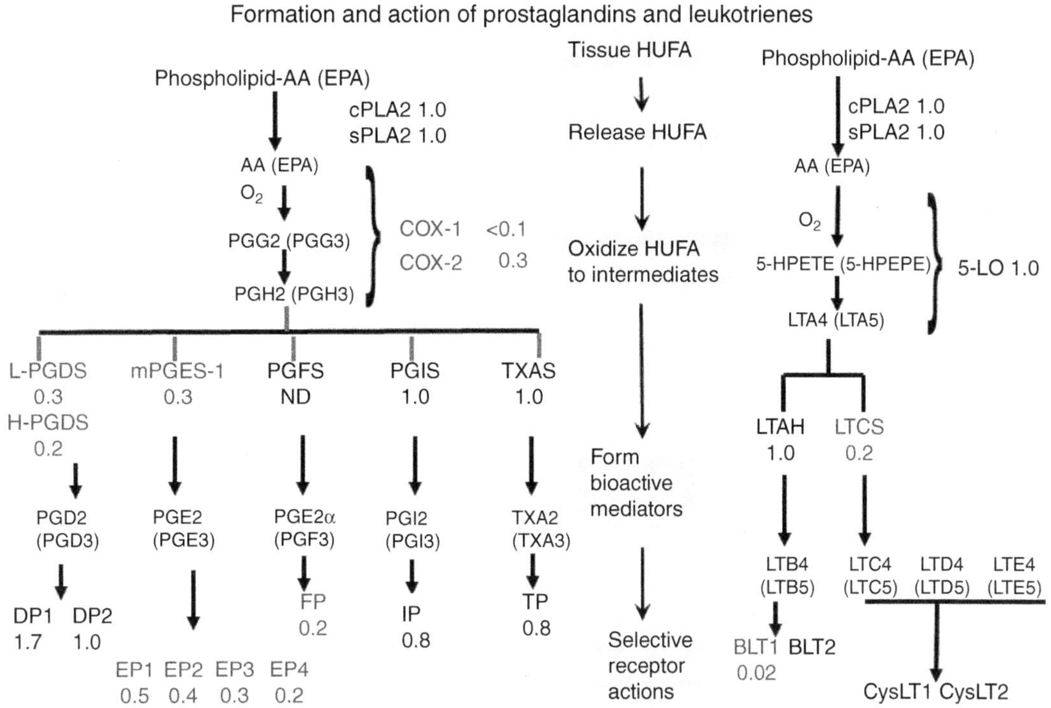

FIGURE 7.6 **Formation and action of prostaglandins and leukotrienes.** Numbers next to enzymes or receptors indicate ratios of the relative intensity of formation or signaling for the n–3/n–6 compounds. The *light gray (red in the web version) color* indicates situations in which the n-6 is much more potent than the n–3 mediator.

phosphoinositidase to give IP_3 plus diglycerides which enhance Ca^{2+} mobilization and stimulate protein kinase C (PKC) activity. Similar Ca^{2+} mobilization and PKC signaling via Gq may occur when the appropriate ligand binds to leukotriene receptors, BLT; $CysLT_1$; $CysLT_2$. Finally, leukotriene BLT_1 and BLT_2 receptors may also signal into the cell via Gi, inhibiting adenylyl cyclase and lowering cAMP stimulation of PKA activity (Yokomizo, 2011).

Undesired eicosanoid receptor signaling is increasingly recognized to give very diverse unwanted health conditions. EP_1 receptor signaling with PGE_2 attenuates the mesocortical dopaminergic pathway and mediates acquisition of social defeat behaviors (Tanaka et al., 2012). These can be less when the EP_1 receptor binds an inhibitor or the less potent PGE_3. The TP receptor mobilization of Ca^{2+} in blood platelets can have fatal consequences in heart attacks, providing the rationale for prophylactic use of low-dose aspirin (or fish oil supplements) to lower the intensity of thromboxane A_2 (TXA_2) formation. The pharmaceutical industry has identified many pathophysiological conditions made worse by excessive n–6 eicosanoid actions (Lands, 2015d). Examples include arthritis, asthma, COPD, cardiovascular diseases (including atherogenesis and thrombosis), metabolic syndrome, back pain, headache, hypertension, bone density loss, cancer proliferation, behavioral disorders, oppositional behaviors, depression, and suicide.

The 100-fold greater intensity of n–6 LTB_4 compared to n–3 LTB_5 acting through the BLT_1 receptor (Lee et al., 1988) makes it clear that food choices can influence inflammatory conditions as LTB stimulates monocyte chemotaxis, adhesion, and activation. The past two decades of biomedical research have made it clear that preventable food-based chronic inflammatory processes underlie much human distress and many serious clinical disorders. The very narrow therapeutic window for n–6 nutrients (Lands, 2014) makes it wise to eat it at the lowest effective level and eat more competing n–3 nutrients to prevent food-related harm.

Inflammation has Many Outcomes

Atherosclerosis is an inflammatory disease that begins with diet-induced vascular endothelial dysfunction (Ross, 1999) which is likely initiated by transient excessive postprandial food energy and release of nonesterified fatty acids. The resulting oxidative stress and suppressed nitric oxide formation lead to accumulated leukocytes which recruit more leukocytes and begin development of chronic inflammatory plaques. The inflammatory plaques begin forming at bifurcations where eddy currents (Ku et al., 1985; Giddens et al., 1993) allow leukocytes, chemokines, and cytokines to have longer residence times and amplify the endothelial dysfunction. This is amplified by the potent chemotactic action of LTB_4 attracting more leukocytes to the area and enhancing their adhesion and activation to release more chemokines. The steady progression of vascular inflammation which eventually limits blood flow in coronary and carotid arteries begins by adolescence and continues in severity year-by-year (Strong et al., 1999). Its prevalence is greater among people with HUFA balance values greater than 50% n–6 in HUFA (Fig. 7.1).

Obesity is much more than accumulated triglyceride in adipocytes. It has a systemic inflammatory aspect as adipose tissue gradually accumulates leukocytes as major cellular components arrayed in crown-like structures around adipocytes (Mohanan et al., 2013). Macrophages are scarce in adipose tissue of people of normal weight, and they increase markedly in morbid obesity. The inflammatory cells release mediators that recruit more inflammatory cells. They become more prevalent in omental/abdominal regions than subcutaneous regions (Cancello et al., 2006), illustrating a basis for the greater CVD risk from "apple" than "pear" body shapes. Macrophages contain the key genes for n–6 enhanced inflammatory signaling pathways acting in morbid obesity (Xu et al., 2003).

The long-standing association between tumor proliferation and cyclooxygenase, n–6 eicosanoids and inflammatory conditions may be due to TXA_2 acting through the TP receptor. This action increases intracellular Ca^{2+} as a critical mediator for tumor-promoting effects of cyclooxygenase-2 (COX-2) (Huang et al., 2014). Blocking the TP receptor arrested cells at the G2/M phase and induced apoptosis. TP also has an important role in pathology of prostate cancer (Nie et al., 2008). Expression of TPα correlated with increasing prostate and breast tissue tumors, and a TXA_2 mimetic promoted both proliferation and migration of the respective prostate- and breast-derived carcinoma cell lines (Keating et al., 2014). The significant rise in prostate cancer deaths in Japan as the HUFA balance of the population rises was mentioned in the Section on *Considering Blood Cholesterol Level*. It is an example of a missed opportunity for constructive preventive nutrition that arranges to NIX the 6 and EAT the 3.

Macrophage-related inflammatory activities contribute to obesity-induced insulin resistance: a chronic inflammatory disorder (Grant and Stephens, 2015). The release of proinflammatory cytokines stimulates lipolysis and enhances insulin resistance, leading to adipose tissue dysfunction and systemic disruptions of metabolism. Li et al. (2015) noted that macrophages can become 40% of the cells in visceral fat of obese people. Other immune cells (lymphocytes, eosinophils, and neutrophils) also add to inflammatory conditions in obesity. Gene knockout mice missing the BLT1 receptor were protected from inflammation and insulin resistance (Spite et al., 2011). LTB_4 directly inhibits about half of the insulin-stimulated glucose transport in myocytes. LTB_4 acts through BLT1 and Gi through a mechanism dependent on c-Jun-N-terminal kinase to interfere with insulin-stimulated protein kinase B phosphorylation and translocation of the glucose transporter type 4 (Li et al., 2015).

HUFA Balance Affects Food Energy Toxicity

Inflammatory mediators released from the macrophages arrayed as crown-like structures around adipocytes contribute much to the pathophysiology of obesity. However, restricting calorie intake reversed inflammation with more than a 75% decrease in crown-like structures and normalized levels of proinflammatory mediators (Bhardwaj et al., 2013). Knowledge of this example of food energy toxicity and its reversal might have constructively altered discussions at the 1984 Consensus Conference on cardiovascular disease noted above. Even though the conference report put strong emphasis on decreasing the causal imbalance in food energy (Consensus, 1985), the conference facilitated a rapid introduction and use of cholesterol-lowering drugs to lower a food energy-related risk factor, (reviewed in Lands, 2008). Fig. 7.2 shows that the ability of blood cholesterol to predict CVD death depends on the extent to which the HUFA balance has more n–6 than n–3 in HUFA. When the balance favors n–3 HUFA, transient postprandial insults appear to become resolved, and when the balance favors n–6 HUFA, the transient insults become transformed into chronic inflammatory vascular injury (Lands, 2014). Eating fewer calories per meal, less n–6 nutrients and more n–3 nutrients can prevent the chronic injury.

TWO CHOICES: PREVENT THE CAUSE OR TREAT SIGNS AND SYMPTOMS

With the growing awareness of food-based mediators of pathophysiology, very important issues arise. Is it ethical to wait for a food-based disease to develop until obvious clinical signs and symptoms appear before applying biomedical information to prevent those signs and symptoms? Is it ethical to diminish clinical signs and symptoms with drugs while the food-based cause of the signs and symptoms is left unchanged, causing a continual need for future medications? Moderating excessive n–6 actions by treatments with expensive selective drugs has been highly profitable, and the costs for treatments have risen dramatically. Can society profit by helping people prevent the need for treatments by making voluntary food choices that lower the n–6 arachidonate availability and increase competing n–3 HUFA substrates? Each person who voluntarily lowers intakes of n–6 nutrients and increases intakes of n–3 nutrients (http://efaeducation.org/?p=226; NIX the 6 and EAT the 3) is free to experience the physiological consequence of a HUFA balance that prevents over-reactions of n–6 eicosanoids.

Fig. 7.4 shows how the response to increased supplies of n–6 nutrient forms a "plateau" and is no longer evident above a certain intake. This saturable phenomenon is also evident when reversing platelet aggregation mediated by the n–6 TXA2. After 4 weeks of supplemental n–3 HUFA, patients with high production of thromboxane showed little reduction in aggregation response, whereas patients with lower production had marked reduction in aggregation sensitivity (Figure 3 in Lands et al., 1985). Risk for 13 morbidity and mortality outcomes (including all causes, coronary heart disease, stroke, cardiovascular disease, homicide, bipolar disorder, and major postpartum depressions) associates with dietary availability of n–3 HUFA in 38 countries (Hibbeln et al., 2006). A healthy intake of n–3 HUFA was estimated at 3.5 g/day for a current United States 2000-kcal diet containing 7 en% n–6 linoleate (Hibbeln et al., 2006). The estimate can be reduced to one-tenth of that amount by consuming fewer n–6 fats. Lowering the supply of n–6 mediators gives a better HUFA balance.

Pain and distress were clearly less when the percentage of n–6 in HUFA was lowered in 3 months in a controlled secondary prevention clinical trial using the tactic of lowering n–6 intakes while raising n–3 intakes (Ramsden et al., 2013). If this type of nutritional intervention to shift HUFA balance succeeds for secondary prevention with people already having disease, it will likely benefit people in a primary prevention mode. Objective measurable outcomes would be a higher sense of well-being and lower annual health-care costs. The open challenge to those who understand the information in this review is to apply the knowledge in balancing their personal daily food choices for eating foods from the land and sea.

TWO ORIGINS OF FOOD: LAND AND SEA

Dietitians and nutritionists often classify foods as plant or animal, but they could direct attention to two different locations from which the food originates: land and sea. In both locations, animals obtain their essential n–3 and n–6 nutrients from the plants around them or from smaller animals that ate those plants. However, the two locations differ in a striking way on the relative supply of n–3 and n–6 nutrients. Major land-based plants have foliage that converts solar energy, carbon dioxide, and minerals into the materials of life. A system of land-based agriculture creates a food chain in which plant products supply needed energy and nutrients for producing chicken, turkey, pork, and beef. Plants make both n–3 and n–6 18-carbon PUFA, and most of their seeds (nuts, grains, and cereals) are rich in n–6 fats. The n–6 fats particularly abundant in seed oils have been used increasingly in "Westernized" foods after the start of the 20th century (Blasbalg et al., 2011). Now, people should regard the narrow therapeutic window for n–6 linoleic acid in preventing deficiency yet not producing harm (Lands, 2014) and consider eating the lowest effective amount to avoid harmful HUFA balances.

In marine environments, aquatic plants, diatoms and algae often contain more n–3 than n–6 fats (Lands, 2015c). Diatoms elongate and desaturate PUFA and form appreciable amounts of HUFA (more n–3 than n–6). They are important food for molluscs, fishes, and copepods, and copepods are also consumed by crustaceans, molluscs, and fishes. The flow of food energy and essential nutrients in the aquatic environment moves through a complex open food web rather than a simple linear food chain. The seas and oceans provide a relatively uncontrolled web of wild foods that humans eat as a rich source of essential n–3 HUFA.

Fishermen are the last of the major hunter–forager groups of humans. In contrast, farmers supply a controlled food chain for farmed animals rather than the open food web that nature provides to fish and seafood in the open seas. Farmers raising seafood often feed much more n–6 than n–3 nutrients than would be available in wild, open environments. This aspect is evident in the increasing proportion of marketed seafood that has been raised in controlled, intensive farming conditions. The consequence of different food supplies affects the animals fed/farmed as well as the humans eating them.

The balance of n–3 and n–6 nutrients in different foods is easily recognized in their omega 3–6 balance scores (Omega 3-6 Balance Apps, 2014). Wild-caught foods will have Scores that reflect the wild environment in which they lived. In contrast, Scores for farmed foods will depend greatly on selections the farmer provides. Typical values for farm-raised meats are negative, indicating more n–6 than n–3 nutrients. These values are mainly due to grains providing the major source of energy and PUFA for the farmed animals. However, foods from the sea have positive scores indicating more n-3 than n-6 nutrients.

Land-based grains now provide much of the food energy and PUFA for humans. Also, legumes are important for their high protein content, as well as a high amount of energy in the fat of soybeans and peanuts. The difference between foods from the land and sea becomes especially striking when the oils extracted from the foods are compared. Many vegetable oils have very negative balance scores: corn oil, −59; peanut oil, −36; rice oil, −36; soybean oil, −59; sunflower oil, −74; wheat oil, −54. They differ greatly from fish oils: cod liver, +140; herring, +86; menhaden, +200; salmon, +263; sardine, +166. The large contrast in Omega 3–6 Balance Scores for food oils from the land and the sea creates very different impacts on the HUFA balance in human tissues and on the health consequences that flow from the HRA biomarker, the percentage of n–6 in HUFA.

Fig. 7.1 illustrates the range of HUFA balance that can occur when people eat different combinations of foods. A significant difference in balance gives a significant difference in health risk. Fig. 7.6 indicates some of the selective processes by which food choices have serious consequences. "Apps" are available to help readers navigate the numbers involved in balancing 11 different n–3 and n–6 nutrients. Readers are free to estimate the impact that a familiar food has on their health risk and make choices in accord with their own personal priorities.

Acknowledgment

The author thanks Dr. N. Schoene for helpful advice on the manuscript.

Abbreviations

CHD	Coronary heart disease
CVD	Cardiovascular disease
COPD	Chronic obstructive pulmonary disease
CoA	Coenzyme A
COX	Cyclooxygenases
ENHANCE	Ezetimibe and simvastatin in hypercholesterolemia enhances atherosclerosis regression trial
en%	Percent of food energy
HRA	Health risk assessment
HUFA	Highly unsaturated fatty acids
MRFIT	Multiple risk factor intervention trial
n–3	Omega-3
n–6	Omega-6
PKA	Protein kinase A
PKC	Protein kinase C
PUFA	Polyunsaturated fatty acids
TP	Thromboxane receptor
TXA2	The n–6 thromboxane A2

References

Bhardwaj, P., Du, B., Zhou, X.K., Sue, E., Harbus, M.D., Falcone, D.J., Giri, D., Hudis, C.A., Kopelovich, L., Subbaramaiah, K., Dannenberg, A.J., 2013. Caloric restriction reverses obesity-induced mammary gland inflammation in mice. Cancer Prev. Res. (Philadelphia). 6 (4), 282–289.

Bergstroem, S., Danielsson, H., Klenberg, D., Samuelsson, B., 1964. The enzymatic conversion of essential fatty acids into prostaglandins. J. Biol. Chem. 239, PC4006–PC4008.

Bergstrom, S., Danielsson, H., Samuelsson, B., 1964. The enzymatic formation of prostaglandin E2 from arachidonic acid prostaglandins and related factors 32. Biochem. Biophys. Acta 90 (1), 207–210.

Bibus, D., Lands, B., 2015. Balancing proportions of competing omega-3 and omega-6 highly unsaturated fatty acids (HUFA) in tissue lipids. Prostagland. Leukotr. Essen. Fatty Acid. 2015. 99, 19–23, http://www.plefa.com/article/S0952-3278(15)00087-3/pdf.

Blasbalg, T.L., Hibbeln, J.R., Ramsden, C.E., Majchrzak, S.F., Rawlings, R.R., 2011. Changes in consumption of omega-3 and omega-6 fatty acids in the United States during the 20th century. Am. J. Clin. Nutr. 93 (5), 950–962.

Burr, G.O., Burr, M.M., 1930. On the nature and role of the fatty acids essential in nutrition. J. Biol. Chem. 86, 587–621.

Calculator 2002. http://efaeducation.org/omega_foods_apps/dietary-balance/

Cancello, R., Tordjman, J., Poitou, C., Guilhem, G., Bouillot, J.L., Hugol, D., Coussieu, C., Basdevant, A., Bar Hen, A., Bedossa, P., Guerre-Millo, M., Clément, K., et al., 2006. Increased infiltration of macrophages in omental adipose tissue is associated with marked hepatic lesions in morbid human obesity. Diabetes 55, 1554–1561.

Carey, J. 2008. Heart disease: not about cholesterol? Business Week. http://www.businessweek.com/bwdaily/dnflash/content/apr2008/db20080414_688906.htm

Consensus conference, 1985. Lowering blood cholesterol to prevent heart disease. JAMA 253 (14), 2080–2086.

Couzin, J., 2008. Cholesterol veers off script. Science 322, 220–223.

Cuthbertson, W.F.J., 1976. Essential fatty acid requirements in infancy. Am. J. Clin. Nutr. 29, 559–568, http://ajcn.nutrition.org/content/29/5/559.long.

Dewailly, E., Blanchet, C., Gingras, S., Lemieux, S., Holub, B.J., 2002. Cardiovascular disease risk factors and n3 fatty acid status in the adult population of James Bay Cree. Am. J. Clin. Nutr. 76 (1), 85–92, http://ajcn.nutrition.org/content/76/1/85.full.pdf+html.

Dewailly, E., Blanchet, C., Lemieux, S., Sauve, L., Gingras, S., Ayotte, P., Holub, B.J., 2001b. n-3 fatty acids and cardiovascular disease risk factors among the Inuit of Nunavik. Am. J. Clin. Nutr. 74 (4), 464–473, http://ajcn.nutrition.org/content/74/4/464.full.pdf+html.

Dewailly, E.E., Blanchet, C., Gingras, S., Lemieux, S., Sauvé, L., Bergeron, J., Holub, B.J., 2001a. Relations between n-3 fatty acid status and cardiovascular disease risk factors among Quebecers. Am. J. Clin. Nutr. Nov. 74 (5), 603–611, PubMed PMID: 11684528. http://ajcn.nutrition.org/content/74/5/603.full.pdf+html.

Giddens, D.P., Zarins, C.K., Glagov, S., 1993. The role of fluid mechanics in the localization and detection of atherosclerosis. J. Biomech. Eng. 115 (4B), 588–594.

Grant, R.W., Stephens, J.M., 2015. Fat in flames: Influence of cytokines and pattern recognition receptors on adipocyte lipolysis. Am. J. Physiol. Endocrinol. Metab.

Hansen, A.E., Wiese, H.F., Boelsche, A.N., Haggard, M.E., Adam, D.J.D., Davis, H., 1963. Role of linoleic acid in infant nutrition. Clinical and chemical study of 428 infants fed on milk mixtures varying in kind and amount of fat. Pediatrics 31, 171–192.

Haytowitz, D.B. 2012 List of Key Foods Based on NHANES 2007–08. http://www.ars.usda.gov/SP2UserFiles/Place/12354500/Data/KeyFoods/Keyfoods_0708.xlsx

Hibbeln, J.R., Nieminen, L.R., Blasbalg, T.L., Riggs, J.A., Lands, W.E., 2006. Healthy intakes of n-3 and n-6 fatty acids: estimations considering worldwide diversity. Am. J. Clin. Nutr. 83 (6 (Suppl.)), 1483S–1493S.

Huang, R.Y., Li, S.S., Guo, H.Z., Huang, Y., Zhang, X., Li, M.Y., Chen, G.G., Zeng, X., 2014. Thromboxane A2 exerts promoting effects on cell proliferation through mediating cyclooxygenase-2 signal in lung adenocarcinoma cells. J. Cancer Res. Clin. Oncol., 2014;140 (3):375–386.

Kastelein, J.J., Akdim, F., Stroes, E.S., Zwinderman, A.H., Bots, M.L., Stalenhoef, A.F., Visseren, F.L., Sijbrands, E.J., Trip, M.D., Stein, E.A., Gaudet, D., Duivenvoorden, R., Veltri, E.P., Marais, A.D., de Groot E., 2008. ENHANCE Investigators. Simvastatin with or without ezetimibe in familial hypercholesterolemia. New England J. Med. 358 (14), 1431–1443.

Keating, G.L., Reid, H.M., Eivers, S.B., Mulvaney, E.P., Kinsella, B.T., 2014. Transcriptional regulation of the human thromboxane A(2) receptor gene by Wilms' tumor (WT)1 and hypermethylated in cancer (HIC) 1 in prostate and breast cancers. Biochem. Biophys. Acta Gene Regul. Mech. 1839 (6), 476–492.

Kobayashi, M., Sasaki, S., Kawabata, T., Hasegawa, K., Akabane, M., Tsugane, S., 2001. Single measurement of serum phospholipid fatty acid as a biomarker of specific fatty acid intake in middle-aged Japanese men. Eur. J. Clin. Nutr. 55, 643–650.

Ku, D.N., Giddens, D.P., Zarins, C.K., Glagov, S., 1985. Pulsatile flow and atherosclerosis in the human carotid bifurcation. Positive correlation between plaque location and low oscillating shear stress. Arteriosclerosis 5 (3), 293–302.

Lands, B., 2008. A critique of paradoxes in current advice on dietary lipids. Prog. Lipid Res. 47 (2), 77–106.

Lands, B., 2012. Consequences of Essential Fatty Acids. Nutrients 4, 1338–1357, http://www.ncbi.nlm.nih.gov/pmc/articles/PMC3475243/pdf/nutrients-04-01338.pdf.

Lands, B., 2014. Historical perspectives on the impact of n-3 and n-6 nutrients on health. Prog. Lipid. Res. 55, 17–29, http://www.sciencedirect.com/science/article/pii/S0163782714000253.

Lands, B., 2015a. Cholesterol: The Most Misunderstood Marker. Handbook of Cholesterol: Biology, function and role in health and diseases. In: Watson, R., Meester, F.D., (Eds.), Wageningen Academic Publishers.

Lands, B., 2015b. Choosing Foods to Balance Competing n-3 and n-6 HUFA and Their Actions, EDP Sciences. http://www.ocl-journal.org/articles/ocl/pdf/first/ocl150008.pdf

Lands, B., 2015c. Essential Fatty Acids: the nature of staple foods. In: Caballero, Finglas, Toldrá (Eds.), Encyclopedia of Food and Health. Elsevier.

Lands, B., 2015d. Omega-3 PUFAs Lower the Propensity for Arachidonic Acid Cascade Overreactions. Biomed Res Int. 2015;2015:285135. http://www.hindawi.com/journals/bmri/aa/285135/.

Lands, B., Lamoreaux, E., 2012. Describing essential fatty acid balance as 3-6 differences rather than 3/6 ratios. Nutr. Metab. 9, 46–54, http://www.nutritionandmetabolism.com/content/pdf/1743-7075-9-46.pdf.

Lands, W.E.M., Culp, B.R., Hirai, A., Gorman, R., 1985. Relationship of thromboxane generation to the aggregation of platelets from humans: effects of eicosapentaenoic acid. Prostaglandins 30, 819–825.

Lands, W.E.M., 1986. Fish and Human Health. Academic Press, Orlando, FL.

Lands, W.E.M., 2005. Fish, Omega-3 and Human Health, Second edition AOCS Press, Champaign, IL.

Lands, W.E.M., 2003a. Diets could prevent many diseases. Lipids 38 (4), 317–321.

Lands, W.E.M., 2003b. Functional foods in primary prevention or nutraceuticals in secondary prevention? Curr. Top Nutraceut. Res. 1 (2), 113–120.

Lands, W.E.M., Libelt, B., Morris, A., Kramer, N.C., Prewitt, T.E., Bowen, P., Schmeisser, D., Davidson, M.H., Burns, J.H., 1992. Maintenance of lower proportions of n-6 eicosanoid precursors in phospholipids of human plasma in response to added dietary n-3 fatty acids. Biochem. Biophys. Acta 1180, 147–162.

Lands, W.E.M., Morris, A.J., Libelt, B., 1990. Quantitative effects of dietary polyunsaturated fats on the composition of fatty acids in rat tissues. Lipids 25, 505–516.

Lee, T.H., Sethi, T., Crea, A.E., Peters, W., Arm, J.P., Horton, C.E., Walport, M.J., Spur, B.W., 1988. Characterization of leukotriene B3: comparison of its biological activities with leukotriene B4 and leukotriene B5 in complement receptor enhancement, lysozyme release and chemotaxis of human neutrophils. Clin. Sci. (London) 74, 467–475.

Leslie, C.C., 2004. Regulation of the specific release of arachidonic acid by cytosolic phospholipase A2. Prostagland. Leukotr. Essen. Fatty Acid. 70 (4), 373–376.

Li, P., Oh, D.Y., Bandyopadhyay, G., Lagakos, W.S., Talukdar, S., Osborn, O., Johnson, A., Chung, H., Mayoral, R., Maris, M., Ofrecio, J.M., Taguchi, S., Lu, M., Olefsky, J.M. 2015. LTB4 promotes insulin resistance in obese mice by acting on macrophages, hepatocytes and myocytes. Nat. Med. 21 (3) :239–247.

Lin, Y.H., Hanson, J.A., Strandjord, S.E., Salem, N.M., Dretsch, M.N., Haub, M.D., Hibbeln, J.R., 2014. Fast transmethylation of total lipids in dried blood by microwave irradiation and its application to a population study. Lipids 49, 839–851.

Marugame, T., Mizuno, S., 2005. Comparison of prostate cancer mortality in five countries: France, Italy, Japan, UK and USA from the WHO Mortality Database (1960–2000). Japan J. Clin. Oncol. 35 (11), 690–691.

Mohanan, S., Horibata, S., McElwee, J.L., Dannenberg, A.J., Coonrod, S.A., 2013. Identification of macrophage extracellular trap-like structures in mammary gland adipose tissue: a preliminary study. Front Immunol. 4 pp. 67.

Mohrhauer, H., Holman, R.T., 1963a. The effect of dose level of essential fatty acids upon fatty acid composition of the rat liver. J. Lipid Res. 4, 151–159.

Mohrhauer, H., Holman, R.T., 1963b. Effect of linolenic acid upon the metabolism of linoleic acid. J. Nutr. 81, 67–74.

Murphy, R.C., Pickett, W.C., Culp, B.R., Lands, W.E.M., 1981. Tetraene and pentaene leukotrienes: selective production from murine mastocytoma cells after dietary manipulation. Prostaglandins 22 (4), 613–622.

National Heart, Lung, and Blood Institute, 2013. Fact book: fiscal year 2012. pages 47. http://www.nhlbi.nih.gov/about/factpdf.htm

Nie, D., Guo, Y., Yang, D., Tang, Y., Chen, Y., Wang, M.T., Zacharek, A., Qiao, Y., Che, M., Honn, K.V., 2008. Thromboxane A2 receptors in prostate carcinoma: expression and its role in regulating cell motility via small GTPase Rho. Cancer Res. 68 (1), 115–121.

Ogushi, Y., Hamazaki, T., Kirihara, Y., 2009. Blood choloesterol as a good marker of health in Japan. World Rev. Nutr. Diet. 100, 63–70.

Omega 3-6 Balance Apps., 2014. http://efaeducation.org/omega-3-6-apps/

Ramsden, C.E., Faurot, K.R., Zamora, D., Suchindran, C.M., Macintosh, B.A., Gaylord, S., Ringel, A., Hibbeln, J.R., Feldstein, A.E., Mori, T.A., Barden, A., Lynch, C., Coble, R., Mas, E., Palsson, O., Barrow, D.A., Mann, J.D., 2013. Targeted alteration of dietary n-3 and n-6 fatty acids for the treatment of chronic headaches: a randomized trial. Pain 154 (11), 2441–2451, http://www.ncbi.nlm.nih.gov/pmc/articles/PMC3850757/pdf/nihms514426.pdf.

Ross, R., 1999. Atherosclerosis—an inflammatory disease. New England J. Med. 340 (2), 115–126, PubMed PMID: 9887164.

Soderstrom, M., Mannervik, B., Garkov, V., Hammarstrom, S., 1992. On the nature of leukotriene C4 synthase in human platelets. Arch. Biochem. Biophys. 294 (1), 70–74.

Spite, M., Claria, J., Serhan, C.N., 2014. Resolvins, specialized proresolving lipid mediators, and their potential roles in metabolic diseases. Cell Metabol. 19 (1), 21–36.

Spite, M., Hellmann, J., Tang, Y., Mathis, S.P., Kosuri, M., Bhatnagar, A., Jala, V.R., Haribabu, B., 2011. Deficiency of the leukotriene B4 receptor, BLT-1, protects against systemic insulin resistance in diet-induced obesity. J. Immunol. 187, 1942–1949.

Stamler, J., Neaton, J.D., Cohen, J.D., Cutler, J., Eberly, L., Grandits, G., Kuller, L.H., Ockene, J., Prineas, R., MRFIT Research Group, 2012. Multiple risk factor intervention trial revisited: a new perspective based on nonfatal and fatal composite endpoints, coronary and cardiovascular, during the trial. J. Am. Heart Assoc.;1 (5): pp. e003640.

Stark, K.D., Mulvad, G., Pedersen, H.S., Park, E.J., Dewailly, E., Holub, B.J., 2002. Fatty acid compositions of serum phospholipids of postmenopausal women: a comparison between Greenland Inuit and Canadians before and after supplementation with fish oil. Nutrition 18 (7–8), 627–630.

Steinberg, D., Vaughan, M., Nestel, P.J., Strand, O., Bergstrom, S., 1964. Effects of the prostaglandins on hormone-induced mobilization of free fatty acids. J. Clin. Investig. 43 (8), 1533–1540.

Strandjord, S.E., Lands, B., Hibbeln, J.R., submitted. Nutr. Metabol. Validation of an equation predicting highly unsaturated fatty acid compositions of human blood fractions from dietary intake.

Strong, J.P., Malcom, G.T., McMahan, C.A., Tracy, R.E., Newman, III, W.P., Herderick, E.E., Cornhill, J.F., 1999. Atherosclerosis in youth study prevention from the pathobiological determinants of adolescents and young adults: implications for prevalence. JAMA 281 (8), 727–735.

Tanaka, K., Furuyashiki, T., Shiho Kitaoka, 1* Yuta Senzai, 1* Yuki Imoto, 2Eri Segi-Nishida, 2 Yuichi Deguchi, 1Richard M. Breyer, 3Matthew D. Breyer, 4 and Shuh Narumiya, S., 2012. Prostaglandin E2-mediated attenuation of mesocortical dopaminergic pathway is critical for susceptibility to repeated social defeat stress in mice. J. Neurosci. 32: pp. 4319–4329.

United States Department of Agriculture (USDA) National Nutrient Database. http://www.nal.usda.gov/fnic/foodcomp/search/

van Dorp, D.A., Beerthuis, R.K., Nugteren, D.H., Vonkeman, H., 1964. The biosynthesis of prostaglandins. Biochem. Biophys. Acta 90 (1), 204–207.

Verschuren, W.M., Jacobs, D.R., Bloemberg, B.P., Kromhout, D., Menotti, A., Aravanis, C., Blackburn, H., Buzina, R., Anastasios, S., Dontas, A.S., Fidanza, F., Karvonen, M.J., Nedelijkovic, S., Nissinen, A., Toshima, H., 1995. Serum total cholesterol and long-term coronary heart disease mortality in different cultures. Twenty-five year follow-up of the seven countries study. JAMA 274 (2), 131–136.

Wada, M., DeLong, C.J., Hong, Y.H., Rieke, C.J., Song, I., Sidhu, R.S., Yuan, C., Warnock, M., Schmaier, A.H., Yokoyama, C., Smyth, E.M., Wilson, S.J., FitzGerald, G.A., Garavito, R.M., Sui, D.X., John, W., Regan, J.W., Smith, W.L., 2007. Enzymes and receptors of prostaglandin pathways with arachidonic acid-derived versus eicosapentaenoic acid derived substrates and products. J. Biol. Chem. 282, 22254–22266, http://www.jbc.org/content/282/31/22254.full.pdf+html.

Xu, H., Barnes, G.T., Yang, Q., Tan, G., Yang, D., Chou, C.J., Sole, J., Nichols, A., Ross, J.S., Tartaglia, L.A., Chen, H., 2003. Chronic inflammation in fat plays a crucial role in the development of obesity-related insulin resistance. J. Clin. Invest. 112 (12), 1821–1830, PubMed PMID: 14679177.

Yokomizo, T., 2011. Leukotriene B4 receptors: novel roles in immunological regulations. Adv. Enzym. Regul. 51, 59–64.

CHAPTER

8

Fish Consumption During Pregnancy and Anthropometric Measures at Birth

R. Ramón Bonache

Life-course Health Promotion and Prevention Department, General Directorate of Public Health, Valencia; Spanish Consortium for Research on Epidemiology and Public Health (CIBERESP), Spain

INTRODUCTION

Fish consumption during pregnancy may be part of a healthy diet as it is a good source of nutrients such as marine omega-3 (n–3) fatty acids, proteins, vitamin D, selenium, and iodine that are important for healthy fetal growth development. Fish is a source of polyunsaturated fatty acids (PUFA), particularly of the elongated marine PUFA, DHA, and EPA, which are considered essential for fetal and infant neurodevelopment (Starling et al., 2015). The n–3 fatty acids are involved in placental flow and the process of parturition, and their intake during pregnancy has been related to fetal growth and longer gestation (Olsen et al., 1993; Olsen et al., 1995; Elias and Innis, 2001). However, other observational studies have reported negative associations between n–3 intake, n–3 plasma levels, or fish oil supplements and fetal growth measures (Grandjean et al., 2001; Oken et al., 2004; Thorsdottir et al., 2004; Brantsaeter et al., 2012). Reported reduced postnatal growth in preterm infants given formula fortified with n–3 fatty acids in feeding trials support the prenatal findings (Carlson et al., 1992; Carlson et al., 1996; Oken et al., 2004), probably indicating that supraphysiologic doses of these nutrients may not be appropriate for health. A role of bioactive peptides released from fish proteins on fetal growth has also been hypothesized since lean fish, with less content in n–3, has been associated with an increase in infant birth weight and head circumference (Ramon et al., 2009a; Brantsaeter et al., 2012).

Despite all of its benefits, fish is also a well-known route of exposure to pollutants such as mercury, specifically methyl mercury (MeHg), and persistent organic pollutants (POPs) that include chemical compounds such as polychlorinated biphenyls (PCBs), dioxins, organochlorine pesticides, and polybrominated diphenyl ethers (PBDEs), which may negatively affect fetal growth and birth outcomes (Ramon et al., 2009a; Karagas et al., 2012). Mercury and POPs readily cross through the placenta into the fetus (Crinnion, 2009) and exposure to low doses of those contaminants may affect fetal growth by means of endocrine disruption (Murphy et al., 2010) or via oxidative stress which stimulate the production of free radicals and impair nutrient transport to the fetus (Houston, 2007; Thomas et al., 2015). MeHg also has effects on platelet aggregation and thromboxane production which may affect blood viscosity and placental flow (Xue et al., 2007).

The effects of fish consumption on pregnancy outcomes are measured in terms of duration of gestation or anthropometric measures at birth. Preterm births (PT) are defined as <259 days of gestation and low birth weight (LBW) as <2500 g and are considered dichotomous data. Fetal growth restriction is generally defined as small for gestational age (SGA) for weight, length, or head circumference defined as below the 10th percentile compared with a standard reference group. Birth weight, birth length, and head circumference can also be used as continuous variables and adjusted for gestational age. Growth characteristics can also be measured in different trimesters of pregnancy by fetal ultrasound examinations in order to assess specific critical periods but this type of data is not frequently used (Heppe et al., 2011).

As a consequence of a balance between beneficial nutrients and deleterious chemical compounds contained in seafood, fish, and shellfish, findings from observational studies about the role of seafood intake during pregnancy on fetal growth have failed to give conclusive results, with reports of either positive, negative or null effects (Leventakou et al., 2014). Differences in findings may be explained by the intake of different fish species with varying content of

Fish and Fish Oil in Health and Disease Prevention. http://dx.doi.org/10.1016/B978-0-12-802844-5.00008-7

nutrients and contaminants as well as factors such as season when fish is caught, fish life stage, and fish provenance. For example, fatty fish may contain larger amounts of n–3 than lean fish, as well as higher levels of contaminants, and population exposure will therefore depend on consumption habits (Legrand et al., 2005).

On the other hand, anthropometric measures attained at birth may have considerable prognostic value for subsequent infant growth and development (Ribas-Fito et al., 2002). Birth length has been associated with psychomotor development and attained length at 12 months and, in a British birth cohort, birthweight and birth length were associated with cognition and educational attainment at different ages until adulthood (Morris et al., 1998; Richards et al., 2002). Moreover, birthweight has been related to an increased risk of chronic diseases in adulthood, such as metabolic syndrome (Barker, 2004; Chen et al., 2009; Roberts and Wood, 2014) although the mechanisms are not completely understood and there are other hypotheses regarding shared genetic mechanisms for fetal growth and later disease in life (Wilcox, 2001).

FISH CONSUMPTION AND BIRTH OUTCOMES: RESULTS FROM OBSERVATIONAL STUDIES

Studies Using Fish Consumption as a Proxy of Exposure

The suggestion that a high intake of seafood rich in long-chain n–3 fatty acids increases birth weight in humans comes from long, ecological and observational studies in countries with a high consumption (Olsen et al., 1986). In Denmark, Olsen and coworkers reported an increase of birth and placental weight and an increase in head circumference with increasing levels of daily fish consumption as a main meal (5 strata from 0 to 5 or more times) but only in nonsmokering women. They found no association between birth length or gestational age and fish consumption (Olsen et al., 1990). Later on, low consumption of fish was reported to be a strong risk factor for preterm delivery and low birth weight in women receiving routine antenatal care in Aarhus, Denmark (Olsen and Secher, 2002).

In 2004, a study from the Project Viva (United States), described an inverse association between total fish consumption assessed at the first and second trimesters and fetal growth z-value after multivariate adjustment, but only significant for the first trimester intake. No association of seafood intake and the risk of LBW, SGA, or PT was found (Oken et al., 2004). In the "ALSPAC" cohort of pregnant women in southwest England (UK), positive outcomes were reported. A decreased risk of intrauterine growth retardation (defined as birth weight adjusted for gestational age below the 10th percentile) with increased intake of seafood (assessed at 32 weeks) was found, with an adjusted odds ratio (OR) of 1.37 [95% Confident Interval (CI): 1.02, 1.84] for women who ate no fish compared with women in the highest percentile of fish intake. No significant associations were found between frequency of fish intake and the occurrence of PT or LBW (Rogers et al., 2004).

In 2006, Olsen and coworkers concluded that never consuming fish in the first two trimesters of pregnancy was a strong risk factor for PT delivery based on data from routine antenatal care. Data came from the same cohort formed in 1992–96 (Olsen and Secher, 2002) but, in this paper, they focused the analysis on women with constant intake using dietary data in two periods in pregnancy (Olsen et al., 2006). In Denmark, using data from the Danish National Birth Cohort, women consuming >60 g fatty fish/day (the highest category) had a higher risk of having infants with a birth weight and length below the 10th percentile than the mothers whose fish consumption was <5 g/day (the lowest category); a small decrease in mean birth weight, length, and head circumference was also observed. This inverse association was explained by consumption of fatty fish (salmon, herring, mackerel, trout, and Greenland halibut) assessed around week 25 of gestation (Halldorsson et al., 2007). In a cohort in Brittany (France), data from the PELAGIE study suggested that different categories of seafood may be differently associated with birth outcomes, mainly fish consumption being associated with increased length of gestation and shellfish with decreased fetal growth. They assessed fish and shellfish by means of a food frequency questionnaire (FFQ) completed during the first trimester, asking about consumption just before pregnancy but they did not obtain detailed information about the different types of fish consumed (Guldner et al., 2007).

In 2011, Brantsaeter and coworkers published the results of the Norwegian Mother and Child Cohort Study (MoBa) where they found a positive association between total fish intake or lean fish intake, measured by FFQ in mid pregnancy, with all birth size measures while shellfish was only associated with birth weight. Fatty fish was not associated with any birth measurements. The relative risk of giving birth to a LBW baby in full term women who consumed >60 g/day (the highest category) was lower than in women who consumed ≤5 g/day (the lowest category) with an OR of 0.56 (CI 95%: 0.35, 0.88). The levels of blood mercury concentrations have been previously described as low in this cohort although no mercury adjustment was done in the mentioned study (Brantsaeter et al., 2012).

Nevertheless, in the Generation R Study conducted in the city of Rotterdam (The Netherlands), no associations of first trimester maternal total-fish, lean-fish, fatty-fish, and shellfish consumption were found with the second and third trimesters fetal growth assessed using standardized ultrasound procedures nor with growth characteristics at birth (PT, LBW, SGA) in a population with relatively low fish intake (Heppe et al., 2011).

Studies Using Fish Consumption and Maternal, Fetal, or Infant Mercury Concentrations as Exposure

Mercury is a naturally occurring metal that is widespread in the environment. Anthropogenic sources from industry, combustion of fossils fuels, and mining activities contribute to the atmospheric burden. Mercury is transformed into methylmercury (MeHg), the organic and most toxic form, by microscopic organisms when atmospheric Hg is deposited on contaminated soils or water surfaces. In this form it is capable of bioaccumulation in the marine food chain (Sanfeliu et al., 2003). The main source of human exposure to mercury is through the consumption of fish contaminated with MeHg, where it binds to proteins in fish muscle and accumulates in the edible part, being unaffected by cooking methods (Dovydaitis, 2008). Maternal and fetal blood or hair levels increase with increasing levels of fish consumption by mothers during different trimesters of pregnancy (Sakamoto et al., 2008; Ramon et al., 2011).

The vulnerability of the fetus to mercury exposure was ascertained during the three unfortunate episodes of massive poisoning in Japan, Iraq, and Guatemala. Exposure to mercury during pregnancy has been widely studied due to its potential negative effects on child neurodevelopment (Grandjean and Landrigan, 2006). There is less available evidence for the effects of MeHg on fetal growth and gestation (Karagas et al., 2012).

The current reference dose (RfD) is an estimate of a daily exposure where no appreciable risk of deleterious effects during a lifetime would occur, for MeHg is an intake of 0.1 μg/kg body weight per day (Food and Drug Administration, 2004), and corresponds to a level of MeHg in whole cord blood of 5.8 μg/L or 1 μg/g in hair (Mahaffey, 2005; Oken et al., 2008b). When population levels are known, this RfD will serve to estimate the percentage of vulnerable population above the recommended dose (Mortensen et al., 2014).

High maternal and offspring MeHg blood concentration were suggested to be associated with low mean birth weight by Foldspang and Hansen in 1990 in Greenland (Foldspang and Hansen, 1990), but later the association was refuted when data was reanalyzed (Bjerregaard and Hansen, 2000). Other studies, conducted in communities with a very high intake, also failed to find an association, although they did not adjust for specific types of fish in their analysis (Grandjean et al., 2001; Lucas et al., 2004). In the POUCH study conducted in Michigan (United States), a maternal hair total Hg level was related to PT deliveries. Women who delivered very preterm babies (before 35 week gestation) were more likely to have their hair T-Hg levels at or above the 90th percentile (≥0.55 μg/g) compared to women delivering at term adjusted for total fish consumption (OR: 3.0; 95% CI: 1.3–6.7); (Xue et al., 2007). In a study published in 2008, about the effects of the World Trade Center disaster in USA on pregnant women, with median cord blood concentrations of T-Hg of 4.3 Lg/L and 32% of newborns with concentrations ≥5.8 μg/L, no significant association between T-Hg and newborn size was found; however, the authors did not consider consumption of different types of fishes but total fish in the analysis (Lederman et al., 2008).

In 2009, in a Spanish population based cohort from Valencia, which is one out of five cohorts that form part of a broader multicenter project, the Childhood and Environmental study (INMA project; Ribas-Fito et al., 2006), a negative association between cord blood mercury and birth weight was reported (Ramon et al., 2009a). Newborns in the highest quartile of total mercury weighed 143.7 g less (95% CI: −251.8, −35.6; *p* for trend = 0.02) and had higher odds of being SGA for length (Odds ratio: 5.3; 95% CI: 1.2, 23.9; *p* from likelihood ratio test = 0.03) without a linear relation (*p* for trend = 0.13) compared with those in the lowest quartile. An increased risk of having a baby SGA for weight was also observed with higher consumption of large fatty fish (≥2 portions/week versus < 1 portion/month) adjusted for T-Hg. In this cohort, levels of cord blood T-Hg were above EPA reference dose in 72% of newborns and large predatory fish (swordfish, bonito, and fresh tuna) was the third type of fish most consumed (17.5% of the total). In the same cohort, positive findings between canned tuna and birth weight as well as a decreased risk of being SGA for weight were found. Moreover, higher consumption of lean fish was also associated with lower risk of being SGA for length (Ramon et al., 2009a). Surprisingly, another cohort of the same INMA project (Sabadell cohort) reported an increased risk of SGA for women consuming >1 serving per week of canned tuna compared with women consuming ≤1 serving per week (OR: 2.49, 95% CI: 1.04, 5.97), although this relationship was attenuated when adjusting for serum levels of several POPs (PCBs, HCB, and DDE) with an OR of 2.39 (95% CI: 0.96, 5.96) (Mendez et al., 2010). They also found an increased risk of SGA for crustacean's consumption and a less clear and nonsignificant relationship with fatty fish. Although both studies used the same FFQ, different groups of fatty fish and frequencies of intake were used in the analysis. In the Sabadell cohort, mercury, and some POPs were included in models but only for adjustment.

In France, in the cohort "EDEN mother–child", seafood intake before pregnancy was associated with higher birth weight (100.52 g of BW for an increase of 1 SD of seafood intake, $p = 0.008$) adjusted for maternal hair T-Hg but only in overweight women. In fact, in nonoverweight women, seafood intake was associated with a lower birth length and head circumference, with an average decrease of 0.19 cm and 0.17 cm, respectively, for an increase of 1 SD of seafood intake ($p < 0.02$). The authors also found a lower gestational length with increasing fish intake, although they interpreted this finding with caution as a possible chance finding (Drouillet-Pinard et al., 2010).

Studies Using Fish Consumption and Maternal or Cord Blood Organochlorine Compounds as Exposure

The main intake of organochlorine compounds like PCBs and PBDEs is through diet and, under unusual circumstances, by inhalation (Ribas-Fito et al., 2002). PCBs and PBDEs are man-made; there are no known natural sources. Exposure to these chemicals is almost always a mixture of multiple chemicals (Dovydaitis, 2008). Fish is the main route of exposure when the consumed fish comes from highly contaminated waters, like the Great Lakes or the Baltic Sea (Rylander et al., 1998). For the general population, other foods of animal origin like meat and dairy products, are believed to account for those exposures more than fish (Schecter et al., 2001). POPs are highly lipophilic and persistent in nature and are influenced by various cooking methods, for example removing skin, internal organs, and fat before cooking can reduce exposure (Lee and Jacobs, 2010). This kind of information is not generally available in epidemiological studies using FFQ to assess dietary intake.

Studies on prenatal exposure to low doses of some POPs like PCBs, HCB, DDE, and PBDEs and birth weight have shown inconsistent results. Some studies have reported lower birth weight and impaired fetal growth (Fein et al., 1984; Rylander et al., 1998; Patandin et al., 1998; Govarts et al., 2012), while other studies have showed no effects (Rogan et al., 1986; Vartiainen et al., 1998; Grandjean et al., 2001; Lignell et al., 2013) or even an increased birth weight (Karmaus and Zhu, 2004; Lignell et al., 2013). A negative association between in utero exposure to PCBs and birth weight has been reported in some populations of high fish eaters in the Lake Michigan area (United States; Fein et al., 1984; Karmaus and Zhu, 2004). In Sweden, exposure to PCB-153 was associated with an increased risk of LBW in high fish consumers (Rylander et al., 1998). In Spain, in a highly polluted area with unusually high atmospheric levels of HCB, a negative association between HCB levels in maternal and cord serum and birth length was found with no effect on birth weight (Ribas-Fito et al., 2002); in this study, the rest of the studied PCBs did not show association with anthropometric measures at birth. Moreover, in this highly exposed population, fish consumption from the water reservoir of the village was associated with high concentrations of HCB and PCBs, probably reflecting the practice of dumping chemical waste into the water reservoir (Sala et al., 1999). In the Netherlands, it has been estimated that fish consumption contributes to up to 26% of total PCB intake and 12% of dioxin intake (Heppe et al., 2011).

More recently, Halldorsson and coworkers found an inverse association between maternal plasma PCBs concentrations and birth weight and placental weight in a Danish cohort. The sum of PCB congeners 105, 118, 138, 153, 156, and 180 was used as exposure. The adjusted mean difference between the 75th and 25th PCB percentiles was −155 g (95% CI: −291, −19) for birth weight and −81 g (95% CI: −135, −26). Levels of PCBs in this population were related to fatty fish intake. The authors reported that the effects were observed at moderate levels of exposure (median PCB −153 70 ng/g lipid) compared to other studies assessing infant neurodevelopment (median 110 ng/g lipid) (Halldorsson et al., 2008). Murphy et al., have reported the association between exposure to specific antiestrogenic PCBs congeners during the critical preconception window and a substantial reduction in birth weight (adjusted $\beta = -470.08$, $p = 0.04$) in a high fish consumption population (Murphy et al., 2010).

A positive association between diortho-PCB (CB−138, 153, 180) exposure and birth weight in male infants has been found in the POPUP study in Uppsala County, Sweden (Lignell et al., 2013). In this study, the positive association was found only after adjustment for maternal prepregnancy BMI, weight gain and, concurrent exposure to tetra- to hexabrominated PBDEs (BDE−47, 99, 100, 153). Moreover, a negative association was found between exposure to PBDEs and birth weight, association that became stronger after adjustment for fish consumption with a β −137 ($p = 0.01$) per 1 unit increase in ln-transformed contaminant concentration in breast milk. It has been suggested that a positive association on birth weight can be due to estrogen effects, in particular p, p'–DDE, and that the effects of PCBs may be masked or missed if exposures of both types of contaminants are not separated in the analysis (Karmaus and Zhu, 2004). The significance and long term consequences of an increased birth weight related to prenatal exposure to some POPs remains unclear (Lignell et al., 2013).

FISH CONSUMPTION DURING PREGNANCY: A GLIMPSE AT INFANT NEURODEVELOPMENT

Fish consumption during pregnancy has been positively associated with fetal and infant neurodevelopment in a more consistent way than with birth outcomes (Starling et al., 2015). An intake during pregnancy of more than 340 g/week has been identified as beneficial by some authors at different endpoints of infant development and questioned the recommendations in United States guidelines, issued in 2004, to pregnant women to not exceeded a threshold of 340 g of fish per week (Hibbeln et al., 2007; Oken et al., 2008a).

Nevertheless, the concomitant exposure to pollutants, especially mercury, that are well known neurotoxicants (Grandjean and Landrigan, 2006) is associated with detrimental effects on neurodevelopment. It is probable that prenatal exposure is more deleterious than postnatal exposure (Karagas et al., 2012). Positive effects of fish consumption are observed in women consuming low mercury content fish which indicates that the type of fish recommended is very important (Oken et al., 2008b). From a practical point of view, choosing fish not highly contaminated and rich in n–3 can be complicated for consumers (Oken et al., 2005). Furthermore, some studies have shown childhood neurodevelopment effects at low levels of prenatal MeHg exposure, and as reported by Oken et al., with data of the Project Viva, *"Our findings suggest that no lower threshold exists for the adverse effects of prenatal mercury exposure"* (Oken et al., 2008b).

Evaluating neurodevelopment is complex, due to the subtlety of neurodevelopment outcomes assessed, the different ages at which development milestones are achieved, the different neurological tests used by the studies, the exposure timing, the precision of the exposure assessment, the confounding, geographical and cultural differences, the modest risk or preventive factors being assessed, and the possibility of nonmonotonic dose–response associations.

INCONSISTENCIES OF EPIDEMIOLOGICAL FINDINGS ON BIRTH OUTCOMES

When beneficial nutrients and harmful contaminants coexist in the same food, inconsistent human data can be expected (Lee and Jacobs, 2010). Fish and shellfish may differ in their fatty acid content as well as in their concentrations of different pollutants. On the other hand, patterns of consumption among populations greatly vary geographically in terms of type of fish and shellfish, amount, and frequency of intake. Therefore, apart from the environmental pollution, human exposure will depend on the local habits of fish consumption, as described in two coastal communities in Canada where highly contaminated fish is not frequently consumed by the population (Legrand et al., 2005). Most of the reviewed studies did not consider consumption of different types of fishes and species in their analysis. Not taking into account these factors in the analysis may underestimate both the positive and negative effects on birth outcomes and lead to inconsistencies among studies.

Moreover, published studies often lacked an adjustment for other food groups that are also related with birth outcomes and/or with fish consumption, so they can act as potential confounders or as independent predictors. Furthermore, internal doses of contaminants were not often measured or, if so, the assessment was done for mercury or for some POPs but rarely for both of them. Therefore, controversial results must be interpreted with caution due to the limitations of the studies to accurately assess either detrimental contaminants or beneficial nutrients. In the cohort of the Faroe Islands, a high fish intake community, the statistical reanalysis of previous data showed an underestimation of the effects of MeHg, the toxic exposure, on infant neurodevelopment due to lack of fish adjustment, the proxy for beneficial nutrients intakes (Budtz-Jorgensen et al., 2007).

When mercury concentrations in blood or hair were available, a wide range of prenatal mercury exposure was observed, with some populations having a high proportion of cord blood levels above 5.8 μg/L, the reference dose used by the US EPA (Mahaffey, 2005), while others showed low concentrations of mercury in matrices with respect to the reference dose (Ramon et al., 2009a; Brantsaeter et al., 2012). It is noteworthy that some adverse outcomes have been described in populations at low levels of prenatal mercury exposure or at intakes of fish or shellfish that are not restricted by public health policies in the current recommendations of fish consumption for pregnant women in United States or Europe (European Food Safety Authority, 2004; US Food and Drug Administration, 2004). Geographically differences in the distribution of different POPs in fish species and shellfish may also account for differences in health outcomes. This has been the case for the association between fish consumption and diabetes, with studies in some populations showing a positive association whereas inverse relationships have been described in China, Japan, and Australia (Ruzzin, 2012).

Individual susceptibility due to gene–environmental interaction may also account for the inconsistent findings. Mercury excretion in the feces and urine vary among individuals and involve glutathione conjugation, process catalyzed by selenium-dependent glutathione S-transferase (GST; Karagas et al., 2012). The glutathione S-transferase M1 (GSTM1) and the glutathione S-transferase T1 (GSTT1) null genes, due to two homozygous deletions, result in a loss of functional activity, and impaired ability for Hg detoxification. In the Mothers and Children's Environmental Health (MOCEH) study conducted in Seoul, Cheonan, and Ulsan (Korea), a negative association between birth weight and Hg exposure was more pronounced in women with both, GSTM1 and GSTT1, null genotypes than in women with the intact genotype or one of the null genotypes (Lee and Jacobs, 2010). Other polymorphisms in glutamyl-cysteine ligase (GCLC) that affect the production of glutathione conjugates may also affect MeHg retention (Custodio et al., 2004).

Finally, residual confounding is a drawback in all observational studies. Uncontrolled confounding factors related with lifestyle always are a possibility for explaining inconsistencies.

FISH CONSUMPTION AND BIRTH OUTCOMES: PLANNING AN EPIDEMIOLOGIC STUDY

When planning an epidemiological study on fish consumption and birth outcomes, it is important to know the context of the pregnant women, their food habits, and specifically the species of fish most frequently consumed as well as levels of contaminants in consumed fish and the prevalence of the birth outcomes to be assessed when available. It is also important to carefully think about potential predictors and confounders which are plausible or already described in other populations.

When data exists about concentrations of pollutants in fish, a possible approach is to link the existing public health and environmental data, a population-based, record–linkage study, in order test hypothesis about exposure to contaminants and health outcomes. Burch and coworkers, in a southeast United States coastal community, tested the hypothesis that "women residing in areas with elevated fish total mercury concentrations had increased odds of delivering a term LBW or PT infant" (Burch et al., 2014). The authors found that women residing in regions with elevated total mercury concentrations in fish may have an increased likelihood of delivering a term LBW infant compared to women living in areas with lower fish total mercury levels, particularly among African–American women. These kind of studies can be used as a starting point to decide if a more detailed study is warranted (Shire et al., 2011).

Careful planning of variables to be recorded and data about the context of the study are necessary:

1. Socio–demographic data. Maternal age, infant sex, parental education level, parental employment status, family income, parental country of origin, ethnic group, type of residence (urban versus rural), height and weight of both parents are among the variables to be recorded. In contrast with other studies in high income countries, fish consumption in the two mentioned Spanish cohorts was not related to socio–economic factors and so less residual confounding could be expected when studying the associations with pregnancy outcomes (Ramon et al., 2009a; Mendez et al., 2010). On the other hand, in United States, subsistence fishing behavior has been described in a Virginian coastal community where African–American women of reproductive age consume more fish, have elevated mercury exposures, and are more exposed than other ethnic groups (Burch et al., 2014). Therefore, it is important to explore how socio–economic variables are related to fish consumption in a given study population in order to better understand exposure.
2. Fish consumption assessment. Food frequency questionnaires are generally used to record dietary data in epidemiological studies (Willet, 1998). Preexisting data on fish intake by pregnant women should guide the questions about different types of fish and shellfish to be recorded and the groups to be made. A useful approach is to record separately the fish species that are object of current recommendations by country or by local fisheries authority. In the study conducted by Ramon and coworkers, although fish groups were separated according to the US recommendations (US Food and Drug Administration, 2004), tuna and swordfish were included in the same group (as large oily fish) and taking into account the high consumption of both species by that population, it was not possible to know which one was implicated in the negative outcome found (Ramon et al., 2009a).

   Dietary assessment can be done at different periods during pregnancy or before pregnancy. The studies used different time windows to assess fish intake. Oken and coworkers found a reduction of fetal growth by increasing intakes of n–3 PUFA was similar regardless of trimester, suggesting a biologic effect of the elongated fatty acids throughout pregnancy (Oken et al., 2004).

   Fish oil supplements should be recorded and considered in the analysis of data. The levels of pollutants may vary significantly in fish oil since some decontamination processes will have different impact on contaminant content than others. Supplementary n–3 intake was associated with negative head circumference in the Norwegian cohort (Brantsaeter et al., 2012). Moreover, other nutrients included in supplements taken during pregnancy, like selenium and vitamin E, have shown to interact with mercury (Castoldi et al., 2008) and should also be recorded in order to explore how they are related to mercury levels.

None of the reviewed studies provided separated evaluation of wild versus farmed fish. Both types of fish will present a different risk profile, farmed salmon and catfish are considered to be a great source of current exposures to PCBs, PBDEs, and other chlorinated pesticides while mercury will accumulate in large wild fish predators (Crinnion, 2009; Jacobs et al., 2014). It will be important to incorporate this kind of information while recording fish intake in future studies to minimize confounding.

3. Mercury exposure assessment. Although mercury in cord blood is, in general, considered the best biomarker of prenatal exposure (Grandjean et al., 2005), there is a good correlation between cord blood concentrations and maternal blood, maternal hair or infant hair levels, and these matrices have also been used in epidemiological studies (Bjornberg et al., 2003; Sakamoto et al., 2008). With respect to the type of mercury, most of the studies used T-Hg as biomarker of exposure instead of MeHg due to costs aspects. It has been estimated that when total blood mercury levels are above 4 μg/L, methyl mercury accounts for more than 90% of total mercury (Mahaffey, 2005); therefore, T-Hg in cord blood can be considered a good proxy of MeHg in populations with high levels of exposure. In less exposed populations, analysis of MeHg should be considered.
4. Persistent organic pollutants exposure assessment. An important drawback of most epidemiological studies is that, due to cost and required amount of blood sample, only a few selected POPs are generally measured and used in the analysis. The importance of PCB congener-specific investigation and the critical time window to be assessed has been underscored (Murphy et al., 2010). This fact should be taken into account when interpreting results of associations in a given study (Lee and Jacobs, 2010). Moreover, to evaluate exposure to POPs, a lifetime diet history seems more appropriate since fish consumption during pregnancy can only explain a small part of serum concentrations, due to their highly lipophilic and persistent nature (Lee and Jacobs, 2010). A study in Sweden suggested that exposures during childhood and adolescence influenced the body burdens of the compounds during pregnancy. The authors ascertained the number of months the women had been nursed during infancy as well as growing up in families involved in commercial or sport–fishing and growing up along the Baltic Sea (Glynn et al., 2007). The offspring of the ongoing cohorts will be an opportunity to study long-term exposure and pregnancy outcomes later in life.
5. Covariates. Lifestyle variables are very important for adjustment. Maternal weight-gain during pregnancy, maternal chronic conditions, toxic habits like smoking, or alcohol intake, caffeine intake, fruit, and vegetables intake, and energy intake. Other food groups may be related with mercury or POPs levels, like chicken due to feeding practices. Season of conception or at delivery should be analyzed, seasonal variations in the potential for methylation of mercury in superficial sediments in lakes and rivers have been described, with there being the greatest potential during summer time and in warmers waters (Korthals and Winfrey, 1987; Weis and Ashley, 2007). Seasonal variation in nutrient in pregnant woman, and significant influence of nutrient intake on birth outcomes in different seasons has been reported (Watson and McDonald, 2007). Physical activity during pregnancy is especially related with maternal health, but should be taken into account for adjustment.
6. Visualizing data. It is helpful to visualize the estimates of effect (β-coefficients or Odds ratio) according to different types of fish and their frequency of consumption when interpreting data. In Fig. 8.1, an increase or decrease of birth weight is shown according to T-Hg and consumption of different types of fish by pregnant women. In Fig. 8.2, odds ratios as a measure of association between T-Hg and consumption of different types of fish with SGA for weight (dichotomous data) are shown.

IMPLICATIONS FOR PREGNANT WOMEN

The results from epidemiological studies on birth outcomes are inconclusive or even controversial and the role of fish consumption during pregnancy remains a matter of debate. Concerning neurodevelopment in childhood, fish consumption during pregnancy appears to be more consistent in conferring a benefit but dependent on the type of fish consumed, because mercury and PCBs exposure, which come along to fish, are known neurotoxicants. The reviewed data highlight the complexities inherent in making public health recommendations concerning fish intake during pregnancy. Meanwhile, health care providers and pregnant women, as consumers, continue to face the dilemma: *what fish to eat during pregnancy to obtain the benefits of fish while minimizing the risks on maternal and pregnancy outcomes?*

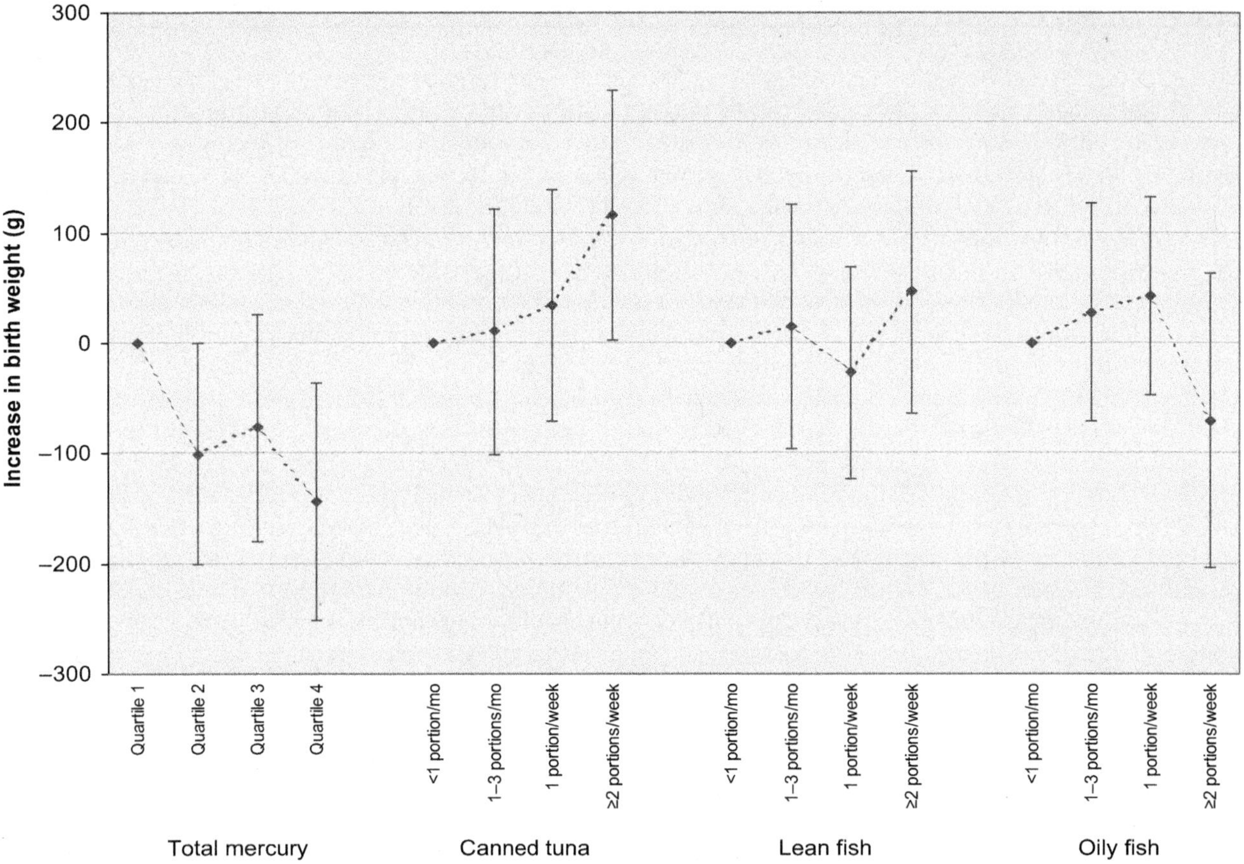

FIGURE 8.1 Associations between total cord blood mercury levels and fish intake by pregnant women with birth weight. Graphics elaborated with data from the Valencia INMA cohort, Spain, 2004–06 (Ramon et al., 2009a). Estimates of effect were simultaneously adjusted for all other variables in the table and for the sum of the other fish consumed, vegetable intake, energy intake, maternal age, prepregnancy weight, paternal height, gestational weight gain, sex of the infant, parity, and smoking status.

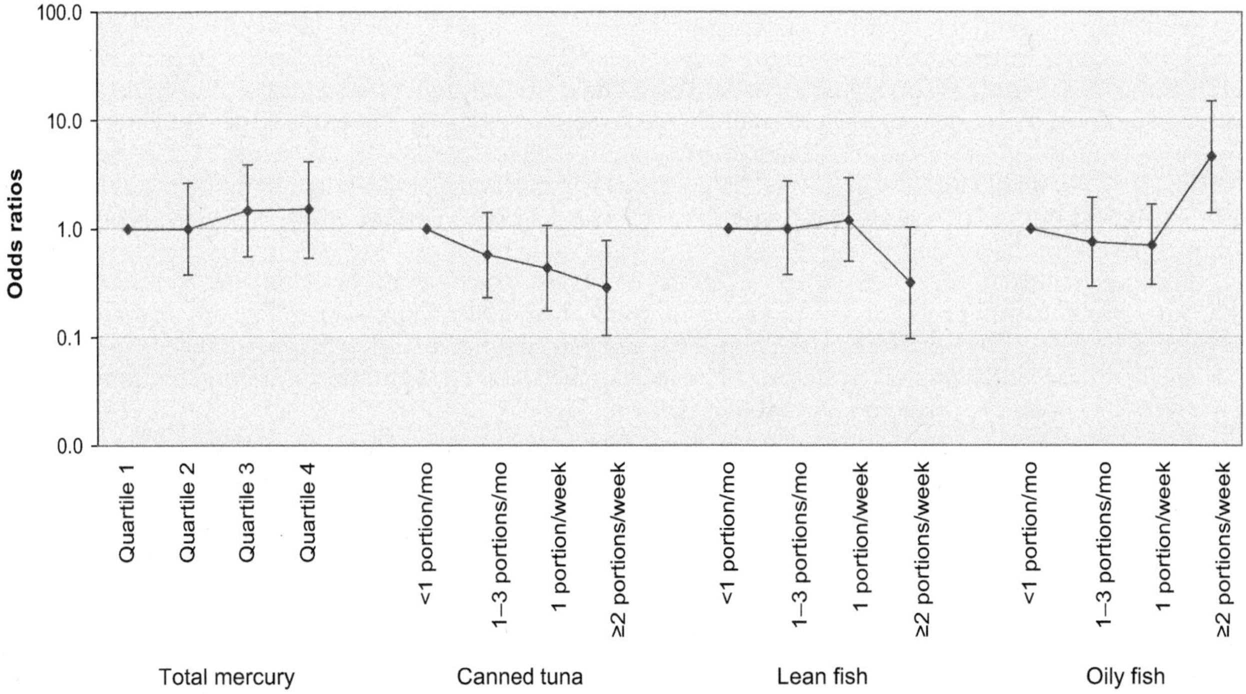

FIGURE 8.2 Associations between total cord blood mercury levels and fish intake by pregnant women with small for gestational age for weight. Graphics elaborated with data from the Valencia INMA cohort, Spain, 2004–06 (Ramon et al., 2009a). Estimates of effect were simultaneously adjusted for all other variables in the table and for the sum of the other fish consumed, vegetable intake, energy intake, maternal age, prepregnancy weight, gestational weight gain, parity, and smoking status.

Pregnant women will benefit from consuming fish with low levels of mercury and other contaminants and high content of nutrients like n–3, but in practical terms that choice is challenging if not impossible. There are available fish consumption advisories in some countries and in some regions where the waterbodies are highly contaminated and could pose health risks, especially during the vulnerable period of pregnancy. Such advisories are intended to provide enough DHA to the fetus while protecting the developing nervous system from mercury neurotoxicity (Oken et al., 2012) and are based on the choice or avoidance of some fish species.

The Food and Drug Administration (FDA) and the Environmental Protection Agency (EPA) are at present reviewing the 2004 advisory regarding fish consumption during pregnancy, breastfeeding, and early childhood, to make the recommendations consistent with those in the Dietary Guidelines for Americans 2010. They recommend eating at least two–three servings of selected fish per week, avoiding certain species, and verifying recommendations for fish caught in local streams (US Food and Drug Administration, 2014). In Europe, the European Food Safety Authority (EFSA) in 2004 recommended that those in vulnerable groups select fish from a wide range of species avoiding large predatory fish likely to contain higher levels of methylmercury (European Food Safety Authority, 2004). Nevertheless, in 2015, the EFSA stated that each country needs to considerer its own pattern of consumption and carefully assess the risk of exceeding a tolerable weekly intake of 1.3 μg/kg bw/week (European Food Safety Authority, 2015). Thus far, effects on fetal growth, exposure to low doses of other POPs or distinction between wild or farmed fish have not been considered when making those recommendations. Moreover, sustainability of fish as a food source is rarely included in guidelines, but, as pointed out by Oken and coworkers, has the potential to benefit all points of view because in one hand the fishing industry depends on the maintenance of fishing stocks, and on the other hand the feasibility to increase or maintain a high fish consumption will depend on sufficient fish supplies (Oken et al., 2012).

Fetal growth is the result of a complex interaction of behavioral, social, environmental, and genetic factors, and all should be taken into account when counseling a pregnant woman. In the complexity of dietary behaviors, fish only represents a part of a balanced diet with potential effects on maternal health and fetal growth. Fruit and vegetables play an essential role in maternal nutrition and have been associated with better anthropometric measures at birth (Ramon et al., 2009b). A diet based on red and processed meat and high-fat diary has been associated with an increased risk for fetal restriction (Knudsen et al., 2008), whereas a healthy pattern in the first trimester has been associated with a lower risk of delivering a fetal growth-restricted infant for weight (Rodriguez-Bernal et al., 2010). Moreover, early life nutrition has been related with better health outcomes in infancy and adulthood (Harding, 2001). A plant based-diet, rich in fruit, vegetables, pulses, and whole grains, limited in products of animal origin and restricted in processed food and processed meat is to be encouraged, and is the diet promoted by the WHO for all life stages in order to prevent noncommunicable diseases (WHO, 2014). It is in this context where fish intake by pregnant women should be placed taking into account local habits and current consumption of different fish species.

Some women are vegetarian or vegan and choose not to eat fish and other foods of animal origin during pregnancy, and still they can have a balanced and healthy diet if carefully planned (Craig and Mangels, 2009). An Adequate Intake has been set for alpha-linolenic acid (ALA), the precursor of n–3 elongated PUFAs, by the Institute of Medicine (IOM) of The National Academies. They have also recommended that approximately 10% of the Acceptable Macronutrient Distribution Range for ALA can be consumed as EPA and/or DHA (Kris-Etherton et al., 2009). There are good sources of ALA in vegetable foods like flaxseed, flaxseed oil, canola, and walnuts, although some authors recommend the intake of long-chain n–3 fatty acids through DHA-rich microalgae in vulnerable periods like pregnancy (Craig and Mangels, 2009). Nevertheless, an increased conversion of ALA to DHA and EPA in vegetarians is postulated and circulating levels of n–3 PUFA have been found to be similar in non-fish eaters and fish eaters (Welch et al., 2010) or at least stable over time of duration of adherence to a vegetarian or vegan diet (Rosell et al., 2005).

Exposure to mercury and POPs through fish consumption only represents a part of the contaminants to which a pregnant woman is exposed to on a daily basis. Brominated flame retardants from bedding, trihalomethanes from chlorinated water, antibacterial soaps with triclosans, cosmetics with parabenes and aluminum, carbon dioxide, cadmium and diesel compounds from cars, volatile organic compounds from upholstery or construction materials, cans releasing bisphenol-A from liners, plastic beverage containers leaching out estrogenic phthalates or BPA, cleaning products, etc., all these products are present in everyday life of pregnant women and also represent prenatal exposures that may pose health risks for the offspring (Genuis, 2009). In this highly contaminated world, the physical and chemical hazards encounter pregnant women via contaminated soil, food, water, and air. The patient environment has been described as comprising three sectors: the home, the community, and the workplace. Providers can use the medical history to characterize pregnant women exposures through diet history including fish consumption: the home, water source, the community, and professional exposures such as at the work place (McDiarmid et al., 2008). Concerning fish choices, the development of a list of fish to eat, and those to minimize or avoid, taking into consideration

TABLE 8.1 When Counselling a Pregnant Women

Home environment: diet history and use of pesticides
Ask about daily consumption of fruits and vegetables
Place fish consumption in a whole diet pattern
Check available recommendations (country and local level)
Inform about avoiding unnecessary pesticide use
Community environment: water source
Work place environment: professional exposures, legal regulations, and rights

other aspects than human health, such as ecological, economic, and sustainability at national or international level, has been proposed and would facilitate the counseling of providers (Oken et al., 2012). Of course, control of emissions and policies to decrease environment contamination will have a higher impact in the long term. Biomonitoring of mercury and other contaminants in vulnerable populations and monitoring contaminants in wild and farmed fish and other foodstuffs will help to evaluate evolution over time Table 8.1.

References

Barker, D.J., 2004. Developmental origins of adult health and disease. J. Epidemiol. Commun. Health 58, 114–115.

Bjerregaard, P., Hansen, J.C., 2000. Organochlorines and heavy metals in pregnant women from the Disko Bay area in Greenland. Sci. Total Environ. 245, 195–202.

Bjornberg, K.A., Vahter, M., Petersson-Grawe, K., Glynn, A., Cnattingius, S., Darnerud, P.O., Atuma, S., Aune, M., Becker, W., Berglund, M., 2003. Methyl mercury and inorganic mercury in Swedish pregnant women and in cord blood: influence of fish consumption. Environ. Health Perspect. 111, 637–641.

Brantsaeter, A.L., Birgisdottir, B.E., Meltzer, H.M., Kvalem, H.E., Alexander, J., Magnus, P., Haugen, M., 2012. Maternal seafood consumption and infant birth weight, length and head circumference in the Norwegian Mother and Child Cohort Study. Br. J. Nutr. 107, 436–444.

Budtz-Jorgensen, E., Grandjean, P., Weihe, P., 2007. Separation of risks and benefits of seafood intake. Environ. Health Perspect. 115, 323–327.

Burch, J.B., Wagner, R.S., Puett, R., Cai, B., Wilkerson, R., Karmaus, W., Vena, J., Svendsen, E., 2014. Mercury in fish and adverse reproductive outcomes: results from South Carolina. Int. J. Health Geogr. 13, 30.

Carlson, S.E., Cooke, R.J., Werkman, S.H., Tolley, E.A., 1992. First year growth of preterm infants fed standard compared to marine oil n-3 supplemented formula. Lipids 27, 901–907.

Carlson, S.E., Werkman, S.H., Tolley, E.A., 1996. Effect of long-chain n-3 fatty acid supplementation on visual acuity and growth of preterm infants with and without bronchopulmonary dysplasia. Am. J. Clin. Nutr. 63, 687–697.

Castoldi, A.F., Johansson, C., Onishchenko, N., Coccini, T., Roda, E., Vahter, M., Ceccatelli, S., Manzo, L., 2008. Human developmental neurotoxicity of methylmercury: impact of variables and risk modifiers. Regul. Toxicol. Pharmacol. 51, 201–214.

Chen, W., Srinivasan, S.R., Berenson, G.S., 2009. Influence of birth weight on white blood cell count in biracial (black-white) children, adolescents, and young adults: the Bogalusa Heart Study. Am. J. Epidemiol. 169, 214–218.

Craig, W.J., Mangels, A.R., 2009. Position of the American Dietetic Association: vegetarian diets. J. Am. Diet Assoc. 109, 1266–1282.

Crinnion, W.J., 2009. Maternal levels of xenobiotics that affect fetal development and childhood health. Altern. Med. Rev. 14, 212–222.

Custodio, H.M., Broberg, K., Wennberg, M., Jansson, J.H., Vessby, B., Hallmans, G., Stegmayr, B., Skerfving, S., 2004. Polymorphisms in glutathione-related genes affect methylmercury retention. Arch. Environ. Health 59, 588–595.

Dovydaitis, T., 2008. Fish consumption during pregnancy: an overview of the risks and benefits. J. Midwifery Womens Health 53, 325–330.

Drouillet-Pinard, P., Huel, G., Slama, R., Forhan, A., Sahuquillo, J., Goua, V., Thiebaugeorges, O., Foliguet, B., Magnin, G., Kaminski, M., Cordier, S., Charles, M.A., 2010. Prenatal mercury contamination: relationship with maternal seafood consumption during pregnancy and fetal growth in the 'EDEN mother-child' cohort. Br. J. Nutr. 104, 1096–1100.

Elias, S.L., Innis, S.M., 2001. Infant plasma trans, n-6, and n-3 fatty acids and conjugated linoleic acids are related to maternal plasma fatty acids, length of gestation, and birth weight and length. Am. J. Clin. Nutr. 73, 807–814.

European Food Safety Authority, 2004. EFSA provides risk assessment on mercury in fish: precautionary advice given to vulnerable groups. http://www.efsa.europa.eu/en/press/news/contam040318

European Food Safety Authority, 2015. Statement on the benefits of fish/seafood consumption compared to the risks of methylmercury in fish/seafood. http://www.efsa.europa.eu/en/efsajournal/pub/3982

Fein, G.G., Jacobson, J.L., Jacobson, S.W., Schwartz, P.M., Dowler, J.K., 1984. Prenatal exposure to polychlorinated biphenyls: effects on birth size and gestational age. J. Pediatr. 105, 315–320.

Foldspang, A., Hansen, J.C., 1990. Dietary intake of methylmercury as a correlate of gestational length and birth weight among newborns in Greenland. Am. J. Epidemiol. 132, 310–317.

Genuis, S.J., 2009. Nowhere to hide: chemical toxicants and the unborn child. Reprod. Toxicol. 28, 115–116.

Glynn, A., Aune, M., Darnerud, P.O., Cnattingius, S., Bjerselius, R., Becker, W., Lignell, S., 2007. Determinants of serum concentrations of organochlorine compounds in Swedish pregnant women: a cross-sectional study. Environ. Health. 6, 2.

Govarts, E., Nieuwenhuijsen, M., Schoeters, G., Ballester F., Bloemen, K., de, B.M., Chevrier, C., Eggesbo, M., Guxens, M., Kramer, U., Legler, J., Martinez, D., Palkovicova, L., Patelarou, E., Ranft, U., Rautio, A., Petersen, M.S., Slama, R., Stigum, H., Toft, G., Trnovec, T., Vandentorren,

S., Weihe, P., Kuperus, N.W., Wilhelm, M., Wittsiepe, J., Bonde, J.P., 2012. Birth weight and prenatal exposure to polychlorinated biphenyls (PCBs) and dichlorodiphenyldichloroethylene (DDE): a meta-analysis within 12 European Birth Cohorts. Environ. Health Perspect. 120, 162–170.

Grandjean, P., Bjerve, K.S., Weihe, P., Steuerwald, U., 2001. Birthweight in a fishing community: significance of essential fatty acids and marine food contaminants. Int. J. Epidemiol. 30, 1272–1278.

Grandjean, P., Budtz-Jorgensen, E., Jorgensen, P.J., Weihe, P., 2005. Umbilical cord mercury concentration as biomarker of prenatal exposure to methylmercury. Environ. Health Perspect. 113, 905–908.

Grandjean, P., Landrigan, P.J., 2006. Developmental neurotoxicity of industrial chemicals. Lancet 368, 2167–2178.

Guldner, L., Monfort, C., Rouget F., Garlantezec, R., Cordier, S., 2007. Maternal fish and shellfish intake and pregnancy outcomes: a prospective cohort study in Brittany, France. Environ. Health 6, 33.

Halldorsson, T.I., Meltzer, H.M., Thorsdottir, I., Knudsen, V., Olsen, S.F., 2007. Is high consumption of fatty fish during pregnancy a risk factor for fetal growth retardation? A study of 44,824 Danish pregnant women. Am. J. Epidemiol. 166, 687–696.

Halldorsson, T.I., Thorsdottir, I., Meltzer, H.M., Nielsen F., Olsen, S.F., 2008. Linking exposure to polychlorinated biphenyls with fatty fish consumption and reduced fetal growth among Danish pregnant women: a cause for concern? Am. J. Epidemiol. 168, 958–965.

Harding, J.E., 2001. The nutritional basis of the fetal origins of adult disease. Int. J. Epidemiol. 30, 15–23.

Heppe, D.H., Steegers, E.A., Timmermans, S., Breeijen, H., Tiemeier, H., Hofman, A., Jaddoe, V.W., 2011. Maternal fish consumption, fetal growth and the risks of neonatal complications: the Generation R Study. Br. J. Nutr. 105, 938–949.

Hibbeln, J.R., Davis, J.M., Steer, C., Emmett, P., Rogers, I., Williams, C., Golding, J., 2007. Maternal seafood consumption in pregnancy and neurodevelopmental outcomes in childhood (ALSPAC study): an observational cohort study. Lancet 369, 578–585.

Houston, M.C., 2007. The role of mercury and cadmium heavy metals in vascular disease, hypertension, coronary heart disease, and myocardial infarction. Altern. Ther. Health Med. 13, S128–S133.

Jacobs, Jr., D.R., Ruzzin, J., Lee, D.H., 2014. Environmental pollutants: downgrading the fish food stock affects chronic disease risk. J. Intern. Med. 276, 240–242.

Karagas, M.R., Choi, A.L., Oken, E., Horvat, M., Schoeny, R., Kamai, E., Cowell, W., Grandjean, P., Korrick, S., 2012. Evidence on the human health effects of low-level methylmercury exposure. Environ. Health Perspect. 120, 799–806.

Karmaus, W., Zhu, X., 2004. Maternal concentration of polychlorinated biphenyls and dichlorodiphenyl dichlorethylene and birth weight in Michigan fish eaters: a cohort study. Environ. Health 3, 1.

Knudsen, V.K., Orozova-Bekkevold, I.M., Mikkelsen, T.B., Wolff, S., Olsen, S.F., 2008. Major dietary patterns in pregnancy and fetal growth. Eur. J. Clin. Nutr. 62, 463–470.

Korthals, E.T., Winfrey, M.R., 1987. Seasonal and spatial variations in mercury methylation and demethylation in an oligotrophic lake. Appl. Environ. Microbiol. 53, 2397–2404.

Kris-Etherton, P.M., Grieger, J.A., Etherton, T.D., 2009. Dietary reference intakes for DHA and EPA. Prostagland. Leukot. Essen. Fatty Acid. 81, 99–104.

Lederman, S.A., Jones, R.L., Caldwell, K.L., Rauh, V., Sheets, S.E., Tang, D., Viswanathan, S., Becker, M., Stein, J.L., Wang, R.Y., Perera, F.P., 2008. Relation between cord blood mercury levels and early child development in a World Trade Center cohort. Environ. Health Perspect. 116, 1085–1091.

Lee, D.H., Jacobs, Jr., D.R., 2010. Inconsistent epidemiological findings on fish consumption may be indirect evidence of harmful contaminants in fish. J. Epidemiol. Comm. Health 64, 190–192.

Legrand, M., Arp, P., Ritchie, C., Chan, H.M., 2005. Mercury exposure in two coastal communities of the Bay of Fundy, Canada. Environ. Res. 98, 14–21.

Leventakou, V., Roumeliotaki, T., Martinez, D., Barros, H., Brantsaeter, A.L., Casas, M., Charles, M.A., Cordier, S., Eggesbo, M., van, E.M., Forastiere F., Gehring, U., Govarts, E., Halldorsson, T.I., Hanke, W., Haugen, M., Heppe, D.H., Heude, B., Inskip, H.M., Jaddoe, V.W., Jansen, M., Kelleher, C., Meltzer, H.M., Merletti F., Molto-Puigmarti, C., Mommers, M., Murcia, M., Oliveira, A., Olsen, S.F., Pele F., Polanska, K., Porta, D., Richiardi, L., Robinson, S.M., Stigum, H., Strom, M., Sunyer, J., Thijs, C., Viljoen, K., Vrijkotte, T.G., Wijga, A.H., Kogevinas, M., Vrijheid, M., Chatzi, L., 2014. Fish intake during pregnancy, fetal growth, and gestational length in 19 European birth cohort studies. Am. J. Clin. Nutr. 99, 506–516.

Lignell, S., Aune, M., Darnerud, P.O., Hanberg, A., Larsson, S.C., Glynn, A., 2013. Prenatal exposure to polychlorinated biphenyls (PCBs) and polybrominated diphenyl ethers (PBDEs) may influence birth weight among infants in a Swedish cohort with background exposure: a cross-sectional study. Environ. Health 12, 44.

Lucas, M., Dewailly, E., Muckle, G., Ayotte, P., Bruneau, S., Gingras, S., Rhainds, M., Holub, B.J., 2004. Gestational age and birth weight in relation to n-3 fatty acids among Inuit (Canada). Lipids 39, 617–626.

Mahaffey, K.R., 2005. Mercury exposure: medical and public health issues. Trans. Am. Clin. Climatol. Assoc. 116, 127–153.

McDiarmid, M.A., Gardiner, P.M., Jack, B.W., 2008. The clinical content of preconception care: environmental exposures. Am. J. Obstet. Gynecol. 199, S357–S361.

Mendez, M.A., Plana, E., Guxens, M., Foradada Morillo, C.M., Albareda, R.M., Garcia-Esteban, R., Goni, F., Kogevinas, M., Sunyer, J., 2010. Seafood consumption in pregnancy and infant size at birth: results from a prospective Spanish cohort. J. Epidemiol. Comm. Health 64, 216–222.

Morris, S.S., Victora, C.G., Barros, F.C., Halpern, R., Menezes, A.M., Cesar, J.A., Horta, B.L., Tomasi, E., 1998. Length and ponderal index at birth: associations with mortality, hospitalizations, development and post-natal growth in Brazilian infants. Int. J. Epidemiol. 27, 242–247.

Mortensen, M.E., Caudill, S.P., Caldwell, K.L., Ward, C.D., Jones, R.L., 2014. Total and methyl mercury in whole blood measured for the first time in the U.S. population: NHANES 2011–12. Environ. Res. 134, 257–264.

Murphy, L.E., Gollenberg, A.L., Buck Louis, G.M., Kostyniak, P.J., Sundaram, R., 2010. Maternal serum preconception polychlorinated biphenyl concentrations and infant birth weight. Environ. Health Perspect. 118, 297–302.

Oken, E., Choi, A.L., Karagas, M.R., Marien, K., Rheinberger, C.M., Schoeny, R., Sunderland, E., Korrick, S., 2012. Which fish should I eat? Perspectives influencing fish consumption choices. Environ. Health Perspect. 120, 790–798.

Oken, E., Kleinman, K.P., Olsen, S.F., Rich-Edwards, J.W., Gillman, M.W., 2004. Associations of seafood and elongated n-3 fatty acid intake with fetal growth and length of gestation: results from a US pregnancy cohort. Am. J. Epidemiol. 160, 774–783.

Oken, E., Osterdal, M.L., Gillman, M.W., Knudsen, V.K., Halldorsson, T.I., Strom, M., Bellinger, D.C., Hadders-Algra, M., Michaelsen, K.F., Olsen, S.F., 2008a. Associations of maternal fish intake during pregnancy and breastfeeding duration with attainment of developmental milestones in early childhood: a study from the Danish National Birth Cohort. Am. J. Clin. Nutr. 88, 789–796.

Oken, E., Radesky, J.S., Wright, R.O., Bellinger, D.C., Amarasiriwardena, C.J., Kleinman, K.P., Hu, H., Gillman, M.W., 2008b. Maternal fish intake during pregnancy, blood mercury levels, and child cognition at age 3 years in a US cohort. Am. J. Epidemiol. 167, 1171–1181.

Oken, E., Wright, R.O., Kleinman, K.P., Bellinger, D., Amarasiriwardena, C.J., Hu, H., Rich-Edwards, J.W., Gillman, M.W., 2005. Maternal fish consumption, hair mercury, and infant cognition in a U.S. Cohort. Environ. Health Perspect. 113, 1376–1380.

Olsen, S.F., Grandjean, P., Weihe, P., Videro, T., 1993. Frequency of seafood intake in pregnancy as a determinant of birth weight: evidence for a dose dependent relationship. J. Epidemiol. Comm. Health 47, 436–440.

Olsen, S.F., Hansen, H.S., Secher, N.J., Jensen, B., Sandstrom, B., 1995. Gestation length and birth weight in relation to intake of marine n-3 fatty acids. Br. J. Nutr. 73, 397–404.

Olsen, S.F., Hansen, H.S., Sorensen, T.I., Jensen, B., Secher, N.J., Sommer, S., Knudsen, L.B., 1986. Intake of marine fat, rich in (n-3)-polyunsaturated fatty acids, may increase birthweight by prolonging gestation. Lancet 2, 367–369.

Olsen, S.F., Olsen, J., Frische, G., 1990. Does fish consumption during pregnancy increase fetal growth? A study of the size of the newborn, placental weight and gestational age in relation to fish consumption during pregnancy. Int. J. Epidemiol. 19, 971–977.

Olsen, S.F., Osterdal, M.L., Salvig, J.D., Kesmodel, U., Henriksen, T.B., Hedegaard, M., Secher, N.J., 2006. Duration of pregnancy in relation to seafood intake during early and mid pregnancy: prospective cohort. Eur. J. Epidemiol. 21, 749–758.

Olsen, S.F., Secher, N.J., 2002. Low consumption of seafood in early pregnancy as a risk factor for preterm delivery: prospective cohort study. BMJ 324, 447.

Patandin, S., Koopman-Esseboom, C., de Ridder, M.A., Weisglas-Kuperus, N., Sauer, P.J., 1998. Effects of environmental exposure to polychlorinated biphenyls and dioxins on birth size and growth in Dutch children. Pediatr. Res. 44, 538–545.

Ramon, R., Ballester F., Aguinagalde, X., Amurrio, A., Vioque, J., Lacasana, M., Rebagliato, M., Murcia, M., Iniguez, C., 2009a. Fish consumption during pregnancy, prenatal mercury exposure, and anthropometric measures at birth in a prospective mother-infant cohort study in Spain. Am. J. Clin. Nutr. 90, 1047–1055.

Ramon, R., Ballester F., Iniguez, C., Rebagliato, M., Murcia, M., Esplugues, A., Marco, A., Garcia de la, H.M., Vioque, J., 2009b. Vegetable but not fruit intake during pregnancy is associated with newborn anthropometric measures. J. Nutr. 139, 561–567.

Ramon, R., Murcia, M., Aguinagalde, X., Amurrio, A., Llop, S., Ibarluzea, J., Lertxundi, A., varez-Pedrerol, M., Casas, M., Vioque, J., Sunyer, J., Tardon, A., Martinez-Arguelles, B., Ballester, F., 2011. Prenatal mercury exposure in a multicenter cohort study in Spain. Environ. Int. 37, 597–604.

Ribas-Fito, N., Ramon, R., Ballester, F., Grimalt, J., Marco, A., Olea, N., Posada, M., Rebagliato, M., Tardon, A., Torrent, M., Sunyer, J., 2006. Child health and the environment: the INMA Spanish Study. Paediatr. Perinat. Epidemiol. 20, 403–410.

Ribas-Fito, N., Sala, M., Cardo, E., Mazon, C., De Muga, M.E., Verdu, A., Marco, E., Grimalt, J.O., Sunyer, J., 2002. Association of hexachlorobenzene and other organochlorine compounds with anthropometric measures at birth. Pediatr. Res. 52, 163–167.

Richards, M., Hardy, R., Kuh, D., Wadsworth, M.E., 2002. Birthweight, postnatal growth and cognitive function in a national UK birth cohort. Int. J. Epidemiol. 31, 342–348.

Roberts, E., Wood, P., 2014. Birth weight and adult health in historical perspective: evidence from a New Zealand cohort, 1907–22. Soc. Sci. Med. 107, 154–161.

Rodriguez-Bernal, C.L., Rebagliato, M., Iniguez, C., Vioque, J., Navarrete-Munoz, E.M., Murcia, M., Bolumar, F., Marco, A., Ballester, F., 2010. Diet quality in early pregnancy and its effects on fetal growth outcomes: the Infancia y Medio Ambiente (Childhood and Environment) Mother and Child Cohort Study in Spain. Am. J. Clin. Nutr. 91, 1659–1666.

Rogan, W.J., Gladen, B.C., McKinney, J.D., Carreras, N., Hardy, P., Thullen, J., Tinglestad, J., Tully, M., 1986. Neonatal effects of transplacental exposure to PCBs and DDE. J. Pediatr. 109, 335–341.

Rogers, I., Emmett, P., Ness, A., Golding, J., 2004. Maternal fish intake in late pregnancy and the frequency of low birth weight and intrauterine growth retardation in a cohort of British infants. J. Epidemiol. Comm. Health 58, 486–492.

Rosell, M.S., Lloyd-Wright, Z., Appleby, P.N., Sanders, T.A., Allen, N.E., Key, T.J., 2005. Long-chain n-3 polyunsaturated fatty acids in plasma in British meat-eating, vegetarian, and vegan men. Am. J. Clin. Nutr. 82, 327–334.

Ruzzin, J., 2012. Public health concern behind the exposure to persistent organic pollutants and the risk of metabolic diseases. BMC Pub. Health 12, 298.

Rylander, L., Stromberg, U., Dyremark, E., Ostman, C., Nilsson-Ehle, P., Hagmar, L., 1998. Polychlorinated biphenyls in blood plasma among Swedish female fish consumers in relation to low birth weight. Am. J. Epidemiol. 147, 493–502.

Sakamoto, M., Kubota, M., Murata, K., Nakai, K., Sonoda, I., Satoh, H., 2008. Changes in mercury concentrations of segmental maternal hair during gestation and their correlations with other biomarkers of fetal exposure to methylmercury in the Japanese population. Environ. Res. 106, 270–276.

Sala, M., Sunyer, J., Otero, R., Santiago-Silva, M., Camps, C., Grimalt, J., 1999. Organochlorine in the serum of inhabitants living near an electrochemical factory. Occup. Environ. Med. 56, 152–158.

Sanfeliu, C., Sebastia, J., Cristofol, R., Rodriguez-Farre, E., 2003. Neurotoxicity of organomercurial compounds. Neurotox. Res. 5, 283–305.

Schecter, A., Cramer, P., Boggess, K., Stanley, J., Papke, O., Olson, J., Silver, A., Schmitz, M., 2001. Intake of dioxins and related compounds from food in the U.S. population. J. Toxicol. Environ. Health A 63, 1–18.

Shire, J.D., Marsh, G.M., Talbott, E.O., Sharma, R.K., 2011. Advances and current themes in occupational health and environmental public health surveillance. Ann. Rev. Pub. Health 32, 109–132.

Starling, P., Charlton, K., McMahon, A.T., Lucas, C., 2015. Fish intake during pregnancy and foetal neurodevelopment--a systematic review of the evidence. Nutrients 7, 2001–2014.

Thomas, S., Arbuckle, T.E., Fisher, M., Fraser, W.D., Ettinger, A., King, W., 2015. Metals exposure and risk of small-for-gestational age birth in a Canadian birth cohort: the MIREC study. Environ. Res. 140, 430–439.

Thorsdottir, I., Birgisdottir, B.E., Halldorsdottir, S., Geirsson, R.T., 2004. Association of fish and fish liver oil intake in pregnancy with infant size at birth among women of normal weight before pregnancy in a fishing community. Am. J. Epidemiol. 160, 460–465.

US Food and Drug Administration, Environmental Protection Agency, 2004. What You Need to Know About Mercury in Fish and Shellfish, 2004. http://www.fda.gov/NewsEvents/Newsroom/PressAnnouncements/2004/ucm108267.htm
US Food and Drug Administration, Environmental Protection Agency, 2014. Fish: What Pregnant Women and Parents Should Know. Draft Updated Advice by FDA and EPA. http://www.fda.gov/Food/FoodborneIllnessContaminants/Metals/ucm393070.htm
Vartiainen, T., Jaakkola, J.J., Saarikoski, S., Tuomisto, J., 1998. Birth weight and sex of children and the correlation to the body burden of PCDDs/PCDFs and PCBs of the mother. Environ. Health Perspect. 106, 61–66.
Watson, P.E., McDonald, B.W., 2007. Seasonal variation of nutrient intake in pregnancy: effects on infant measures and possible influence on diseases related to season of birth. Eur. J. Clin. Nutr. 61, 1271–1280.
Weis, P., Ashley, J.T., 2007. Contaminants in fish of the Hackensack Meadowlands, New Jersey: size, sex, and seasonal relationships as related to health risks. Arch. Environ. Contam. Toxicol. 52, 80–89.
Welch, A.A., Shakya-Shrestha, S., Lentjes, M.A., Wareham, N.J., Khaw, K.T., 2010. Dietary intake and status of n-3 polyunsaturated fatty acids in a population of fish-eating and non-fish-eating meat-eaters, vegetarians, and vegans and the product-precursor ratio [corrected] of alpha-linolenic acid to long-chain n-3 polyunsaturated fatty acids: results from the EPIC-Norfolk cohort. Am. J. Clin. Nutr. 92, 1040–1051.
WHO, Regional Office for Europe, 2014. European Food and Nutrition Action Plan 2015. Available from: (http://www.euro.who.int/__data/assets/pdf_file/0008/253727/64wd14e_FoodNutAP_140426.pdf).
Wilcox, A.J., 2001. On the importance--and the unimportance--of birthweight. Int. J. Epidemiol. 30, 1233–1241.
Willet, W., 1998. Nutritional Epidemiology. NY: Oxford University Press, New York.
Xue, F., Holzman, C., Rahbar, M.H., Trosko, K., Fischer, L., 2007. Maternal fish consumption, mercury levels, and risk of preterm delivery. Environ. Health Perspect. 115, 42–47.

CHAPTER

9

Fish Oil and The Retinopathy of Prematurity

S. Beken, E.U. Kabataş***

*Department of Neonatology, Acıbadem University School of Medicine, Istanbul, Turkey;
**Department of Ophthalmology, Dr Sami Ulus Maternity and Children Training and Research Hospital, Ankara, Turkey

RETINOPATHY OF PREMATURITY

Retinopathy of prematurity (ROP) is a preventable cause of blindness which primarily affects premature infants (Chen et al., 2011). The most important risk factors leading to the development of ROP are the infant's gestational age, birth weight, and immaturity (Araz-Ersan et al., 2013). Infants with a gestational age of <32 weeks and birth weight of <1500 g appear to be at high risk for ROP and must be screened for ROP development (SOAAP, 2006).

Pathogenesis of ROP

Retinal vascularization is completed at the 32nd gestational week in the nasal region and at the 40th gestational week in the temporal region (Chen and Smith, 2007). ROP development occurs in two phases in a preterm infant. At birth, retinal vascularization is not completed and in phase-1 preterm the infant or baby encounters a hyperoxic environment. This hyperoxia suppresses VEGF which is necessary for normal vascularization. Otherwise, the insulin-like growth factor (IGF-1) level that passes through the placenta is low in premature babies. This phase continues up to the 31st week. The second phase occurs between the 31st–45th week and is characterized with hypoxia. Because the retina is avascular, it becomes hypoxic with ever-growing metabolic needs. This hypoxia causes abnormal secretion of Vascular endothelial growth factor (VEGF), causes abnormal angiogenesis, and tractional retinal detachment at the end of this phase (Chen and Smith, 2007; Palmer et al., 1991).

Angiogenesis is the formation of new vessels from the existing ones. The mechanisms of angiogenesis (Kumar et al., 2015) include:

1. Secretion of angiogenic factors induced by hypoxia (the most important one is VEGF).
2. Binding of the angiogenic factors to their receptors in the endothelium (VEGF binds to its tyrosine kinase receptor).
3. Receptor activation and signal delivery to the nucleus; after VEGF binds to its receptor, the signal is transported to the nucleus by MAP kinase (mitogene-activated protein) enzyme. This leads to secretion of proteolytic enzymes.
4. The endothelium-derived proteolytic enzymes are matrix metalloproteinases (MMPs) and plasminogen activator.
5. The proteolytic enzymes break down the basal membranes of pericytes around the endothelium. As a result, endothelial cells are separated and vascular permeability increases.
6. Endothelial cells migrate to the area where angiogenic factors are secreted.
7. Cell adhesion molecules (especially integrins) help the mechanic attraction of the endothelial cells to the hypoxic area.

Fish and Fish Oil in Health and Disease Prevention. http://dx.doi.org/10.1016/B978-0-12-802844-5.00009-9

8. MMPs destroy the tissue in front of the endothelial cell.
9. Endothelial cell sprouts form vessel tubes by coming together.
10. The new vessel is stabilized by the pericyte migration.

It is known that n–3 reduces the pathologic neovascularization and slows down the progression of ROP. Favorable effects of n–3 in diabetic retinopathy and macular degeneration in adults have been shown but the underlying mechanism is still unclear.

FISH OIL

The essential fatty acids (EFAs) alpha-linolenic acid and linoleic acid cannot be synthesized in humans because of the lack of delta 15 and delta 22 desaturase enzymes (San Giovanni and Chew, 2005). After they are taken in by diet they are converted into long chain polyunsaturated fatty acids (LCPUFAs) in the endoplasmic reticulum of liver and retina. Alpha linolenic acid is a precursor for docosahexaenoic acid (DHA) a long chain n–3 fatty acid and its substrate eicosapentaenoic acid (EPA); linoleic acid (LA) is a precursor for arachidonic acid (ARA) an omega-6 (n–6) fatty acid (San Giovanni and Chew, 2005). The active anti-inflammatory metabolites of DHA are neuroprotectin and resolvin D, whereas the active metabolite of EPA is resolvin E (Salem et al., 2001; Serhan and Savill, 2005). All these active metabolites are anti-inflammatory (Connor et al., 2007).

Because these lipids pass through the placenta, especially during the third trimester, premature babies have a deficiency of these lipids (Joseph, 2012). It's known that these fatty acids, especially n-3 PUFAs, have a protective effect against ischemia and inflammation (Connor et al., 2007; Joseph, 2012).

Positive relationships between n–3 PUFAs and visual function have been shown by previous research. Omega-3 PUFAs constitute nearly half of the retinal fatty acids replaced in the outer membrane of the retinal photoreceptor layer. Omega-3 PUFAs affect the thickness, fluidity, and permeability of the photoreceptor membranes. At the same time, they play a role in rhodopsin regeneration and signal transduction by increasing the amounts of membrane dependent retinal proteins (San Giovanni and Chew, 2005).

FISH OIL AND RETINOPATHY OF PREMATURITY

ROP is characterized by abnormal angiogenesis (Palmer et al., 1991). The stimulation factors of angiogenesis can be lipid or protein derived; the lipid-derived factors are the mediators that are formed by cyclooxygenase (COX) and lipoxygenase (LOX) enzymes and protein-derived factors are cytokines and growth factors (San Giovanni and Chew, 2005).

The angiogenic factors which are formed from arachidonic acid by COX enzyme are: ThromboxaneA_2 (TXA_2), ProstaglandinE_2 (PgE_2), Prostacyclin (PgI_2), and the angiogenic factor which is formed by LOX enzyme is Leukotriene B_4 (LTB_4) (Rose and Connolly, 2000). It is thought that these factors stimulate endothelial cell proliferation, migration, and tube formation steps of angiogenesis (Rose and Connolly, 2007). Otherwise, the angiogenic effect of the ARA metabolites have been proven by studies about selective COX-2 inhibitors to inhibit experimentally generated neovascularization (Wilkinson-Berka et al., 2003). Ringbom et al. (2001) showed that DHA and EPA inhibits the COX enzyme in vitro.

LTB_4 is a mediator that can cause increased tumor necrosis factor-alpha (TNF-α) concentration (Talvani et al., 2002). It has been shown that this mediator could play a role in diabetic retinopathy (Limb et al., 1996) and ROP development by increasing the cell adhesion molecules like vascular cell adhesion molecule-1 (VCAM-1) and intercellular adhesion molecule (ICAM-1) both of which play a role in angiogenesis (Yossuck et al., 2001). Furthermore, TNF-α deficient mice have less oxygen-induced retinopathy, which supports the angiogenic effect of these mediators (Gardiner et al., 2005). DHA reduces angiogenesis by inhibition of LTB_4 and TNF-α synthesis (Collie-Duguid and Wahle, 1996; De Caterina et al., 2000). It has been shown that the expression of adhesion molecules (VCAM-1, ICAM-1, and E-selectin) and their role in angiogenesis is decreased when DHA and EPA was added to the adult saphenous vein endothelial cell culture (Collie-Duguid and Wahle, 1996; De Caterina et al., 2000). This finding also supports the antiangiogenic effect of DHA.

Phospholipase A (PLA) is an enzyme that plays a role in ARA synthesis and increases in ischemia (Kolko et al., 2002; Phillis and O'Regan, 2003), inflammation (Bazan et al., 2002) and with the increase of free oxygen radicals (Hutcheson, 2003). Furthermore, there are some reports that PLA increases retinal ischemia and plays a role in

ROP pathogenesis (Kohner and Chibber, 2001). DHA has been shown to suppress PLA (Martin, 1998). So, it can be deduced that DHA inhibits the angiogenesis by suppressing PLA enzyme.

VEGF, which is an important growth factor in angiogenesis, shows it's effect through the MAP kinase enzyme. EPA has been shown to reduce the activity of MAP kinase via VEGF (Yang et al., 1998; Kanayasu et al., 1991). EPA also inhibits the activation of urokinase-type plasminogen activator (u-PA) which allows for the separation and migration of endothelial cells during angiogenesis (du Toit et al., 1996). Another effect of EPA on angiogenesis is inhibition of NF-KB transcription factor (angiogenetic factor), by increasing COX-2 expression and ICAM synthesis (von Knethen et al., 1999). Additionally, it's been shown that EPA inhibited the tube formation of endothelial cells experimentally (Murota et al., 2000).

MMPs play a role in angiogenesis and inflammation. TNF-α, Interleukin-1 (IL-1), VEGF, Fibroblast growth factor-beta (FGFβ), and free oxygen radicals contribute to the angiogenesis by increasing MMPs. MMP-2 and MMP-9 both play a role in angiogenesis by destructing type 4 collagen in the endothelial basal membrane. The increase of this enzyme has also shown to have an effect on ROP development (Sivak and Fini, 2002). A decrease in MMPs levels has been observed in mice fed with foods containing DHA (Harris et al., 2001). Finally, DHA has been shown to provide a direct anti-angiogenic effect via peroxisome proliferator-activated receptor -gamma (PPAR-γ) (Rezende et al., 2014).

Besides these experimental data, there are a few clinical trials assessing the effects of n–3 on ROP development. In their study, Pawlik et al. (2011) evaluated 84 preterm infants who weighed below 1250 g and received parenteral nutrition from the first day of their lives. Of these, 40 infants received fish oil lipid emulsions with soybean and olive oil compared with historical cohort of 44 infants who received soybean and olive oil emulsions. They reported that 13 infants from the fish oil group and 16 infants from soybean and olive oil group developed ROP and no difference was found between groups; however, in the first group, 3 infants required laser therapy whereas 12 infants in the second group required laser therapy and it was statistically significant. In their second study Pawlik et al. (2014) randomized 130 infants below 1250 g to two groups: the first group consisted of 60 infants that received soybean, olive oil, and fish oil emulsion, and a control group of 70 infants that was given a parenteral soybean and olive oil emulsion. They reported that 19 infants from the fish oil group and 26 infants from control group developed ROP and no difference was found between groups; however, 9 infants in the fish oil group required laser therapy for ROP compared with 22 infants in the standard control group. They concluded that IV fat emulsion with incorporated fish oil decreases the severity of ROP.

Beken et al. (2014) randomized 80 infants weighing below 1500 g and receiving parenteral nutrition from the first day of life to two groups: the first group of 40 infants who received fish oil-based lipid emulsions and a control group of 40 infants who received soybean oil based lipid emulsions. Two infants from the fish oil group and 13 infants from soybean oil group developed ROP and this was found to be statistically significant. In each group, at least one patient required laser therapy. They concluded that fish oil lipid emulsions from the first day of life might be preventive treatment for ROP development in preterm infants.

In conclusion, n–3 PUFAs and their metabolites inhibit angiogenesis experimentally. Few randomized, controlled trials support this data and further studies are needed to assess this effect in preterm infants.

References

Araz-Ersan, B., Kir, N., Akarcay, K., et al., 2013. Epidemiological analysis of retinopathy of prematurity in a referral centre in Turkey. Br. J. Ophthalmol. 97, 15–17.

Bazan, N.G., Colangelo, V., Lukiw, W.J., 2002. Prostaglandins and other lipid mediators in Alzheimer's disease. Prostagland. Other Lipid Mediat. 68–69, 197–210.

Beken, S., Dilli, D., Fettah, N.D., Kabataş, E.U., Zenciroğlu, A., Okumuş, N., 2014. The influence of fish oil lipid emulsions on retinopathy of prematurity in very low birth weight infants: arandomized controlled trial. Early Human Dev. 90 (1), 27–31.

Chen, J., Smith, L.E., 2007. Retinopathy of prematurity. Angiogenesis 10, 133–140.

Chen, J., Stahl, A., Hellstrom, A., Smith, L.E., 2011. Current update on retinopathy of prematurity: screening and treatment. Curr. Opin. Pediatr. 23 (2), 173–178.

Collie-Duguid, E.S., Wahle, K.W., 1996. Inhibitory effect of fish oil N-3 polyunsaturated fatty acids on the expression of endothelial cell adhesion molecules. Biochem. Biophys. Res. Comm. 27 (3), 969–974, 220.

Connor, K.M., SanGiovanni, J.P., Lofqvist, C., Aderman, C.M., Chen, J., Higuchi, A., Hong, S., Pravda, E.A., Majchrzak, S., Carper, D., Hellstrom, A., Kang, J.X., Chew, E.Y., Salem, Jr., N., Serhan, C.N., Smith, L.E., 2007. Increased dietary intake of omega-3-polyunsaturated fatty acids reduces pathological retinal angiogenesis. Nat. Med. 13 (7), 868–873.

De Caterina, R., Liao, J.K., Libby, P., 2000. Fatty acid modulation of endothelial activation. Am. J. Clin. Nutr. 71 (Suppl. 1), 213S–223S.

du Toit, P.J., van Aswegen, C.H., du Plessis, D.J., 1996. The effect of essential fatty acids on growth and urokinase-type plasminogen activator production in human prostate DU-145 cells. Prostagland. Leukot. Essen. Fatty Acid. 55 (3), 173–177.

Gardiner, T.A., Gibson, D.S., de Gooyer, T.E., de la Cruz, V.F., McDonald, D.M., Stitt, A.W., 2005. Inhibition of tumor necrosis factor-a improves physiological angiogenesis and reduces pathological neovascularization in ischemic retinopathy. Am. J. Pathol. 166 (2), 637–644.

Harris, M.A., Hansen, R.A., Vidsudhiphan, P., Koslo, J.L., Thomas, J.B., Watkins, B.A., Allen, K.G., 2001. Effects of conjugated linoleic acids and docosahexaenoic acid on rat liver and reproductive tissue fatty acids, prostaglandins and matrix metalloproteinase production. Prostagland. Leukot. Essen. Fatty Acid. 65 (1), 23–29.

Hutcheson, K.A., 2003. Retinopathy of prematurity. Curr. Opin. Ophthalmol. 14 (5), 286–290.

Joseph, N., 2012. Gastroenterology and Nutrition, Neonatology Questions And Controversies, Second ed., Elsevier Saunders, Chapter 12, Sheila M. Innis, PhD. Lipids for neonates, pp:183–202.

Kanayasu, T., Morita, I., Nakao-Hayashi, J., Asuwa, N., Fujisawa, C., Ishii, T., Ito, H., Murota, S., 1991. Eicosapentaenoic acid inhibits tube formation of vascular endothelial cells in vitro. Lipids 26 (4), 271–276.

Kohner, E.M., Chibber, R., 2001. Retinal ischemia. Schachat, A.P. (Ed.), Retina, vol. 2, Third ed. St. Mosby, Louis, pp. 982–994.

Kolko, M., de Turco, E.B., Diemer, N.H., Bazan, N.G., 2002. Secretory phospholipase A2 mediated neuronal cell death involves glutamate ionotropic receptors. Neuroreport 13 (15), 1963–1966.

Kumar, Vinay, Abbas Abul, K., Aster Jon, C., 2015. Robbins and Cotran Pathologic Basis of Disease, Ninth ed. Elsevier Saunders, p:104–105.

Limb, G.A., Chignell, A.H., Green, W., LeRoy, F., Dumonde, D.C., 1996. Distribution of TNF alpha and its reactive vascular adhesion molecules in fibrovascular membranes of proliferative diabetic retinopathy. Br. J. Ophthalmol. 80, 168–173.

Martin, R.E., 1998. Docosahexaenoic acid decreases phospholipase A2 activity in the neurites/nerve growth cones of PC12 cells. J. Neurosci. Res. 15 (6), 805–813, 54.

Murota, S.I., Onodera, M., Morita, I., 2000. Regulation of angiogenesis by controlling VEGF receptor. Ann. NY Acad. Sci. 902, 208–212, discussion 212-3.

Palmer, E.A., Flynn, J.T., Hardy, R.J., Phelps, D.L., Phillips, C.L., Schaffer, D.B., Tung, B., 1991. Incidence and early course of retinopathy of prematurity. The cryotherapy for retinopathy of prematurity cooperative group. Ophthalmology 98, 1628–1640.

Pawlik, D., Lauterbach, R., Turyk, E., 2011. Fish-oil fat emulsion supplementation may reduce the risk of severe retinopathy in VLBW infants. Pediatrics 127, 223–228.

Pawlik, D., Lauterbach, R., Walczak, M., Hurkala, J., Sherman, M.P., 2014. Fish-oil fat emulsion supplementation reduces the risk of retinopathy in very low birth weight infants: a prospective, randomized study. J. Parenter. Enteral. Nutr. 38 (6), 711–716.

Phillis, J.W., O'Regan, M.H., 2003. The role of phospholipases, cyclooxygenases, and lipoxygenases in cerebral ischemic/traumatic injuries. Crit. Rev. Neurobiol. 15 (1), 61–90.

Rezende, F.A., Lapalme, E., Qian, C.X., Smith, L.E., SanGiovanni, J.P., Sapieha, P., 2014. Omega 3 supplementation combined with anti vascular endothelial growth factor lowers vitreal levels of vascular endothelial growth factor in wet age-related macular degeneration. Am. J. Ophthalmol. 158 (5), 1071–1078.

Ringbom, T., Huss, U., Stenholm, A., Flock, S., Skattebol, L., Perera, P., Bohlin, L., 2001. COX-2 inhibitory effects of naturally occurring and modified fatty acids. J. Nat. Prod. 64, 745–749.

Rose, D.P., Connolly, J.M., 2000. Regulation of tumor angiogenesis by dietary fatty acids and eicosanoids. Nutr. Cancer. 37 (2), 119–127.

Salem, Jr., N., Litman, B., Kim, H.Y., Gawrisch, K., 2001. Mechanisms of action of docosahexaenoic acid in the nervous system. Lipids 36 (9), 945–959.

San Giovanni, J.P., Chew, E.Y., 2005. The role of omega-3 long- chain polyunsaturated fatty acids in health and disease of the retina. Prog. Retin. Eye Res. 24 (1), 87–138.

Section on Ophthalmology American Academy of Pediatrics; American Academy of Ophthalmology; American Association for Pediatric Ophthalmology and Strabismus. Screening examination of prematüre infants for retinopathy of prematurity. Pediatrics. 2006; 117: 572–576.

Serhan, C.N., Savill, J., 2005. Resolution of inflammation: the beginning programs the end. Nat. Immunol. 6 (12), 1191–1197.

Sivak, J.M., Fini, M.E., 2002. MMPs in the eye: emerging roles formatrix metalloproteinases in ocular physiology. Prog. Retin. Eye Res. 21 (1), 1–14.

Talvani, A., Machado, F.S., Santana, G.C., Klein, A., Barcelos, L., Silva, J.S., Teixeira, M.M., 2002. Leukotriene B(4) induces nitric oxide synthesis in *Trypanosoma cruzi*-infected murine macrophages and mediates resistance to infection. Infect. Immun. 70 (8), 4247–4253.

von Knethen, A., Callsen, D., Brüne, B., 1999. Superoxide attenuates macrophage apoptosis by NF-kappa B and AP-1 activation that promotes cyclooxygenase-2 expression. J. Immunol. 163 (5), 2858–2866.

Wilkinson-Berka, J.L., Alousis, N.S., Kelly, D.J., Gilbert, R.E., 2003. COX-2 inhibition and retinal angiogenesis in a mouse model of retinopathy of prematurity. Invest. Ophthalmol. Vis. Sci. 44 (3), 974–979.

Yang, S.P., Morita, I., Murota, S.I., 1998. Eicosapentaenoic acid attenuates vascular endothelial growth factor-induced proliferation via inhibiting Flk-1 receptor expression in bovine carotid artery endothelial cells. J. Cell Physiol. 176 (2), 342–349.

Yossuck, P., Yan, Y., Tadesse, M., Higgins, R.D., 2001. Dexamethasone alters TNF-alpha expression in retinopathy. Mol. Genet. Metab. 72 (2), 164–167.

CHAPTER

10

Fish Oil for Physical Performance in Athletes

G.E. Peoples, P.L. McLennan

School of Medicine, University of Wollongong, Wollongong, New South Wales, Australia

INTRODUCTION

Physical performance is an innate requirement of competitive athletes. In fact, for those who classify themselves as professional athletes, performance is the single measure that is a benchmark of a successful career. Engagement in physical work, training or competition, is physiologically stressful. Multiple body systems including cardiovascular, respiratory, and skeletal muscle are repetitively subjected to acute bouts of strain and as a consequence these physiologically adapt leading to functional improvement. Dietary practices form a central part of an athlete's regime and include both whole foods and added supplements. Often the primary concern of the athlete is carbohydrate intake to replenish muscle glycogen stores, balanced against a background of dietary fat (Burke et al., 2004). Dietary fat, in a loading sense, has been differentially recognized as a possible factor that can modulate metabolism during exercise (Jeukendrup et al., 1998) although it has not been transferable in the sense of athletic performance (Burke, 2006). However, dietary fats are a complex grouping of nonessential and essential fatty acid chains, including the polyunsaturated fatty acids (PUFA) characterized into discrete families according to the first placed double bond. On the basis of their diverse structures, there are equally diverse physiological roles supported by these differing fatty acids beyond simply being available for the production of aerobic ATP. In fact, survey data of elite athletes reflects high rates of supplement use, including fish oil, and indicate they do consider single dietary components, such as, fatty acids, essential for training and competition (Ronsen et al., 1999; Lun et al., 2012) warranting clarification of their role in the athlete's diet.

DIETARY FISH OIL: PROVISION OF LONG-CHAIN OMEGA-3 POLYUNSATURATED FATTY ACIDS

Long-chain omega-3 polyunsaturated fatty acids (LC n–3 PUFA) have emerged as showing potential for supporting physical exertion. Fatty fish especially provides the LC n–3 PUFA eicosapentaenoic acid (EPA) and docosahexaenoic acid (DHA). Dietary intakes of foods high in preformed DHA, such as fish oils, are essential to increase the concentration of LC n–3 PUFA in the body as conversion of short-chain alpha-linolenic acid (ALA) to EPA and DHA is inefficient (Leonard et al., 2004; Gibson et al., 2013). In fact, fish consumption is now recognized as critical in the human diet to optimize health (Gogus and Smith, 2010) and physical capacity over a lifetime (Abbatecola et al., 2009). For example, in the cardiovascular system fish consumption contributes to reduced risk of primary cardiac arrest (Mozaffarian and Rimm, 2006; James et al., 2014) including primary prevention of sudden cardiac death (Siscovick et al., 1995). Underpinning the cardiovascular risk, the low median Omega-3 Index (EPA% + DHA%) of Western populations is in turn indicative of low dietary fish or fish oil consumption (Colquhoun et al., 2008). Despite the intense focus on nutrition for elite athletes, the low consumption of LC n–3 PUFA appears to be no different from the rest of the population. In a recent study of elite German endurance athletes where the dietary exposure to EPA

Fish and Fish Oil in Health and Disease Prevention. http://dx.doi.org/10.1016/B978-0-12-802844-5.00010-5

and DHA was measured using the red blood cell membranes (von Schacky et al., 2014), only one athlete (out of 106) obtained an Omega-3 Index in the range 8–11%, associated with the lowest cardiovascular risk. Moreover, the mean Omega-3 Index in the group was <5% and therefore one in three athletes screened were classified in the highest risk category for cardiac disease for this biomarker (<4%) (Harris and von Schacky, 2004). There is a move to have LC n–3 PUFA EPA and DHA recognized as essential for reducing responses to the stresses of cardiovascular disease by establishing a set of dietary reference intakes including allowance for adequate intake for healthy individuals (Flock et al., 2013). Given the significant and repeated stress placed upon the cardiovascular system during athletic endeavor, it is intriguing to speculate upon the physiological impact that a low systemic LC n–3 PUFA concentration may eventually have, not only on the heart, but also on multiple body systems including the skeletal muscle, nervous, and immune systems.

DIETARY FISH OIL AND PERFORMANCE: A REEMERGING THEME

Limits to performance, particularly endurance, have inherent physiological links to oxygen conductance, diffusion and efficiency, where cardiac output and vascular resistance are primary control variables. Leaf and Rauch (1988) were first to propose that elite athletes may benefit from increasing the intake of EPA and DHA via dietary fish oil on the basis of enhancing aerobic energy supply. Alexander Leaf's (1920–12) initial findings, although debatable, relate to a potential increase in maximal oxygen consumption after consuming an oil rich in EPA. Specifically, Leaf and Rauch (1988) proposed that a reported enhanced fluidity of the red blood cell membranes to increase cell deformability from EPA in the diet (Cartwright et al., 1985) would translate to improve blood (mass) flow, or conductance, and therefore oxygen delivery to the working skeletal muscle. Nonetheless, despite significant short fallings in the data analysis, it must be stated that Leaf's publication has not been awarded the historical recognition in the current literature related to dietary fish oil and exercise. Arguably, his contribution has stimulated the discussions and thinking that has led to many of the most recent advances in the understanding of fish oil and exercise. In essence, the basis for oxygen being central to the mechanism of dietary fish oil supporting physical work was partly correct. Therefore, this chapter will dedicate the first of the proposed mechanism categories to the cellular modulation of oxygen consumption and impact on physical performance in athletes.

Dietary fish oil has also been closely linked to the modulation of inflammatory responses in health and disease (Calder, 2006). Exercise, in its extreme form, is commonly associated with susceptibility to acute and chronic inflammatory (Margeli et al., 2005) and immune cell proliferation (Gleeson et al., 2004). Ernst et al., 1991 first posed the significant question that the provision of fish oil in the diet, and as a result LC n–3 PUFA, could aid in the attenuation of postexercise inflammatory response immunomodulation. Their early findings that acute phase proteins in the plasma can be altered after consuming fish oil for three weeks (Ernst et al., 1991) has formed the scientific ground work to continue this line of investigation over the last 25 years. The initial hypothesis, in the context of exercise induced inflammation, centered upon the LC n–3 PUFA, in particular EPA, 'competing' against and reducing tissue arachidonic acid and as such the production of proinflammatory leukotrienes (Calder, 2013). However, the emergence that DHA derived resolvins play an integral role in the resolution of inflammation (Serhan, 2005) open new hypotheses in regards to the dose requirements to achieve such effects. Therefore, the impact of fish oil on exercise related inflammation, immunity and by extension oxidative stress will be separately addressed in this chapter.

SETTING A FRAMEWORK AROUND "ATHLETES"

Recently, there have been several reviews that have focused on dietary fish oil supporting or optimizing physical performance (Simopoulos, 2007; Tiryaki-Sonmez et al., 2011; Shei et al., 2014). However, in the cases of both Tiryaki-Sonmez et al. (2011) and Shei et al. (2014) their papers have been drawn-out to include role of dietary fish oil in populations including trained, sedentary, and severe pathology. Although this has provided a general overview of the topic, there is yet to be a focused discussion that critically appraises the impact that dietary fish oil may have on supporting physical performance in trained athletes per se. Simopoulos (2007) was able to limit her review to athletes in the context of sports performance and recommended fish oil at 1–2 g per day in training and competition, essentially just matching these doses to those meeting general health recommendations. Nevertheless, arguably due to the recent surge of interest and publications, an up to date discussion is required that specifically addresses the role of fish oil in the diet of athletes. This chapter will focus upon the emerging roles of EPA and/or DHA when provided in the diet in the context of physically active and trained individuals. As such, a clear framework for this current discussion will include: first, performance related studies that apply inclusion criteria involving humans and must report the participants' maximal aerobic capacity, maximal aerobic power, or current physical activity status in line with published definitions (De Pauw et al., 2013). Second, and in addition, animal studies will be included so as to provide mechanistic explanations or comparative species examples for either performance measures or physiology to highlight the effects of EPA and DHA or their potential effects on physical performance. Third, studies that report on the effects of dietary fish oil and physical capacity and/or performance in pathology groups will only be discussed to highlight possible mechanisms that help to design future studies in athletic populations. The current chapter will therefore address the premise that fish oil, delivering LC n–3 PUFA, is an essential component of the athlete's diet for physical performance.

DIETARY FISH OIL AND ITS PHYSIOLOGICAL CONTRIBUTION TO PHYSICAL PERFORMANCE

Physical work capacity is the ability to sustain ongoing muscle contraction in the face of fatigue processes ultimately against a background of oxidative ATP availability (Hogan et al., 1992). Therefore, the rate of work production, or performance, is expressed as the combined interaction of aerobic and anaerobic energy supply and the product of the gross mechanical efficiency in the system (Joyner and Coyle, 2008). On this basis, two themes are now established that provide a potential physiological basis for fish oil supporting physical performance. The first theme is underpinned by the cellular incorporation of EPA and DHA into tissues including red blood cells, heart and skeletal muscle that make up the delivery and efficient use of oxygen to supply ongoing energy demand of the contractile proteins. The second theme is concerned with the temporal inflammatory, immunomodulation and oxidative stress responses to acute and chronic exercise that have collectively been associated with engagement in prolonged or intense physical exhaustion (Fisher-Wellman and Bloomer, 2009). These themes and their components will be separately critiqued in the following section against a background of evidence supporting improvements in physical performance.

FISH OIL AND OXYGEN MODULATION

Skeletal muscle fatigue is tightly coupled with oxygen supply and demand (Gladden et al., 1978; Gorman et al., 1988; Hogan et al., 1992; Barclay, 1993) and skeletal muscle rapidly adjusts developed force when oxygen is limiting or demand is increased well before tissue levels of ATP decline (Hogan et al., 1996). Therefore, available oxygen and its cellular use underpin repetitive and sustained skeletal muscle force production. To date, studies that have supplemented the diet of trained populations with fish oil have considered several key steps in the oxygen demand and supply of the metabolically active skeletal muscle.

BLOOD FLOW

Dietary fish oil increases erythrocyte membrane LC n–3 PUFA and thereby attenuates the loss of membrane fluidity and erythrocyte deformability in pathological conditions such as in animals with sickle cell disease (Wandersee et al., 2015). In untrained healthy humans, increased intake of EPA (3 g/day) is also reported to decrease whole blood viscosity (Terano et al., 1983; Cartwright et al., 1985). From this, it was first hypothesized that such effects would enhance blood flow and oxygen delivery to working skeletal muscle (Table 10.1). Leaf and Rauch (1988), despite reasoning that this change would occur, in fact did not measure red blood cell fluidity. Raastad et al. (1997) and Oostenbrug et al., (1997) reinvestigated the potential for rheological changes following 10 weeks and 3 weeks of fish oil supplementation respectively. In neither study was there evidence that either erythrocyte osmotic gradients (Raastad et al., 1997) or deformability (Oostenbrug et al., 1997) was altered, despite using high doses that could only be considered as therapeutic and difficult to attain in a balance diet. To date, only one study has demonstrated that fish oil can alter erythrocyte fluidity in the context of exercise performance. This was observed rather as attenuation of the negative impact of hypoxic exposure on red blood cell deformability in recreational trained subjects (Guezennec et al., 1989) like the effects seen in sickle cell disease. In line with potential to promote improved blood flow, LC n–3 PUFA have been demonstrated to promote flow mediated dilation in cyclists (Zebrowska et al., 2014) and limit vascular reactivity (Walser et al., 2006); however, direct measurement of vascular resistance in animal models indicates

TABLE 10.1 Intervention Studies to Determine the Effect of Fish Oil Supplementation on Oxygen Consumption and Performance in Trained Subjects

Author/year	Subjects	EPA/DHA (mg/day)	Primary physiological measures	Performance measure
BLOOD FLOW				
Leaf and Rauch (1988)	12 trained athletes	High–4200/1800 Low–2100/900 42 days	RBC deformability not reported	↑estimated $\dot{V}O_{2max}$ in the low group only
Guezennec et al. (1989)	14 recreational trained males	1080/720 42 days	Attenuated RBC deformability loss during hypoxia	↑$\dot{V}O_{2max}$ during hypoxia
Raastad et al. (1997)	28 trained soccer players	1600/1040 70 days	↔RBC osmotic fragility	↔$\dot{V}O_{2max}$, max aerobic power ↔Running performance
Oostenbrug et al. (1997)	24 trained athletes	1020/720 21 days	↔RBC deformability	↔$\dot{V}O_{2max}$ ↔70% $\dot{V}O_{2max}$ cycling time trial
Zebrowska et al. (2014)	13 well-trained cyclists	660/440 21 days	↑ FMD, ↑ nitric oxide release	↑$\dot{V}O_{2max}$, ↑max aerobic power
CARDIAC				
[a]Peoples et al. (2008)	16 well-trained cyclists	560/2160 56 days	↓f_c, $\dot{V}O_2$, RPP during cycling 60% $\dot{V}O_{2max}$	↔$\dot{V}O_{2max}$ ↔Time to fatigue (60% $\dot{V}O_{2max}$)
[a]Buckley et al. (2009)	25 well-trained football players	360/1560 35 days	↓f_c, during 10 km treadmill run	↔Time to complete 2.2 km run
[a]Macartney et al. (2014)	28 trained athletes	140/540 56 days	↓ submaximal f_c, faster heart rate recovery	↔6 × 30 s power output ↔5 min cycling time trial

FMD, flow mediated dilation; *RBC*, red blood cell; $\dot{V}O_{2max}$, maximal aerobic capacity; f_c, heart rate; *RPP*, rate pressure product.
[a]*Studies that have monitored red blood cell fatty acid profiles across the dietary intervention.*

that blood flow may even decrease during active muscle metabolism, subject to LC n–3 PUFA enhanced efficiency of oxygen use, showing that skeletal muscle blood flow is driven by muscle oxygen demand (Henry et al., 2015). Evidently muscle blood flow supports but does not drive performance per se, as it is tightly regulated in line with work capacity (Saltin et al., 1998). An increase in efficiency might be expected to increase vasodilator reserve and cardiac output reserve and support increased exercise driven oxygen demand.

CARDIAC FUNCTION

Heart rate is coupled with exercise intensity (Vokac et al., 1975) and is a strong predictor of myocardial oxygen consumption (Kitamura et al., 1972). Metaanalysis of randomized controlled trails reports that fish oil intake reduces resting heart rate (Mozaffarian et al., 2005). More recently, studies using trained athletes have also demonstrated that heart rate is lower following dietary provision of fish oil. Most evidently, these studies are unique in that the fish oil used was predominately comprised of DHA and delivered very little EPA (Peoples et al., 2008; Buckley et al., 2009; Macartney et al., 2014). Peoples et al. (2008) supplemented well-trained cyclists with a therapeutic dose of fish oil over 8 weeks and significantly elevated the Omega-3 Index. As a consequence, during submaximal cycling at 60% $\dot{V}O_{2max}$ to the point of fatigue, heart rate and rate pressure product were significantly reduced. Buckley et al. (2009), using Australian football players, also reported lower heart rates while completing a 10 km treadmill run after 6 weeks of DHA-rich fish oil supplementation. In the most recent study, Macartney et al. (2014) reduced the total dose of fish oil to be equivalent to one to two fatty fish meals per week, easily achievable in the human diet. The Omega-3 index was still increased by this low dose of DHA-rich oil over 8 weeks, with lower submaximal heart rate and improved heart rate recovery observed after a maximal 5 min cycling time trail. There was no further reduction in the already very low resting heart rates of the trained athletes, however most interestingly, the altered heart rate variability suggested that the fish oil supplemented group were less reliant on vagal tone for their low heart rate at rest. Similarly, heart rate recovery improved without change in vagal tone. Together both results indicated that fish oil, via alterations in the myocardial membranes toward a higher DHA concentration, is working directly in the heart to slow the rate and improve efficiency (McLennan, 2014) where stroke volume is also documented to be enhanced (Walser and Stebbins, 2008). This is exemplified by observation using a human neurally "isolated heart" model, the heart transplant patient, in whom LC n–3 PUFA reduces resting heart rate in the absence of neural tone input (Harris et al., 2006).

OXYGEN EFFICIENCY

Modulation of whole body oxygen consumption following provision of fish oil is not evident during rest (Gerling et al., 2014) despite stored intramuscular triglycerides rapidly shifting to LC n–3 PUFA (McGlory et al., 2014) and this concept is supported by animal studies (Peoples and McLennan, 2010; Henry et al., 2015). However, when metabolic demand is elevated during sustained exercise a different picture emerges. In untrained, although healthy participants, provision of EPA has been reported to both enhance exercise economy (Kawabataa et al., 2014) or alternatively not effect energy efficiency (Bortolotti et al., 2007). Nonetheless, therapeutic doses of DHA-rich fish oil (8 g/day) were shown to reduce whole body oxygen consumption in well-trained cyclists, suggesting possible improved exercise economy beyond the effects on heart alone (Peoples et al., 2008). Structural membrane composition directly impacts on cellular function (Gorjao et al., 2009). When dietary fish oil increases membrane LC n–3 PUFA in tissues such as myocardium (McLennan et al., 1988; Charnock et al., 1992; McLennan et al., 1996; Pepe and McLennan, 1996), function is enhanced, particularly in the face of compromised oxygen supply or declining contractility (Pepe and McLennan, 2002; Abdukeyum et al., 2008). Skeletal muscle membranes also incorporate DHA to well above the dietary and circulating concentrations (Charnock et al., 1992; Pan and Storlien, 1993; Ayre and Hulbert, 1996; Peoples and McLennan, 2010). Improved muscle function, on the basis of enhanced economy, is supported by tightly controlled animal physiology experiments when DHA is the predominant LC n–3 PUFA in the diet (Peoples and McLennan, 2010). As such, this translates directly into resistance to muscle fatigue and sustained steady state of contraction (Peoples and McLennan, 2014; Henry et al., 2015) in line with a "peripheral governor" of skeletal muscle contractile force production (MacIntosh and Shahi, 2011). Importantly, fatigue resistance has been achieved using dietary achievable nutritional doses of fish oil (Henry et al., 2015).

The mechanism by which dietary fish oil may provide improved skeletal muscle function, likely involves the mitochondria, further supporting the theory of oxygen modulation. In humans, 12 weeks of fish oil supplementation increases DHA concentration in the skeletal muscle mitochondrial membranes and as a physiological consequence both the ADP sensitivity and reactive oxygen species emissions increased in these mitochondria with no evidence of oxidative damage (Herbst et al., 2014). Thus, when membrane DHA concentrations are optimized in skeletal muscle, and therefore the mitochondria, there is a similar improvement in oxygen efficiency as reported in metabolically active heart (Pepe and McLennan, 2002; Abdukeyum et al., 2008) and is most evident when oxygen demand is increased such as during exercise (Peoples et al., 2008). Nevertheless, there is a further need to conduct future, well-designed studies in humans, linking the biological plausibility of DHA in particular, with oxygen modulation, particularly when physiological strain is high.

OXYGEN MODULATION AND PHYSICAL PERFORMANCE

Despite physiological evidence that dietary fish oil can modify and support the oxygen requirements during exercise, there is no established evidence to date that this translates to improved performance in trained individuals, and this includes indirect measures such as maximal aerobic power and direct measures such as endurance performance.

MAXIMAL OXYGEN CONSUMPTION

The initial claim by Leaf and Rauch (1988) that maximal aerobic capacity was increased after provision of fish oil, has clearly been rejected by all (Oostenbrug et al., 1997; Raastad et al., 1997; Peoples et al., 2008) bar one recent study (Zebrowska et al., 2014). Careful consideration of the individual subject data in the original manuscript, by Leaf and Rauch (1988), shows that the improvement in mean estimated maximal oxygen consumption with the low dose fish oil intervention, was driven by one subject, who despite not reaching volitional fatigue in the baseline assessments, was retained in the pre–post supplement comparison. In omitting this subject's data, the outcome no longer supports any effects on maximal aerobic capacity. The other more recent study to claim that maximal aerobic capacity is enhanced (Zebrowska et al., 2014) also has several significant shortcomings that make for cautious interpretation. The authors implemented a crossover study design where subjects were provided with both control and fish oil supplements, however, the wash out period between treatments was short and no long-term tissues markers were measured. In addition, nitric oxide production, the physiological mechanism hypothesized to primarily underpin the improvement in maximal aerobic capacity, only explained 20% of the variation rendering the effects due to LC n–3 PUFA weak in terms of cause and effect, a broad issue in nutrition physiology (Lands, 2008).

ENDURANCE AND EXERCISE PERFORMANCE

Exercise endurance can be measured by a variety of protocols including: time to fatigue; completion time of a set distance; or work completed in a set time period. To date, there have been no measurable effects on endurance performance when athletes have been supplemented within the range of 2–12 g/day fish oil for as long as 70 days (Table 10.1). Peoples et al. (2008) reported no change in time to fatigue of well-trained cyclists when cycling at 60% $\dot{V}O_{2max}$, supporting similar observations by Oostenbrug et al., 1997 (at 70% $\dot{V}O_{2max}$). Time to complete a set running distance was also unaltered in soccer (Raastad et al., 1997) and Australian Football players (Buckley et al., 2009), the latter using a DHA-rich supplement. In addition, Macartney et al. (2014) reported that a DHA-rich supplement had no measurable effect on work capacity in cyclists under significant physiological strain, where they were required to complete a 5 min cycling time trial immediately after a fatiguing, 6 × 30 s, Wingate sprint protocol. Finally, in the most recent applied sports science study of recreational athletes, EPA and DHA provided over 21 days, in the form of seal oil, had no measureable nor statistical effect on a range of physiological assessments including isometric strength, Wingate cycling and time trial (Table 10.2) despite the authors' claims that muscle activation was enhanced (nonstatistical) compared to the loss experience in the olive oil placebo group (Lewis et al., 2015).

FISH OIL AND INFLAMMATION, IMMUNE, AND OXIDATIVE STRESS

In a series of recent publications relating to applied sports science (Table 10.2), an enriched-DHA sports drink consumed over 8 weeks of training was reported to increase red blood cell DHA in soccer players (Capo et al., 2015). In this same group of soccer players, the authors also reported that DHA lowered acute inflammation (Capo et al., 2014)

TABLE 10.2 Intervention Studies to Determine the Effect of Fish Oil Supplementation During Sports Simulation in Trained Subjects

Author/year	Subjects	EPA/DHA (mg/day)	Primary physiological measures	Performance measure
APPLIED SPORTS SCIENCE				
Guzman et al. (2011)	34 well trained soccer players	0/3500 28 days	↓ complex reaction time ↑ decision efficiency	↑ neuromotor function
[a]Capo et al. (2014)	15 trained soccer players	0/1140 56 days	↓ TNF-α, IL-6 after acute Exercise	Not measured
[a]Capo et al. (2015)	15 trained soccer players	0/1140 56 days	↑ RBC DHA, ↑UCP3 ↑ SOD, ↓ROS	Not measured
[a]Martorell et al. (2014)	15 trained soccer players	0/1140 56 days	↑ plasma PGE2 ↔ROS of neutrophils	Not measured
[a]Martorell et al. (2015)	15 trained soccer players	0/1140 56 days	↑ SOD in erythrocytes ↓ exercise peroxidative damage	Not measured
Santos et al. (2013)	21 well trained marathon runners	300/1500 60 days	↓ TNF-α, IL-2, IL-10 at baseline in Con-A stimulated lymphocytes	↔marathon time
Lewis et al. (2015)	31 recreationally trained subjects	375/510 21 days	↑ plasma EPA ↔muscle activation	↔MVC, cycling time trial or Wingate

MVC, maximal voluntary contraction; *PGE2*, prostaglandin E2; *ROS*, reactive oxygen stress; *SOD*, superoxide dismutase; *TBARS*, thiobarbituric acid reactive substances; *TNF-α*, tumor necrosis factor-α; *UCP3*, uncoupling protein 3.
[a]*All derived from the same and small pool of participants after a single intervention (DHA supplemented N = 9, control supplemented N = 6).*

whilst paradoxically increasing plasma PGE_2 (Martorell et al., 2014) and decreasing reactive oxygen stress markers (Capo et al., 2015; Martorell et al., 2015). The limitations of field-based research are certainly apparent in the series of publications steaming from the study, namely: the small sample size ($n = 9$ fish oil; $n = 6$ control), variability in exercise intensity during training-induced exercise stimulation and the large number of measured blood markers which raises the risk of type 1 statistical error. Nonetheless, marathon runners provided with 3 g/day of DHA-rich fish oil for 10 weeks were also reported to improve lymphocyte function (Santos et al., 2013) although this time a control placebo was not used in the study and limits relevance of interpretation (Table 10.2). Nevertheless, given the acknowledged interaction of essential fatty acids with human immunology and inflammation, there has emerged a line of research, with varying level of first principles study design, that warrant interpretative discussion against the background of applied sports science.

INFLAMMATION AND IMMUNE MODULATION

In trained subjects, Andrade et al. (2007) demonstrated a reduction in inflammatory markers after fish oil supplementation. Swimmers consuming high EPA fish oil for 6 weeks recorded decreased plasma concentrations of PGE_2 and TNF-α while plasma IL-2 increased (Andrade et al., 2007). However, in direct contrast, several studies have demonstrated that fish oil only influenced resting inflammation in trained athletes (Bloomer et al., 2009), had no effect on acute phase cytokines post-exercise in runners (Toft et al., 2000), no alteration in leukocytes, C-reactive protein, creatine kinase, salivary IgA in cyclists (Nieman et al., 2009), and no measurable effect on oxidative stress after exercise (Filaire et al., 2011) where notably, the subject populations were well trained (Table 10.3).

In contrast, recreationally trained athletes (Table 10.3) supplemented with a high EPA fish oil for 6 weeks moderately increase *superoxide dismutase* in response to cycling one hour at 60% VO_{2max} (Poprzecki et al., 2009), similar to Capo et al., who also reported catalase increased during recovery (Capo et al., 2015). In further agreement, a high EPA fish oil supplement for 6 weeks increased peripheral blood mononuclear cell (PBMC) IL-2 and natural killer cell activity in 16 recreationally trained males after 60-min cycling at 70% VO_{2max}, although other inflammatory or immune markers were unchanged (Gray et al., 2012) (Table 10.3). More recently, in recreationally trained males and females (no gender effect) provision of a phospholipid dense krill oil over 6 weeks increased PBMC IL-2 and natural killer cell activity at 3 h postexercise (70% VO_2) (Da Boit et al., 2015). On this occasion, erythrocyte Omega-3 Index was measured and shown to increase after intake of the krill oil. However, the Omega-3 Index also indicated some subjects were already consuming dietary LC n–3 PUFA and potentially confounding interpretation. Equally, some caution should be raised given the study design failed to include presupplementation blood levels, and group differences may simply be a reflection individual response to exercise with limited cause and effect support (Lands, 2008).

Fish oil's potential to attenuate inflammation seems most likely when an underlying pathological state already exists. Mickleborough et al. (2003) supplemented 20 trained runners and cyclists presenting with underlying exercise-induced asthma, itself an inflammatory process in (Table 10.2). Over 3 weeks the runners were randomly assigned to consume what can only be described as a high therapeutic dose of either 20 g of fish oil or a control oil. Impressively, the very high dose of EPA rich fish oil was able to reduce a range of inflammatory markers such as LTE_4 and TNF-α that are normally elevated in exercise-induced asthma (Mickleborough et al., 2003) similar to how high therapeutic doses are required for clinical management of rheumatoid arthritis (Cleland et al., 2006).

In summary, the interaction of dietary fish oil and immune response to exercise appears partly dependent upon the extent of physical activity engagement, that is training status, or underlying pathology driving baseline inflammation in the case of athletes with sensitivity to exercise induced asthma. Although, the current discussion has been limited to studies of physically active participants, there is obviously still a continuum between recreationally trained and elite athletes. Exercise, when undertaken regularly, projects its own endogenous upregulation of antiinflammatory effects (Gleeson et al., 2011), whereas baseline immune markers, including acute phase proteins, are reduced in physically active humans as part of the exercise based adaptation (Horn et al., 2015). Many of the studies reporting positive effects of omega-3 supplements have engaged recreationally trained individuals where training status is known to interact with acute inflammation, likely due to differing body composition, not the skeletal muscle per se (Olesen et al., 2015). At this point in time, the effects of LC n–3 PUFA on immune and inflammation are preliminary and not broadly supported by all concerned (Walsh et al., 2011) particularly when athletes are highly trained.

TABLE 10.3 Intervention Studies to Determine the Effect of Fish Oil Supplementation on Inflammatory Response to Exercise in Trained Subjects

Author/year	Subjects	EPA/DHA (mg/day)	Primary physiological measures	Performance measure
Toft et al. (2000)	20 well-trained runners	1836/1116 42 days	↔ acute cytokines post exercise	Not measured
Mickleborough et al. (2003)	20 trained runners, cyclists	3600/2200 21 days	↓ LT(E4), 9α, 11β PE F2, TNF-α interleikin-1β in EIA subjects	Not reported
Andrade et al. (2007)	20 well-trained swimmers	950/500 42 days	↓ plasma AA, PGE2, TNF- α ↑ IL-2	Not measured
Poprzecki et al. (2009)	24 recreationally trained subjects	390/260 42 days	↑ SOD (cycling 1h (60% $\dot{V}O_{2max}$) ↑ CAT activity in recovery	↔$\dot{V}O_{2max}$ reported
Nieman et al. (2009)	23 trained cyclists	3000/400 42 days	↔leukocytes, CRP, CK, salivary IgA myeloperoxidase (baseline or recovery)	↔10 km cycling time trial
Bloomer et al. (2009)	14 trained athletes	2224/2208 42 days	↓ resting inflammation~ inflammation/oxidative stress post exercise	Not measured
McAnulty et al. (2010)	11 trained cyclists	2000/400 42 days	↑ F2-isoprostane post 3 days intense exercise (60% $\dot{V}O_{2max}$)	10 km cycling time trial not reported
Filaire et al. (2011)	36 trained	600/400 42 days	↑ oxidative stress at rest ↔ oxidative stress post exercise	Not measured
Gray et al. (2012)	16 recreationally trained subjects	1300/300 42 days	↑ PBMC IL-2/NK cell post 60 min cycling (70% $\dot{V}O_{2max}$)	Not measured
Da Boit et al. (2015)	37 recreationally trained subjects	240/120† 42 days	↑ O3I, ↑ PBMC IL-2/NK cell 3 h Post cycling time trial (approximately 80 mins)	↔cycling time trial (elicit 70% $\dot{V}O_{2max}$)

AA, arachidonic acid; *LT E4*, leukotriene E4; *11β PE F2*, 11β prostaglandin F2; *TNF-α*, tumor necrosis factor- α; *PGE2*, prostaglandin E2; *IL-2*, interleukin 2; *CRP*, C-reactive protein; *CK*, creatine kinase; *PBMC*, peripheral blood mononuclear cell; *NK*, natural killer; and † = krill oil.

SKELETAL MUSCLE DAMAGE AND OXIDATIVE STRESS

Engagement in nonaccustomed physical activity results in delayed onset muscle soreness (DOMS) which is particularly evident after eccentric muscle contractions. Provision of dietary fish oil prior to the exercise stimulus has mainly focused on nontrained populations where markers of both inflammation and oxidative stress as well as perceived pain is reported to be improved (Phillips et al., 2003; Jouris et al., 2011; Tartibian et al., 2011; Dilorenzo et al., 2014). However, translation of these studies into physically active and trained populations is of mixed result. Currently there are only several studies that have supplemented fish oil, and predominately with EPA, into the diets of physically active or trained participants (Table 10.4).

Atashak et al. (2013) randomly assigned 20 trained collegiate male handball players to either an unnamed placebo control or a fish oil intervention (3 g) providing 540 mg EPA and 350 mg DHA for only 7 days. Notably, the eccentric protocol for lower limb muscle damage was not conducted at baseline, rather only after the completion of the fish oil supplementation. In addition, no biological marker of either EPA or DHA was reported, casting doubt upon the efficacy of the supplement or the compliance of the subjects. The authors claimed that levels of plasma marker of muscle damage creatine kinase and fatty acid oxidation marker MDA were both attenuated in the fish oil group, although many other indices demonstrate no treatment effect (Atashak et al., 2013).

Gray et al. (2014) randomly assigned 20 recreationally trained participants to 3 g/day of either olive oil control, or EPA-rich fish oil, providing 1300 mg EPA and 300 mg DHA for 6 weeks (Table 10.3). Eccentric damage of the quadriceps muscles was induced at baseline and following intervention. The fish oil group reduced H_2O_2-induced lymphocyte damage immediately after exercise and reduced plasma TBARS at 48 and 72 h. The authors concluded that the results were reflective of fish oil attenuating the oxidative stress response to eccentric muscle damage (Gray et al., 2014); however, this was not accompanied by any effect on either maximal voluntary contraction or muscle soreness.

TABLE 10.4 Intervention Studies to Determine the Effect of Fish Oil Supplementation on Delayed Onset Muscle Soreness and ROS in Trained Subjects

Author/year	Subjects	EPA/DHA (mg/day)	Primary physiological measures	Performance measure
SKELETAL MUSCLE DAMAGE				
Atashak et al. (2013)	20 trained collegiate handball players	540/360 7 days	Attenuating ↑ MDA, CK, CRP	ΔMVC not measured
Gray et al. (2014)	20 recreational trained subjects	1300/300 42 days	↓ TBARS, DNA damage following eccentric exercise	↔MVC
Mickleborough et al. (2015)	32 recreational trained subjects	464/352 26 days	↓ troponin I, CK, TNF-α over 4 days post downhill running	Cycling time trial (20 min) not reported; ↑ quadriceps twitch potentiation post fatigue

CK, creatine kinase; *CRP*, C-reactive protein; *MDA*, malondialdehyde; *MVC*, maximal voluntary contraction; *ROS*, reactive oxygen stress; *TBARS*, thiobarbituric acid reactive substances; *TNF-α*, tumor necrosis factor-α.

In the most recent study, Mickleborough et al., 2015 supplemented their participants for 26 days with marine oil derived from New Zealand green mussel. The relative concentration of EPA/DHA in the oil was very low and therefore 8 g/day in the treatment group still only amounted to 464 mg EPA and 352 mg DHA per day. Although the authors identified their participants as untrained (Mickleborough et al., 2015), the study has been included for the purpose of this discussion, as their characteristics allowed them to be classified as recreationally trained. Muscle damage was induced using a downhill running protocol. Several markers of damage, including troponin I, creatine kinase and a marker of inflammation, TNF-α were attenuated and muscle soreness was reportedly less in the treatment group compared to controls.

Oxidative stress is not confined to skeletal muscle damage. It has also been shown to increase in response to physical exertion where oxygen consumption is significantly elevated. In a single study, fish oil supplemented subjects exercising at 60% VO_{2max} exhibited increased oxidative stress, measured as F_2-isoprostane concentrations (McAnulty et al., 2010). This anomaly might well be explained on the basis of measurement variability derived as a "spot" sample after three consecutive days of moderate intensity cycling. Isoprostanes, as markers of oxidative stress, are subject to a complex function of both appearance and clearance where the timing, frequency and tissue sample, whether it be plasma or urine, will systematically influence the interpretive outcomes (Halliwell and Lee, 2010) on the background that F_2-isoprostanes are omega-6 derived rather than omega-3 fatty acids. The multiple double bonds in LC n–3 PUFA make them highly prone to oxidation and potentially promotors of oxidative damage. However, animal research shows that LC n–3 PUFA through producing low-level nondamaging oxidation, upregulate endogenous antioxidant systems (Abdukeyum et al., 2016) and fish oil paradoxically protects the heart during exercise or ischemia/reperfusion oxidative stress (Castillo et al., 2014). As yet only a single small human athlete study (Martorell et al., 2015) has sought to replicate these observations and reports a similar increase in antioxidant defenses in red blood cells after fish oil supplementation.

INFLAMMATION, REACTIVE OXYGEN STRESS, AND PHYSICAL PERFORMANCE

Studies concerning fish oil and its modulation of inflammatory, immune or oxidative stress responses have lacked quantitative measures of physical performance (Tables 10.2 and 10.3). Only three studies have directly measured either performance or fatigue. Nieman et al. (2009), supplemented cyclists with high-EPA fish oil for 6 weeks, then subjected both control and intervention groups to 3 hours of cycling at 70% $\dot{V}O_{2max}$ over 3 consecutive days, followed by 10 km of cycling time trial. When the times to complete 10 km were averaged over the 3 days, there were no measurable differences between the control and fish oil groups. Similarly, Da Boit et al. (2015) supplemented recreationally trained males and females with krill oil for 6 weeks and also reported no effect on cycling time trial lasting >80 min. Finally, Mickleborough et al. (2015) assessed skeletal muscle fatigue 4 days after downhill running. The LC n–3 PUFA supplemented group demonstrated an attenuation of decline in quadriceps twitch force potentiation following a 20 min cycling time trail. The authors reported these findings as improved muscle function, underpinned by the reduced inflammatory response previously discussed. However, these results should be interpreted cautiously given that some critical results were not transparent, including the sustained power output of both the control and the marine oil groups during the time trail where a difference would more than likely be a stronger influence of quadriceps twitch force production. Nonetheless, assuming the cycling workloads were equivalent, an alternative interpretation could be provided. Eccentric exercise preferentially recruits type II muscle fibers and the demonstrated reduction in maximal voluntary contraction could be a reflection of low frequency fatigue, where calcium handling of the sarcoplasmic reticulum is a primary mechanism (Allen et al., 2008). In the myocardium LC n–3 PUFA act directly to improve cellular processes including calcium handling (McLennan, 2014) and in skeletal muscle attenuate fatigue-related decline in maximum rates of contraction and relaxation (Peoples and McLennan, 2014; Henry et al., 2015) which are also indicative of improved calcium cycling.

EPA VERSUS DHA: DOES IT MATTER AND HOW MUCH IS ENOUGH?

The principle question of whether the individual LC n–3 PUFA EPA and DHA, provide the same or complementary effects is often considered in the context of the cardiovascular system (Mozaffarian and Wu, 2012) and directed toward pathophysiological conditions. The establishment of both dose and specific biological roles of EPA and DHA in the trained athlete is yet to be fully considered, although, some interpretation can be applied to the studies identified in the current discussion. This includes the effective dose and specificity for membrane incorporation, the relevance of therapeutic doses and finally, the inherent question of whether LC n–3 PUFA, being achievable through normally dietary patterns, can improve performance where carbohydrate and protein consumption is optimized.

First, many of the identified studies, listed in this discussion, have used "off the shelf" fish oil products high in EPA. In fact, recent evidence suggests that the fish oil in those products simply may not meet the concentrations listed on their labels (Albert et al., 2015). Furthermore, uncertainty of dose concentrations of either EPA or DHA in supplements, is compounded by a consistent failure to measure medium to long-term tissue incorporation, as reported by red blood cell incorporation, questioning actual LC n–3 PUFA provision across the majority of experiments. More concerning is the influence of control groups in interpreting these results where background intake is rarely monitored via tissues, leading to considerable but unspecified overlap between control and treated groups in clinical trials (James et al., 2014). It is entirely possible that control groups already have adequate LC n–3 PUFA intake for physiological optimization. Equally, it is clear that little attention has been paid to the duration of interventions, ranging from 1 week to 10 weeks. Therapeutic doses of fish oil, beyond intakes reasonably achievable in the human diet, dominate the studies in trained athletes, especially those most concerned with inflammation, immune, and oxidative stress. Arguably, there is a physiological basis that EPA would provide greater efficacy, given the biochemical competition with omega-6 fatty acid, linoleic acid, for production of inflammation products (Calder, 2006). Nonetheless, in light of newly discovered roles of DHA in regards to the formation of resolvins and protectins derived from DHA (Serhan, 2005) a greater emphasis is recommended toward eventually seeing therapeutic doses of fish be reduced to more obtainable daily amounts coupled with relevant biological end points. In cardiovascular health and disease, high dose effects on inflammatory conditions such as atherosclerosis may be derived through EPA or DHA whereas DHA is selectively incorporated into myocardial membranes and appears responsible for low dose direct alterations in cardiac physiology such as heart rate lowering and arrhythmia prevention (McLennan, 2014).

The effective fish oil dose for altering systems physiology is evident in the series of studies that have focused on oxygen modulation (Table 10.1). Firstly, the total provision of fish oil has progressively reduced overtime from therapeutic doses (Leaf and Rauch, 1988) to doses achievable as whole fish in the human diet (Macartney et al., 2014). Secondly, EPA has been removed from the effective dose where physiological change, such as heart rate reduction, is biologically linked to DHA-rich fish oil. In fact, monitoring incorporation of EPA and DHA over the course of interventions and to associate biological change is best exemplified by several studies in Table 10.1 (Peoples et al., 2008; Buckley et al., 2009; Macartney et al., 2014). The principle of monitoring background and long-term exposure of LC n–3 PUFA should not be underestimated given the known temporal difference in red blood cell and plasma concentrations (Harris et al., 2013). Macartney et al. (2014), in trained males, demonstrated that DHA incorporation into erythrocyte membranes significantly increased (with little change in EPA) and primarily underpinned the omega-3 index increase to 6.3% in the fish oil group from the provision of only 4900 mg of EPA + DHA per week. As a 100 g serving of salmon contains up to 2000 mg of EPA (~550 mg) plus DHA (~1450 mg) (USDA, 2009) and a typical salmon portion is 150–250 g (3000–5000 mg EPA + DHA), only one to two salmon meals per week would be needed to deliver the LC n–3 PUFA equivalent of the study. Therefore, the supplemental dose used by Macartney et al. (2014) could readily be achieved through the normal diet. Notably, the control supplement in the study was soy oil, containing α-linolenic acid (ALA), and did not affect the omega-3 index. This supports the finding that minimal de novo synthesis of DHA in humans occurs from dietary ALA (Pawlosky et al., 2001). Furthermore, the control supplemental delivery of 1 g/day of omega-6 linoleic acid produced no change in erythrocyte fatty acids, indicative of a high background omega-6 PUFA dietary intake and already maximal membrane incorporation.

Summary evaluation of epidemiology and randomized control trials collectively indicates that 250 mg/day of EPA + DHA is the optimum required for cardiac health and preventing cardiac disease (Mozaffarian and Rimm, 2006). It is not possible to justify a similar claim for exercise performance simply because such low intakes have never been tested and to date there is no equivocal evidence that performance in athletes is altered following administration of dietary LC n–3 PUFA. In terms of supporting the associated physiological strain of physical exercise, there is no doubt that an adequate intake of EPA + DHA should support skeletal muscle and cardiac function more so than low or no intake and consuming EPA and DHA equivalent to one to two fatty fish meals per week may be sufficient.

FUTURE FOCUS: UNCOVERING THE POTENTIAL EFFECTS OF DIETARY FISH OIL ON PERFORMANCE

Despite the physiological effects of dietary fish oil associated with exercise in healthy, well-trained individuals, there is very little evidence that either EPA or DHA can improve physical performance. There are a number of factors that may be contributing to these inconsistent outcomes. To date, very few investigations (Peoples et al., 2008; Buckley et al., 2009; Macartney et al., 2014) have retrospectively met the study design recommendations underpinning the potential to demonstrate physiological change (von Schacky, 2011; James et al., 2014), or the physical performance outcomes. Maximum dose effects in cardiovascular disease (Mozaffarian and Rimm, 2006), benefits of low (one to two fish meals per week) versus none and animal studies demonstrating effectiveness of very low intakes versus none (Henry et al., 2015) all point to performance benefits of correcting deficiency in those athletes with inadequate intake. Erythrocyte membranes are a reliable biomarker for the uptake of DHA into other membranes, such as myocardial and skeletal muscle (Metcalf et al., 2007). Therefore, future investigations must aim to recruit well trained participants with a habitually low diet of LC n–3 PUFA, use red blood cell incorporation as a marker of baseline omega-3 status, and then monitor compliance to the fish oil intervention and ultimately LC n–3 PUFA tissue incorporation (von Schacky, 2011). This will collectively improve the consistency and opportunity to demonstrate that dietary fish oil can both physiologically support athletes and ultimately determine if measurably enhanced performance in elite athletes is possible.

FISH OIL AND EXERCISE INTOLERANCE: AN INSIGHT TO STUDY DESIGN

Dietary fish oil has been considered as a nutritional approach in populations restricted in their capacity to effectively deal with fatigue during activities of daily living. This has included COPD (Broekhuizen et al., 2005) and peripheral artery disease patients (Madden et al., 2007). Although it is irresponsible to directly extend these findings to healthy athletes to whom they bare little physiological resemblance, the mechanisms of action uncovered may provide particular clues to conditions experienced during exhaustive exercise. As such, future studies in athletes, in light of the physiological benefits of fish oil consumption, can indeed become purposely focused on hypothesis driven and physiologically viable study designs. This will ultimately consider if there are clear and accepted performance benefits, not unlike carbohydrate provision, when dietary LC n–3 PUFA EPA and DHA concentrations are raised in the body's tissues including heart, blood, skeletal muscle and nervous system.

NUTRITIONAL PRECONDITIONING IN HYPOXIC ENVIRONMENTS

Exercise is compromised under conditions of sustained low oxygen delivery, or hypoxia (Gore et al., 1997). Acute exposure to hypoxic conditions, such as altitude, impacts on multiple physiological systems, most commonly reported as alterations in cardiovascular and respiratory function (Peltonen et al., 2001) implicating oxygen supply to the contractile tissue as a primary factor. However, skeletal muscle contractile function is compromised independently of the reduced oxygen delivery (Perrey and Rupp, 2009). Therefore, improved work economy of skeletal muscle has emerged as an important adaptive process to sustain exercise tolerance under hypoxic stress (Gore et al., 2007). On the basis that membrane DHA is emerging as a modulator of skeletal muscle oxygen consumption, there is substantial evidence that athletes may benefit from combined altitude exposure and nutritional pre-conditioning with fish oil.

In animals, the provision of LC n–3 PUFA (in combination with vitamin E) to high altitude rescue dogs improved rescue times (exercise performance), lowered heart rates and reduced expression of oxidative stress makers (Grandjean et al., 1998) where acute hypoxia is known to accelerate their production (Ottenheijm et al., 2006). In addition, DHA protects against loss of nerve conduction velocity during chronic altitude exposure in rats (Erken et al., 2013). This opens up avenues to further explore the potential for LC n–3 PUFA to support reaction time (Guzman et al., 2011) and neuromuscular function (Lewis et al., 2015) in trained athletes (Table 10.2) including involvement of the central nervous system where the interaction of fish oil branch chain amino acid has been shown to reduce free tryptophan/BCAA recreational trained males and females although no improvement in endurance performance occurred (Huffman et al., 2004). As discussed previously, in humans, fish oil supplementation prior to acute altitude exposure blunted the expected detrimental increase in blood viscosity, however disappointingly, no meaningful exercise performance measures were collected (Guezennec et al., 1989). Nonetheless, in COPD patients, not unlike chronic heart failure animals (Holdsworth et al., 2014), where skeletal muscle mitochondrial dysfunction and hypoxia (Meyer et al., 2013) contribute to exercise intolerance, the provision of fish oil in conjunction with exercise training improved exercise capacity (Broekhuizen et al., 2005). This shows potential for the nutritional application of DHA in muscle pathogenesis underpinned by poor economy of oxygen-use, not unlike an athlete first exposed to altitude training.

Optimizing the concentrations of DHA in excitable cells exposed to hypoxia, occurs also independent of diet. For example, in rats, left ventricular membrane concentrations of DHA (and total n–3 PUFA) were increased after 8 weeks of simulated altitude, while linoleic acid (18:2n-6) concentrations decreased (Jezková et al., 2002). Equally, oxygen management, through PUFA modification, is also reported in migrating birds, exposed to altitude (McWilliams et al., 2004) and seals required to perform muscle contractions during extended breath hold diving (Kanatous et al., 1999) both cases highlighting the combined relationship of adaption to physical performance under low oxygen stress. The collective evidence supports dietary fish oil providing a pre-conditioning effect for excitable cells, where improved use of oxygen is a central theme. It is intriguing to speculate how DHA may interplay with whole body capacity at altitude or in fact partly explain individual and varied response to altitude exposure (Chapman et al., 1998). Future research should be directed toward the theme of combining altitude training and the optimal provision of DHA in the diets of athletes to focus on the non-hematological underpinnings of exercise economy.

FISH OIL SUPPORTING SUPRA-MAXIMAL EXERCISE

When physical performance has been measured in relation to dietary fish oil, the exercise stimulus has been predominantly submaximal. In other words, there has been little attention given to engagement in severe conditions known to rapidly decrease contractile activity such as repeat bout supra-maximal exercise that will engage the large skeletal muscle motor units associated with, high power and rapid fatigue (Bentley et al., 2000). Fast twitch, type II fibers, densely packed with sarcoplasmic reticulum and expressing high sarcoplasmic reticulum Ca^{2+}ATPase (SERCA) concentration, a requirement to sustain rapid force production and relaxation. Highly effective SERCA, like those in the powerful muscle fibers, rely on the phospholipid environment to carry out rapid removal of calcium against its concentration gradient (Infante, 1987). There is accumulating evidence that when DHA makes up a high proportion of the membrane fatty acids, this process of Ca^{2+} pumping is optimized, thus sustaining force production in the periods of rapid fatigue. A high incorporation of DHA into faster compared to slow muscle types is emphasized in species such as the rattlesnake and the hummingbird, which possess muscle groups of even more extreme contrast in contraction speed within the one animal (Infante et al., 2001). In a move designed to evaluate effects of nutritionally relevant intakes a study of rats fed a DHA-rich fish oil, equivalent to one to two fatty fish meals per week, found greater membrane DHA concentration in skeletal muscles dominated by type II fibers compared to fatigue resistant type I rich muscle and heart ventricle (Henry et al., 2015). Physiologically, when the muscles were stimulated to contract, increased skeletal muscle membrane DHA attenuated muscle fatigue represented as sustained contractile tension rates of force development and relaxation. At the elite level of sports performance, exercise intensity is often sustained above 85% of maximal oxygen consumption. Slight alterations in the balance of ATP derived from aerobic and anaerobic energy supply coupled with oxygen economy have major implications on volitional fatigue (Joyner and Coyle, 2008) and future emphasis of LC n–3 PUFA should be directed toward exercise performance underpinned by sustained contraction of fast twitch muscle fibers, a comparative observation in the natural world where increased DHA is associated with sustained high contractile forces (Lindstedt et al., 1998; Infante et al., 2001). In addition, the preliminary reported evidence that complex reaction times are improved in female soccer players (Guzman et al., 2011) suggests that loss of neuromuscular function may be attenuated following provision of fish oil (Lewis et al., 2015) (Table 10.2). Future research should consider supra-maximal exercise involving repeated bouts of fatiguing contractions.

MAINTAINING SKELETAL MUSCLE MASS

The role of LC n–3 PUFA in maintaining or supporting muscle mass in athletes is largely unexplored. To date, the theoretical concepts that dietary fish oil may either alter pathways of anabolic metabolism or testosterone production have been restricted to the elderly (Molfino et al., 2014). At population level in the aged, dietary intake of fatty fish is associated with improved grip strength (Robinson et al., 2008) and physical function (Abbatecola et al., 2009). Dietary fish oil supplementation in elderly women enhanced strength gains in lower limb muscles associated with resistance training (Rodacki et al., 2012). In part, the enhanced effects of strength gains have been attributed to an increased rate of protein synthesis in the elderly (Smith et al., 2011) although, preliminary evidence in trained athletes suggests dietary fish oil does not alter muscle protein synthesis (McGlory et al., 2016). Nonetheless, these effects on muscle mass and functional changes need to be contextualized based upon the age-related loss of muscle mass and skeletal muscle metabolism. Physical activity promotes skeletal muscle function compared to age match sedentary individuals. Therefore, if there are physiological foundations for dietary fish oil to support skeletal muscle mass in athletes, it seems plausible only when the maintenance of skeletal muscle cross sectional area is significantly challenged. For example, elite athletes competing through middle age can experience reduction in skeletal muscle contractile power ahead of noticeable loss in specifically Type II fiber number (Faulkner et al., 2008). Testosterone, a steroid hormone, acts directly on skeletal muscle to upregulate anabolic effects (Pearlman and Crepy, 1967). Circulating testosterone has previously been shown to be negatively correlated with the PUFA/SFA ratio (Volek et al., 1997) indicating that the fatty acid content in the diet should be considered more closely, where protein and carbohydrate have been the central focus to date (Tarnopolsky, 2008). Equally, overtraining is associated with altered circulating testosterone (Maso et al., 2004) and in some circumstance, such as extreme endurance, there is perhaps a role for LC n–3 PUFA in the diet to attenuate acute decline in muscle mass. The behavioral nature of diet modification, coupled with the achievable dose required to elicit membrane phospholipid incorporation, means that this would be a worth-while and interesting avenue of research.

LONG-TERM MONITORING AND OPTIMIZATION OF LC N–3 PUFA IN ATHLETES

Dietary LC n–3 PUFA alter tissue fatty acid profiles, in particular the cellular membrane composition. Nonetheless, independent of diet, exercise also provides a stimulus by which membranes, particularly skeletal muscle, can be modulated. This remodeling, mostly in the direction of PUFA, has been demonstrated in animals (Helge et al., 1999) and humans (Helge et al., 2001b), where the predominance of eccentric muscle contractions alone provides a unique approach to altering the membrane fatty acid profile (Helge et al., 2001a). Elite athletes, training almost daily and competing year round, have this added and independent physiological stimulus that must interplay with the dietary sources of fatty acids. There are currently no long-term investigations that have addressed the role of dietary fish oil on protracted physiological stress, performance markers and outcomes in athletes during a full cycle of training and competition. No doubt the themes explored in this discussion would form a reasonable premise for monitoring tissue omega-3 status in athletes over the longer term. In the first instance, the interrelationships between training loads, detailed and repeated measures of both intake and maintenance of tissue LC n–3 PUFA and physiological measures of both performance and strain would be intriguing. In addition, given that the dose of fish oil required to raise the omega-3 status is equivalent to one or two fish meals per week, easily attainable without compromising the intake of valuable carbohydrates or other macronutrients, it is recommended that future studies focus on long term, randomized control trials that project over full training and competition cycles.

CONCLUSIONS

The important role of nutrition in exercise has directed research to uncover both the physiological and performance benefits of optimizing the athlete's diet. Dietary fish oil, providing EPA and DHA, has emerged as an important nutritional component and is worthy of recognition alongside other triggers for exercise adaptations (Stellingwerff, 2014). Fig. 10.1 is a summary of outcomes from supplementing the diet of trained athletes. Fish oil is yet to establish any measurable effects to athletic performance, yet there are multiple avenues to still pursue including limiting factors in performance physiology. Nonetheless, there is strong physiological basis that body systems including the cardiovascular system and skeletal muscle will positively respond, via oxygen modulation, to exposure of DHA at concentrations that are achievable as whole foods in the diet (Fig. 10.1). Dietary intake of DHA, as little as 500 mg/day in physically trained subjects, has been shown to elevate the erythrocyte omega-3 index. This dose is in agreement

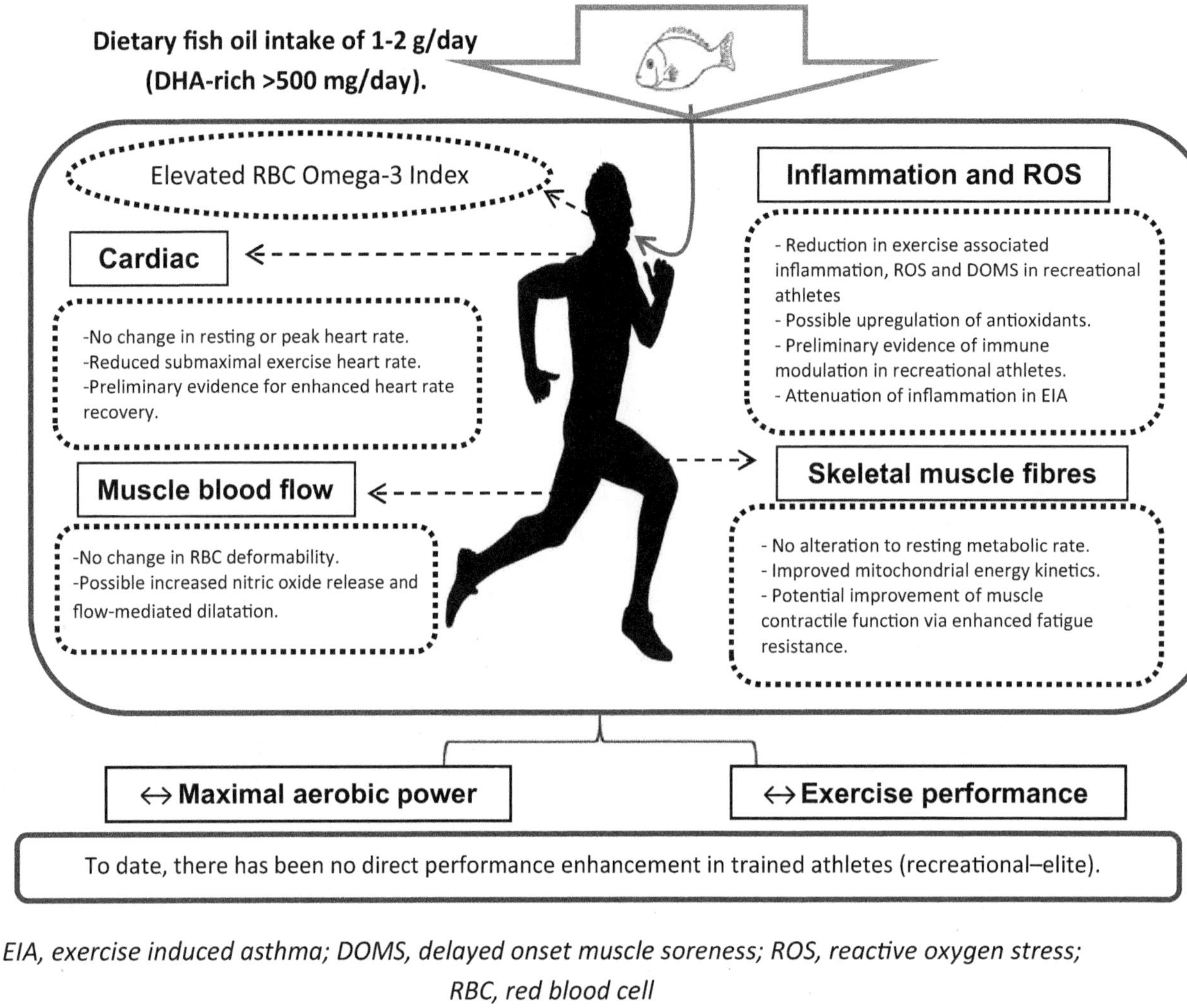

FIGURE 10.1 **Summary of the physiological and performance effects of dietary fish oil supplementation in trained populations.**

with animal tissues where 1.25% or down to as little as 0.3% of overall diet provided as DHA-rich fish oil is above a critical threshold for cell membrane incorporation of DHA into heart (Slee et al., 2010) and skeletal muscle (Henry et al., 2015). Given the apparent essential nature of DHA for some physiological function, it is reasonable to predict that performance gain might only be achieved in athletes whose dietary intake is inadequate, which on the basis of the low median intake of LC n–3 PUFA amongst the general population, is likely to be a considerable proportion. The role of circulating EPA has primarily focused upon immune and inflammatory support, including muscle damage, where there is some evidence for attenuation in less trained athletes (Fig. 10.1). Future studies will need to consider the biological differences that DHA can offer in these fields in context to the adaptations that exercise independently offers. Given that there is plausible evidence that enhancing LC n–3 PUFA, via intake of dietary fish oil, does not need to compromise carbohydrate or protein requirements in the balanced diet, there are many future opportunities to explore the limits of physical performance.

References

Abbatecola, A., Cherubini, A., Guralnik, J., Lacueva, C., Ruggiero, C., Maggio m, Bandinelli, S., Paolisso, G., Ferrucci, L., 2009. Plasma polyunsaturated fatty acids and age related physical performance decline. Rejuvenation Res. 12, 25–32.

Abdukeyum, G., Owen, A., McLennan, P., 2008. Dietary (n-3) long chain polyunsaturated fatty acids inhibit ischemia and reperfusion arrhythmias and infarction in rat heart not enhanced by ischemic preconditioning. J. Nutr. 138, 1902–1909.

Abdukeyum, G.G., Owen, A.J., Larkin, T.A., McLennan, P.L., 2016. Up-regulation of mitochondrial antioxidant superoxide dismutase underpins persistent cardiac nutritional-preconditioning by n-3 long chain polyunsaturated fatty acids in the rat. J. Clin. Med. 5 (3), 1–13.

Albert, B.B., Cameron-Smith, D., Hofman, P.L., Tumanov, S., Villas-Boas, S.G., Garg, M.L., Cutfield, W.S., 2015. Fish oil supplements in New Zealand are highly oxidised and do not meet label content of n-3 PUFA. Sci. Rep. 5, pp. 1–6.

Allen, D., Lamb, G., Westerblab, H., 2008. Skeletal muscle fatigue: cellular mechanisms. Physiol. Rev. 88, 287–332.

Andrade, P.M.M., Ribeiro, B.G., Bozza, M.T., Rosa, L., do Carmo, M.G.T., 2007. Effects of the fish-oil supplementation on the immune and inflammatory responses in elite swimmers. Prostagland. Leukotr. Essen. Fatty Acid. 77, 139–145.
Atashak, S., Sharafi, H., Azarbayjani, M.A., Stannard, S.R., Goli, M.A., Haghighi, M.M., 2013. Effect of omega-3 supplementation on blood levels of oxidative stress, muscle dammage and inflammation markers after acute resistance exercise in young athletes. Kinesiology 45, 22–29.
Ayre, K., Hulbert, A., 1996. Dietary fatty acid profile influences the composition of skeletal muscle phospholipids in rats. J. Nutr. 126, 653–662.
Barclay, J.K., 1993. A delivery-independant blood flow effect on skeletal muscle fatigue. J. Appl. Physiol. 74, 2294–2300.
Bentley, D., Smith, P., Davie, A., Zhou, S., 2000. Muscle activation of the knee extensors following high intensity endurance exercise in cyclists. Eur. J. Appl. Physiol. 81, 297–302.
Bloomer, R.J., Larson, D.E., Fisher-Wellman, K.H., Galpin, A.J., Schilling, B.K., 2009. Effect of eicosapentaenoic and docosahexaenoic acid on resting and exercise-induced inflammatory and oxidative stress biomarkers: a randomized, placebo controlled, cross-over study. Lipids Health Dis. 8 (36), 1–12. doi: 10.1186/1476-511x-8-36.
Bortolotti, M., Tappy, L., Schneiter, P., 2007. Fish oil supplementation does not alter energy efficiency in healthy males. Clin. Nutr. 26, 225–230.
Broekhuizen, R., Wouters, E., Creutzberg, E., Weling-Scheepers, C., Schols, A., 2005. Polyunsaturated fatty acids improve exercise capacity in chronic obstructive pulmonary disease. Thorax 60, 376–382.
Buckley, J.D., Burgess, S., Murphy, K.J., Howe, P.R.C., 2009. DHA-rich fish oil lowers heart rate during submaximal exercise in elite Australian Rules footballers. J. Sci. Med. Sport 12, 503–507.
Burke, L.M., 2006. Fat adaptation" for athletic performance: the nail in the coffin? J. Appl. Physiol. 100, 7–8.
Burke, L.M., Kiens, B., Ivy, J.L., 2004. Carbohydrates and fat for training and recovery. J. Sports Sci. 22, 15–30.
Calder, P.C., 2006. n-3 polyunsaturated fatty acids, inflammation, and inflammatory diseases. Am. J. Clin. Nutr. 83, 1505S–1519S.
Calder, P.C., 2013. Omega-3 polyunsaturated fatty acids and inflammatory processes: nutrition or pharmacology? Br. J. Clin. Pharmacol. 75, 645–662.
Capo, X., Martorell, M., Llompart, I., Sureda, A., Tur, J.A., Pons, A., 2014. Docosahexanoic acid diet supplementation attenuates the peripheral mononuclear cell inflammatory response to exercise following LPS activation. Cytokine 69, 155–164.
Capo, X., Martorell, M., Sureda, A., Llompart, I., Tur, J.A., Pons, A., 2015. Diet supplementation with DHA-enriched food in football players during training season enhances the mitochondrial antioxidant capabilities in blood mononuclear cells. Eur. J. Nutr. 54, 35–49.
Cartwright, I.J., Pockley, A.G., Galloway, J.H., Greaves, M., Preston, F.E., 1985. The effects of dietary omega-3 polyunsaturated fatty-acids on erthrocyte-membrane phospholipids, erythrocyte deformability and blood viscosity in healthy volunteers. Atherosclerosis 55, 267–281.
Castillo, R.L., Arias, C., Farías, J.G., 2014. Omega 3 chronic supplementation attenuates myocardial ischaemia-reperfusion injury through reinforcement of antioxidant defense system in rats. Cell Biochem. Funct. 32, 274–281.
Chapman, R., Stray-Gunndersen, J., Levine, B., 1998. Individual variation in response to altitude training. J. Appl. Physiol. 85, 1448–1456.
Charnock, J.S., Abeywardena, M.Y., Poletti, V.M., McLennan, P.L., 1992. Differences in fatty acid composition of various tissues of the marmoset monkey after different lipids supplement diets. Compar. Biochem. Physiol. 101A, 387–393.
Cleland, L.G., James, M.J., Proudman, S.M., 2006. Fish oil: what the prescriber needs to know. Arthritis Res. Therapy 8, 202.
Colquhoun, D., Ferreira, J., A, Udell, T., Eden, B., 2008. Committee of the Heart Foundation Review of evidence: fish, fish oils, n-3 PUFA and cardiovascular health, vol. 2013. Foundation NH, Sydney. www.heartfoundation.org.au/images/uploads/main/For_professionals/Fish-FishOils-revie-of-evidence.pdf
Da Boit, M., Mastalurova, I., Brazaite, G., McGovern, N., Thompson, K., Gray, S., 2015. The effect of krill oil supplementation on exercise performance and markers of immune function. PLoS ONE, 10.
De Pauw, K., Roelands, B., Cheung, S.S., de Geus, B., Rietjens, G., Meeusen, R., 2013. Guidelines to classify subject groups in sport-science research. Int. J. Sports Physiol. Perf. 8, 111–122.
Dilorenzo, F.M., Drager, C.J., Rankin, J.W., 2014. Docosahexaenoic acid affects markers of inflammation and muscle damage after eccentric exercise. J. Str. Condition. Res. 28, 2768–2774.
Erken, H.A., Erken, G., Colak, R., Genc, O., 2013. Exercise and DHA prevent the negative effects of hypoxia on EEG and nerve conduction velocity. High Altitude Med. Biol. 14, 360–366.
Ernst, E., Saradeth, T., Achhammer, G., 1991. N-3 fatty-acids and acute phase proteins. Eur. J. Clin. Investig. 21, 77–82.
Faulkner, J.A., Davis, C.S., Mendias, C.L., Brooks, S.V., 2008. The aging of elite male athletes: age-related changes in performance and skeletal muscle structure and function. Clin. J. Sport Med. 18, 501–507.
Filaire, E., Massart, A., Rouveix, M., Portier, H., Rosado, F., Durand, D., 2011. Effects of 6 weeks of n-3 fatty acids and antioxidant mixture on lipid peroxidation at rest and postexercise. Eur. J. Appl. Physiol. 111, 1829–1839.
Fisher-Wellman, K., Bloomer, R.J., 2009. Acute exercise and oxidative stress: a 30 year history. Dyn. Med. 8, 1.
Flock, M., Harris, W., Kris-Etherton, P., 2013. Long-chain omega-3 fatty acids: time to establish a dietary reference intake. Nutr. Rev. 71, 692–707.
Gerling, C.J., Whitfield, J., Mukai, K., Spriet, L.L., 2014. Variable effects of 12 weeks of omega-3 supplementation on resting skeletal muscle metabolism. Appl. Physiol. Nutr. Metabol. Physiol. Appl. Nutr. Et Metabol. 39, 1083–1091.
Gibson, R.A., Neumann, M.A., Lien, E.L., Boyd, K.A., Tu, W.C., 2013. Docosahexaenoic acid synthesis from alpha-linolenic acid is inhibited by diets high in polyunsaturated fatty acids. Prostagland. Leukotr. Essen. Fatty Acid. 88, 139–146.
Gladden, L.B., McIntosh, B.R., Stainsby, W.N., 1978. Oxygen uptake and developed tension during and after fatigue, curare block, and ischemia. J. Appl. Physiol. 45, 751–756.
Gleeson, M., Nieman, D.C., Pedersen, B.K., 2004. Exercise, nutrition and immune function. J. Sports Sci. 22, 115–125.
Gleeson, M., Bishop, N.C., Stensel, D.J., Lindley, M.R., Mastana, S.S., Nimmo, M.A., 2011. The anti-inflammatory effects of exercise: mechanisms and implications for the prevention and treatment of disease. Nature Rev. Immunol. 11, 607–615.
Gogus, U., Smith, C., 2010. n-3 Omega fatty acids: a review of current knowledge. Int. J. Food Sci. Technol. 45, 417–436.
Gore, C., Little, S., Hahn, A., 1997. Reduced performance of male and female athletes at 580 m altitude. Eur. J. Appl. Physiol. 75, 136–143.
Gore, C., Clark, S., Saunders, P., 2007. Nonhematological mechanisms of improved sea-level performance after hypoxic exposure. Med. Sci. Sports Exercise 39, 1600–1609.
Gorjao, R., Azevedo-Martins, A., Rodrigues, H., Abdulkader, F., Arcisio-Miranda, M., Procopio, J., Curi, R., 2009. Comparative effects of DHA and EPA on cell function. Pharmacol. Therapeut. 122, 56–64.
Gorman, M.W., Barclay, J.K., Sparks, H.V., 1988. Effects of ischemia on VO_2 tension and vascular resistance in contracting canine skeletal muscle. J. Appl. Physiol. 65, 1075–1081.

Grandjean, D., Sergheraert, R., Valette, J., Driss, F., 1998. Biological and nutrional consequences of work at high altitude in search and rescue dogs: the scientific expedition chiens des cimes-licancabur 1996. Nutr. Health 128, 2694S–2697S.

Gray, P., Gabriel, B., Thies, F., Gray, S., 2012. Fish oil supplementation augments post-exercise immune function in young males. Brain Behavior Immun., 1265–1272.

Gray, P., Chappell, A., Jenkinson, A., Thies, F., Gray, S.R., 2014. Fish oil supplementation reduces markers of oxidative stress but not muscle soreness after eccentric exercise. Int. J. Sport Nutr. Exer. Metab. 24, 206–214.

Guezennec, C., Nadaud, J., Satabin, P., Leger, F., Lafargue, P., 1989. Influence of polyunsaturated fatty acid diet on the hemorreological response to exercise in hypoxia. Int. J. Sport Med. 10, 286–291.

Guzman, J., Esteve, H., Pablos, C., Blasco, C., Villegras, J., 2011. DHA-rich fish oil improves complex reaction time in female elite soccer players. J. Sports Sci. Med. 10, 301–305.

Halliwell, B., Lee, C.Y.J., 2010. Using isoprostanes as biomarkers of oxidative stress: some rarely considered issues. Antioxidants Redox Signal. 13, 145–156.

Harris, W.S., von Schacky, C., 2004. The Omega-3 Index: a new risk factor for death from coronary heart disease? Preventive Med. 39, 212–220.

Harris, W.S., Gonzales, M., Laney, N., Sastre, A., Borkon, A.M., 2006. Effects of Omega-3 Fatty acids on heart rate in cardiac transplant recipients. Am. J. Cardiol. 98, 1393–1395.

Harris, W.S., Varvel, S.A., Pottala, J.V., Warnick, G.R., McConnell, J.P., 2013. Comparative effects of an acute dose of fish oil on omega-3 fatty acid levels in red blood cells versus plasma: implications for clinical utility. J. Clin. Lipidol. 7, 433–440.

Helge, J.W., Ayre, K.J., Hulbert, A.J., Kiens, B., Storlien, L.H., 1999. Regular exercise modulates muscle membrane phospholipid profile in rats. J. Nutr. 129, 1636–1642.

Helge, J., Therkildsen, K., Jorgensen, T., Wu, B., Storlien, L., Asp, S., 2001a. Eccentric contractions affect muscle membrane phospholipid acid composition in rats. Experiment. Physiol. 86, 599–604.

Helge, J.W., Wu, B.J., Willer, M., Daugaard, J.R., Storlien, L.H., Kiens, B., 2001b. Training affects muscle phospholipid fatty acid compostion in humans. J. Appl. Physiol. 90, 670–677.

Henry, R., Peoples, G.E., McLennan, P.L., 2015. Muscle fatigue-resistance in the rat hindlimb in vivo from low dietary intakes of tuna fish oil that selectively increase phospholipid omega-3 docosahexaenoic acid according to muscle fibre type. Br. J. Nutr. 114, 873–884.

Herbst, E.A.F., Paglialunga, S., Gerling, C., Whitfield, J., Mukai, K., Chabowski, A., Heigenhauser, G.J.F., Spriet, L.L., Holloway, G.P., 2014. Omega-3 supplementation alters mitochondrial membrane composition and respiration kinetics in human skeletal muscle. J. Physiol. London 592, 1341–1352.

Hogan, M.C., Arthur, P.G., Bebout, P.D., Hochachka, P.W., Wagner, P.D., 1992. Role of O_2 in regulating tissue respiration in dog muscle working in situ. J. Appl. Physiol. 73, 728–736.

Hogan, M.C., Kurdak, S.S., Arthur, P.G., 1996. Effect of gradual reduction in O_2 delivery on intracelullar homeostasis in contracting skeletal muscle. J. Appl. Physiol. 80, 1313–1321.

Holdsworth, C., Copp, S., Hirai, D., Ferguson, S., Sims, G., Hageman, K., Stebbins, C., Poole, D., Musch, T., 2014. The effects of dietary fish oil on exercising skeletal muscle vascular and metabolic control in chronic heart failure rats. Appl. Physiol. Nutr. Metabol. 39, 299–307.

Horn, P.L., West, N.P., Pyne, D.B., Koerbin, G., Lehtinen, S.J., Fricker, P.A., Cripps, A.W., 2015. Routine exercise alters measures of immunity and the acute phase reaction. Eur. J. Appl. Physiol. 115, 407–415.

Huffman, D., Altena, T., Mawhinney, T., Thomas, T., 2004. Effect of n-3 fatty acids on free tryptophan and exercise fatigue. Eur. J. Appl. Physiol. 92, 584–591.

Infante, J.P., 1987. Docosahexaenoate-containing phospholipids in sarcoplasmic-reticulum and retinal photoreceptors: a proposal for a role in Ca2 + -ATPase calcium-transport. Mol. Cell. Biochem. 74, 111–116.

Infante, J., Kirwan, R., Brenna, J., 2001. High levels of docosahexaenoic acid (22:6 n-3)- containing phospholipids in high-frequency contraction muscles of hummingbirds and rattlesnakes. Comp. Biochem. Physiol. 130, 291–298.

James, M., Sullivan, T., Metcalf, R., Cleland, L., 2014. Pitfalls in the use of randomised controlled trials for fish oil studies with cardiac patients. Br. J. Nutr. 112, 812–820.

Jeukendrup, A.E., Thielen, J.J., Wagenmakers, A.J.M., Brouns, F., Saris, W.H.M., 1998. Effect of MCT and carbohydrate ingestion on substrate utilization and cycling performance. Am. J. Clin. Nutr. 67, 397–404.

Jezková, J., Nováková, O., Kolá, F., Tvrzická, E., Necká, J., Novák, F., 2002. Chronic hypoxia alters fatty acid composition of phospholipids in right and left ventricular myocardium. Mol. Cell. Biochem. 232, 49–56.

Jouris, K., McDaniel, J., Weiss, E., 2011. The effect of omega-3 fatty acid supplementation on the inflammatory response to eccentric strength exercise. J. Sports Sci. Med. 10, 432.

Joyner, M., Coyle, E., 2008. Endurance exercise performance: the physiology of champions. J. Physiol. 586, 35–44.

Kanatous, S.B., DiMichele, L.V., Cowan, D.F., Davis, R.W., 1999. High aerobic capacities in the skeletal muscles of pinnipeds: adaptations to diving hypoxia. J. Appl. Physiol. 86, 1247–1256.

Kawabataa, F., Neyab, M., Hamazakic, K., Watanabeb, Y., Kobayashid, S., Tsujia, T., 2014. Supplementation with eicosapentaenoic acid-rich fish oil improves exercise economy and reduces perceived exertion during submaximal steady-state exercise in normal healthy untrained men. Biosci. Biotechnol. Biochem. 78 (12), 2081–2088.

Kitamura, K., Jorgensen, C.R., Gobel, F.L., Taylor, H.L., Wang, Y., 1972. Hemodynamic correlates of myocardial oxygen consumption during upright exercise. J. Appl. Physiol. 32, 516–522.

Lands, B., 2008. A critique of paradoxes in current advice on dietary lipids. Prog. Lipid Res. 47, 77–106.

Leaf, A., Rauch, C., 1988. Omega-3 supplementation and estimation of VO_{2max}: a double blind randomised controlled trial in athletes. Annals Sports Med. 4, 37–40.

Leonard, A.E., Pereira, S.L., Sprecher, H., Huang, Y.S., 2004. Elongation of long-chain fatty acids. Prog. Lipid Res. 43, 36–54.

Lewis, E.J.H., Radonic, P.W., Wolever, T.M.S., Wells, G.D., 2015. 21 days of mammalian omega-3 fatty acid supplementation improves aspects of neuromuscular function and performance in male athletes compared to olive oil placebo. J. Int. Soc. Sports Nutr. 12 (28), 1–11.

Lindstedt, S.L., McGlothlin, T., Percy, E., Pifer, J., 1998. Task-specific design of skeletal muscle: balancing muscle structural composition. Compar. Biochem. Physiol. B 120, 35–40.

Lun, V., Erdman, K., Fung, T., Reimer, R., 2012. Dietary Supplementation Practices in Canadian High-Performance Athletes. Int. J. Sport Nutr. Exercise Metabol. 22, 31–37.

Macartney, M., Hingley, L., Brown, M., Peoples, G., McLennan, P.L., 2014. Intrinsic heart rate recovery after dynamic exercise is improved with increased omega-3 index in healthy males. Br. J. Nutr. 112, 1984–1992.

MacIntosh, B.R., Shahi, M.R.S., 2011. A peripheral governor regulates muscle contraction. Appl. Physiol. Nutr. Metabol. Physiol. Appl. Nutr. Metabol. 36, 1–11.

Madden, J., Brunner, A., Dastur, N.D., Tan, R.M., Nash, G.B., Rainger, G.E., Shearman, C.P., Calder, P.C., Grimble, R.F., 2007. Fish oil induced increase in walking distance, but not ankle brachial pressure index, in peripheral arterial disease is dependent on both body mass index and inflammatory genotype. Prostagland. Leukotr. Essen. Fatty Acid. 76, 331–340.

Margeli, A., Skenderi, K., Tsironi, M., Hantzi, E., Matalas, A.L., Vrettou, C., Kanavakis, E., Chrousos, G., Papassotiriou, I., 2005. Dramatic elevations of interleukin-6 and acute-phase reactants in athletes participating in the ultradistance foot race spartathlon: Severe systemic inflammation and lipid and lipoprotein changes in protracted exercise. J. Clin. Endocrinol. Metabol. 90, 3914–3918.

Martorell, M., Capo, X., Sureda, A., Batle, J.M., Llompart, I., Argelich, E., Tur, J.A., Pons, A., 2014. Effect of DHA on plasma fatty acid availability and oxidative stress during training season and football exercise. Food Funct. 5, 1920–1931.

Martorell, M., Capo, X., Bibiloni, M.M., Sureda, A., Mestre-Alfaro, A., Batle, J.M., Llompart, I., Tur, J.A., Pons, A., 2015. Docosahexaenoic acid supplementation promotes erythrocyte antioxidant defense and reduces protein nitrosative damage in male athletes. Lipids 50, 131–148.

Maso, F., Lac, G., Filaire, E., Michaux, O., Robert, A., 2004. Salivary testosterone and cortisol in rugby players: correlation with psychological overtraining items. Br. J. Sports Med. 38, 260–263.

McAnulty, S.R., Nieman, D.C., Fox-Rabinovich, M., Duran, V., McAnulty, L.S., Henson, D.A., Jin, F.X., Landram, M.J., 2010. Effect of n-3 fatty acids and antioxidants on oxidative stress after exercise. Med. Sci. Sports Exer. 42, 1704–1711.

McGlory, C., Galloway, S.D.R., Hamilton, D.L., McClintock, C., Breen, L., Dick, J.R., Bell, J.G., Tipton, K.D., 2014. Temporal changes in human skeletal muscle and blood lipid composition with fish oil supplementation. Prostagland. Leukotr. Essen. Fatty Acid. 90, 199–206.

McGlory, C., Wardle, S.L., Macnaughton, L.S., Witard, O.C., Scott, F., Dick, J., Gordon Bell, J., Phillips, S.M., Galloway, S.D.R., Hamilton, L., Tipton, K.D., 2016. Fish oil supplementation suppresses resistance exercise and feeding-induced increases in anabolic signalling without affecting myofibrillar protein synthesis in young men. Physiol. Rep. 4 (6), e12715.

McLennan, P.L., 2014. Cardiac physiology and clinical efficacy of dietary fish oil clarified through cellular mechanisms of omega-3 polyunsaturated fatty acids. Eur. J. Appl. Physiol. 114, 1333–1356.

McLennan, P., Abeywardena, M.Y., Charnock, J.S., 1988. Dietary fish oil prevents ventricular fibrillation following coronary artery occlusion and reperfusion. Am. Heart J. 116, 709–717.

McLennan, P., Howe, P., Abeywardena, M., Muggli, R., Raederstorff, D., Mano, M., Rayner, T., Head, R., 1996. The cardiovascular protective role of docosahexaenoic acid. Eur. J. Pharmacol. 300, 83–89.

McWilliams, S.R., Guglielmo, C., Pierce, B., Klaassen, M., 2004. Flying, fasting, and feeding in birds during migration: a nutritional and physiological ecology perspective. J. Avian Biol. 35, 377–393.

Metcalf, R.G., James, M.J., Gibson, R.A., Edwards, J.R., Stubberfield, J., Stuklis, R., Roberts-Thomson, K., Young, G.D., Cleland, L.G., 2007. Effects of fish-oil supplementation on myocardial fatty acids in humans. Am. J. Clin. Nutr. 85, 1222–1228.

Meyer, A., Zoll, J., Charles, A., Charloux, A., de Blay, F., Diemmunsch, P., Sibilia, J., Piquard, F., Geny, B., 2013. Skeletal muscle mitochondrial dysfunction during chronic obstructive pulmonary disease: central actor and theraputic target. Experiment. Physiol. 98, 1063–1078.

Mickleborough, T.D., Murray, R.L., Ionescu, A.A., Lindley, M.R., 2003. Fish oil supplementation reduces severity of exercise-induced bronchoconstriction in elite athletes. Am. J. Respirat. Critical Care Med. 168, 1181–1189.

Mickleborough, T., Sinex, J., Platt, D., Chapman, R., Hirt, M., 2015. The effects PCSO-524®, a patented marine oil lipid and omega-3 PUFA blend derived from the New Zealand green lipped mussel (*Perna canaliculus*), on indirect markers of muscle damage and inflammation after muscle damaging exercise in untrained men: a randomized, placebo controlled trial. J. Int. Soc. Sports Nutr., 12.

Molfino, A., Gioia, G., Fanelli, F.R., Muscaritoli, M., 2014. The role for dietary omega-3 fatty acids supplementation in older adults. Nutrients 6, 4058–U4667.

Mozaffarian, D., Rimm, E., 2006. Fish intake, contaminants, and human health: evaluating the risks and the benefits. J. Am. Med. Assoc. 296, 1885–1889.

Mozaffarian, D., Wu, J.H., 2012. (n-3) fatty acids and cardiovascular health: are effects of EPA and DHA shared or complementary? J. Nutr. 142, 614S–625S.

Mozaffarian, D., Geelen, A., Brouwer, I., Geleijnse, J., Zock, P., Katan, M., 2005. Effect of fish oil on heart rate: a meta-analysis of randomised controlled trials. Circulation 112, 1945–1952.

Nieman, D., Henson, D., McAnulty, S., Jin, F., Maxwell, K., 2009. n-3 polyunsaturated fatty acids do not alter immune and inflammation measures in endurance athletes. Int. J. Sport Nutr. Exer. Metabol. 19, 536–546.

Olesen, J., Bienso, R.S., Meinertz, S., van Hauen, L., Rasmussen, S.M., Gliemann, L., Plomgaard, P., Pilegaard, H., 2015. Impact of training status on LPS-induced acute inflammation in humans. J. Appl. Physiol. 118, 818–829.

Oostenbrug, G.S., Hardeman, M., De Vries, T., Brouns, F., Hornstra, G., 1997. Exercise performance, red blood cell deformability, and lipid peroxidation: effects of fish oil and vitamin E. J. Appl. Physiol. 83, pp. 746–752.

Ottenheijm, C., Heunks, L., Geraedts, M., Dekhuijzen, P., 2006. Hypoxia induced skeletal muscle fibre dysfunction:role for reactive nitrogen species. Am. J. Physiol. 290, L127–L135.

Pan, D., Storlien, L.H., 1993. Dietary lipid profile is a determinate of tissue phospholipids fatty acid composition and rate weight gain in rats. J. Nutr. 123, 512–519.

Pawlosky, R.J., Hibbeln, J.R., Novotny, J.A., Salem, Jr., N., 2001. Physiological compartmental analysis of alpha-linolenic acid metabolism in adult humans. J. Lipid Res. 42, 1257–1265.

Pearlman, W.H., Crepy, O., 1967. Steriod-protein interaction with particualr reference to testosterone binding human serum. J. Biol. Chem. 242, 182–189.

Peltonen, J., Tikkanen, H., Rusko, H., 2001. Cardiorespiratory responses to exercise in acute hypoxia, hyperoxia and normoxia. Eur. J. Appl. Physiol. 85, 82–88.

Peoples, G., McLennan, P., 2010. Dietary fish oil reduces skeletal muscle oxygen consumption, provides fatigue resistance and improves contractile recovery in the rat in vivo hindlimb. Br. J. Nutr. 104, 1771–1779.

Peoples, G., McLennan, P., 2014. Long-chain n-3 DHA reduces the extent of skeletal muscle fatigue in the rat in vivo hindlimb model. Br. J. Nutr. 111, 996–1003.

Peoples, G., McLennan, P., Howe, P., Groeller, H., 2008. Fish oil reduces heart rate and oxygen consumption during exercise. J. Cardio. Pharmacol. 52, 540–547.

Pepe, S., McLennan, P., 1996. Dietary fish oil confers direct antiarrhythmic properties on the myocardium of rats. J. Nutr. 126, 34–42.

Pepe, S., McLennan, P.L., 2002. Cardiac membrane fatty acid composition modulates mycardial oxygen consumption and postischemic recovery of contractile function. Circulation 105, 2303–2308.

Perrey, S., Rupp, T., 2009. Altitude-induced changes in muscle contractile properties. High Altitude Med. Biol. 10, 175–182.

Phillips, T., Childs, A.C., Dreon, D.M., Phinney, S., Leeuwenburgh, C., 2003. A dietary supplement attenuates IL-6 and CRP after eccentric exercise in untrained males. Med. Sci. Sports Exer. 35, 2032–2037.

Poprzecki, S., Zajac, A., Chalimoniuk, M., Waskiewicz, Z., Langfort, J., 2009. Modification of blood antioxidant status and lipid profile in response to high-intensity endurance exercise after low doses of omega-3 polyunsaturated fatty acids supplementation in healthy volunteers. Int. J. Food Sci. Nutr. 60, 67–79.

Raastad, T., Hostmark, A.T., Stromme, S.B., 1997. Omega-3 fatty acid supplementation does not improve maximal aerobic power, anaerobic threshold and running performance in well trained soccer players. Scandinavian J. Med. Sci. Sports 7, 25–31.

Robinson, S.M., Jameson, K.A., Batelaan, S.F., Martin, H.J., Syddall, H.E., Dennison, E.M., Cooper, C., Sayer, A.A., Hertfordshire Cohort Study, G., 2008. Diet and its relationship with grip strength in community-dwelling older men and women: the hertfordshire cohort study. J. Am. Geriatrics Soc. 56, 84–90.

Rodacki, C., Rodacki, A., Pereira, G., Naliwaiko, K.C., Pequito, I., Fernandes L, D., 2012. Fish-oil supplementation enhances the effects of strength training in elderly women. Am. J. Clin. Nutr. 95, 428–436.

Ronsen, O., Sundgot-Borgen, J., Maehlum, S., 1999. Supplement use and nutritional habits in Norwegian elite athletes. Scandinavian J. Med. Sci. Sports 9, 28–35.

Saltin, B., Radegran, G., Koskolou, M.D., Roach, R.C., 1998. Skeletal muscle blood flow in humans and its regulation during exercise. Acta Physiol. Scandinavica 162, 421–436.

Santos, V.C., Levada-Pires, A.C., Alves, S.R., Pithon-Curi, T.C., Curi, R., Cury-Boaventura, M.F., 2013. Effects of DHA-rich fish oil supplementation on lymphocyte function before and after a marathon race. Int. J. Sport Nutr. Exer. Metabol. 23, 161–169.

Serhan, C.N., 2005. Novel eicosanoid and docosanoid mediators: resolvins, docosatrienes, and neuroprotectins. Curr. Opinon Clin. Nutr. Metabol. Care 8, 115–121.

Shei, R.J., Lindley, M.R., Mickleborough, T.D., 2014. Omega-3 polyunsaturated fatty acids in the optimization of physical performance. Military Med. 179, 144–156.

Simopoulos, A.P., 2007. Omega-3 fatty acids and athletics. Curr. Sports Med. Rep. 6, 230–236.

Siscovick, D.S., Raudgunathan, T.E., Weinmann, S., Wicklund, K.G., Albright, J., Bovbjerg, V., Arbogast, P., Smith, H., Kushi, L.H., Cobb, L.A., Copass, M.K., Psaty, B.M., Lemaitre, R., Retzlaff, B., Childs, M., Knopp, R.H., 1995. Dietary intake and cell membrane levels of long-chain n-3 polyunsaturated fatty acids and risk of primary cardiac arrest. JAMA 274, 1363–1367.

Slee, E., McLennan, P., Owen, A., Theiss, M., 2010. Low dietary fish-oil threshold for myocardial membrane n-3 PUFA enrichment independent of n-6 PUFA intake in rats. J. Lipid Res. 51, 1841–1848.

Smith, G., Atherton, P., Reeds, D., Mohammed, S., Rankin, D., Rennie, M., Mittendorfer, B., 2011. Dietary omega-3 fatty acid supplementation increases the rate of muscle protein synthesis in older adults: a randomized controlled trial. Am. J. Clin. Nutr. 93, 402–412.

Stellingwerff, T., 2014. Nutrtional triggers to adaptation and performance. Appl. Physiol. Nutr. Metabol. 39, v–v10.

Tarnopolsky, M.A., 2008. Nutritional consideration in the aging athlete. Clin. J. Sport Med. 18, 531–538.

Tartibian, B., Maleki, B., Abbasi, A., 2011. Omega-3 fatty acids supplementation attenuates inflammatory markers after eccentric exercise in untrained men. Clin. J. Sports Med. 21, 131–137.

Terano, T., Hirai, A., Hamazaki, T., Kobayashi, S., Fujita, T., Tamura, Y., Kumagai, A., 1983. Effects of oral administration of highly purified eicosapentaenoic acid on platelet function, blood viscosity and red cell deformability in healthy human subjects. Atherosclerosis 46, 321–331.

Tiryaki-Sonmez, G., Schoenfeld, B., Vatensever-Ozen, S., 2011. Omega-3 fatty acids and exercise: a review of thier combined effects on body composition and physical performance. Biomed. Human Kinetics 3, 23–29.

Toft, A.D., Thorn, M., Ostrowski, K., Asp, S., Molller, K., Iversen, S., Hermann, C., Sondergaard, S.R., Pedersen, B.K., 2000. N-3 polyunsaturated fatty acids do not affect cytokine response to strenuous exercise. J. Appl. Physiol. 89, 2401–2406.

USDA, 2009. National Nutrient Database for Standard Reference, vol. 2013.

Vokac, Z., Bell, H., Bautz Holter, E., Rodahl, K., 1975. Oxygen uptake/heart rate relationship in leg and arm exercise, sitting and standing. J. Appl. Physiol. 39, 54–59.

Volek, J.S., Kraemer, W.J., Bush, J.A., Incledon, T., Boetes, M., 1997. Tesosterone and cortisol in relationship to dietary nutrients and resistance exercise. J. Appl. Physiol. 82, 49–54.

von Schacky, C., 2011. The omega-3 index as a risk factor for cardiovascular diseases. Prostagland. Other Lipid Mediators 96, 94–98.

von Schacky, C., Kemper, M., Haslbauer, R., Halle, M., 2014. Low omega-3 index in 106 German elite winter endurance athletes: a pilot study. Int. J. Sport Nutr. Exer. Metabol. 24, 559–564.

Walser, B., Stebbins, C., 2008. Omega-3 fatty acid supplementation enhances stroke volume and cardiac output during dynamic exercise. Eur. J. Appl. Physiol. 104, 455–461.

Walser, B., Giordano, R., Stebbins, C., 2006. Supplementation with omega-3 polyunsaturated fatty acids augments brachial artery dilation and blood flow during forearm contraction. Eur. J. Appl. Physiol. 97, 347–354.

Walsh, N.P., Gleeson, M., Pyne, D.B., Nieman, D.C., Dhabhar, F.S., Shephard, R.J., Oliver, S.J., Bermon, S., Kajeniene, A., 2011. Position statement part two: maintaining immune health. Exer. Immunol. Rev. 17, 64–103.

Wandersee, N.J., Maciaszek, J.L., Giger, K.M., Hanson, M.S., Zheng, S.L., Guo, Y.H., Mickelson, B., Hillery, C.A., Lykotrafitis, G., Low, P.S., Hogg, N., 2015. Dietary supplementation with docosahexanoic acid (DHA) increases red blood cell membrane flexibility in mice with sickle cell disease. Blood Cells Molecules Dis. 54, 183–188.

Zebrowska, A., Mizia-Stec, K., Mizia, M., Gasior, Z., Poprzecki, S., 2014. Omega-3 fatty acids supplementation improves endothelial function and maximal oxygen uptake in endurance-trained athletes. Eur. J. Sport Sci. 15, 305–314.

CHAPTER

11

Fish Intake and Strength in the Elderly

L.C. Fernandes

Physiology Department, University Federal of Paraná, Curitiba, Paraná, Brazil

AGING

It has been estimated that by the end of 2020, there will be a population of 45 million people above 65 years old. Clearly this will be accompanied by socioeconomic challenges in every country (Etzioni et al., 2003).

Aging is associated with an increase in the likelihood of musculoskeletal-related disabilities such as a decrease in mobility and a direct reduction in muscle strength. Also, aging is characterized by difficulties in homeostasis maintenance, leading to decreased physical fitness caused by a time-progressive decline in the ability of aged persons to adapt to the environmental stress. Therefore, as time goes on, these individuals may face age-related loss of skeletal muscle (SM) mass which may have many consequences (Jin et al., 2015). In fact, sarcopenia, which means "a reduction in SM mass with aging" was a term coined in 1989 (Rosenbert, 1989) which is considered a major public health problem because of its direct impact on physical function, dramatically reducing the quality of life of aged people(Clarck and Manini, 2010). Sarcopenia is a major contributor to physical frailty in older adults (Pel-Little et al., 2009).

Beginning in middle age and affecting up to 50% of those over 80 years of age (Baumgartner et al., 1998), the progressive decline in SM mass will result in impairment in lifting, walking, and stair climbing, resulting in a substantially higher risk of falls (Yu et al., 2007). The decline in SM mass between 40–80 years is estimated to be between 30% and 50% with reported losses in functional capacity amounting to as much as 3% each year beyond the age of 60 (Masanes et al., 2012). This decrease in volume is mostly due to a decline in fiber numbers along with fiber atrophy, particularly in the type II glycolytic muscle fibers (Lexell et al., 1986). In addition to these morphological alterations, increased fat, and connective tissue infiltration is commonly observed in SM of the elderly. The physiological mechanisms underlying age-associated decline in SM mass are not fully known. A very plausible cause could be an imbalance in SM protein turnover (ChaleRush et al., 2009). The rate of muscle loss or gain is the simple product of protein synthesis and breakdown. With aging, the capacity of SM to properly respond with an increase in the rate of tissue protein synthesis in response to anabolic stimuli is lost or greatly reduced (Kumar et al., 2009). This is, in part, due to defects in the signaling pathway in muscle which may be mediated by increased inflammatory activity. Anabolic stimuli to a healthy, active, older adult shows postabsorptive net protein balance comparable with that of healthy and younger individuals. When they are challenged with the combined anabolic effect of elevated amino acid and insulin concentrations they are less responsive (Smith et al., 2011). SM mass begins to decline at a rate of approximately 0.5–1.0% per year, normally during middle age (the 40s). These alterations will negatively affect muscle strength and power, resulting in a 2–3% decline of muscle function per year. Although these numbers do not seem impressive, it sometimes results in a significant increase in effort needed to perform very basic daily living tasks (Dela and Kjaer, 2006). Given that muscle mass is essential for locomotion and is a critical regulator of glucose and fatty acid uptake and their utilization, it is important to understand how environmental factors such as diet and exercise affect the maintenance of SM function. Importantly, strength and muscle mass are inversely associated with all causes of mortality including degenerative diseases; in particular, cancer and cardiovascular disease (Schiesel et al., 2015).

Obviously, reducing activities of daily living directly impacts physical activity levels, which in turn, aggravates fat-free mass loss. Therefore, exercise is considered an important tool for attenuating sarcopenia in the elderly and resistance training (RT) has been gaining popularity due to its role in attenuating or even reversing the age-related deleterious effects of sarcopenia. Resistance training enhances muscular strength and increases muscle mass to a

Fish and Fish Oil in Health and Disease Prevention. http://dx.doi.org/10.1016/B978-0-12-802844-5.00011-7

much greater extent than other forms of exercise. It contributes to the reduction of metabolic risk factors correlated with reduced muscle mass in advancing age, markedly improving body composition with reductions in body fat and increases in muscle mass. Also, RT improves muscle mass and strength which directly affect functional ability (Strasser et al., 2009; Peterson et al., 2010).

FISH OIL

In order to maintain adequate muscle mass and physical fitness throughout life, both adequate diet and regular exercise are required. Regarding older adults, diet is not generally a problem but exercising regularly might be challenging for different reasons. Some strategies to reduce the effects of aging, such as therapy with testosterone, growth hormone, and dehydroepiandrosterone (DHEA) are normally used to increase muscle mass and function (Baker et al., 2011; Giannoulis et al., 2006). However, due to undesirable side effects their use is limited. Considering these factors, health professionals have been seeking new approaches to slow age-related loss of muscle mass and function. N-3 fatty acid supplementation has been providing some evidence of efficacy and the results from the past five years are quite promising. For example, data obtained from patients with cancer, rheumatoid arthritis who perform resistance–training has shown that fish oil can stimulate muscle growth, strength, and functionality (Rondanelli et al., 2015).

Fatty acids are molecules found in fat and oils where the structure is of hydrocarbon chain having a methyl (CH_3) at one end and a carboxyl (COO^-) at the other end. The carbon numbers range from 4 to 30 but the most common are from 12 to 22. Also they can have no double bonds (saturated), one double bond (monounsaturated) two or more double bonds (polyunsaturated). There are two important families of PUFA named according to the position of the first bond from the CH_3 (Fig. 11.1). The n–3 PUFA family is metabolized from α-linolenic acid (18:3 n–3) by a series of desaturation and elongation reactions to yield the most important long chain n–3 PUFA eicosapentaenoic acid (EPA 20:5 n–3) and docosahexaenoic acid (DHA 22:6 n–3). The n–6 PUFA family is metabolized from linoleic acid (18:2 n–6) also by the same enzymes yielding the long-chain n-6 PUFA arachidonic acid (20:4 n–6). The long chain n–3 PUFA is found in fatty fish, shellfish, fish from cold waters, and particularly in fish oil. Over the past 200 years, human beings have significantly increased their consumption of saturated and n–6 PUFA, while reducing the intake of n–3 PUFA (Hwang, 1989; Calder et al., 1994).

Western diets typically are rich in n–6 PUFA and low in n–3 PUFA and usually the n–6: n–3 ratio is about 20–30:1. Such an environment allows increases in the concentration of arachidonic acid metabolites, specifically the 2-series of prostaglandins (PG) and thromboxanes (TX) and also 4-series leukotrienes (LT), which have been associated with chronic diseases due to their proinflammatory properties. Intake of long-chain n–3 PUFA, on the other hand, will decrease the production of the inflammatory PG and LT as well as the production of inflammatory cytokines (IL-1, IL-6, and TNF-α) because they increase the production of 3-series of prostaglandins and thromboxanes and 5-series of leukotrienes. Therefore, n–3 PUFAs are considered antiinflammatory (Yan et al., 2013).

As we age the metabolism or relationship between anabolism versus catabolism is not balanced. Catabolism prevails leading to the so called "anabolic resistance" because even with nutritional or mechanical stimuli, as well as anabolic hormones, the muscle protein synthesis (MPS) response is impaired (Rennie, 2009). This feature is also

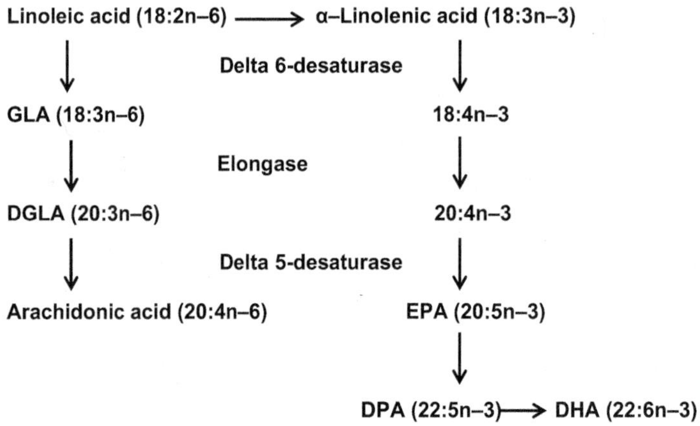

FIGURE 11.1 Metabolism of n–3 and n–6 polyunsaturated fatty acids from both essential fatty acids. From EPA to DHA two elongations take place followed by the action of a delta 6-desaturase (24:6 n–3) and one β-oxidation yields DHA.

present in other conditions such as cancer–cachexia, malnutrition, type 2 diabetes, and overweightness (Muscaritoli et al., 2010). Sedentary individuals and elderly people have a low grade of inflammation contributing to SM loss due to the increase of protein catabolism (Rieux et al., 2009). Since n–3 PUFA have anti-inflammatory and also anticachectic effects they are important tools for combatting the effects of aging (Bougnoux et al., 2010). Smith and coworkers conducted a very interesting study aiming to investigate the effect of n–3 PUFA (Lovaza-acid ethyl esters) supplementation on muscle protein synthesis in older people (Smith et al., 2010). To do so they assigned one group to receive n–3 PUFA and the other corn oil (n–6 PUFA) for eight weeks. Either corn oil or n–3 PUFA had no effect on the muscle protein synthesis at basal rate, but when they induced hyperaminoacidemia–hyperinsulinemia the muscle protein synthesis increased significantly above basal levels. This was accompanied by an increase of muscle mammalian target of rapamycin/ribosomal protein kinase 6 phosphorylation which is involved in the signaling pathway that controls muscle cell growth. This is an interesting finding because in other work (Smith et al., 2011) it was reported that younger adults, compared to older adults, have doubled the muscle protein synthesis above basal levels, corroborating anabolic resistance associated with aging. Therefore, the presence of n–3 PUFA changes the SM physiology in older adults which becomes more responsive to anabolic stimuli (Zérouga et al., 1991). Due to its antiinflammatory properties perhaps n–3 PUFA might assuage the anabolic resistance in muscle from older subjects. We already know of many age-related diseases that take place and the n–3 PUFA might have protective effects, especially on the central nervous system, due to the high concentration of complex lipids (Yeshuda et al., 1999).

Aging causes alterations in the neuromuscular system such as reduction in fiber muscle size and neural degenerative disorders (Lexell et al., 1988; Scaglioni et al., 2003; Johnson et al., 2008). As a consequence, the ability of SM to generate torque is reduced. Among the anabolic stimuli, the physical activity possibly is the most important and powerful to increase muscle protein metabolism (Peterson et al., 2010). At first, neural adjustments occur followed by increasing in muscle crosssectional area (Peterson et al., 2010). It has been demonstrated that fish oil (FO) supplementation is able to increase nerve conduction velocity (Johnson et al., 2008), modulate sarcolemma ion channels (Supari et al., 1995) and improve heart contractility (Holquin et al., 2005) in elderly. Therefore, because FO can improve both heart function and nerve conduction velocity, it is reasonable to hypothesize that exercise associated with n–3 PUFA might add or potentiate muscle strength and function. To investigate this hypothesis, we assigned randomly three groups of elderly women (aged 64.6 ± 1.4 years). One performed strength training (ST); group two received 2 g/day of FO throughout 90 days of strength training (ST90). Group 3 was supplemented 60 days before training and follows the same training protocol (ST150). EPA and DHA plasma concentrations were higher in both ST90 and ST150 groups indicating that in the cell membrane of central nervous system and SM the long-chain fatty acids were incorporated. The metabolism of such fatty acids will yield eicosanoids which modulate signal transduction pathways, facilitating channel opening (Supari et al., 1995). From pre- to post-training muscle strength increased in all three groups. The inclusion of FO enhances SM activation and force; however, FO supplementation before period training did not add any further effect. We also measured the immune response in circulating immune cells. RT and FO supplementation increased phagocytosis, lisossomal volume, peroxide hydrogen, and superoxide anion by neutrophils, CD4 and CD8 lymphocytes and reduced the concentration of inflammatory cytokine TNF-α (Rodacki et al., 2015). Concluding FO supplementation combined with a strength training program in elderly women did induce a higher improvement in muscle strength and function, as well as in the immune system when compared with strength training alone. This finding in SM was further corroborated by the study of Hutchins-Wiese et al., 2013 which supplied half of the dose (1 g/day FO) used by the Rodackís group (2 g/day FO). Even so, they reported positive and significant interaction between FO supplementation and physical performance. They also measured the DHA/ARA ratio in erythrocytes where the supplemented group had a higher content of DHA which was associated with a better walking speed, meaning reduced frailty. Both doses of FO supplementation caused significant anabolic effects on muscle.

Another study for elderly people was done in a 6-month long, double-blind, randomized control trial (RCT) to evaluate the effect of n–3 PUFA therapy on muscle volume, strength, and average isokinetic power in 60–85 year-old men and women (Smith et al., 2015). In this study, the subjects consumed 1.86 g EPA and 1.50 g DHA/day. The results show that 6 months of n–3 PUFA therapy had significant beneficial effects on thigh muscle volume, hand grip strength, and on one repetition maximum muscle strength of upper-and lower-body and did not significantly increase the isokinetic leg muscle power. Changes in muscle mass and function induced by n–3 PUFA therapy in these subjects were less than those reported for Rodackís group with exercise training, but were the same or greater than those achieved with testosterone, GH or DHEA therapy in older adults and clearly has clinical relevance. The difference in muscle volume between the n–3 PUFA and control groups at 6 months may, in theory (Smith et al., 2015), prevent 2–3 years of normal age-associated losses in muscle mass (0.5–1.0% per year) and function (~2–3% per year). The exact mechanisms by which FO therapy increases muscle mass are not completely known but they likely involve alteration in both anabolic and catabolic pathways. FO-derived n-3 PUFA therapy increases the rate of muscle protein synthesis

(Smith et al., 2010) and studies with n–3 PUFAs in isolated mouse muscles showed attenuated muscle protein breakdown (Whitehouse et al., 2001). Studies conducted in cell cultures and animal models indicated that FO, rich in n–3 PUFA, stimulate SM mitochondrial biosynthesis and function, and also reduce total muscle lipid content. It is possible that FO therapy ameliorates muscle by its well-known protective and motor-neuron excitability properties. Clearly FO therapy provokes important changes in muscle anabolism causing physical performance improvements in older adults. Additional studies must be done in older subjects with clinical impairment of physical function to subsequently determine the magnitude of response of SM compared to healthy ones. All of these data raise important questions to compare younger and older adults such as: What is the best amount of FO supplementation? For how long should someone intake and how quickly do they get in? Are they well retained? Do EPA and DHA have the same pattern? What is the best time of intervention? We must keep in mind that demand for long chain n–3 PUFA may vary between individuals, between tissues within an individual and with stages of the life cycle.

Recently, Huang et al. (2015) found in an older Japanese community (434 people age ≥ 70 years) that high circulating adiponectin concentration may be an indicator of decreased physical performance, specifically muscle strength in older adults. Perhaps this hormone may serve as a new biomarker of muscle strength in an older population.

MOLECULAR EFFECTS OF n–3 PUFA

Several molecular mechanisms for n–3 PUFA have been demonstrated as chemopreventive and chemosuppressive in different diseases, particularly in heart disease, diabetes, immune system disorders, and cancers (Calder and Grimble, 2002), but regarding sarcopenia few studies have addressed that. The mammalian target of rapamycin/ribosomal protein kinase 6 (mTOR-p70s6k) is a signaling pathway known to modify SM mass, particularly under conditions of mechanical stimulation (Drummond et al., 2009). The mTOR-p70s6k pathway activation was first observed by supplying long-chain n–3 PUFA to bovine (Gingras et al., 2007) and the same was observed in humans (Smith et al., 2010).

Supplementation with fish oil provokes higher DHA content in cell membranes which stimulates the protein kinase C pathway leading to enhanced translational activity and muscle protein synthesis (Smith et al., 2010; Rodacki et al., 2012; Van Dyke et al., 2014). Protein/amino acid intake, insulin and physical activity associated with FO supplementation in elderly individuals improve MPS by increasing the mass and function of skeletal muscle (Rondanelli et al., 2015). Other molecular effects of n–3 PUFA are on transcription factor activity, gene expression and signal transduction. Among them cyclooxygenase-2 is over expressed in many pathological conditions; *nuclear transcription factor kB-* is involved in gene expression, cellular adhesion, cell cycle activation, apoptosis, carcinogenesis and inflammation; transcription factors PPAR- are also involved in cell proliferation and differentiation, as well as inflammation; *ras* oncogenes are genes activated in tumors. All of these factors have their expression reduced by the presence of EPA and DHA (Mund et al., 2007; Monk et al., 2011; Da Silva Pedroza et al., 2015). Aging is a chronic inflammatory condition. ARA yields eicosanoids which are proinflammatory and carcinogenic. Thus, the suppression of arachidonic acid-derived eicosanoid biosynthesis is a potential target to ameliorate aging inflammatory conditions. Fish oil supplementation reduced inflammation, angiogenesis and altered immune response (Mund et al., 2007). Free radicals and reactive oxygen species and their metabolites can damage DNA (Mund et al., 2007). Double bond fatty acids are easy to oxidize and several studies have shown that n–3 fatty acids have protective effect against producing free radicals by suppressing inflammation (Calder and Grimble, 2002). Other mechanisms have also been proposed such as the effect on cell membrane fluidity which changes characteristics of membranes. The receptors of excitatory neurotransmitter acetylcholine, as well as from PG and tromboxanes, are on the cell membranes and stimulate the MAPK pathway. The alteration in the fluidity of membranes from the nervous system and SM, caused by the presence of n–3 PUFA, positively affects membrane fusion and neurotransmitter release leading to faster conduction velocity and better impulse transmission, thus enhancing the speed of muscle contraction (Rodacki et al., 2012).

Also insulin sensitivity will be improved by these changes in the membrane fluidity due to receptor response and glucose transporter-4 incorporation. Also a potential target for future investigation should be p53 which is a tumor suppressor protein which plays an important role in cellular stress signals, including DNA damage, apoptosis and cellular senescence (Yang et al., 2015). Growth factors and their receptors are also modulated by n–3 fatty acids (Liu et al., 2015).

N–3 fatty acid supplementation could potentially provide a safe, simple and low-cost intervention to counteract muscle loss and its complications in clinical conditions associated with sarcopenia. Aging is a low-grade inflammatory stage therefore the study of such cytokines and their effects upon n–3 fatty acids effects on aging has a bright future.

References

Baker, W.L., Karan, S., Kenny, A.M., 2011. Effect of dehydroepiandrosterone on muscle strength and physical function in older adults: a systematic review. J. Am. Geriatrics Soc. 59, 997–1002.

Baumgartner, R.N., Koehler, K.M., Gallagher, D., Romero, L., Heymsfield, S.B., Ross, R.R., Garry, P.J., Lindeman, R.D., 1998. Epidemiology of sarcopenia among the elderly in New Mexico. Am. J. Epidemiol. 147, 755–763.

Bougnoux, P., Haijajin, N., Maheo, K., Couet, C., Chevalier, S., 2010. Fatty acid and breast cancer sensitization to treatments and prevention of metastatic growth. Prog. Lipid Res. 49, 76–86.

Calder, P.C., Grimble, R.F., 2002. Polyunsaturated fatty acids, inflammation and immunity. Eur. J. Clin. Nutr. 56 (3), S14–S19.

Calder, P.C., Yaqoob, P., Harvey, D.J., Watt, S.A., Newsholme, E.A., 1994. The incorporation of fatty acids by lymphocytes and the effect on fatty acid composition and membrane fluidity. Biochem. J. 300 (Pt2), 509–518.

ChaleRush, A., Morris, E.P., Kendal, T.L., Brooks Ne, Fielding, R.A., 2009. Effects of chronic overload on muscle hypertrophy and mTOR signaling in young adult and aged rats. J. Gerontol. Ser. A 64A, 1232–1239.

Clarck, B.C., Manini, T.M., 2010. Functional consequences of sarcopenia and dynapenia in the elderly. Curr. Opin. Clin. Nutr. Metabol. Care 13 (3), 271–276.

Da Silva Pedroza, A.A., Lopes, A., Mendes da Silva, R.F., Braz, G.R., Nascimento, L.P., Ferreira, D.S., Dos Santos, A.A., Batista-de-Oliveira-Hornsby, M., Lagranha, C.J., 2015. Can fish oil supplementation and physical training improve oxidative metabolism in ageing rat hearts? Life Sci. 137, 133–141.

Dela, F., Kjaer, M., 2006. Resistance training insulin sensitivity and muscle function in the elderly. Essays Biochem. 42, 75–88.

Drummond, M.J., Dreyer, H.C., Fry, C.S., Glynn, E.L., Rasmussen, B.B., 2009. Nutritional and contractile regulation of human skeletal muscle protein synthesis and mTORC1 signaling. J. Appl. Physiol. 106, 1374–1384.

Etzioni, D.A., Liu, J.H., Maggard, M.A., Ko, C.Y., 2003. The aging population and its impact on the surgery workforce. Annal. Surg. 238 (2), 170–177, 2003.

Giannoulis, M.G., Sonksen, P.H., Umpleby, M., Breen, L., Pentecost, C., Whyte, M., McMillan, C.V., Bradley, C., Martin, F.C., 2006. The effects of growth hormone and/or testosterone in healthy elderly men: a randomized controlled trial. J. Clin. Endocrinol. Metabol. 91, 477–484.

Gingras, A.A., White, R.J., Chouinard, P.Y., Julien, P., Davis, T.A., Dombrowski, L., Couture, Y., Dubreuil, P., Myre, A., Bergeron, K., Marette, A., Thivierge, M.C., 2007. Long chain omega-3 fatty acids regulate bovine whole-body protein metabolism by promoting muscle insulin signaling to the akt-mTOR-s6k1 pathway and insulin sensitivity. J. Physiol. 579 (pt1), 269–284.

Holquin, F., Tellez-Rojo, M.M., Lazo, M., Mannino, D., Schwartz, J., Hernández, M., Romieu, I., 2005. Cardiac autonomic changes associated with fish oil vs soy oil supplementation in the elderly. Chest 127 (4), 1102–1107.

Huang, C., Yomata, Y., Kakizak, M., Sugawara, Y., Hozawa, A., Momma, H., Tsuji, I., Nagatomi, R., 2015. High circulating adiponectin levels predicted decreased muscle strength among older adults aged 70 years and over: a prospective cohor study. Nutr. Metabol. Cardiovascul. Dis. 25 (6), 594–601.

Hutchins-Wiese, H.L., Kleppinger, A., Annis, K., Liva, E., Lammi-Keefe, C.J., Durham, H.A., Kenny, A.M., 2013. The impact of supplemental n-3 long chain polyunsaturated fatty acids and dietary antioxidants on physical performance in postmenopausal women. J. Nutr. Health Aging 17, 76–80.

Hwang, D., 1989. Essential fatty acids and the immune response. FASEB J. 3 (9), 2052–2061.

Jin, E.H., Park, S., So, J.M., 2015. The effect of muscle power training with elastic band on blood glucose, cytokine, and physical function in elderly women with hyperglycemia. J. Exercise Nutr. Biochem. 19 (1), 19–24.

Johnson, E.J., McDonald, K., Caldarella, S.M., Chung, H.Y., Troen, A.M., Snodderly, D.M., 2008. Cognitive findings of an exploratory trial of docosahexaenoic acid and lutein supplementation in older women. Nutr. Neurosci. 11, 75–83.

Kumar, V., Selby, A., Ranki, D., Patel, R., Atherton, P., Hildebrandt, W., Williams, J., Smith, K., Seynnes, O., Hiscock, N., Rennie, M.J., 2009. Age related differences in the dose-response relationship of muscle protein synthesis to resistance exercise in young and old men. J. Physiol. 507 (pt1), 211–217.

Lexell, J., Downham, D., Sjostrom, M., 1986. Distribution of different type of fibre types in human skeletal muscles. Fibre type arrangement in m. vastus lateralis from three groups of healthy men between 15 and 83 years. J. Neurol. Sci. 72, 211–222.

Lexell, J., Taylor, C.C., Sjostrom, M., 1988. What is the cause of the ageing atrophy? J. Neurol. Sci. 84, 275–294.

Liu, Z., Hopkins, M.M., Zhang, Z., Quisenberry, C.B., Fix, L.C., Galvan, B.M., Meier, K.E., 2015. Omega-3 fatty acids and other FFA4 agonists inhibit growth factor signaling in human prostate cancer cells. J. Pharmacol. Exp. Therapeutics 352 (2), 380–394.

Masanes, F., Lulla, A., Navarro-Gonzales, M., Sacanella, E., Lopes-Soto, A., 2012. Prevalence of sarcopenia in healthy community-dwelling elderly in an urban area of Barcelona (Spain). J. Nutr. Health Aging 16 (2), 184–187.

Monk, J.M., Hou, T.Y., Chapkin, R.S., 2011. Recent advances in the field of nutritional immunology: nutritional immunology: role in health and diseases carefree. Expert Rev. Clin. Immunol. 7 (6), 747–749.

Mund, R.C., Pizato, N., Bonatto, S., Nunes, E.A., Vicenzi, T., Tanhoffer, R., de Oliveira, H.H., Curi, R., Calder, P.C., Fernandes, L.C., 2007. Decreased tumor growth in Walker 256 tumor-bearing rats chronically supplemented with fish oil involves COX-2 and PGE2 reduction associated with apoptosis and increased peroxidation. Prostagland. Leukotr. Essen. Fatty Acid. 76 (2), 113–120.

Muscaritoli, M., Anker, S.D., Argilés, J., Aversa, Z., Bauer, J.M., Biolo, G., Boirie, Y., Bosaeus, I., Cederholm, T., Costelli, P., Fearon, K.C., Laviano, A., Maggio, M., Rossi Fanelli, F., Schneider, S.M., Schols, A., Sieber, C.C., 2010. Consensus definition of sarcopenia, cachexia and precachexia. Joint document elaborated by Special Interest Groups (SIG) "cachexia-anorexia in chronic wasting diseases" and "nutrition in geriatrics". Clin. Nutr. 29 (2), 154–159.

Pel-Little, R.E., Schuurmans, M.J., Emmelot-Vonk, M.H., Verhaar, H.J., 2009. Frailty: defining and measuring of a concept. J. Nutr. Health Aging 13 (4), 390–394.

Peterson, M.D., Rhea, M.R., Sen, A., Gordon, P.M., 2010. Resistance exercise for muscular strength in older adults: a meta-analysis. Ageing Res. Rev. 9 (3), 226–237.

Rennie, M.J., 2009. Anabolic resistance: the effects of aging, sexual dimorphism, and immobilization on human muscle protein turnover. Appl. Physiol. Nutr. Metab. 34 (3), 377–381.

Rieux, I., Magne, H., Savary-Auzeloux, I., Averous, J., Bos, C., Peyron, M.A., Combaret, L., Dardevet, D., 2009. Reduction of low grade inflammation restores blunting of postprandial muscle anabolism and limits sarcopenia in old rats. J. Physiol. 587, 5483–5492.

Rodacki, C.L.N., Rodacki, A.L.F., Pereira, G., Naliwaiko, K., Coelho, I., Pequito, D., Fernandes, L.C., 2012. Fish-oil supplementation enhances the effects of strength training in elderly women. Am. J. Clin. Nutr. 95, 428–436.

Rodacki, C.L.N., Rodacki, A.L.F., Coelho, I., Pequito, D., Krause, M., Bonato, S., Naliwaiko, K., Fernandes, L.C., 2015. Influence of fish oil supplementation and strength training on some functional aspects of immune cells in healthy elderly women. Br. J. Nutr. 114 (1), 43–52.

Rondanelli, M., Faliva, M., Monteferrario, F., Peroni, G., Repaci, E., Allieri, F., Perna, S., 2015. Novel insights on nutrient management of sarcopenia in elderly. Biomed. Res. Int. Article ID 524948.

Rosenbert, I., 1989. Summary comments. Am. J. Clin. Nutr. 50, 1231–1233.

Scaglioni, G., Narci, M.V., MaFiuletti, N.A., Pensini, M., Martin, A., 2003. Effects of ageing on the electrical and mechanical properties of human slues motor unit activated by the H reflex and M wave. J. Physiol. 548, 649–661.

Schiesel, D.L., Yamazaki, R.K., Kryczyk, M., Coelho, I., Yamaguchi, A.A., Pequito, D.C., Brito, G.A., Borghetti, G., Fernandes, L.C., 2015. A-Linolenic fatty acid supplementation decreases tumor growth and cachexia parameters in Walker 256 tumor-bearing rats. Nutr. Cancer 67 (5), 839–846.

Smith, G.I., Atherton, P., Reeds, D.N., Mohammed, B.S., Rankin, D., Rennie, M.J., Mittendorfer, B., 2010. Dietary omega-3 fatty acid supplementation increases the rate of muscle protein synthesis in older adults: a randomized controlled trial. Am. J. Clin. Nutr. 93, 402–412.

Smith, G.I., Atherton, P., Reed, D.N., Mohammed, B.S., Rankin, D., Rennie, M.J., Mittendorfer, B., 2011. Omega-3 polyunsaturated fatty acids augment the muscle protein anabolic response to hyperinsulinemia-hyperaminoacidemia in healthy young and middle-aged men and women. Clin. Sci. (London) 121, 267–278.

Smith, G.I., Julliand, S., Reeds, D.N., Sinacore, D.R., Klein, S., Mittendorfer, B., 2015. Fish oil-derived n-3 PUFA therapy increases muscle mass and function in healthy older adults. Am. J. Clin. Nutr. 102 (1), 115–122.

Strasser, B., Kenrad, M., Haber, P., Schobersberger, W., 2009. Efficacy of systematic endurance and resistance training on muscle strength and endurance performance in elderly adults – a randomized controlled trial. Wiener Klinische Wochenschrift 121, 757–764.

Supari, F., Ungerer, T., Harrison, D.G., Williams, J.K., 1995. Fish oil treatment decreased superoxide anions in the myocardium and coronary arteries of atheroschlerotic monkeys. Circulation 91, 1102–1007.

Van Dyke, J.M., Bain, J.L., Riley, D.A., 2014. Stretch activated signaling is modulated by stretch magnitude and contraction. Muscle Nerve 49, 98–107.

Whitehouse, A.S., Smith, H.J., Drake, J.L., Tisdale, M.J., 2001. Mechanisms of attenuation of skeletal muscle protein catabolism in cancer cachexia by eicosapentaenoic acid. Cancer Res. 16, 3604–3609.

Yan, Y., Jiang, W., Spinetti, T., Tardivel, A., Castillo, R., Bourquin, C., Guarda, G., Tian, Z., Tschopp, J., Zhou, R., 2013. Omega-3 fatty acids prevent inflammation and metabolic disorder through inhibition of NLRP3 inflammasome activation. Immunity 38 (6), 1154–1163.

Yang, K., Li, H., Dong, J., Dong, Y., Wang, C.Z., 2015. Expression profile of polyunsaturated fatty acid in colorectal cancer. World J. Gastroenterol. 21 (8), 2405–2412.

Yeshuda, S., Rabinovitz, S., Mostofsky, D.I., 1999. Essential fatty acids are mediators of brain biochemistry and cognitive functions. J. Neurosci. Res. 56, 565–570.

Yu, F., Hedstrom, M., Cristea, A., Dalen, N., Larsson, L., 2007. Effects of ageing and gender on contractile properties in human skeletal muscle and singlefires. Acta Physiol. (Oxford) 190, 229–241.

Zérouga, M., Beauge, F., Niel, E., Durand, G., Bourre, J.M., 1991. Interactive effects of dietary (n-3) polyunsaturated fatty acids and chronic ethanol intoxication on synaptic membrane lipid composition and fluidity in rats. Biochimica et. Biophysica Acta (BBA) Lipids and Lipids Metabolism 1086 (3), 295–304.

CHAPTER

12

Fish and Fish Oil for the Aging Brain

C.M. Butt*, N. Salem Jr.**

*HNH-Biological Models, DSM Nutritional Products, Boulder, Colorado, United States;
**Nutritional Lipids, DSM Nutritional Products, Columbia, Maryland, United States

INTRODUCTION

Adverse environmental and other external factors are believed to be involved in the breakdown of repair processes that lead to the aging and degradation of the brain (Krstic et al., 2013). In addition, aging of the brain is associated with processes very similar to those exhibited by Alzheimer's disease (AD), although aging occurs at a much slower rate. As such, the "Alzheimerization," or aging of the brain, is essentially a steady disconnection of progressively lower brain centers that results in the loss of cognitive function and eventually more basic functions (Bartzokis, 2011). Fortunately, at least one of the environmental factors over which individuals have some control is their diet (Vahid et al., 2015). Dietary factors likely have nutrigenomic effects on brain signaling and function, which could be keys to combating impaired brain energy metabolism (Gomez-Pinilla and Tyagi, 2013) as well as chronic neuroinflammation and its neurodegenerative sequelae (Krstic et al., 2013; Mohajeri et al., 2015). Fish contain several components that have the potential to slow the aging of the brain.

Fish oil is a complex mixture of nutrients and lipids that is derived from fish flesh or fish livers. The composition of fish oil varies widely between fish species, fish diets, and the season in which the fish were caught. Despite these variations, fish and fish oil are generally considered part of a healthy diet and primary sources of the omega-3 long-chain polyunsaturated fatty acids (LC-PUFA) of docosahexaenoic acid (DHA; 22:6n-3) and eicosapentaenoic acid (EPA; 20:5n-3) and of vitamins A, D, and E (Moffat and McGill, 1993). A recent analysis of ten different fish oils indicates that its LC-PUFA concentrations can range between ~35–645 mg of DHA and ~40–510 mg of EPA per gram of oil (Yi et al., 2014). Vitamin A ranges between 10 and 50,000 μg retinol equivalents per g oil depending on the fish species from which it was harvested. Vitamin D contents of many fish oils are <0.05 μg/g oil, but cod liver oils can have up to 2.5 μg/g oil [United States Department of Agriculture (USDA), 2015]. Vitamin E concentrations have been measured between 10–750 μg/g oil (Moffat and McGill, 1993). However, vitamin E has antioxidant properties that fish oil manufacturers often take advantage of and thus they add it to their oils during processing to obtain enhanced preservation.

Given the wide content ranges described above, regulatory bodies such as the Food and Drug Administration (FDA), the European Food Safety Administration (EFSA), as well as many advisory committees (eg, Institute of Medicine, National Academies of the United States, Food and Nutrition Board) have provided guidance on the recommended daily intakes for the nutrients in fish oil. Nonetheless, most populations do not have adequate intake of most vitamins (Troesch et al., 2012), DHA or EPA (Salem and Eggersdorfer, 2015). Appropriate use of fish oil or its equivalents may assuage these circumstances.

The purpose of this chapter is to align the functional data that are available for the chief components of fish oil (DHA, EPA, and vitamins A, D and E) with their dietary intake data. Deficits in the appropriate intake of these nutrients likely play into subclinical effects on brain function that eventually contribute to age-related dementia or Alzheimer's disease (Mohajeri et al., 2015). Each fish oil component will be addressed individually with regards to its general function in the brain and how its mechanisms could mitigate the effects of aging on the brain. Potential interactions between the nutrients will also be considered, and a recommendation as to how much fish oil an individual would require to offset perceived dietary deficiencies will be proposed in the chapter's concluding remarks.

Fish and Fish Oil in Health and Disease Prevention. http://dx.doi.org/10.1016/B978-0-12-802844-5.00012-9

VITAMIN A

Vitamin A cannot be synthesized de novo, making it an essential nutrient for vision, growth and development, fertility, healthy epithelia, and appropriate immune function. It is known chemically as retinol, but it is most commonly ingested as retinyl palmitate esters from animal food products or as its precursor, β-carotene, from vegetables. The recommended daily intake and upper limits of vitamin A intake are detailed in Table 12.1.

Vitamin A deficiency is less common in the adult populations of Westernized societies because it can be sourced not only from fish, but also from eggs, butter, milk, and cheese, as well as β-carotene from vegetables such as carrots, spinach, and broccoli (Ross and Harrison, 2007). Despite this array of vitamin A sources, deficiency still occurs in a significant portion of Western adults (Troesch et al., 2012), and it can present as problems with eyesight, epithelial lesions and impaired immune function due to a decrease in the metabolites of vitamin A, 11-cis-retinal and all-trans-retinoic acid (ATRA). The general functions of these two metabolites have been reviewed in detail elsewhere as they have been studied since the early 1900's (Ross and Harrison, 2007).

Aging is associated with a reduction in retinol metabolism and a concomitant decrease of ATRA levels in the rodent brain (Touyarot et al., 2013). Similarly, better cognitive function in elderly humans has been correlated with better carotenoid status in the blood and brain (Johnson et al., 2013). Approximately 50–75% of American adults do not consume enough vitamin A equivalents in comparison to the recommendations (700 μg/day for women; 900 μg/day for men; Table 12.1). Similarly, the average vitamin A intakes for British women are 612 μg/day and 809 μg/day for men, while the median intakes are 521 μg/day for women and 604 μg/day for men (Troesch et al., 2012).

TABLE 12.1 Recommended Intakes of Vitamin A (retinol equivalents/day) Versus its Delivery by Fish Oils and Fish

Age range	EAR[a]		RDA/AI[b]		UL[c]	
31–50 years	μg	IU[d]	μg	IU	μg	IU
Males	625	2,100	900	3,000	3,000	10,000
Females	500	1,700	700	2,300	3,000	10,000
50–70 years						
Males	625	2,100	900	3,000	3,000	10,000
Females	500	1,700	700	2,300	3,000	10,000
>70 years						
Males	625	2,100	900	3,000	3,000	10,000
Females	500	1,700	700	2,300	3,000	10,000

Fish oil (1 g)[e]			
Cod Liver		**Others[f]**	
μg	IU	μg	IU
300	1000	0	0

Cooked fish (70g ≈ 2.5 oz.)[d]			
Anchovy		**Cod**	
μg	IU	μg	IU
8	28	10	33
Salmon		**Tuna (Bluefin)**	
μg	IU	μg	IU
104	347	530	1764

[a]*Estimated Average Requirements for 50% of the United States population, Institute of Medicine, 2001.*
[b]*Recommended Daily Allowance/Adequate Intake for 97.5% of the United States population, Institute of Medicine, 2001.*
[c]*Tolerable Upper intake Levels in United States, Institute of Medicine, 2001.*
[d]*International Units.*
[e]*United States Department of Agriculture (USDA) National Nutrient Database for Standard Reference Release 27.*
[f]*Averages of herring, menhaden, salmon, and sardine oils.*

The vitamin A intakes of the elderly are likely lower due to age-related declines in appetite, overall food intake (Mohajeri et al., 2015), and possibly reduced carotenoid processing (Touyarot et al., 2013). One study in the United States indicated that approximately 10% of the elderly population involved did not reach adequate intakes of vitamin A (Wardwell et al., 2008). Reducing this 100–300 μg/day intake gap is important because vitamin A replenishment can reverse the cognitive and biochemical repercussions of vitamin A deficiency (Misner et al., 2001; Ono and Yamada, 2012; Sodhi and Singh, 2014; Touyarot et al., 2013).

Consumption of fish or fish oil could mitigate the gaps in vitamin A intake. As Table 12.1 illustrates, cod liver oil has a high amount of vitamin A in comparison to other fish oils. One gram of cod liver oil per day would bridge the largest average gap of ~300 μg/day without exceeding the 3000-μg upper limit of intake. According to the USDA, other fish oils carry virtually no vitamin A, but it should also be noted that fish oil processing removes significant amounts of vitamin A in comparison to crude fish oil (USDA, 2015). For example, crude Menhaden oil has approximately 6 μg vitamin A per gram of oil, but refined, bleached, deodorized and stabilized Menhaden oil has only ~1 μg/g oil (Scott and Latshaw, 1991). It is not clear whether the fish oil compositions published by the USDA are specific to crude oils or processed oils. However, crude fish oil generally lacks palatability in terms of taste and smell. Thus, it could be presumed that most fish oils are processed, and these are the basis of the USDA data.

Cooked Bluefin tuna may be a better source in terms of typical daily dose or serving (1 g oil or 70 g fish; USDA, 2015). One serving of cooked Bluefin tuna (530 μg vitamin A) or three servings of cooked salmon (~100 μg vitamin A each) would bridge the largest average vitamin A deficiency in the United States, while only one serving of cooked salmon per day would cover the smallest average disparity. Another possibility is eating raw vegetables as sources of β-carotene. One 10-oz. (284 g) package of spinach contains over 1300 μg of retinol equivalents, while 1 cup (~100 g) of carrots carries 835 μg of retinol equivalents (USDA, 2015). Clearly, a balanced diet that includes fish or fish oil, as well as vegetables, will maintain appropriate vitamin A levels, but the role of vitamin A in the aging adult nervous system is just emerging.

The lipophilic properties of retinol make it bioavailable to nearly all tissues of the body, but retinol must be converted to ATRA for use by the brain. In rodents, the brain astrocytes (Wang et al., 2011) or meningeal epithelial cells are responsible for absorbing retinol from the bloodstream and performing its conversion to ATRA. In contrast, human neurons, particularly in the hippocampus, express all of the retinaldehyde dehydrogenases necessary for ATRA production (Fragoso et al., 2012). The ATRA then acts through the retinoid-X- and retinoid-A-receptor systems (RXR and RAR, respectively) as homodimer or heterodimer transcription factors that can modulate the migration of neuronal stem cells (Chen et al., 2007), the differentiation of those stem cells (Környei et al., 2007), circadian rhythms and sleep (Ransom et al., 2014). The RXR can also heterodimerize with peroxisome proliferator-activated receptors (PPAR) or liver X receptors (LXR), lending support to estimates that 15% of the protein-coding genes in humans are affected by retinoid signaling (Olson and Mello, 2010). Interestingly, expression of all of these nuclear receptors are upregulated in some fashion as part of antiinflammatory and neurotrophic processes in models of demyelination, spinal cord injury, multiple sclerosis, ischemia (König et al., 2012) and AD (Ono and Yamada, 2012). Nuclear receptors also have affinity for DHA, EPA, and vitamin D, making interactions of vitamin A with these other nutrients possible.

The topic of receptor interaction is connected to the other side of vitamin A status that has not yet been discussed: the risk of toxicity associated with hypervitaminosis A. Vitamin A toxicity can result acutely in headache, liver swelling, and gastrointestinal stress, and manifest itself chronically as mood disorders or cognitive dysfunction (de Oliveira, 2015; Myhre et al., 2003; O'Reilly et al., 2008). The mechanisms by which these symptoms occur are not clear, but they involve overwhelming the normal metabolism of vitamin A, over-activation of vitamin A signaling pathways, and possibly increased oxidative stress in mitochondria (de Oliveira, 2015; Zhong et al., 2012). Despite these potential problems, vitamin A is used therapeutically at large doses for low birth weight, acne and leukemia (eg, 150,000–300,000 IU/day for leukemia; de Oliveira, 2015). The risk of toxicity is only associated with preformed retinol and its derivatives. There are no reports of vitamin A toxicity due to high intake of β-carotene because of its lower degree of absorption. Furthermore, the third National Health and Nutrition Examination Survey in the United States indicated that some women, and approximately 75% of children, taking vitamin A supplements regularly exceed the upper limit of vitamin A intake without any adverse effects. Indeed, the no adverse effect level in women of reproductive age has been estimated at 4,500 μg of retinol equivalents per day, and the lowest intake known to cause adverse effects in children aged 1–3 years is 6,000 μg of retinol equivalents per day (Allen and Haskell, 2002). Thus, although the higher levels of vitamin A present in cod liver oil (Table 12.1) are available as retinol, it is unlikely that intake of fish or fish oil will result in toxicity. Nonetheless, caution should be exercised, particularly if an individual is already taking vitamin A supplements.

VITAMIN D

Unlike vitamin A, the active form of vitamin D, vitamin D_3 (1_α,25-dihydroxyvitamin D_3; calcitriol), can be synthesized de novo in the skin from its cholesterol-based precursors, along with the assistance of ultraviolet light from the sun. Thus, given the downstream functions of calcitriol, vitamin D is technically a hormone precursor, not a vitamin. Nonetheless, vitamin D is important for the metabolism of calcium and phosphorus and accordingly essential for normal bone development and maintenance. Vitamin D also has a known role in stimulating the proliferation and activity of peripheral immune cells, and its actions in the brain are also being established. It is most commonly ingested as vitamin D_3 from egg yolks and oily fish, but plant products, such as mushrooms, can serve as a source of its vitamin D_2 (ergocalciferol) precursor. Milk and butter are typically also thought of as appreciable sources of vitamin D, but they require fortification to be so (Norman and Henry, 2007). The recommended daily intake and upper limits of Vitamin D intake are detailed in Table 12.2.

As with vitamin A, deficiency of vitamin D occurs in a significant portion of Westernized populations (Troesch et al., 2012), and it affects more than 1 billion people worldwide (Annweiler et al., 2013b). The prevalence of this deficiency is primarily due to people residing in northern latitudes that have significantly reduced access to the sun in comparison to more southern latitudes (Fernandes de Abreu et al., 2009). Vitamin D deficiency in adults can commonly exhibit itself as osteoporosis and osteomalacia (Norman and Henry, 2007). However, the associations of vitamin D deficiency with mood and seasonal affective disorder (Barnard and Colón-Emeric, 2010; Kerr et al., 2015; Gloth et al., 1999), as well as the presence of functional vitamin D receptors and 1_α-hydroxylase in the brain, argue that vitamin D has extra-skeletal effects on brain function and that the brain can locally synthesize calcitriol from 25-hydroxyvitamin D_3, the status of which varies with diet (Eyles et al., 2005),

Deficiency in vitamin D is associated with increasing age, decreased vitamin D intake, reduced time spent outdoors, poor skin integrity and cognitive decline (Meehan and Penckofer, 2014; Mohajeri et al., 2015). Furthermore,

TABLE 12.2 Recommended Intakes of Vitamin D (cholecalciferol equivalents/day) Versus its Delivery by Fish Oils and Fish

Age range	EAR[a]		RDA/AI		UL	
31–50 years	μg	IU	μg	IU	μg	IU
Males	10	400	15	600	100	4000
Females	10	400	15	600	100	4000
50–70 years						
Males	10	400	15	600	100	4000
Females	10	400	15	600	100	4000
>70 years						
Males	10	400	20	800	100	4000
Females	10	400	20	800	100	4000

Fish oil (1 g)			
Cod Liver		**Others**	
μg	IU	μg	IU
2.5	100	0.02	0.83
Cooked fish (70g ≈ 2.5 oz.)			
Anchovy		**Cod**	
μg	IU	μg	IU
1.2	48	0.8	32
Salmon		**Tuna (Bluefin)**	
μg	IU	μg	IU
0	0	0	0

[a]*All abbreviations are the same as those in Table 12.1.*
Source for recommended intakes is Institute of Medicine, 2011.

blood plasma levels of 25-hydroxyvitamin D_3 <20 nmol/L have been correlated with reduced processing speeds and attention as well as increased risks of cognitive decline, dementia, AD, and depression (Annweiler et al., 2013b; Meehan and Penckofer, 2014). Such findings are compelling in light of the fact that more than 75% of American and British adults do not consume adequate amounts of vitamin D. In Britain, the average vitamin D intakes for men are 3.5 μg/day and 2.6 μg/day for women, while the median intakes are 3.1 μg/day for men and 2.1 μg/day for women (Troesch et al., 2012). Similar to vitamin A, vitamin D intakes of the elderly are likely lower due to age-related declines in appetite and overall food intake (Mohajeri et al., 2015), but vitamin D is impacted further by the less time spent outdoors by older individuals (Meehan and Penckofer, 2014). This suggestion is supported by data from an elderly American population in that only 4% of the individuals studied had adequate intakes of vitamin D from the diet alone, while 69% achieved adequate vitamin D intake when taking supplements (Wardwell et al., 2008). Overall, these findings suggest an intake gap of 13–18 μg/day that, if addressed appropriately, could potentially increase the quality of life for aging individuals and possibly protect them from mood disorders and neurodegeneration.

Some fish and some fish oils contain vitamin D, but it is not clear whether their consumption would completely bridge the intake gap. Earlier versions of the USDA Nutrient Database reported higher levels of vitamin D in cooked fish and cod liver oil, such that a typical serving size would deliver ≥90% of the adult RDA for vitamin D at the time (10 μg/day; Norman and Henry, 2007). The current version of the USDA Nutrient Database indicates that the vitamin D contents of fish and fish oil have decreased, while the daily requirements for intake have increased (Table 12.2). At present, ~4–7 g of the average cod liver oil per day would be necessary to completely cover the largest average gap of ~18 μg/day. Other fish-related sources of vitamin D would require larger consumption amounts. In addition, fish oil processing removes approximately 80% of the vitamin D in crude fish oil. Crude Menhaden oil has 27 μg vitamin D per gram of oil on average, but only 5 μg/g oil remains after refining, bleaching, deodorizing, and stabilization (Scott and Latshaw, 1991). Despite these findings, consumption of cod liver oil to any extent would significantly reduce an individual's degree of vitamin D deficiency, but care must be taken in avoiding overconsumption of vitamin A.

The classical functions and metabolism of vitamin D have been established and reviewed elsewhere (Norman and Henry, 2007), while less is known about its role in the adult and aging brain. The most prevalent form carried in the blood is 25-hydroxyvitamin D_3, and blood levels of this form vary with diet, while those of calcitriol are tightly controlled. Interestingly, upon arrival in the brain, the presence 1_α-hydroxylase likely allows for local conversion to calcitriol, which can then be bound by two different types of vitamin D receptors (Eyles et al., 2005). Nongenomic actions of increase calcium influx and activation of second-messenger cascades are mediated by the membrane-associated rapid–response steroid (MARRS) receptor, while the vitamin D receptor (VDR) initiates heterodimerization with the RXR nuclear receptor family (the same used by ATRA) and subsequent actions as a transcription factor. The VDR is expressed throughout the brain by all cell types, and it is involved in upregulating the expression of choline acetyltransferase (ChAT), tyrosine hydroxylase (TH), nerve growth factor (NGF), neurotrophin-3 (NT-3), glial-derived neurotrophic factor (GDNF), the p75 neurotrophin receptor, transforming growth factor-β (TGF-β), and calbindin. In contrast, vitamin D downregulates inducible nitric oxide synthase (iNOS) and L-type calcium channel activity (Fernandes de Abreu et al., 2009).

The gene regulating activities of vitamin D are very important during neurodevelopment, and the available data are replete with problems linked to vitamin D deficiency during this critical period (eg, monoamine neurotransmitter disturbances, mitochondrial dysfunction, enlarged brain ventricles, reduced adult hippocampal neurogenesis, schizophrenia, and reduced cognitive performance). By some accounts, the most consistent preclinical effects that vitamin D has on adult brain function, notwithstanding juvenile deficiencies, is that of increasing ChAT or TH, and, by extension, the synthesis of acetylcholine and catecholamine neurotransmitters, under pathological conditions (Eyles et al., 2013). These findings provide support to the clinical effects of vitamin D that have been described for mood (Annweiler et al., 2013b). They have also given promise towards vitamin D-related therapies directed at Parkinson's disease and AD because of the associations of low vitamin D levels exhibited by individuals affected by these diseases. However, many interventional studies of vitamin D for AD, cognition and depression have failed, suggesting that adverse effects induced by developmental deficiency may be irreversible (Elyes et al., 2013).

Studies assessing the effects of vitamin D on neuroanatomical measures of myelin maintenance or immune function in adult tissues have experienced more recent success. Reduced vitamin D status has been implicated in multiple sclerosis (Yadav et al., 2015), all-cause dementia, AD, stroke, white matter abnormalities associated with cerebrovascular disease in the elderly (Buell et al., 2010), reduced cognitive performance and white matter volume in aging humans (Hooshmand et al., 2014), reduced volume of the optic chiasm (Annweiler et al., 2013a), and thinning of the adult cerebral cortex (Walhovd et al., 2014). The data are mixed as to whether vitamin D supplementation can decrease the impacts of multiple sclerosis, but it appears that vitamin D intervention during adolescence may inhibit the activation of peripheral helper T cells by interferon-γ (IFNγ; Adzemovic et al., 2013; Fernandes de Abreu et al., 2009; Grishkan et al., 2013).

VITAMIN E

Vitamin E can only be made by plants, so its presence in humans, fish and other animals is entirely dependent on their respective diets. It is a biological antioxidant that protects genomic material, lipids, and proteins from oxidation, and it is a collective term that includes 4 isoforms of tocopherol (α, β, γ, δ), 4 isoforms of tocotrienols (α, β, γ, δ) and all of their respective isomers (Brigelius-Flohe and Traber, 1999). The α-tocopherol form is the most abundant (Burton et al., 1983), but interactions between its activity and bioavailability with those of the other isoforms can occur (*e.g.* δ-tocopherol; Jiang et al., 2001). The complexity of vitamin E is increased further by the knowledge that RRR-α-tocopherol is most the effective isomer of α-tocopherol (Traber, 2007), but that a mix of the isoforms (tocopherols and tocotrienols) may confer the largest benefit (Brigelius-Flohe et al., 2002; Mangialasche et al., 2010; Wu and Meydani, 2008). Despite these known complexities, the recommended daily intake and upper limits of collective vitamin E intake have been studied to a large extent and are detailed in Table 12.3.

Vitamin E deficiency is difficult to detect in healthy individuals because adipose tissue is the chief storage site, and it does not reflect dietary changes in vitamin E intake for up to 2 years. Young children, individuals with inefficient fat absorption (eg, in cystic fibrosis), or people carrying mutations in the α-tocopherol transport protein are the most susceptible to the symptoms of vitamin E deficiency. These symptoms can include hemolysis, weakened connective and muscle tissues, or cerebellar ataxia. The muscle weakness and ataxia are due to the loss of myelinated sensory nerve axons in the peripheral and central nervous systems (Traber, 2007). Although gross deficiencies in vitamin E are not apparent in the general populace, significant differences exist between recommended intakes and actual intakes.

As with vitamin D, more than 75% of American adults do not consume enough Vitamin E. British citizens are similar in that they only consume 8.0–10.5 mg of vitamin E per day on average (Troesch et al., 2012). In a study of elderly Americans, only 13% of the people involved consumed adequate amounts of vitamin E from their diets alone, but supplementation

TABLE 12.3 Recommended Intakes of Vitamin E (RRR-α-Tocopherol equivalents/day) Versus its Delivery by Fish Oils and Fish

Age range	EAR[a]		RDA/AI		UL	
31–50 years	mg	IU	mg	IU	mg	IU
Males	12	18	15	23	1000	1500
Females	12	18	15	23	1000	1500
50-70 years						
Males	12	18	15	23	1000	1500
Females	12	18	15	23	1000	1500
>70 years						
Males	12	18	15	23	1000	1500
Females	12	18	15	23	1000	1500

Fish oil (1 g)			
Cod liver		**Others**	
mg	IU	mg	IU
0	0	0	0
Cooked fish (70 g ≈ 2.5 oz.)			
Anchovy		**Cod**	
mg	IU	mg	IU
2.3	3.5	0.6	0.9
Salmon		**Tuna (Bluefin)**	
mg	IU	mg	IU
0	0	0	0

[a]*All abbreviations are the same as those in Table 12.1.*
Source for recommended intakes is Institute of Medicine, 2000.

allowed for 74% of the population studied to achieve adequate intake (Wardwell et al., 2008). Such intake levels and intake rates, combined with the increased risks of nervous system damage and the reduced overall food intake, make the elderly particularly vulnerable to the problems related to vitamin E insufficiency. Indeed, low plasma levels of vitamin E are associated with increased risk for AD and mild cognitive impairment (La Fata et al., 2014; Mohajeri et al., 2015).

Consumption of some types of fish or fish oil may alleviate the differences between vitamin E intakes versus the recommendations. As Table 12.3 shows, cooked cod and anchovies can be a source of vitamin E in the diet, but other commonly consumed fish products contain virtually no vitamin E. As with vitamins A and D, fish oil processing removes a large amount of the vitamin E that is normally found in crude fish oil. The vitamin E content in crude Menhaden oil is ~117 μg/g oil, but refined, bleached, deodorized and stabilized Menhaden oil has only ~63 μg/g oil (Scott and Latshaw, 1991). Sardine oil has even less: 25.3 μg/g in the crude oil versus 14.3 μg/g in the refined (Irianto, 1994). Such microgram quantities are far from the 15-mg requirements, but some fish- or algae-based oil concentrates contain 400–3000 ppm of mixed tocopherols for stabilization purposes. However, only ~18% of these tocopherols are RRR-α-tocopherol (~72–540 μg/g oil; DSM Nutritional Products product factsheets), making these oils sources of vitamin E, but they certainly do not meet the definitions of good or excellent sources of the vitamin.

Higher vitamin E status in the plasma has been associated with reduced cognitive decline (Mangialasche et al., 2012; Morris et al., 2002a; Ravaglia et al., 2008), reduced risk for AD (Corrada et al., 2005; Morris et al., 2002b), and increased life expectancy (Hemila and Kaprio, 2011; Xu et al., 2009). These effects have largely been attributed to the antioxidative effects of vitamin E, which can include the protection of LC-PUFAs, such as DHA (Mohajeri et al., 2015). Normal cellular function results in the production of reactive oxygen species (ROS) that need to be sequestered. These ions can be handled by superoxide dismutase, glutathione peroxidase, and catalase, but vitamin E also assists by being one of the most effective lipid-soluble antioxidants in biological membranes (Meydani, 1995; Niki and Traber, 2012; Mocchegiani et al., 2014). The high PUFA contents of brain cells and immune cells make their membranes susceptible to oxidation that can alter their function significantly (Mocchegiani et al., 2014). For example, the age-related decline in T-cell function can be reduced by vitamin E blocking the propagation of ROS across LC-PUFAs or their associated membrane proteins (Molano and Meydani, 2012). In the brain, vitamin E protects against injury and neurodegeneration by inhibiting lipid peroxidation in three ways: classical absorption of ROS, inhibition of peroxidative enzymes such as 12-lipoxygenase, and inhibition of the pro-inflammatory cascades such as those involving NF-κB (Frank et al., 2012).

Vitamin E also protects the myelin membranes of oligodendrocytes. Peroxide insults to oligodendrocytes *in vitro* result in a loss of MBP expression that is inhibited by vitamin E analogs (Perfeito et al., 2007). Similarly, in vitro oxysterol stress induces cell death, mitochondrial dysfunction and apoptosis in oligodendrocytes that can all be reduced by vitamin E, and these protective functions involve protein kinase B (also known as AkT), glycogen synthase kinase-3β (GSK3β) and caspase-3 (Ragot et al., 2011; Vejux et al., 2009). In vivo studies suggest that vitamin E and vitamin E analogues protect myelin and oligodendrocytes in models of multiple sclerosis by reducing demyelination (Blanchard et al., 2013; Goudarzvand et al., 2010) and microglial activation (Blanchard et al., 2013), most likely through the mechanisms described above in vitro. Interestingly, low levels of vitamin E are found in multiple sclerosis patients in comparison to matched controls, but interventional clinical trials have not been undertaken to date (Torkildsen et al., 2013).

DOCOSAHEXAENOIC ACID (DHA) AND EICOSAPENTAENOIC ACID (EPA)

Like some other nutrients (eg, lycopene and vitamin A from β-carotene), DHA and EPA can be synthesized de novo from a common precursor. In the cases of DHA and EPA, α-linolenic acid (ALA; 18:3n-3) is the precursor. The precursor conversion rate for DHA synthesis in humans is generally considered as low (≤0.1%; Lin et al., 2010; Pawlosky and Salem, 2004; Plourde and Cunnane, 2007), but some studies suggest that it can be as high as 3.8% (Emken et al., 1994). Thus, ingestion of the preformed LC-PUFAs is the recommended manner for delivery to the body and brain (Brenna et al., 2009). Optimal development of the brain requires DHA (Innis, 2008; McNamara and Carlson, 2006), and it is the most important omega-3 PUFA in the CNS from a quantitative perspective (Dyall, 2015). Both DHA and EPA enter the brain at the same rate, but brain EPA levels are held at ~250-fold lower levels than those of DHA due to β-oxidation and reduced accretion into membranes (Chen and Subbaiah, 2013; Ouellet et al., 2009). Along these lines, dietary ingestion of EPA, which can be converted to DHA, changes only EPA levels in the blood (Arterburn et al., 2006; Brenna et al., 2009). Individual roles for DHA and EPA in the adult or aging brain have not been completely elucidated, but data that differentiate the two are beginning to emerge (Dyall, 2015). DHA seems to be necessary for maintaining the optimal function of membrane-bound receptors/enzymes (Mitchell et al., 2012; Niu et al., 2004; Polozova and Litman, 2000; Salem et al., 2001) and to serve as a differentiation factor in adult neurogenesis, while EPA, EPA metabolites and DHA metabolites likely have neuroprotective and anti-inflammatory roles in the brain and peripheral vasculature (Bazan, 2013).

Adult humans most commonly ingest DHA and EPA through fish, fish oils, or supplements based on marine algae. Fish oil contains DHA and EPA because the fish ingest the marine algae (Salem and Eggersdorfer, 2015). The DHA and EPA contents of fish and fish oil are dependent on the fish diets, and seasonal variations in these contents are common (Bandarra et al., 1997; Bell et al., 1985; Shirai et al., 2002a,b). In addition, dietary linoleic acid (LA; 18:2n-6) prevents formation of EPA and DHA and their accumulation by competitive inhibition of the desaturase system required for ALA conversion (Emken et al., 1994; Mohrhauer and Holman, 1963). Thus, the shifts in Western diets to low ALA consumption (~1.5 g/day) and high ingestion of LA (~15 g/day), taken together with their low average fish intake, have led to the relatively low omega-3 status in Westerners (Blasbalg et al., 2011). Dietary recommendations for adults are not established in the US for DHA and EPA. However, EFSA and several other expert recommendations suggest that 250–500 mg of DHA + EPA should be consumed per day (EFSA, 2012; Gebauer et al., 2006).

Increased omega-3 status is linked to reduced risk of cognitive disorders in adulthood (Mohajeri and Winwod, 2012), reduced development of dementia or AD (Muldoon et al., 2010; Wurtman et al., 2010), and maintenance of cognitive performance with age (Yurko-Mauro et al., 2010). However, only DHA status, not EPA status or ALA status, has been linked specifically to better cognitive skills in adults (reviewed by Mohajeri et al., 2015). Similarly, a larger omega-3 index in red blood cells has been associated with larger volumes of the brain's hippocampal region that is important for memory formation (Pottala et al., 2014), but only blood DHA levels have been significantly correlated with total brain volume (Tan et al., 2012). Given these findings, it is concerning that the intakes of DHA and EPA are so low in Westernized societies. Adult American males consume an average of only 40 mg of EPA per day and 80 mg of DHA per day. American women have average intakes of 30 mg EPA and 60 mg DHA per day (USDA, 2012). A study in elderly Americans indicated that only 6% of the people studied had adequate intake of DHA + EPA from their diets, and only 13% of the study participants taking supplements had adequate intake of DHA and EPA (Wardwell et al., 2008). Similarly, a study of elderly Canadians showed that their daily intake of DHA + EPA was only 70 mg (Fratesi et al., 2009). In Germany, adult women ingest approximately 125 mg/day of DHA + EPA (Bauch et al., 2006), and Dutch men get an average of 140 mg/day of DHA + EPA (Kuratko and Salem, 2013; Schuurman et al., 1999). These findings indicate an intake gap for DHA + EPA on the order of 360–410 mg/day. Since fish and fish oils typically contain DHA and EPA (Table 12.4), it is clear that regular consumption of them would bridge the intake gap for these two nutrients and likely reduce the risks of age-related brain problems. For example, consumption of 0.5–3 servings of unfried fish per week has been associated with decreased risk of stroke (Bouzan et al., 2005; He et al., 2002; Larsson and Orsini, 2011; Virtanen et al., 2008; Wang et al., 2006).

Preclinical models of injury to the peripheral nerves (Gladman et al., 2012), spinal cord (Hall et al., 2012; Paterniti et al., 2014) and brain (Mills et al., 2011; Wu et al., 2014), as well as in models of stroke (Belayev et al., 2011) and AD (Calon, 2011; Green et al., 2007) provide converging evidence that DHA, EPA, or their metabolites protect the adult nervous system and its myelin (reviewed by Michael-Titus and Priestley, 2014). For example, recent reports suggest that some neuroprotective effects of DHA may involve its specialized proresolving mediator (SPM) derivatives (Buckley et al., 2014), such as protectins (Bazan et al., 2012), lipoxins (Luo et al., 2013), and resolvins. The DHA-derived resolvin D1, but not the EPA-derived resolvin E1, significantly preserved motor and cognitive function in a mouse model of traumatic brain injury (Harrison et al., 2015). Similarly, the DHA-derived neuroprotectin D1 improved performance in a neurological test after the induction of stroke in rats (Bazan et al., 2012). These findings provide support to the concept that sufficient DHA and EPA consumption may provide prophylactic benefits to the aging brain by acting on elements that are shared by aging and these damaging ailments or injuries.

The physical properties of DHA and its presence in brain cell membranes allow for one of its most established functions: increasing the activity of transmembrane proteins. The length of DHA (22 carbons), and the degree of desaturation (6 double bonds), increase the deformability, permeability and free volume of the plasma membrane

TABLE 12.4 Average DHA and EPA Contents of Fish Oils (1 g) and Fish (70 g ≈ 2.5 oz.)

Cod liver oil[a] (mg PUFA)		Other fish oils[b] (mg PUFA)		Anchovy[c] (mg PUFA)		Cod[c] (mg PUFA)		Salmon[c] (mg PUFA)		Tuna (Bluefin)[c] (mg PUFA)	
DHA	EPA	DHA	EPA	DHA	EPA	DHA	EPA	DHA	EPA	DHA	EPA
105	75	255	230	630	420	70	trace	490	420	630	210

[a]*Adapted from Nordic Naturals Arctic Cod Liver Oil supplement factsheet.*
[b]*Adapted from Yi et al., 2014.*
[c]*Adapted from Lewin et al., 2005.*

and result in greater motional freedom for membrane proteins to change their conformations after being activated (Gawrisch et al., 2008; Niu et al., 2004; Stillwell et al., 2005). Rhodopsin requires more than the vitamin A metabolite cis-11-retinal for its function. The light receptor also needs DHA in the membrane for optimization of its activity (Mitchell et al., 2012; Niu et al., 2004; Polozova and Litman, 2000; Salem et al., 2001). As the percentage of DHA in the retina increases, the sensitivity of the retinal response also increases (Jeffrey et al., 2001; Weisinger et al., 1999). Similarly, the activity and membrane translocation of phosphatidylinositol-3-kinase (PI3K) is highest when DHA is present, but PI3K activity is reduced when DHA is substituted by docosapentaenoic acid (DPA; 22:5n-6), another LC-PUFA that has only one less double bond than DHA. In contrast, EPA partitions into membranes differently and has less of an effect on neuronal signaling than DHA (Crawford et al., 2013; Williams et al., 2012).

As with vitamins A, D, and E, DHA sufficiency and its interactions with PI3K are associated with AkT activation and subsequent inhibition of GSK3β (Akbar et al., 2005), reduced expression of tau, reduced accumulation of amyloid-β (Aβ; Calon, 2011; Green et al., 2007), inhibition of caspase-3 (Akbar et al., 2005) and activation of the mammalian target of rapamycin (mTOR; Narayanan et al., 2009). These AkT activities promote the survival of cells under the metabolic stress that occurs during brain injury and neurodegenerative diseases (Giza and Hovda, 2001; Gomez-Pinilla and Tyagi, 2013). It is also interesting that, just like omega-3 sufficiency (Akbar et al., 2005; Bach et al., 2014; Pan et al., 2009), NGF and brain-derived neurotrophic factor (BDNF) increase PUFA-derived neuroprotectins (Mukherjee et al., 2007) and activate AkT/mTOR (Gururajan and van den Buuse, 2014), the Src/Fyn kinase pathway (Bartlett and Wang, 2013), and the ERK/MAPK/CREB pathway. In addition, the ERK pathway is activated by other DHA receptors such as gpr40 (Boneva and Yamashima, 2012; Zamarbide et al., 2014) and gpr120 (Wellhauser and Belsham, 2014), and the RXR system has also been implicated in these processes (Akbar et al., 2005; Michael-Titus and Priestley, 2014).

The mechanisms described above are the likely basis for why LC-PUFA supplementation of AD patients improves their omega-3 status and some biomarkers of the condition. However, as with the vitamins, potential problems with lipid processing in both AD and aging (Vandal et al., 2014) seem to contribute to an overall lack of effect of supplementation after AD has been diagnosed (Quinn et al., 2010). It is therefore interesting that the ApoE4 isoform of the apolipoprotein lipid carrier transports DHA less efficiently than the ApoE2 and ApoE3 isoforms and that ApoE4 is associated with increased risk of AD (Barberger-Gateau et al., 2011), reduced outcomes after TBI, increased tau and low DHA status (Mahley and Huang 2012; Mills et al., 2011; Zhou et al., 2008). In contrast, a randomized, controlled clinical trial has demonstrated that 900 mg/d DHA for 6 months improved mild cognitive impairment in adults that have not been diagnosed with any neurodegenerative disorder (Yurko-Mauro et al., 2010), suggesting that prevention of age-related brain problems may be possible to some extent via proper nutrition. This suggestion is supported by a recent meta-analysis of six randomized controlled trials that found that dosing DHA + EPA (400–1800 mg/day), over 3–40 months, significantly reduced the rate of cognitive decline in the elderly as measured by the minimental status exam (Zhang et al., 2015). Furthermore, a prospective follow-up to the Framingham Heart Study found that the top quartile of plasma phosphatidylcholine-DHA levels was associated with a significant reduction (47%) in the probability of developing dementia (Schaefer et al., 2006).

THE AGING BRAIN, MYELIN MAINTENANCE, AND NUTRIENTS FROM FISH

One proposed model of brain aging ties the commonalities of energy metabolism, histopathology, biochemical signaling and the effects of environmental insults between brain injury, inflammation, aging, and AD all together within the context of myelin maintenance and its metabolic expense. The myelin maintenance model postulates that aging and AD-related pathologies can be characterized as the developmental myelination pattern in reverse. Maintenance of brain health throughout life, and particularly its myelin, is energetically expensive. Most of the enzymes that maintain brain function use adenosine triphosphate (ATP) as a source of chemical energy to power their activities. Oligodendrocytes consume two to three times more energy than neurons, making age-related or injury-related imbalances in energy, or environmental challenges and genetic defects in nutrient processing or repair mechanisms, particularly impactful on these myelinating cells of the brain (Bartzokis, 2011; Connor and Menzies, 1996). These notions are supported in that white matter integrity is the first casualty of neurodegeneration (Goodenowe et al., 2007).

When the brain is damaged by blunt trauma, cells engage in hyperglycolysis that attempts to compensate for an induced loss of ATP production. The loss of ATP is caused by excessive calcium influx to damaged cells or to others that are nearby damaged cells. Excessive calcium ultimately causes depolarization of the mitochondrial membrane that damages its integral role in ATP production. With reduced ATP, a cell cannot maintain the voltage potentials of sodium and potassium across the plasma membrane, compromising its function. When a cell no longer functions it becomes necrotic or is targeted for apoptosis (Giza and Hovda, 2001). Vitamin D combats these processes by inhibiting calcium channel activity and upregulating calcium-sequestering proteins (Fernandes de Abreu et al., 2009). The association of retinoids with better glucose uptake (Berti et al., 2015) may also confer some benefits before damage, but after damage ATRA may contribute to hyperglycolysis (Olson and Mello, 2010).

Neurodegeneration and AD exhibit reductions in the uptake of glucose (Henderson, 2008) and lipid-related energy sources to the brain (Vandal et al., 2014) that eventually result in necrosis or apoptosis. Interestingly, the repair processes that occur after such events are also centered on glucose metabolism that can be modified by fish oil nutrients. Myelin repair slows or halts the transport of mitochondria and nutrients in the axon for their delivery to the damaged area, and this process is regulated by β-amyloid cleaving enzyme (BACE1) and γ-secretase enzyme, the same enzymes that produce Aβ, the classical hallmark of AD. The slowing of axonal transport is marked by hyperphosphorylated tau, swelling of the axon, Aβ deposition, and the potential starving and death of neurons, all of which are biomarkers for aging, neurodegeneration and AD (Medhi and Chakrabarty, 2013) as well as myelin repair (Bartzokis, 2011). Furthermore, these biomarkers are downstream from the activation of glycogen synthase kinase-3β (GSK3β). All of the fish oil nutrients that have been discussed, when supplied in sufficient quantities, result in the inhibition of GSK3β (Akbar et al., 2005; Briones and Darwish, 2014; Calon, 2011; Green et al., 2007; Keeney et al., 2013; König et al., 2012; Latimer et al., 2014; Puttagunta and Di Giovanni, 2011; Ragot et al., 2011; Sodhi and Singh, 2014; Vejux et al., 2009; Wu et al., 2010). Thus, glucose uptake and storage are increased, and tau phosphorylation is reduced (Folsom and Fatemi, 2013).

The metabolic stress and hyperglycolysis induced by age-related damage can also lead to the production of ROS. As described earlier, ROS can damage membrane lipids, DNA, and proteins that are important for repair, maintenance or function. The chief function of vitamin E is to inhibit this process and protect the double-bonds of LC-PUFA in the membrane. It is therefore possible that the sparing of DHA by vitamin E may explain the connection of vitamin E to the PI3K/AkT/GSK3β pathway (Ragot et al., 2011; Vejux et al., 2009; Wu et al., 2010). In fact, the combination of DHA with vitamin E is more protective of oligodendroctyes in vitro than vitamin E alone or DHA alone (Nury et al., 2015). However, ROS also increases the production of protective docosanoid and eicosanoid metabolites of DHA and EPA, respectively, and these metabolites inhibit inflammatory cascades (Bazan, 2013).

The external environment presents inflammatory stress to the brain over time. The brain's main defense against environmental stress is the blood-brain barrier (BBB). However, the effectiveness of the BBB is reduced by age, infections, trauma, and AD (Farkas et al., 2006; Spielman et al., 2014), and it has been suggested that inflammation arising from such chronic insults can lead to cytoskeletal impairments that can spread through the axonal tracts of the brain (Krstic et al., 2013). The processes by which chronic neuroinflammation causes progressive damage/aging of the brain are not completely understood, but they clearly involve dysregulated microglia. Microglia are the immune cells of the brain that are similar to peripheral macrophages. These cells normally serve to remove cellular debris or are used for synapse pruning during development. Some studies suggest that peripheral inflammation can spread to the brain via tumor necrosis factor-α (TNF-α) or interleukin-1 (IL-1) signaling across the BBB to activate the brain-resident microglia (Denes et al., 2011; Galic et al., 2012). Others suggest that excessive cytokine and ROS stimulation can put microglial activation into a positive feedback loop that causes a cycle of healthy brain tissue destruction and more microglial activation.

Retinoids, vitamin D, vitamin E, DHA, EPA, docosanoids, and eicosanoids have been proposed as therapies for aging and AD because they all downregulate pro-inflammatory pathways or ROS. Retinoids reduce peripheral interferon-γ (IFNγ) and the subsequent invasion of activated helper T-cells into the CNS that occurs in demyelinating models of multiple sclerosis (Zhan et al., 2013). Brain microglia are also activated by IFNγ, invade demyelinating regions, and damage oligodendrocytes with their proinflammatory signals (Peferoen et al., 2015), but they are inhibited by TGF-β (Zhou et al., 2015), which happens to be upregulated by vitamin D (Fernandes de Abreu et al., 2009). The vitamin D receptor (VDR) also attenuates iNOS, which can activate microglia (Keeney et al., 2013). Vitamin E and vitamin E analogues protect myelin and oligodendrocytes in vivo by reducing microglial activation (Blanchard et al., 2013), most likely through the inhibition of ROS and proinflammatory signals (Mocchegiani et al., 2014). In addition, vitamin E supplementation protects from the losses of superoxide dismutase and energy-sensing sirtuins (Wu et al., 2010), while blocking the increases of Aβ deposition and isoprostane generation (Conte et al., 2004), after traumatic brain injury. The metabolites of DHA and EPA activate PPARγ and inhibit NFKB in peripheral immune cells and brain microglia which results in important antiinflammatory benefits (Bazan, 2013; Farooqui et al., 2007; Michael-Titus and Priestley, 2014), and the most established role for EPA is to be a source of the anti-inflammatory eicosanoids (Dyall, 2015). Recently, a mechanism that employs DHA binding to the gpr120 receptor in the brain has also exhibited anti-inflammatory effects. These gpr120-mediated actions were independent from AkT, ERK, and PPARγ, but instead engaged TGF- β-activated kinase 1, which was similar to the activities of gpr120 in the periphery (Wellhauser and Belsham, 2014).

Beyond inflammation, there are multiple overlaps in the function of fish oil nutrients at increasing the function of receptor systems after brain damage has occurred. After demyelination, the activation of RXRγ by the ATRA isomer, cis-9-retinoic acid, increases myelin basic protein (MBP) expression in vitro and remyelination in aged rats in vivo (Huang et al., 2011). Similarly, ATRA acting through RARβ increases neurite outgrowth after spinal cord injury (Puttagunta and Di Giovanni, 2011). Vitamin D interacts with the VDR and RXR systems to increase dopamine and glutamate receptors as well as neurotransmitter recycling, which are important for synaptic transmission and memory formation during aging. In addition, vitamin D increases contactins, which decrease with age but serve to anchor myelin to the axon (Fernandes de Abreu et al., 2009; Latimer et al., 2014). These mechanisms may also explain why axogenesis and myelination are implicated in the benefits conferred by vitamin D in models of peripheral nerve damage (Chabas et al., 2013). Vitamin E analogs protect oligodendrocytes from peroxide insults in vitro that would otherwise result in a loss of MBP (Perfeito et al., 2007). DHA increases the function of several transmembrane receptors (Mitchell et al., 2012; Niu et al., 2004; Poloz.ova and Litman, 2000; Salem et al., 2001), but it might also activate RXR with subsequent heterodimerization with RAR or PPAR. While some questions exist regarding the physiological relevance of the micromolar DHA levels needed to activate these transcription factor complexes (Lengqvist et al., 2004), the host of genes promoted and likely interactions with the above indicate that proteins related to growth, synaptogenesis and myelination (Bazan et al., 2011; Kim and Spector, 2013; Michael-Titus and Priestley, 2014; van Neerven et al., 2008) can be modulated positively by appropriate supply of fish oil nutrients.

SUMMARY AND CONCLUSIONS

Interactions between the neuron, oligodendrocytes, and signals related to the immune system are necessary for the maintenance and repair of nervous system circuitry (Jakovcevski et al., 2009; Lee and Fields, 2009). The existing data support the premise that the downstream signaling of the fish-related nutrients of vitamin A, vitamin D, vitamin E, DHA, and EPA, when supplied at adequate levels, can support processes that combat age-related damage to the brain. Each nutrient can have individual effects on age-related brain functions, but many of these functions can overlap or interact between the nutrients. The experiments necessary to understand these interactions have, for the most part, not been performed and may be quite complex. What is clear is that many human populations exhibit significant gaps in their intakes of these nutrients in comparison to what is considered adequate, and elderly individuals are generally more vulnerable to the development of nutrient deficiencies and their consequences. No single fish product consumed at everyday levels can meet the intake requirements of all five nutrients at levels set forth by the regulatory agencies. For example, three grams of cod liver oil per day may come the closest to bridging the 100–300-μg gap in daily vitamin A intake, the 13–18-μg gap in daily vitamin D intake, and the 360–410-mg gap in daily DHA + EPA intake by providing 900 μg of vitamin A, 7.5 μg of vitamin D, and 540 mg of DHA + EPA. However, even cod liver oil falls short by not quite covering the entire vitamin D gap, by not having any appreciable levels of vitamin E, and by increasing the risk of having too much vitamin A. Thus, a balanced diet that includes fish, fish oil, and vegetables is necessary to meet the requirements. However, if the entire world was attempting to concurrently meet only the DHA + EPA intake recommendations, the present fish catch and aquaculture production would be insufficient. Moreover, we have reached a plateau in the fish available for wild catch and the resultant fish oil, which is available primarily for aquaculture. Therefore, algal-derived nutrients and vitamin fortification are likely necessary to ultimately meet the nutritional demands of the world's population (Salem and Eggersdorfer, 2015).

References

Adzemovic, M.Z., Zeitelhofer, M., Hochmeister, S., Gustafsson, S.A., Jagodic, M., 2013. Efficacy of vitamin D in treating multiple sclerosis-like neuroinflammation depends on developmental stage. Exp. Neurol. 249, 39–48.

Akbar, M., Calderon, F., Wen, Z., Kim, H.Y., 2005. Docosahexaenoic acid: a positive modulator of Akt signaling in neuronal survival. Proc. Natl. Acad. Sci. USA 102, 10858–10863.

Allen, L.H., Haskell, M., 2002. Estimating the potential for vitamin A toxicity in women and young children. J. Nutr. 132, 2907S–2919S.

Annweiler, C., Beauchet, O., Bartha, R., Graffe, A., Milea, D., Montero-Odasso, M., 2013a. Association between serum 25-hydroxyvitamin D concentration and optic chiasm volume. J. Am. Geriatr. Soc. 61, 1026–1028.

Annweiler, C., Llewellyn, D.J., Beauchet, O., 2013b. Low serum vitamin D concentrations in Alzheimer's disease: a systematic review and meta-analysis. J. Alzheimers Dis. 33, 659–674.

Arterburn, L.M., Hall, E.B., Oken, H., 2006. Distribution, interconversion, and dose response of n-3 fatty acids in humans. Am. J. Clin. Nutr. 83, 1467S–1476S.

Bach, S.A., de Siqueira, L.V., Muller, A.P., Oses, J.P., Quatrim, A., Emanuelli, T., Vinade, L., Souza, D.O., Moreira, J.D., 2014. Dietary omega-3 deficiency reduces BDNF content and activation NMDA receptor and Fyn in dorsal hippocampus: implications on persistence of long-term memory in rats. Nutr. Neurosci. 17, 186–192.

Bandarra, N.M., Batista, I., Nunes, M.L., Empis, J.M., Christie, W.W., 1997. Seasonal changes in lipid composition of sardine (*Sardina pilchardus*). J. Food Sci. 62, 40–42.

Barberger-Gateau, P., Samieri, C., Feart, C., Plourde, M., 2011. Dietary omega 3 polyunsaturated fatty acids and Alzheimer's disease: interaction with apolipoprotein E genotype. Curr. Alzheimer Res. 8, 479–491.

Barnard, K., Colón-Emeric, C., 2010. Extraskeletal effects of vitamin D in older adults: cardiovascular disease, mortality, mood, and cognition. Am. J. Geriatr. Pharmacother. 8, 4–33.

Bartlett, T.E., Wang, Y.T., 2013. The intersections of NMDAR-dependent synaptic plasticity and cell survival. Neuropharmacology 74, 59–68.

Bartzokis, G., 2011. Alzheimer's disease as homeostatic responses to age-related myelin breakdown. Neurobiol. Aging 32, 1341–1371.

Bauch, A., Lindtner, O., Mensink, G.B., Niemann, B., 2006. Dietary intake and sources of long-chain n-3 PUFAs in German adults. Eur. J. Clin. Nutr. 60, 810–812.

Bazan, N.G., 2013. The docosanoid neuroprotectin D1 induces homeostatic regulation of neuroinflammation and cell survival. Prostagland. Leukotr. Essen. Fatty Acid. 88, 127–129.

Bazan, N.G., Eady, T.N., Khoutorova, L., Atkins, K.D., Hong, S., Lu, Y., Zhang, C., Jun, B., Obenaus, A., Fredman, G., Zhu, M., Winkler, J.W., Petasis, N.A., Serhan, C.N., Belayev, L., 2012. Novel aspirin-triggered neuroprotectin D1 attenuates cerebral ischemic injury after experimental stroke. Exp. Neurol. 236, 122–130.

Bazan, N.G., Molina, M.F., Gordon, W.C., 2011. Docosahexaenoic acid signalolipidomics in nutrition: significance in aging, neuroinflammation, macular degeneration, Alzheimer's, and other neurodegenerative diseases. Annu. Rev. Nutr. 31, 321–351.

Belayev, L., Khoutorova, L., Atkins, K.D., Eady, T.N., Hong, S., Lu, Y., Obenaus, A., Bazan, N.G., 2011. Docosahexaenoic acid therapy of experimental ischemic stroke. Transl. Stroke Res. 2, 33–41.

Bell, M.V., Henderson, R.J., Sargent, J.R., 1985. Changes in the fatty acid composition of phospholipids from turbot (*Scophthalmus maximus*) in relation to dietary polyunsaturated fatty acid deficiencies. Comp. Biochem. Physiol. B 81, 193–198.

Berti, V., Murray, J., Davies, M., Spector, N., Tsui, W.H., Li, Y., Williams, S., Pirraglia, E., Vallabhajosula, S., McHugh, P., Pupi, A., de Leon, M.J., Mosconi, L., 2015. Nutrient patterns and brain biomarkers of Alzheimer's disease in cognitively normal individuals. J. Nutr. Health Aging 19, 413–423.

Blanchard, B., Heurtaux, T., Garcia, C., Moll, N.M., Caillava, C., Grandbarbe, L., Klosptein, A., Kerninon, C., Frah, M., Coowar, D., Baron-Van Evercooren, A., Morga, E., Heuschling, P., Nait Oumesmar, B., 2013. Tocopherol derivative TFA-12 promotes myelin repair in experimental models of multiple sclerosis. J. Neurosci. 33, 11633–11642.

Blasbalg, T.L., Hibbeln, J.R., Ramsden, C.E., Majchrzak, S.F., Rawlings, R.R., 2011. Changes in consumption of omega-3 and omega-6 fatty acids in the United States during the 20th century. Am. J. Clin. Nutr. 93, 950–962.

Boneva, N.B., Yamashima, T., 2012. New insights into "GPR40-CREB interaction in adult neurogenesis" specific for primates. Hippocampus 22, 896–905.

Bouzan, C., Cohen, J.T., Connor, W.E., Kris-Etherton, P.M., Gray, G.M., Konig, A., Lawrence, R.S., Savitz, D.A., Teutsch, S.M., 2005. A quantitative analysis of fish consumption and stroke risk. Am. J. Prev. Med. 29, 347–352.

Brenna, J.T., Salem, Jr., N., Sinclair, A.J., Cunnane, S.C., 2009. alpha-Linolenic acid supplementation and conversion to n-3 long-chain polyunsaturated fatty acids in humans. Prostagland. Leukotr. Essent. Fatty Acid. 80, 85–91.

Brigelius-Flohe, R., Kelly, F.J., Salonen, J.T., Neuzil, J., Zingg, J.M., Azzi, A., 2002. The European perspective on vitamin E: current knowledge and future research. Am. J. Clin. Nutr. 76, 703–716.

Brigelius-Flohe, R., Traber, M.G., 1999. Vitamin E: function and metabolism. FASEB J. 13, 1145–1155.

Briones, T.L., Darwish, H., 2014. Decrease in age-related tau hyperphosphorylation and cognitive improvement following vitamin D supplementation are associated with modulation of brain energy metabolism and redox state. Neuroscience 262, 143–155.

Buckley, C.D., Gilroy, D.W., Serhan, C.N., 2014. Proresolving lipid mediators and mechanisms in the resolution of acute inflammation. Immunity 40, 315–327.

Buell, J.S., Dawson-Hughes, B., Scott, T.M., Weiner, D.E., Dallal, G.E., Qui, W.Q., Bergethon, P., Rosenberg, I.H., Folstein, M.F., Patz, S., Bhadelia, R.A., Tucker, K.L., 2010. 25-Hydroxyvitamin D, dementia, and cerebrovascular pathology in elders receiving home services. Neurology 74, 18–26.

Burton, G.W., Joyce, A., Ingold, K.U., 1983. Is vitamin E the only lipid-soluble, chain-breaking antioxidant in human blood plasma and erythrocyte membranes? Arch. Biochem. Biophys. 221, 281–290.

Calon, F., 2011. Omega-3 polyunsaturated fatty acids in Alzheimer's disease: key questions and partial answers. Curr. Alzheimer Res. 8, 470–478.

Chabas, J.F., Stephan, D., Marqueste, T., Garcia, S., Lavaut, M.N., Nguyen, C., Legre, R., Khrestchatisky, M., Decherchi, P., Feron, F., 2013. Cholecalciferol (vitamin D(3)) improves myelination and recovery after nerve injury. PLoS One 8, e65034.

Chen, S., Subbaiah, P.V., 2013. Regioisomers of phosphatidylcholine containing DHA and their potential to deliver DHA to the brain: role of phospholipase specificities. Lipids 48, 675–686.

Chen, Y., Kundakovic, M., Agis-Balboa, R.C., Pinna, G., Grayson, D.R., 2007. Induction of the reelin promoter by retinoic acid is mediated by Sp1. J. Neurochem. 103, 650–665.

Connor, J.R., Menzies, S.L., 1996. Relationship of iron to oligodendrocytes and myelination. Glia 17, 83–93.

Conte, V., Uryu, K., Fujimoto, S., Yao, Y., Rokach, J., Longhi, L., Trojanowski, J.Q., Lee, V.M., McIntosh, T.K., Pratico, D., 2004. Vitamin E reduces amyloidosis and improves cognitive function in Tg2576 mice following repetitive concussive brain injury. J. Neurochem. 90, 758–764.

Corrada, M.M., Kawas, C.H., Hallfrisch, J., Muller, D., Brookmeyer, R., 2005. Reduced risk of Alzheimer's disease with high folate intake: the Baltimore Longitudinal Study of Aging. Alzheimers Dement. 1, 11–18.

Crawford, M.A., Broadhurst, C.L., Guest, M., Nagar, A., Wang, Y., Ghebremeskel, K., Schmidt, W.F., 2013. A quantum theory for the irreplaceable role of docosahexaenoic acid in neural cell signalling throughout evolution. Prostagland. Leukotr. Essent. Fatty Acid. 88, 5–13.

de Oliveira, M.R., 2015. Vitamin A and Retinoids as Mitochondrial Toxicants. Oxid. Med. Cell Longev. 2015, 140267.

Denes, A., Pinteaux, E., Rothwell, N.J., Allan, S.M., 2011. Interleukin-1 and stroke: biomarker, harbinger of damage, and therapeutic target. Cerebrovasc. Dis. 32, 517–527.

Dyall, S.C., 2015. Long-chain omega-3 fatty acids and the brain: a review of the independent and shared effects of EPA, DPA and DHA. Front Aging Neurosci. 7, 52.

EFSA Panel on Dietetic Products, N.a.A.N., 2012. Scientific Opinion related to the Tolerable Upper Intake Level of eicosapentaenoic acid (EPA), docosahexaenoic acid (DHA) and docosapentaenoic acid (DPA); 10.

Emken, E.A., Adlof, R.O., Gulley, R.M., 1994. Dietary linoleic acid influences desaturation and acylation of deuterium-labeled linoleic and linolenic acids in young adult males. Biochem. Biophys. Acta 1213, 277–288.

Eyles, D.W., Burne, T.H., McGrath, J.J., 2013. Vitamin D, effects on brain development, adult brain function and the links between low levels of vitamin D and neuropsychiatric disease. Front Neuroendocrinol. 34, 47–64.

Eyles, D.W., Smith, S., Kinobe, R., Hewison, M., McGrath, J.J., 2005. Distribution of the vitamin D receptor and 1 alpha-hydroxylase in human brain. J. Chem. Neuroanat. 29, 21–30.

Farkas, O., Lifshitz, J., Povlishock, J.T., 2006. Mechanoporation induced by diffuse traumatic brain injury: an irreversible or reversible response to injury? J. Neurosci. 26, 3130–3140.

Farooqui, A.A., Horrocks, L.A., Farooqui, T., 2007. Modulation of inflammation in brain: a matter of fat. J. Neurochem. 101, 577–599.

Fernandes de Abreu, D.A., Eyles, D., Feron, F., 2009. Vitamin D, a neuro-immunomodulator: implications for neurodegenerative and autoimmune diseases. Psychoneuroendocrinology 34 (Suppl. 1), S265–277.

Folsom, T.D., Fatemi, S.H., 2013. The involvement of Reelin in neurodevelopmental disorders. Neuropharmacology 68, 122–135.

Fragoso, Y.D., Shearer, K.D., Sementilli, A., de Carvalho, L.V., McCaffery, P.J., 2012. High expression of retinoic acid receptors and synthetic enzymes in the human hippocampus. Brain Struct. Funct. 217, 473–483.

Frank, J., Chin, X.W., Schrader, C., Eckert, G.P., Rimbach, G., 2012. Do tocotrienols have potential as neuroprotective dietary factors? Ageing Res. Rev. 11, 163–180.

Fratesi, J.A., Hogg, R.C., Young-Newton, G.S., Patterson, A.C., Charkhzarin, P., Block Thomas, K., Sharratt, M.T., Stark, K.D., 2009. Direct quantitation of omega-3 fatty acid intake of Canadian residents of a long-term care facility. Appl. Physiol. Nutr. Metab. 34, 1–9.

Galic, M.A., Riazi, K., Pittman, Q.J., 2012. Cytokines and brain excitability. Front Neuroendocrinol. 33, 116–125.

Gawrisch, K., Soubias, O., Mihailescu, M., 2008. Insights from biophysical studies on the role of polyunsaturated fatty acids for function of G-protein coupled membrane receptors. Prostagland. Leukotr. Essent. Fatty Acid. 79, 131–134.

Gebauer, S.K., Psota, T.L., Harris, W.S., Kris-Etherton, P.M., 2006. n-3 fatty acid dietary recommendations and food sources to achieve essentiality and cardiovascular benefits. Am. J. Clin. Nutr. 83, 1526S–1535S.

Giza, C.C., Hovda, D.A., 2001. The neurometabolic cascade of concussion. J. Athl. Train 36, 228–235.

Gladman, S.J., Huang, W., Lim, S.N., Dyall, S.C., Boddy, S., Kang, J.X., Knight, M.M., Priestley, J.V., Michael-Titus, A.T., 2012. Improved outcome after peripheral nerve injury in mice with increased levels of endogenous omega-3 polyunsaturated fatty acids. J. Neurosci. 32, 563–571.

Gloth, 3rd, F.M., Alam, W., Hollis, B., 1999. Vitamin D vs broad spectrum phototherapy in the treatment of seasonal affective disorder. J. Nutr. Health Aging 3, 5–7.

Gomez-Pinilla, F., Tyagi, E., 2013. Diet and cognition: interplay between cell metabolism and neuronal plasticity. Curr. Opin. Clin. Nutr. Metab. Care 16, 726–733.

Goodenowe, D.B., Cook, L.L., Liu, J., Lu, Y., Jayasinghe, D.A., Ahiahonu, P.W., Heath, D., Yamazaki, Y., Flax, J., Krenitsky, K.F., Sparks, D.L., Lerner, A., Friedland, R.P., Kudo, T., Kamino, K., Morihara, T., Takeda, M., Wood, P.L., 2007. Peripheral ethanolamine plasmalogen deficiency: a logical causative factor in Alzheimer's disease and dementia. J Lipid Res 48, 2485–2498.

Goudarzvand, M., Javan, M., Mirnajafi-Zadeh, J., Moz.afari, S., Tiraihi, T., 2010. Vitamins E and D3 attenuate demyelination and potentiate remyelination processes of hippocampal formation of rats following local injection of ethidium bromide. Cell Mol Neurobiol 30, 289–299.

Green, K.N., Martinez-Coria, H., Khashwji, H., Hall, E.B., Yurko-Mauro, K.A., Ellis, L., LaFerla, F.M., 2007. Dietary docosahexaenoic acid and docosapentaenoic acid ameliorate amyloid-beta and tau pathology via a mechanism involving presenilin 1 levels. J. Neurosci. 27, 4385–4395.

Grishkan, I.V., Fairchild, A.N., Calabresi, P.A., Gocke, A.R., 2013. 1,25-Dihydroxyvitamin D3 selectively and reversibly impairs T helper-cell CNS localization. Proc. Natl. Acad. Sci. USA 110, 21101–21106.

Gururajan, A., van den Buuse, M., 2014. Is the mTOR-signalling cascade disrupted in Schizophrenia? J. Neurochem. 129, 377–387.

Hall, J.C., Priestley, J.V., Perry, V.H., Michael-Titus, A.T., 2012. Docosahexaenoic acid, but not eicosapentaenoic acid, reduces the early inflammatory response following compression spinal cord injury in the rat. J. Neurochem. 121, 738–750.

Harrison, J.L., Rowe, R.K., Ellis, T.W., Yee, N.S., O'Hara, B.F., Adelson, P.D., Lifshitz, J., 2015. Resolvins AT-D1 and E1 differentially impact functional outcome, post-traumatic sleep, and microglial activation following diffuse brain injury in the mouse. Brain Behav Immun 47, 131–140.

He, K., Rimm, E.B., Merchant, A., Rosner, B.A., Stampfer, M.J., Willett, W.C., Ascherio, A., 2002. Fish consumption and risk of stroke in men. JAMA 288, 3130–3136.

Hemila, H., Kaprio, J., 2011. Vitamin E may affect the life expectancy of men, depending on dietary vitamin C intake and smoking. Age Ageing 40, 215–220.

Henderson, S.T., 2008. Ketone bodies as a therapeutic for Alzheimer's disease. Neurotherapeutics 5, 470–480.

Hooshmand, B., Lokk, J., Solomon, A., Mangialasche, F., Miralbell, J., Spulber, G., Annerbo, S., Andreasen, N., Winblad, B., Cedazo-Minguez, A., Wahlund, L.O., Kivipelto, M., 2014. Vitamin D in relation to cognitive impairment, cerebrospinal fluid biomarkers, and brain volumes. J Gerontol A Biol Sci Med Sci 69, 1132–1138.

Huang, J.K., Jarjour, A.A., Nait Oumesmar, B., Kerninon, C., Williams, A., Krezel, W., Kagechika, H., Bauer, J., Zhao, C., Baron-Van Evercooren, A., Chambon, P., Ffrench-Constant, C., Franklin, R.J., 2011. Retinoid X receptor gamma signaling accelerates CNS remyelination. Nat Neurosci 14, 45–53.

Innis, S.M., 2008. Dietary omega 3 fatty acids and the developing brain. Brain Res 1237, 35–43.

Institute of Medicine, 2000. Dietary reference intakes for vitamin C, vitamin E, selenium, and carotenoids. National Academy Press, Washington, DC, pp. 8–9.

Institute of Medicine, 2001. Dietary reference intakes for vitamin A, vitamin K, arsenic, boron, chromium, copper, iodine, iron, manganese, molybdenum, nickel, silicon, vanadium, and zinc. National Academy Press, Washington, DC, pp. 8–9.

Institute of Medicine, 2011. Dietary reference intakes for calcium and vitamin D. National Academy Press, Washington, DC, p. 9.

Irianto, H.E., 1994. Effects of resin refining on the chemical and physical stability of sardine oils. Indonesian Food Nutr. Prog. 1, 22–27.

Jakovcevski, I., Filipovic, R., Mo, Z., Rakic, S., Zecevic, N., 2009. Oligodendrocyte development and the onset of myelination in the human fetal brain. Front. Neuroanat. 3 (5), 1–15.

Jeffrey, B.G., Weisinger, H.S., Neuringer, M., Mitchell, D.C., 2001. The role of docosahexaenoic acid in retinal function. Lipids 36, 859–871.

Jiang, Q., Christen, S., Shigenaga, M.K., Ames, B.N., 2001. gamma-tocopherol, the major form of vitamin E in the US diet, deserves more attention. Am. J. Clin. Nutr. 74, 714–722.

Johnson, E.J., Vishwanathan, R., Johnson, M.A., Hausman, D.B., Davey, A., Scott, T.M., Green, R.C., Miller, L.S., Gearing, M., Woodard, J., Nelson, P.T., Chung, H.Y., Schalch, W., Wittwer, J., Poon, L.W., 2013. Relationship between Serum and Brain Carotenoids, alpha-Tocopherol, and Retinol Concentrations and Cognitive Performance in the Oldest Old from the Georgia Centenarian Study. J Aging Res 2013, 951786.

Keeney, J.T., Forster, S., Sultana, R., Brewer, L.D., Latimer, C.S., Cai, J., Klein, J.B., Porter, N.M., Butterfield, D.A., 2013. Dietary vitamin D deficiency in rats from middle to old age leads to elevated tyrosine nitration and proteomics changes in levels of key proteins in brain: implications for low vitamin D-dependent age-related cognitive decline. Free Radic Biol Med 65, 324–334.

Kerr, D.C., Zava, D.T., Piper, W.T., Saturn, S.R., Frei, B., Gombart, A.F., 2015. Associations between vitamin D levels and depressive symptoms in healthy young adult women. Psychiatry Res 227, 46–51.

Kim, H.Y., Spector, A.A., 2013. Synaptamide, endocannabinoid-like derivative of docosahexaenoic acid with cannabinoid-independent function. Prostagland. Leukotr. Essent. Fatty Acid. 88, 121–125.

König, R., Stillfried, M., Aperdannier, P., Clarner, T., Beyer, C., Kipp, M., Mey, J., 2012. Expression of retinoid X receptor beta is induced in astrocytes during corpus callosum demyelination. J. Chem. Neuroanat. 43, 120–132.

Környei, Z., Gocza, E., Ruhl, R., Orsolits, B., Voros, E., Szabo, B., Vagovits, B., Madarasz, E., 2007. Astroglia-derived retinoic acid is a key factor in glia-induced neurogenesis. FASEB J 21, 2496–2509.

Krstic, D., Pfister, S., Notter, T., Knuesel, I., 2013. Decisive role of Reelin signaling during early stages of Alzheimer's disease. Neuroscience 246, 108–116.

Kuratko, C.N., Salem, N., 2013. Docosahexaenoic acid from algal oil. Eur. J. Lipid Sci. Technol. 115, 965–976.

La Fata, G., Weber, P., Mohajeri, M.H., 2014. Effects of vitamin E on cognitive performance during ageing and in Alzheimer's disease. Nutrients 6, 5453–5472.

Larsson, S.C., Orsini, N., 2011. Fish consumption and the risk of stroke: a dose-response meta-analysis. Stroke 42, 3621–3623.

Latimer, C.S., Brewer, L.D., Searcy, J.L., Chen, K.C., Popovic, J., Kraner, S.D., Thibault, O., Blalock, E.M., Landfield, P.W., Porter, N.M., 2014. Vitamin D prevents cognitive decline and enhances hippocampal synaptic function in aging rats. Proc. Natl. Acad. Sci. USA 111, E4359–4366.

Lee, P.R., Fields, R.D., 2009. Regulation of myelin genes implicated in psychiatric disorders by functional activity in axons. Front Neuroanat 3, 4.

Lengqvist, J., Mata De Urquiza, A., Bergman, A.C., Willson, T.M., Sjovall, J., Perlmann, T., Griffiths, W.J., 2004. Polyunsaturated fatty acids including docosahexaenoic and arachidonic acid bind to the retinoid X receptor alpha ligand-binding domain. Mol Cell Proteomics 3, 692–703.

Lewin, G.A., Schachter, H.M., Yuen, D., Merchant, P., Mamaladze, V., Tsertsvadze, A., 2005. Effects of omega-3 fatty acids on child and maternal health. Evid. Rep. Technol. Assess. (Summ.) 118, 1–11.

Lin, Y.H., Llanos, A., Mena, P., Uauy, R., Salem, Jr., N., Pawlosky, R.J., 2010. Compartmental analyses of 2H5-alpha-linolenic acid and C-U-eicosapentaenoic acid toward synthesis of plasma labeled 22:6n-3 in newborn term infants. Am. J. Clin. Nutr. 92, 284–293.

Luo, C.L., Li, Q.Q., Chen, X.P., Zhang, X.M., Li, L.L., Li, B.X., Zhao, Z.Q., Tao, L.Y., 2013. Lipoxin A4 attenuates brain damage and downregulates the production of pro-inflammatory cytokines and phosphorylated mitogen-activated protein kinases in a mouse model of traumatic brain injury. Brain Res 1502, 1–10.

Mahley, R.W., Huang, Y., 2012. Apolipoprotein e sets the stage: response to injury triggers neuropathology. Neuron 76, 871–885.

Mangialasche, F., Kivipelto, M., Mecocci, P., Rizzuto, D., Palmer, K., Winblad, B., Fratiglioni, L., 2010. High plasma levels of vitamin E forms and reduced Alzheimer's disease risk in advanced age. J Alzheimers Dis 20, 1029–1037.

Mangialasche, F., Xu, W., Kivipelto, M., Costanzi, E., Ercolani, S., Pigliautile, M., Cecchetti, R., Baglioni, M., Simmons, A., Soininen, H., Tsolaki, M., Kloszewska, I., Vellas, B., Lovestone, S., Mecocci, P., 2012. Tocopherols and tocotrienols plasma levels are associated with cognitive impairment. Neurobiol Aging 33, 2282–2290.

McNamara, R.K., Carlson, S.E., 2006. Role of omega-3 fatty acids in brain development and function: potential implications for the pathogenesis and prevention of psychopathology. Prostagland. Leukotr. Essent. Fatty Acid. 75, 329–349.

Medhi, B., Chakrabarty, M., 2013. Insulin resistance: an emerging link in Alzheimer's disease. Neurol Sci 34, 1719–1725.

Meehan, M., Penckofer, S., 2014. The Role of Vitamin D in the Aging Adult. J Aging Gerontol 2, 60–71.

Meydani, M., 1995. Vitamin E. Lancet 345, 170–175.

Michael-Titus, A.T., Priestley, J.V., 2014. Omega-3 fatty acids and traumatic neurological injury: from neuroprotection to neuroplasticity? Trends Neurosci 37, 30–38.

Mills, J.D., Hadley, K., Bailes, J.E., 2011. Dietary supplementation with the omega-3 fatty acid docosahexaenoic acid in traumatic brain injury. Neurosurgery 68, 474–481, discussion 481.

Misner, D.L., Jacobs, S., Shimizu, Y., de Urquiza, A.M., Solomin, L., Perlmann, T., De Luca, L.M., Stevens, C.F., Evans, R.M., 2001. Vitamin A deprivation results in reversible loss of hippocampal long-term synaptic plasticity. Proc. Natl. Acad. Sci. USA 98, 11714–11719.

Mitchell, D.C., Niu, S.L., Litman, B.J., 2012. Quantifying the differential effects of DHA and DPA on the early events in visual signal transduction. Chem Phys Lipids 165, 393–400.

Mocchegiani, E., Costarelli, L., Giacconi, R., Malavolta, M., Basso, A., Piacenza, F., Ostan, R., Cevenini, E., Gonos, E.S., Franceschi, C., Monti, D., 2014. Vitamin E-gene interactions in aging and inflammatory age-related diseases: implications for treatment. A systematic review. Ageing Res. Rev. 14, 81–101.

Moffat, C.F., McGill, A.S., 1993. Variability of the composition of fish oils: significance for the diet. Proc Nutr Soc 52, 441–456.

Mohajeri, M.H., Troesch, B., Weber, P., 2015. Inadequate supply of vitamins and DHA in the elderly: implications for brain aging and Alzheimer-type dementia. Nutrition 31, 261–275.

Mohajeri, M.H., Winwood, R.J., 2012. The role of DHA in cognitive performance of children. AgroFOOD industry hi-tech 23, 22–24.

Mohrhauer, H., Holman, R.T., 1963. Effect of Linolenic Acid Upon the Metabolism of Linoleic Acid. J Nutr 81, 67–74.

Molano, A., Meydani, S.N., 2012. Vitamin E, signalosomes and gene expression in T cells. Mol Aspects Med 33, 55–62.

Morris, M.C., Evans, D.A., Bienias, J.L., Tangney, C.C., Wilson, R.S., 2002a. Vitamin E and cognitive decline in older persons. Arch Neurol 59, 1125–1132.

Morris, M.C., Evans, D.A., Bienias, J.L., Tangney, C.C., Bennett, D.A., Aggarwal, N., Wilson, R.S., Scherr, P.A., 2002b. Dietary intake of antioxidant nutrients and the risk of incident Alzheimer disease in a biracial community study. JAMA 287, 3230–3237.

Mukherjee, P.K., Chawla, A., Loayza, M.S., Bazan, N.G., 2007. Docosanoids are multifunctional regulators of neural cell integrity and fate: significance in aging and disease. Prostagland. Leukotr. Essent. Fatty Acid. 77, 233–238.

Muldoon, M.F., Ryan, C.M., Sheu, L., Yao, J.K., Conklin, S.M., Manuck, S.B., 2010. Serum phospholipid docosahexaenonic acid is associated with cognitive functioning during middle adulthood. J Nutr 140, 848–853.

Myhre, A.M., Carlsen, M.H., Bohn, S.K., Wold, H.L., Laake, P., Blomhoff, R., 2003. Water-miscible, emulsified, and solid forms of retinol supplements are more toxic than oil-based preparations. Am. J. Clin. Nutr. 78, 1152–1159.

Narayanan, S.P., Flores, A.I., Wang, F., Macklin, W.B., 2009. Akt signals through the mammalian target of rapamycin pathway to regulate CNS myelination. J. Neurosci. 29, 6860–6870.

Niki, E., Traber, M.G., 2012. A history of vitamin E. Ann Nutr Metab 61, 207–212.

Niu, S.L., Mitchell, D.C., Lim, S.Y., Wen, Z.M., Kim, H.Y., Salem, Jr., N., Litman, B.J., 2004. Reduced G protein-coupled signaling efficiency in retinal rod outer segments in response to n-3 fatty acid deficiency. J Biol Chem 279, 31098–31104.

Nury, T., Zarrouk, A., Mackrill, J.J., Samadi, M., Durand, P., Riedinger, J.M., Doria, M., Vejux, A., Limagne, E., Delmas, D., Prost, M., Moreau, T., Hammami, M., Delage-Mourroux, R., O'Brien, N.M., Lizard, G. 2015. Induction of oxiapoptophagy on 158N murine oligodendrocytes treated by 7-ketocholesterol-, 7beta-hydroxycholesterol-, or 24(S)-hydroxycholesterol: Protective effects of alpha-tocopherol and docosahexaenoic acid (DHA; C22:6 n-3). Steroids.

Olson, C.R., Mello, C.V., 2010. Significance of vitamin A to brain function, behavior and learning. Mol Nutr Food Res 54, 489–495.

Ono, K., Yamada, M., 2012. Vitamin A and Alzheimer's disease. Geriatr Gerontol Int 12, 180–188.

O'Reilly, K., Bailey, S.J., Lane, M.A., 2008. Retinoid-mediated regulation of mood: possible cellular mechanisms. Exp Biol Med (Maywood) 233, 251–258.

Ouellet, M., Emond, V., Chen, C.T., Julien, C., Bourasset, F., Oddo, S., LaFerla, F., Bazinet, R.P., Calon, F., 2009. Diffusion of docosahexaenoic and eicosapentaenoic acids through the blood-brain barrier: An in situ cerebral perfusion study. Neurochem Int 55, 476–482.

Pan, H.C., Kao, T.K., Ou, Y.C., Yang, D.Y., Yen, Y.J., Wang, C.C., Chuang, Y.H., Liao, S.L., Raung, S.L., Wu, C.W., Chiang, A.N., Chen, C.J., 2009. Protective effect of docosahexaenoic acid against brain injury in ischemic rats. J Nutr Biochem 20, 715–725.

Paterniti, I., Impellizzeri, D., Di Paola, R., Esposito, E., Gladman, S., Yip, P., Priestley, J.V., Michael-Titus, A.T., Cuzzocrea, S., 2014. Docosahexaenoic acid attenuates the early inflammatory response following spinal cord injury in mice: in-vivo and in-vitro studies. J Neuroinflammation 11, 6.

Pawlosky, R.J., Salem, Jr., N., 2004. Perspectives on alcohol consumption: liver polyunsaturated fatty acids and essential fatty acid metabolism. Alcohol 34, 27–33.

Peferoen, L.A., Vogel, D.Y., Ummenthum, K., Breur, M., Heijnen, P.D., Gerritsen, W.H., Peferoen-Baert, R.M., van der Valk, P., Dijkstra, C.D., Amor, S., 2015. Activation status of human microglia is dependent on lesion formation stage and remyelination in multiple sclerosis. J Neuropathol Exp Neurol 74, 48–63.

Perfeito, R., Pereira, J., Oliveira, C.R., Bettencourt-Relvas, J., Rego, A.C., 2007. Trolox protection of myelin membrane in hydrogen peroxide-treated mature oligodendrocytes. Free Radic Res 41, 444–451.

Plourde, M., Cunnane, S.C., 2007. Extremely limited synthesis of long chain polyunsaturates in adults: implications for their dietary essentiality and use as supplements. Appl. Physiol. Nutr. Metab. 32, 619–634.

Polozova, A., Litman, B.J., 2000. Cholesterol dependent recruitment of di22:6-PC by a G protein-coupled receptor into lateral domains. Biophys J 79, 2632–2643.

Pottala, J.V., Yaffe, K., Robinson, J.G., Espeland, M.A., Wallace, R., Harris, W.S., 2014. Higher RBC EPA + DHA corresponds with larger total brain and hippocampal volumes: WHIMS-MRI study. Neurology 82, 435–442.

Puttagunta, R., Di Giovanni, S., 2011. Retinoic acid signaling in axonal regeneration. Front Mol Neurosci 4, 59.

Quinn, J.F., Raman, R., Thomas, R.G., Yurko-Mauro, K., Nelson, E.B., Van Dyck, C., Galvin, J.E., Emond, J., Jack, Jr., C.R., Weiner, M., Shinto, L., Aisen, P.S., 2010. Docosahexaenoic acid supplementation and cognitive decline in Alzheimer disease: a randomized trial. JAMA 304, 1903–1911.

Ragot, K., Delmas, D., Athias, A., Nury, T., Baarine, M., Lizard, G., 2011. alpha-Tocopherol impairs 7-ketocholesterol-induced caspase-3-dependent apoptosis involving GSK-3 activation and Mcl-1 degradation on 158N murine oligodendrocytes. Chem Phys Lipids 164, 469–478.

Ransom, J., Morgan, P.J., McCaffery, P.J., Stoney, P.N., 2014. The rhythm of retinoids in the brain. J. Neurochem. 129, 366–376.

Ravaglia, G., Forti, P., Lucicesare, A., Pisacane, N., Rietti, E., Mangialasche, F., Cecchetti, R., Patterson, C., Mecocci, P., 2008. Plasma tocopherols and risk of cognitive impairment in an elderly Italian cohort. Am. J. Clin. Nutr. 87, 1306–1313.

Ross, A.C., Harrison, E.H., 2007. Vitamin A: Nutritional aspects of retinoids and carotenoids. In: Zempleni, J., Rucker, R.B., McCormick, D.B., Suttie, J.W. (Eds.), Handbook of Vitamins. fourth ed. Taylor & Francis Group, Boca Raton, FL, USA, pp. 1–39.

Salem, Jr., N., Eggersdorfer, M., 2015. Is the world supply of omega-3 fatty acids adequate for optimal human nutrition? Curr. Opin. Clin. Nutr. Metab. Care 18, 147–154.

Salem, Jr., N., Litman, B., Kim, H.Y., Gawrisch, K., 2001. Mechanisms of action of docosahexaenoic acid in the nervous system. Lipids 36, 945–959.

Schaefer, E.J., Bongard, V., Beiser, A.S., Lamon-Fava, S., Robins, S.J., Au, R., Tucker, K.L., Kyle, D.J., Wilson, P.W., Wolf, P.A., 2006. Plasma phosphatidylcholine docosahexaenoic acid content and risk of dementia and Alzheimer disease: the Framingham Heart Study. Arch. Neurol. 63, 1545–1550.

Schuurman, A.G., van den Brandt, P.A., Dorant, E., Brants, H.A., Goldbohm, R.A., 1999. Association of energy and fat intake with prostate carcinoma risk: results from The Netherlands Cohort Study. Cancer 86, 1019–1027.

Scott, K.C., Latshaw, J.D., 1991. Effects of commercial processing on the fat-soluble vitamin content of menhaden fish oil. J. Am. Oil Chem. Soc. 68, 234–236.

Shirai, N., Suzuki, H., Tokairin, S., Ehara, H., Wada, S., 2002a. Dietary and seasonal effects on the dorsal meat lipid composition of Japanese (*Silurus asotus*) and Thai catfish (*Clarias macrocephalus* and hybrid *Clarias macrocephalus* and *Clarias galipinus*). Comp. Biochem. Physiol. A Mol. Integr. Physiol. 132, 609–619.

Shirai, N., Terayama, M., Takeda, H., 2002b. Effect of season on the fatty acid composition and free amino acid content of the sardine *Sardinops melanostictus*. Comp. Biochem. Physiol. B Biochem. Mol. Biol. 131, 387–393.

Sodhi, R.K., Singh, N., 2014. Retinoids as potential targets for Alzheimer's disease. Pharmacol. Biochem. Behav. 120, 117–123.

Spielman, L.J., Little, J.P., Klegeris, A., 2014. Inflammation and insulin/IGF-1 resistance as the possible link between obesity and neurodegeneration. J. Neuroimmunol. 273, 8–21.

Stillwell, W., Shaikh, S.R., Zerouga, M., Siddiqui, R., Wassall, S.R., 2005. Docosahexaenoic acid affects cell signaling by altering lipid rafts. Reprod. Nutr. Dev. 45, 559–579.

Tan, Z.S., Harris, W.S., Beiser, A.S., Au, R., Himali, J.J., Debette, S., Pikula, A., Decarli, C., Wolf, P.A., Vasan, R.S., Robins, S.J., Seshadri, S., 2012. Red blood cell omega-3 fatty acid levels and markers of accelerated brain aging. Neurology 78, 658–664.

Torkildsen, O., Loken-Amsrud, K.I., Wergeland, S., Myhr, K.M., Holmoy, T., 2013. Fat-soluble vitamins as disease modulators in multiple sclerosis. Acta Neurol. Scand. Suppl., 16–23.

Touyarot, K., Bonhomme, D., Roux, P., Alfos, S., Lafenetre, P., Richard, E., Higueret, P., Pallet, V., 2013. A mid-life vitamin A supplementation prevents age-related spatial memory deficits and hippocampal neurogenesis alterations through CRABP-I. PLoS One 8, e72101.

Traber, M.G., 2007. Vitamin E. In: Zempleni, J., Rucker, R.B., McCormick, D.B., Suttie, J.W. (Eds.), Handbook of Vitamins. fourth ed. Taylor & Francis Group, Boca Raton, FL, USA, pp. 153–174.

Troesch, B., Hoeft, B., McBurney, M., Eggersdorfer, M., Weber, P., 2012. Dietary surveys indicate vitamin intakes below recommendations are common in representative Western countries. Br. J. Nutr. 108, 692–698.

United States Department of Agriculture, Agricultural Research Service, 2012. Nutrient intakes from food: mean amounts consumed per individual, by gender and age, what we eat in America, NHANES 2009–2010. http://www.ars.usda.gov/SP2UserFiles/Place/80400530/pdf/0910/Table_1_NIN_GEN_09.pdf.

United States Department of Agriculture, Agriculture Research Service, 2015. USDA nutrient database for standard reference, Release 27. http://ndb.nal.usda.gov/ndb/search.

Vahid, F., Zand, H., Nosrat-Mirshekarlou, E., Najafi, R., Hekmatdoost, A., 2015. The role dietary of bioactive compounds on the regulation of histone acetylases and deacetylases: a review. Gene 562, 8–15.

van Neerven, S., Kampmann, E., Mey, J., 2008. RAR/RXR and PPAR/RXR signaling in neurological and psychiatric diseases. Prog. Neurobiol. 85, 433–451.

Vandal, M., Alata, W., Tremblay, C., Rioux-Perreault, C., Salem, Jr., N., Calon, F., Plourde, M., 2014. Reduction in DHA transport to the brain of mice expressing human APOE4 compared to APOE2. J. Neurochem. 129, 516–526.

Vejux, A., Guyot, S., Montange, T., Riedinger, J.M., Kahn, E., Lizard, G., 2009. Phospholipidosis and down-regulation of the PI3-K/PDK-1/Akt signalling pathway are vitamin E inhibitable events associated with 7-ketocholesterol-induced apoptosis. J. Nutr. Biochem. 20, 45–61.

Virtanen, J.K., Siscovick, D.S., Longstreth, Jr., W.T., Kuller, L.H., Moz.affarian, D., 2008. Fish consumption and risk of subclinical brain abnormalities on MRI in older adults. Neurology 71, 439–446.

Walhovd, K.B., Storsve, A.B., Westlye, L.T., Drevon, C.A., Fjell, A.M., 2014. Blood markers of fatty acids and vitamin D, cardiovascular measures, body mass index, and physical activity relate to longitudinal cortical thinning in normal aging. Neurobiol. Aging 35, 1055–1064.

Wang, C., Harris, W.S., Chung, M., Lichtenstein, A.H., Balk, E.M., Kupelnick, B., Jordan, H.S., Lau, J., 2006. n-3 Fatty acids from fish or fish-oil supplements, but not alpha-linolenic acid, benefit cardiovascular disease outcomes in primary- and secondary-prevention studies: a systematic review. Am. J. Clin. Nutr. 84, 5–17.

Wang, C., Kane, M.A., Napoli, J.L., 2011. Multiple retinol and retinal dehydrogenases catalyze all-trans-retinoic acid biosynthesis in astrocytes. J. Biol. Chem. 286, 6542–6553.

Wardwell, L., Chapman-Novakofski, K., Herrel, S., Woods, J., 2008. Nutrient intake and immune function of elderly subjects. J. Am. Diet Assoc. 108, 2005–2012.

Weisinger, H.S., Vingrys, A.J., Bui, B.V., Sinclair, A.J., 1999. Effects of dietary n-3 fatty acid deficiency and repletion in the guinea pig retina. Invest Ophthalmol. Vis Sci. 40, 327–338.

Wellhauser, L., Belsham, D.D., 2014. Activation of the omega-3 fatty acid receptor GPR120 mediates anti-inflammatory actions in immortalized hypothalamic neurons. J. Neuroinflammation 11, 60.

Williams, J.A., Batten, S.E., Harris, M., Rockett, B.D., Shaikh, S.R., Stillwell, W., Wassall, S.R., 2012. Docosahexaenoic and eicosapentaenoic acids segregate differently between raft and nonraft domains. Biophys. J. 103, 228–237.

Wu, A., Ying, Z., Gomez-Pinilla, F., 2010. Vitamin E protects against oxidative damage and learning disability after mild traumatic brain injury in rats. Neurorehabil. Neural Repair 24, 290–298.

Wu, A., Ying, Z., Gomez-Pinilla, F., 2014. Dietary strategy to repair plasma membrane after brain trauma: implications for plasticity and cognition. Neurorehabil. Neural Repair 28, 75–84.

Wu, D., Meydani, S.N., 2008. Age-associated changes in immune and inflammatory responses: impact of vitamin E intervention. J. Leukoc. Biol. 84, 900–914.

Wurtman, R.J., Cansev, M., Sakamoto, T., Ulus, I., 2010. Nutritional modifiers of aging brain function: use of uridine and other phosphatide precursors to increase formation of brain synapses. Nutr. Rev. 68 (Suppl 2), S88–101.

Xu, Q., Parks, C.G., DeRoo, L.A., Cawthon, R.M., Sandler, D.P., Chen, H., 2009. Multivitamin use and telomere length in women. Am. J. Clin. Nutr. 89, 1857–1863.

Yadav, S.K., Mindur, J.E., Ito, K., Dhib-Jalbut, S., 2015. Advances in the immunopathogenesis of multiple sclerosis. Curr. Opin. Neurol. 28, 206–219.

Yi, T., Li, S.M., Fan, J.Y., Fan, L.L., Zhang, Z.F., Luo, P., Zhang, X.J., Wang, J.G., Zhu, L., Zhao, Z.Z., Chen, H.B., 2014. Comparative analysis of EPA and DHA in fish oil nutritional capsules by GC-MS. Lipids Health Dis. 13, 190.

Yurko-Mauro, K., McCarthy, D., Rom, D., Nelson, E.B., Ryan, A.S., Blackwell, A., Salem, Jr., N., Stedman, M., 2010. Beneficial effects of docosahexaenoic acid on cognition in age-related cognitive decline. Alzheimers Dement. 6, 456–464.

Zamarbide, M., Etayo-Labiano, I., Ricobaraza, A., Martinez-Pinilla, E., Aymerich, M.S., Luis Lanciego, J., Perez-Mediavilla, A., Franco, R., 2014. GPR40 activation leads to CREB and ERK phosphorylation in primary cultures of neurons from the mouse CNS and in human neuroblastoma cells. Hippocampus 24, 733–739.

Zhan, X.X., Liu, Y., Yang, J.F., Wang, G.Y., Mu, L., Zhang, T.S., Xie, X.L., Wang, J.H., Liu, Y.M., Kong, Q.F., Li, H.L., Sun, B., 2013. All-trans-retinoic acid ameliorates experimental allergic encephalomyelitis by affecting dendritic cell and monocyte development. Immunology 138, 333–345.

Zhang, X.W., Hou, W.S., Li, M., Tang, Z.Y., 2015. Omega-3 fatty acids and risk of cognitive decline in the elderly: a meta-analysis of randomized controlled trials. Aging Clin. Exp. Res.

Zhong, M., Kawaguchi, R., Kassai, M., Sun, H., 2012. Retina, retinol, retinal and the natural history of vitamin A as a light sensor. Nutrients 4, 2069–2096.

Zhou, W., Xu, D., Peng, X., Zhang, Q., Jia, J., Crutcher, K.A., 2008. Meta-analysis of APOE4 allele and outcome after traumatic brain injury. J. Neurotrauma 25, 279–290.

Zhou, X., Zoller, T., Krieglstein, K., Spittau, B., 2015. TGFbeta1 inhibits IFNgamma-mediated microglia activation and protects mDA neurons from IFNgamma-driven neurotoxicity. J. Neurochem.

P A R T I I I

FISH AND FISH OILS IN HEALTH PROMOTION AND DISEASE PREVENTION AND TREATMENT

CHAPTER

13

Farmed Fish: A Valuable Source of Lipid Based Nutrients

M.J. Picklo

United States Department of Agriculture, Agricultural Research Service, Grand Forks Human Nutrition Research Center, Grand Forks, North Dakota, United States

The domestication of terrestrial plants and animals between 8,000 and 10,000 years ago is an achievement that allowed for prevention of hunger, growth of communities, and growth of the overall population (Bruford et al., 2003; Naderi et al., 2008; Teletchea and Fontaine, 2014). Today, except for seafood (shellfish and finfish, marine, and freshwater), domesticated terrestrial plants and animals comprise all but a small fraction of total food consumed globally and are the dominant sources of macronutrients and micronutrients needed for good health.

Seafood consumption, on the other hand, is derived from harvesting wild sources (predominantly marine) as well as "farmed", aquaculture sources of marine and freshwater nature. There are several historical antecedents of small scale aquaculture; however, the industrial scaling of aquacultural practices has only blossomed within the past 50 years (Teletchea and Fontaine, 2014). In 2012, aquaculture-derived seafood comprised 42% of total global seafood output at 66 million tons with a value of US$ 137.7 billion (FAO, 2014). Asian aquaculture accounts for nearly 90% of this output. Of the total aquaculture, two-thirds is inland production and one-third is marine-based (FAO, 2014).

For nearly 3 billion people, seafood represents 20% of protein intake and in some African countries over 50% (FAO, 2014). Given the growing world population and that most capture fisheries are either over-harvested or harvested at capacity, aquaculture is becoming the dominant source of many types of seafood for provision of protein and other nutrients (FAO, 2014; HLPE, 2014). The role of aquaculture in fulfilling protein requirements is of eminent concern in developing countries with burgeoning populations. The geographical and economic influences upon aquacultural production are outside the scope of this chapter and have been reviewed by others (Kawarazuka and Béné, 2011; Khan et al., 2011; Pinstrup-Andersen and Pandya-Lorch, 1998; Tacon and Metian, 2008). Certainly, environmental and sustainability issues influence the discussion of aquacultural practices, particularly with regard to omega-3 (n-3) fatty acids, and cover a broad range of thinking (Byelashov and Griffin, 2014; Chauton et al., 2015; Deutsch et al., 2007; Liland et al., 2013; Miller et al., 2008; Naylor et al., 2009; Sarker et al., 2013; Shepherd and Bachis, 2014).

In this chapter, the role of aquaculture-derived fish as sources of fat soluble nutrients will be reviewed. The chapter focuses primarily upon improving levels of long chain n–3 fatty acids (LCn3) in farmed oily fish like salmon and trout. In addition, the role of farmed fish in supplying other nutrients is discussed.

FISH: A SOURCE OF FAT SOLUBLE NUTRIENTS

Fish are often classified as lean or oily depending on their fat content. Fish like mackerel, salmon, trout, and sardines are considered oily fish as opposed to the leaner fish like tilapia and catfish. Of the oily fish, farmed Atlantic salmon (*Salmo salar*) and rainbow trout (*Oncorhynchus mykiss*) have undergone domestication and farming resulting in the production of *S. salar* at 2 million tons in 2013 (>50% of total commercial salmon) and *O. mykiss* production at 0.8 million tons in 2013 (FAO, 2015).

Oily fish reside in cool or cold waters and the intramuscular lipids are enriched in polyunsaturated fatty acids (PUFA), especially the LCn3 fatty acids eicosapentaenoic acid (EPA; 20:5n3), docosapentaenoic acid (DPA; 22:5n3)

Fish and Fish Oil in Health and Disease Prevention. http://dx.doi.org/10.1016/B978-0-12-802844-5.00013-0

and docosahexaenoic acid (DHA: 22:6n3). In addition to LCn3, oily fish contain lipid soluble nutrients including vitamin D and carotenoids.

An advantage of aquacultural production of fish is the ability to feed diets of known composition that is not subject to variation in climate, food quality or food availability. As outlined below, aquacultural practices for salmon and trout have the potential to be modified for enhanced levels of LCn3 and other nutrients for optimal human health.

DETERMINANTS OF LCn3 CONTENT

Consumption of LCn3 is linked to several positive health outcomes. The clinical and experimental data linking fish consumption, LCn3 and reduction of cardiovascular disease risk have been reviewed extensively and is presented in other chapters of this book (Mozaffarian and Rimm, 2006; Mozaffarian and Wu, 2012; Raatz et al., 2013b). In addition to reducing CVD risk, LCn3 are critical for cognitive development and association data indicate a relationship between DHA and mood disorders (Brenna and Carlson, 2014; McNamara et al., 2015; Scholtz et al., 2013). Furthermore, EPA and DHA are precursors to a number of antiinflammatory products, termed resolvins and protectins, that assist with the resolution of inflammatory processes (Serhan and Chiang, 2008).

The LCn3 content of farmed Atlantic salmon and rainbow trout is determined by the fatty acid content of the feed and the activity of the enzymes necessary for the conversion of the dietary n–3 fatty acids α-linolenic acid (ALA; 18:3n3) and hexadecatrienoic acid (16:3n3; HTA) to LCn3. Like other vertebrates, salmonids lack the capacity to synthesize these smaller n–3 PUFA, the starting substrates for the elongation and desaturation processes yielding EPA and DHA. Thus, endogenously synthesized LCn3 results from the elongation and desaturation of dietary HTA and ALA, derived from microalgae which is consumed and then converted to LCn3 in plankton and by small fish (Dunstan et al., 1992). In the larger salmonids, a substantial portion of LCn3 is accrued through the bioaccumulation process of consuming the LCn3 present in smaller fish.

Salmonids require dietary lipid for proper growth. Historically, the aquacultural production of salmonids (including Atlantic salmon and rainbow trout) has relied upon the provision of fish by-products and fish oil as dietary lipid sources (including LCn3) in the feed (Bibus, 2015; Miller et al., 2008; Shepherd and Bachis, 2014; Stone et al., 2011). However, the economic influences of higher global demand and higher prices have directed significant research into use of terrestrial, plant-based oils as dietary lipids (Chauton et al., 2015; Deutsch et al., 2007; Liland et al., 2013). ALA-rich oils like flaxseed oil and camelina oil have been used to raise LCn3 content in Atlantic salmon and rainbow trout (Hixson et al., 2014a; Hixson et al., 2014b; Hixson et al., 2014c; Wijekoon et al., 2014). The use of plant oils as a lipid source has been the focus of significant investigation and has been extensively reviewed (Miller et al., 2008; Turchini et al., 2009b).

Since terrestrial oils lack LCn3, it is not unexpected that lack of LCn3 fish oil in the diet reduces fillet content of LCn3 (Bell et al., 2004; Hixson et al., 2014b; Hixson et al., 2014c). Thus, there is significant need for study on how to maintain or increase LCn3 in the face of reduced fish oil use with increased plant oil use. This need has led to the investigation of means of optimizing LCn3 content through novel feeding regimens and novel breeding strategies, and research into the processes of PUFA metabolism and disposition in Atlantic salmon and rainbow trout.

Use of terrestrial, plant-derived, vegetable oils in salmonid production has stimulated investigation into the teleostic processes of ALA elongation and desaturation to LCn3. In mammals and salmonids, ALA undergoes a series of desaturation steps (by delta 6 desaturase and delta 5 desaturase) and elongation steps (by elongase 2 and elongase 5) to form EPA and DHA (Gregory and James, 2014). Like mammals, this process is dependent on multiple micronutrients (Giri et al., 2015). In mammals, linoleic acid (18:2n6; LNA) competes with ALA in this pathway to form arachidonic acid (20:4n6) (Tu et al., 2010). Results by Emery and coworkers suggest that this is not the case in rainbow trout (Emery et al., 2013). Furthermore, delta 6 desaturase activity appears to not be rate limiting to LCn3 synthesis in rainbow trout unlike mammals. (Cleveland et al., 2012).

In addition to LCn3 conversion, ALA has other metabolic pools, namely storage in glycerolipids (triacylglycerides and phospholipids), beta-oxidation for ATP and carbon sources (Barcelo-Coblijn and Murphy, 2009). In rainbow trout, a substantial portion (58%) of ALA is stored, and approximately 30% undergoes beta-oxidation (Turchini and Francis, 2009a). In mammals, ALA conversion to LCn3 is estimated to be >1% (Barcelo-Coblijn and Murphy, 2009). In contrast, conversion of ALA to LCn3 in rainbow trout is estimated to be between 12 and 25% but only about 6% in Atlantic cod (*Gaddus gaddus*) (Hixson et al., 2014c; Turchini et al., 2009b). The reasons for this elevated conversion level are not clear. The variation in these metabolic pools perhaps may be exploited through breeding strategies to enhance LCn3 synthesis.

Other efforts are being focused upon selection of traits allowing for increased formation of LCn3 or deposition of LCn3 into muscle. Research by Overturf and coworkers shows that genetic variation exists between rainbow trout families in their ability to accrete LCn3 (Overturf et al., 2013). Other data by Picklo and coworkers suggest that mature, triploid female rainbow trout accrete higher levels of LCn3 and total fatty acids in fillets than female, diploid trout (Picklo et al., 2013). The basis for these variations, whether the result of altered distribution amongst metabolic pools or altered trafficking of LCn3 amongst tissues, is under investigation. The establishment of rainbow trout lines and mapping of the rainbow trout genome will assist in identifying means to increase LCn3 content in rainbow trout and other salmonids (Thorgaard et al., 2002).

When the lipid source of the diet consists of vegetable oils alone, farmed salmonids accumulate less than half of the levels of LCn3 fed on a fish oil-containing diet (Bell et al., 2005; Bell et al., 2003). Rather than providing growing fish until harvest with fish oil supplemented feed, use of fish oil is reduced by using a combination of vegetable oils (eg, canola, flaxseed, or soybean) and fish oil or by using a finishing diet process (Torstensen et al., 2008; Torstensen et al., 2005). In a finishing strategy, fish are fed initially with a diet that uses vegetable-based oil as a fat source for the majority of the time until post smolting. Three to five months prior to harvest, a second "finishing" diet is provided that contains significant amounts fish oil from which EPA and DHA are accreted in the flesh.

Research into finishing diet strategies indicate that the ability to accrete LCn3 in tissue depends on the type of oils used during the initial growth phase and length of the finishing diet prior to harvest. Research by Bell and coworkers demonstrated that feeding a fish oil finishing diet for 20 weeks increases LCn3 content in fillets of Atlantic salmon fed a 100% flaxseed oil or canola oil-based diet for 50 weeks prior (Bell et al., 2003). However, LCn3 content was still 20% less than salmon fed a fish oil diet. Furthermore, it was found that levels of linoleic acid (18:2n6) were higher in the plant oil fed fish perhaps as a result of reduced turnover of linoleic acid. Similar results are observed in rainbow trout (Thanuthong et al., 2011). Work by Codabaccus et al. (2011) indicates that a period of food restriction prior to implementing the finishing diet may enhance final LCn3 content in Atlantic salmon (Codabaccus et al., 2011). It has been estimated that the duration of the finishing diet should allow for doubling of the animal weight (Turchini et al., 2009b).

While the use of a finishing diet reduces the need for LCn3-containing fish oil, it does not eliminate its use and while the ratio of fish oil in fish feed has declined, this decline is greatly offset by the total increase in production (Naylor et al., 2009). The use of novel sources of LCn3-rich oil from algal and modified terrestrial, plant-based oils to replace fish oil is under investigation. While various species of algae are able to synthesize EPA and DHA, the use of algal-derived oils for large scale aquaculture is likely cost prohibitive (Shields and Lupatsch, 2012).

In an effort to increase LCn3 content in Atlantic salmon, Betancour and coworkers fed Atlantic salmon an EPA-enriched oil derived from transgenic *Camelina sativa* (Betancor et al., 2015). This *C. sativa* was genetically engineered with a series of microalgal genes resulting in the production of an oil that was 20% EPA and 11% ALA. In these studies, post smolt Atlantic salmon were fed a 7-week diet with lipid derived from either fish oil, high-ALA camelina oil, or high-EPA camelina oil. Resulting fillets from fish oil-fed salmon had twice the DHA content of the high-ALA or high-EPA camelina-fed groups while the high EPA-fed salmon had similar EPA and three fold higher EPA than the fish oil and ALA-fed groups, respectively. These data show that transgenic plant oils have the potential to replace fish oil as an LCn3 source in aquaculture.

The use of genetically-modified plants in fish feed can be controversial as reviewed by Sissener et al. (2011). Several concerns have been raised on the basis that there may be "harmful" interactions from novel expressed genes or that the transgenes may incorporate into the fish genome. Use of LCn3-rich oil derived from terrestrial sources limit these possibilities since the oil is extracted from the seeds separating out the protein and nucleic acids. In the high-EPA camelina oil experiments described above, the presence of camelina-based transgenes was not observed (Betancor et al., 2015).

LCn3 FROM AQUACULTURE TO HUMAN HEALTH

As would be expected, LCn3 from farm raised Atlantic salmon are bioavailable. Studies by Raatz and coworkers demonstrated that twice weekly consumption of 90 g of farmed raised Atlantic salmon, with resulting intakes of about 1000 mg each of EPA and DHA weekly, was sufficient to increase and saturate the plasma phospholipid fatty acid (PLFA) pool of DHA. Higher intakes (180 g and 270 g twice weekly) elevated the EPA content in PLFA (Raatz et al., 2013a).

The ability to customize the fatty acid content of fillets led to research investigating the relationship of fillet fatty acid composition and resulting health outcomes. In a study by Seierstad et al. (2005), patients with coronary heart disease were fed 700 g of salmon per week for 6 weeks. The salmon was grown on diets containing (1) fish oil, (2) fish oil and canola (50:50) or (3) 100% canola oil resulting in patients consuming 2.9 g, 1.5 g, or 0.5 g of LCn3 daily. Positive outcomes for inflammatory markers were observed only among individuals eating salmon raised with fish oil, but not the canola oil alone (Seierstad et al., 2005). Other studies performed in mice indicate that daily consumption of Atlantic salmon raised on soybean oil alone can lead to increases in metabolic syndrome and obesity (Alvheim et al., 2013; Midtbo et al., 2015; Midtbo et al., 2013). However, in one study, salmon was the only protein source and was fed as part of an existing obesogenic diet (Midtbo et al., 2013). None the less, these studies indicate that the LCn3 content of the fillet is critical to health outcomes.

There is concern among many that fat-soluble pollutants like dioxins and polychlorinated biphenyls (PCB) can accumulate in wild-caught oily fish or in farmed fish raised with fish oil in their diets throughout production or as a finishing diet. Data derived using farm-raised salmon and farm-raised rainbow trout demonstrate that reducing or eliminating fish oil (with replacement by flaxseed and canola oils) from the diet reduces levels of PCBs and dioxins (Bell et al., 2005; Bethune et al., 2006; Drew et al., 2007). However, LCn3 levels are also reduced. Such data suggest that use of terrestrial derived LCn3-rich oils in fish diets can yield farm raised fish with optimal fillet levels of LCn3 and reduced organic pollutants. Moreover, these data highlight the potential need for analysis of organic pollutants in terrestrial and marine-based oils.

While a majority of research regarding LCn3 enrichment is focused upon salmonids, leaner farmed fish like tilapia have the capacity to accrue LCn3. Tilapia production occurs in over 135 countries worldwide (FAO 2014). Studies by Teoh and coworkers indicate that LCn3 can be accumulated in whole Nile tilapia or red hybrid tilapia (Teoh et al., 2011). Other studies have shown that ALA-rich flaxseed oil can be used as a feed to increase the EPA and DHA content of tilapia fillets to 25 mg/g (2.5%) of the total lipid (Visentainer et al., 2005). Given the low fat content of the fillets (approx. 1%), the fillet itself is a relatively poor source of LCn3. Tilapia constitutes a large portion of aquaculture produced fish for commercial sale and is promoted for small shareholders in many communities, particularly in areas with limited protein sources and undernutrition (Dey et al., 2013; Kaliba et al., 2006). Determining the extent to which tilapia may be bred for higher fat content as well as higher LCn3 accumulation would be of potential benefit for health.

OTHER LIPID SOLUBLE NUTRIENTS

Carotenoids

The flesh of wild caught salmon and rainbow trout have a pink/orange color due to the presence of the carotenoids astaxanthin and canthaxanthin that are deposited in the muscle (Torrissen and Christiansen, 1995). In the wild, these pigments are obtained through the food chain (Torrissen and Christiansen, 1995). Given consumer desire for fillets with optimal visual color qualities, astaxanthin, and canthaxanthin are added to feeds of aquaculture-derived Atlantic salmon and rainbow trout (Torrissen, 1996). Some data indicate that these carotenoids can have beneficial biological activity; however, the levels present in the fillet cannot be an appreciable source of these carotenoids in the human diet (Brizio et al., 2013). Other carotenoids such as β-carotene, lutein, and zeaxanthin are associated with eye health (SanGiovanni and Neuringer, 2012). However, these carotenoids are not appreciably absorbed by salmonids (Schiedt et al., 1985). Lutein and zeaxanthin are absorbed by catfish and the use of lutein-containing corn-based feeds can cause a yellow coloration in farmed catfish *Ictalurus punctatus* (Li et al., 2011; Li et al., 2007). Again, however, even with lutein-rich feed, the fillets do not contain appreciable amounts of these carotenoids (>120 μg/100g fillet) compared to the mg/serving quantities found in several vegetables (Li et al., 2011; USDA, 2015).

Vitamin D

Vitamin D is a nutrient necessary for optimal bone health and a growing literature demonstrates the role of vitamin D for prevention of other chronic diseases (Wacker and Holick, 2013). It is estimated that 30–50% of the population is vitamin D deficient and does not meet the recommended daily allowance of 600 IU for adults (IOM, 2011; Wacker and Holick, 2013).

Vitamin D (as vitamin D3 or vitamin D2) is not synthesized in fish but is accumulated through the food chain from initial synthesis in plankton (Lock et al., 2010). Analogous to other vertebrates, vitamin D has essential functions in fish. That vitamin D is fat soluble and stored in adipose suggests that fish can be a dietary source of vitamin D.

The USDA National Nutrient Database lists the vitamin D content of numerous fish and many commercially available fish have >400 IU vitamin D per 3 oz. portion; however, designations as wild versus farmed are not often apparent and farmed Atlantic salmon is not listed (USDA, 2015) (Lock et al., 2010). In one study of commercially available fish, vitamin D content in wild caught fish flesh ranged from 988 IU/3.5 oz. in wild salmon (species not reported) to 404 IU/3.5 oz. in Ahi tuna, to 104 IU/3.5 oz. in cod (Lu et al., 2007). On the other hand, farmed salmon (species not reported) had a vitamin D content of 240 IU/3.5 oz. Furthermore, there exists considerable intersample variation (>50% in many cases) in vitamin D content (Lu et al., 2007). The reason for this variation, observed in this study and others, has not been explained and requires further research.

Limited studies exist regarding maximizing vitamin D content in farmed fish. Data by Matilla and coworkers demonstrates that vitamin D content in the muscle of mature farmed rainbow trout is saturable and does not increase following 4 month of feeding of diets with elevated vitamin D content (Mattila et al., 1999). It is not known whether vitamin D accumulation in the intramuscular lipids is age-dependent. Data derived from juvenile farmed Atlantic salmon suggest vitamin D can accumulate in these depots (Graff et al., 2002).

That farmed salmon may have less vitamin D than wild caught salmon is the likely function of the amount of vitamin D present in the feed. Recommendations of optimal vitamin D content in fish feed for various species of fish are known (Lock et al., 2010). However, these recommendations are for the adequate growth of the fish, not for optimal vitamin D levels for subsequent human consumption. Subsequent data are needed to determine the extent to which and the processes under which vitamin D can be elevated in farmed fish (Atlantic salmon, rainbow trout, tilapia, or catfish) and the cost-effectiveness of enriching the fish diet with vitamin D.

CONCLUSIONS

Seafood derived from aquaculture plays an important role in supplying nutrients for optimal human health. Data show that the LCn3 content of oily fish is a major contributor to its health benefits. The extent to which the LCn3 content in oily fish can be maximized in the face of a decline of fish oil in the fish diets needs more research, but LCn3-enriched oils from transgenic plants offer an alternative. The extent to which other lipid soluble vitamins like vitamin D can be enhanced for human nutritional needs remains to be explored.

Acknowledgments

This material is based upon work that is supported by the National Institute of Food and Agriculture, United States Department of Agriculture, under award number 2014-67017-21758 and through USDA-ARS project 5450-51000-048-00D. Any opinions, findings, conclusions, or recommendations expressed in this publication are those of the author(s) and do not necessarily reflect the view of the United States Department of Agriculture. The United States Department of Agriculture, Agricultural Research Service, Plains Area is an equal opportunity/affirmative action employers and all agency services are available without discrimination. Mention of trade names or commercial products in this article is solely for providing specific information and does not imply recommendation or endorsement by the United States Department of Agriculture.

References

Alvheim, A.R., Torstensen, B.E., Lin, Y.H., Lillefosse, H.H., Lock, E.J., Madsen, L., Hibbeln, J.R., Malde, M.K., 2013. Dietary linoleic acid elevates endogenous 2-arachidonoylglycerol and anandamide in Atlantic salmon (*Salmo salar* L.) and mice, and induces weight gain and inflammation in mice. Br. J. Nutr. 109, 1508–1517.

Barcelo-Coblijn, G., Murphy, E.J., 2009. Alpha-linolenic acid and its conversion to longer chain n-3 fatty acids: benefits for human health and a role in maintaining tissue n-3 fatty acid levels. Prog. Lipid Res. 48, 355–374.

Bell, J.G., Henderson, R.J., Tocher, D.R., Sargent, J.R., 2004. Replacement of dietary fish oil with increasing levels of linseed oil: modification of flesh fatty acid compositions in Atlantic salmon (*Salmo salar*) using a fish oil finishing diet. Lipids 39, 223–232.

Bell, J.G., McGhee, F., Dick, J.R., Tocher, D.R., 2005. Dioxin and dioxin-like polychlorinated biphenyls (PCBs) in Scottish farmed salmon (*Salmo salar*): effects of replacement of dietary marine fish oil with vegetable oils. Aquaculture 243, 305–314.

Bell, J.G., Tocher, D.R., Henderson, R.J., Dick, J.R., Crampton, V.O., 2003. Altered fatty acid compositions in atlantic salmon (*Salmo salar*) fed diets containing linseed and rapeseed oils can be partially restored by a subsequent fish oil finishing diet. J. Nutr. 133, 2793–2801.

Betancor, M., Sprague, M., Usher, S., Sayanova, O., Campbell, P., Napier, J.A., Tocher, D.R., 2015. A nutritionally-enhanced oil from transgenic *Camelina sativa* effectively replaces fish oil as a source of eicosapentaenoic acid for fish. Scientif. Rep. 5, 1–10.

Bethune, C., Seierstad, S.L., Seljeflot, I., Johansen, O., Arnesen, H., Meltzer, H.M., Rosenlund, G., Froyland, L., Lundebye, A.K., 2006. Dietary intake of differently fed salmon: a preliminary study on contaminants. Eur. J. Clin. Invest. 36, 193–201.

Bibus, D.M., 2015. Long-chain omega-3 from low-trophic-level fish provides value to farmed seafood. Lipid Tech. 27, 55–58.

Brenna, J.T., Carlson, S.E., 2014. Docosahexaenoic acid and human brain development: evidence that a dietary supply is needed for optimal development. J. Hum. Evol. 77, 99–106.

Brizio, P., Benedetto, A., Righetti, M., Prearo, M., Gasco, L., Squadrone, S., Abete, M.C., 2013. Astaxanthin and Canthaxanthin (Xanthophyll) as Supplements in Rainbow Trout Diet: In Vivo Assessment of Residual Levels and Contributions to Human Health. J. Ag. Food Chem. 61, 10954–10959.

Bruford, M.W., Bradley, D.G., Luikart, G., 2003. DNA markers reveal the complexity of livestock domestication. Nature Rev. Genet. 4, 900–910.

Byelashov, O.A., Griffin, M.E., 2014. Fish In, fish out: perception of sustainability and contribution to public health. Fisheries 39, 531–535.

Chauton, M.S., Reitan, K.I., Norsker, N.H., Tveterås, R., Kleivdal, H.T., 2015. A techno-economic analysis of industrial production of marine microalgae as a source of EPA and DHA-rich raw material for aquafeed: research challenges and possibilities. Aquaculture 436, 95–103.

Cleveland, B.J., Francis, D.S., Turchini, G.M., 2012. Echium oil provides no benefit over linseed oil for (n-3) long-chain PUFA biosynthesis in rainbow trout. J. Nutr. 142, 1449–1455.

Codabaccus, M.B., Bridle, A.R., Nichols, P.D., Carter, C.G., 2011. Restoration of fillet n-3 long-chain polyunsaturated fatty acid is improved by a modified fish oil finishing diet strategy for Atlantic salmon (*Salmo salar* L.) smolts fed palm fatty acid distillate. J. Ag. Food Chem. 60, 458–466.

Deutsch, L., Gräslund, S., Folke, C., Troell, M., Huitric, M., Kautsky, N., Lebel, L., 2007. Feeding aquaculture growth through globalization: exploitation of marine ecosystems for fishmeal. Global Environ. Change 17, 238–249.

Dey, M.M., Spielman, D.J., Haque, A.M., Rahman, M., Valmonte-Santos, R., 2013. Change and diversity in smallholder rice–fish systems: recent evidence and policy lessons from Bangladesh. Food Pol. 43, 108–117.

Drew, M.D., Ogunkoya, A.E., Janz, D.M., Van Kessel, A.G., 2007. Dietary influence of replacing fish meal and oil with canola protein concentrate and vegetable oils on growth performance, fatty acid composition and organochlorine residues in rainbow trout (*Oncorhynchus mykiss*). Aquaculture 267, 260–268.

Dunstan, G., Volkman, J., Jeffrey, S., Barrett, S., 1992. Biochemical composition of microalgae from the green algal classes Chlorophyceae and Prasinophyceae. 2. Lipid classes and fatty acids. J. Exp. Marine Biol. Ecol. 161, 115–134.

Emery, J.A., Hermon, K., Hamid, N.K., Donald, J.A., Turchini, G.M., 2013. Δ-6 Desaturase substrate competition: dietary linoleic acid (18: 2n-6) has only trivial effects on α-linolenic acid (18: 3n-3) bioconversion in the teleost rainbow trout. PloS One 8, e57463.

FAO, 2014. The State of the World Fisheries and Aquaculture. Food and Agriculture Organization of the United Nations, Rome.

FAO, 2015. Cultured Aquatic Species Information Programme (Online). http://www.fao.org/fishery/culturedspecies/search/en.

Giri, S.S., Graham, J., Hamid, N.K., Donald, J.A., Turchini, G.M., 2015. Dietary micronutrients and in vivo n– 3 LC-PUFA biosynthesis in Atlantic salmon. Aquaculture.

Graff, I., Waagbø, R., Fivelstad, S., Vermeer, C., Lie, Ø., Lundebye, A., 2002. A multivariate study on the effects of dietary vitamin K, vitamin D3 and calcium, and dissolved carbon dioxide on growth, bone minerals, vitamin status and health performance in smolting Atlantic salmon *Salmo salar* L. J. Fish Dis. 25, 599–614.

Gregory, M.K., James, M.J., 2014. Rainbow trout (*Oncorhynchus mykiss*) Elovl5 and Elovl2 differ in selectivity for elongation of omega-3 docosapentaenoic acid. Biochem. Biophys. Acta 1841, 1656–1660.

Hixson, S.M., Parrish, C.C., Anderson, D.M., 2014a. Changes in tissue lipid and fatty acid composition of farmed rainbow trout in response to dietary camelina oil as a replacement of fish oil. Lipids 49, 97–111.

Hixson, S.M., Parrish, C.C., Anderson, D.M., 2014b. Full substitution of fish oil with camelina (*Camelina sativa*) oil, with partial substitution of fish meal with camelina meal, in diets for farmed Atlantic salmon (*Salmo salar*) and its effect on tissue lipids and sensory quality. Food Chem. 157, 51–61.

Hixson, S.M., Parrish, C.C., Anderson, D.M., 2014c. Use of camelina oil to replace fish oil in diets for farmed salmonids and Atlantic cod. Aquaculture 431, 44–52.

HLPE, 2014. High Level Panel of Experts - Sustainable fisheries and aquaculture for food security and nutrition. Summary and recommendations. Food and Agriculture Organization of the United Nations. Rome, Italy.

IOM, 2011. DRI Dietary Reference Intakes: Calcium Vitamin D Institute of Medicine. The National Academies Press, Washington, D.C.

Kaliba, A.R., Osewe, K.O., Senkondo, E.M., Mnembuka, B.V., Quagrainie, K.K., 2006. Economic analysis of Nile tilapia (*Oreochromis niloticus*) production in Tanzania. J. World. Aquacult. Soc. 37, 464–473.

Kawarazuka, N., Béné, C., 2011. The potential role of small fish species in improving micronutrient deficiencies in developing countries: building evidence. Public Health Nutr. 14, 1927–1938.

Khan, M., Khan, S., Miyan, K., 2011. Aquaculture as a food production system: a review. Biol. Med. 3, 291–302.

Li, M.H., Robinson, E.H., Oberle, D.F., Lucas, P.M., Peterson, B.C., Bates, T.D., 2011. Clearance of yellow pigments lutein and zeathanxin in channel catfish, Ictalurus punctatus, reared at different water temperatures. J. World Aquacult. Soc. 42, 105–110.

Li, M.H., Robinson, E.H., Oberle, D.F., Zimba, P.V., 2007. Effects of various dietary carotenoid pigments on fillet appearance and pigment absorption in channel catfish, *Ictalurus punctatus*. J. World Aquacult. Soc. 38, 557–563.

Liland, N., Rosenlund, G., Berntssen, M., Brattelid, T., Madsen, L., Torstensen, B., 2013. Net production of Atlantic salmon (FIFO, Fish in Fish out < 1) with dietary plant proteins and vegetable oils. Aquacult. Nutr. 19, 289–300.

Lock, E.J., Waagbø, R., Wendelaar Bonga, S., Flik, G., 2010. The significance of vitamin D for fish: a review. Aquacult. Nutr. 16, 100–116.

Lu, Z., Chen, T., Zhang, A., Persons, K., Kohn, N., Berkowitz, R., Martinello, S., Holick, M., 2007. An evaluation of the vitamin D 3 content in fish: is the vitamin D content adequate to satisfy the dietary requirement for vitamin D? J. Steroid Biochem. Mol. Biol. 103, 642–644.

Mattila, P., Piironen, V., Hakkarainen, T., Hirvi, T., Uusi-Rauva, E., Eskelinen, P., 1999. Possibilities to raise vitamin D content of rainbow trout (Oncorhynchus mykiss) by elevated feed cholecalciferol contents. J. Sci. Food Ag. 79, 195–198.

McNamara, R.K., Vannest, J.J., Valentine, C.J., 2015. Role of perinatal long-chain omega-3 fatty acids in cortical circuit maturation: mechanisms and implications for psychopathology. World J. Psychiatry 5, 15–34.

Midtbo, L.K., Borkowska, A.G., Bernhard, A., Ronnevik, A.K., Lock, E.J., Fitzgerald, M.L., Torstensen, B.E., Liaset, B., Brattelid, T., Pedersen, T.L., Newman, J.W., Kristiansen, K., Madsen, L., 2015. Intake of farmed Atlantic salmon fed soybean oil increases hepatic levels of arachidonic acid-derived oxylipins and ceramides in mice. J. Nutr. Biochem. 26, 585–595.

Midtbo, L.K., Ibrahim, M.M., Myrmel, L.S., Aune, U.L., Alvheim, A.R., Liland, N.S., Torstensen, B.E., Rosenlund, G., Liaset, B., Brattelid, T., Kristiansen, K., Madsen, L., 2013. Intake of farmed Atlantic salmon fed soybean oil increases insulin resistance and hepatic lipid accumulation in mice. PloS One 8, e53094.

Miller, M.R., Nichols, P.D., Carter, C.G., 2008. n-3 Oil sources for use in aquaculture–alternatives to the unsustainable harvest of wild fish. Nutr. Res. Rev. 21, 85–96.

Mozaffarian, D., Rimm, E.B., 2006. Fish intake, contaminants, and human health: evaluating the risks and the benefits. JAMA 296, 1885–1899.

Mozaffarian, D., Wu, J.H., 2012. (n-3) fatty acids and cardiovascular health: are effects of EPA and DHA shared or complementary? J. Nutr. 142, 614S–625S.

Naderi, S., Rezaei, H.-R., Pompanon, F., Blum, M.G., Negrini, R., Naghash, H.-R., Balkız, Ö., Mashkour, M., Gaggiotti, O.E., Ajmone-Marsan, P., 2008. The goat domestication process inferred from large-scale mitochondrial DNA analysis of wild and domestic individuals. Proc. Nat. Acad. Sci. 105, 17659–17664.

Naylor, R.L., Hardy, R.W., Bureau, D.P., Chiu, A., Elliott, M., Farrell, A.P., Forster, I., Gatlin, D.M., Goldburg, R.J., Hua, K., 2009. Feeding aquaculture in an era of finite resources. Proc. Nat. Acad. Sci. 106, 15103–15110.
Overturf, K., Welker, T., Barrows, F., Towner, R., Schneider, R., LaPatra, S., 2013. Variation in rainbow trout, *Oncorhynchus mykiss*, to biosynthesize eicosapentaenoic acid and docosahexaenoic acid when reared on plant oil replacement feeds. J. World Aquacult. Soci. 44, 326–337.
Picklo, M.J., Raatz, S.K., Cleveland, B., Rexroad, III, C., 2013. Evaluation of long-chain n3 fatty acid content in diploid and triploid rainbow trout. FASEB J. 27, 1079.1015.
Pinstrup-Andersen, P., Pandya-Lorch, R., 1998. Food security and sustainable use of natural resources: a 2020 vision. Ecol. Econ. 26, 1–10.
Raatz, S.K., Rosenberger, T.A., Johnson, L.K., Wolters, W.W., Burr, G.S., Picklo, Sr., M.J., 2013a. Dose-dependent consumption of farmed atlantic salmon (*Salmo salar*) increases plasma phospholipid n-3 fatty acids differentially. J. Acad. Nutr. Diet 113, 282–287.
Raatz, S.K., Silverstein, J.T., Jahns, L., Picklo, M.J., 2013b. Issues of fish consumption for cardiovascular disease risk reduction. Nutrients 5, 1081–1097.
SanGiovanni, J.P., Neuringer, M., 2012. The putative role of lutein and zeaxanthin as protective agents against age-related macular degeneration: promise of molecular genetics for guiding mechanistic and translational research in the field. Am. J. Clin. Nutr. 96, 1223S–1233S.
Sarker, P.K., Bureau, D.P., Hua, K., Drew, M.D., Forster, I., Were, K., Hicks, B., Vandenberg, G.W., 2013. Sustainability issues related to feeding salmonids: a Canadian perspective. Rev. Aquacult. 5, 199–219.
Schiedt, K., Leuenberger, F., Vecchi, M., Glinz, E., 1985. Absorption, retention and metabolic transformations of carotenoids in rainbow trout, salmon and chicken. Pure Appl. Chem. 57, 685–692.
Scholtz, S.A., Colombo, J., Carlson, S.E., 2013. Clinical overview of effects of dietary long-chain polyunsaturated fatty acids during the perinatal period. Nestle Nutr. Inst. Workshop Ser. 77, 145–154.
Seierstad, S.L., Seljeflot, I., Johansen, O., Hansen, R., Haugen, M., Rosenlund, G., Froyland, L., Arnesen, H., 2005. Dietary intake of differently fed salmon; the influence on markers of human atherosclerosis. Eur. J. Clin. Invest. 35, 52–59.
Serhan, C.N., Chiang, N., 2008. Endogenous pro-resolving and anti-inflammatory lipid mediators: a new pharmacologic genus. Br. J. Pharmacol. 153, S200–215.
Shepherd, J., Bachis, E., 2014. Changing supply and demand for fish oil. Aquacult. Econ. Manage 18, 395–416.
Shields, R.J., Lupatsch, I., 2012. Algae for aquaculture and animal feeds. J. Anim. Sci. 21, 23–37.
Sissener, N.H., Sanden, M., Krogdahl, Å., Bakke, A.-M., Johannessen, L.E., Hemre, G.-I., 2011. Genetically modified plants as fish feed ingredients. Can. J. Fisheries Aquatic Sci. 68, 563–574.
Stone, D., Oliveira, A., Plante, S., Smiley, S., Bechtel, P., Hardy, R., 2011. Enhancing highly unsaturated ω-3 fatty acids in phase-fed rainbow trout (*Oncorhynchus mykiss*) using Alaskan fish oils. Aquacult Nutr. 17, e501–e510.
Tacon, A.G., Metian, M., 2008. Global overview on the use of fish meal and fish oil in industrially compounded aquafeeds: trends and future prospects. Aquaculture 285, 146–158.
Teletchea, F., Fontaine, P., 2014. Levels of domestication in fish: implications for the sustainable future of aquaculture. Fish Fisher. 15, 181–195.
Teoh, C.-Y., Turchini, G.M., Ng, W.-K., 2011. Genetically improved farmed Nile tilapia and red hybrid tilapia showed differences in fatty acid metabolism when fed diets with added fish oil or a vegetable oil blend. Aquaculture 312, 126–136.
Thanuthong, T., Francis, D.S., Senadheera, S.D., Jones, P.L., Turchini, G.M., 2011. Fish oil replacement in rainbow trout diets and total dietary PUFA content: I) Effects on feed efficiency, fat deposition and the efficiency of a finishing strategy. Aquaculture 320, 82–90.
Thorgaard, G.H., Bailey, G.S., Williams, D., Buhler, D.R., Kaattari, S.L., Ristow, S.S., Hansen, J.D., Winton, J.R., Bartholomew, J.L., Nagler, J.J., 2002. Status and opportunities for genomics research with rainbow trout. Compar. Biochem. Physiol. B 133, 609–646.
Torrissen, O., 1996. Effective use of carotenoids for salmon flesh pigmentation. Can. Feed Ind. Assoc.
Torrissen, O., Christiansen, R., 1995. Requirements for carotenoids in fish diets. J. Appl. Ichthyol. 11, 225–230.
Torstensen, B., Espe, M., Sanden, M., Stubhaug, I., Waagbø, R., Hemre, G.-I., Fontanillas, R., Nordgarden, U., Hevrøy, E., Olsvik, P., 2008. Novel production of Atlantic salmon (*Salmo salar*) protein based on combined replacement of fish meal and fish oil with plant meal and vegetable oil blends. Aquaculture 285, 193–200.
Torstensen, B.E., Bell, J.G., Rosenlund, G., Henderson, R.J., Graff, I.E., Tocher, D.R., Lie, Ø., Sargent, J.R., 2005. Tailoring of Atlantic salmon (*Salmo salar* L.) flesh lipid composition and sensory quality by replacing fish oil with a vegetable oil blend. J. Ag. Food Chem. 53, 10166–10178.
Tu, W.C., Cook-Johnson, R.J., James, M.J., Muhlhausler, B.S., Gibson, R.A., 2010. Omega-3 long chain fatty acid synthesis is regulated more by substrate levels than gene expression. Prost. Leuk. Essen. Fatty Acid. 83, 61–68.
Turchini, G.M., Francis, D.S., 2009a. Fatty acid metabolism (desaturation, elongation and β-oxidation) in rainbow trout fed fish oil-or linseed oil-based diets. Br. J. Nutr. 102, 69–81.
Turchini, G.M., Torstensen, B.E., Ng, W.K., 2009b. Fish oil replacement in finfish nutrition. Rev. Aquacult. 1, 10–57.
USDA. 2015. USDA National Nutrient Database for Standard Reference, Release 27 (Online). http://www.ars.usda.gov/ba/bhnrc/ndl
Visentainer, J.V., de Souza, N.E., Makoto, M., Hayashi, C., Franco, M.R.B., 2005. Influence of diets enriched with flaxseed oil on the α-linolenic, eicosapentaenoic and docosahexaenoic fatty acid in Nile tilapia (*Oreochromis niloticus*). Food. Chem. 90, 557–560.
Wacker, M., Holick, M.F., 2013. Vitamin D—effects on skeletal and extraskeletal health and the need for supplementation. Nutrients 5, 111–148.
Wijekoon, M.P., Parrish, C.C., Mansour, A., 2014. Effect of dietary substitution of fish oil with flaxseed or sunflower oil on muscle fatty acid composition in juvenile steelhead trout (*Oncorhynchus mykiss*) reared at varying temperatures. Aquaculture 433, 74–81.

CHAPTER

14

Fish and Fish Oil and the Metabolic Syndrome

C. Tørris

Department of Behavioural Sciences, Faculty of Health Sciences, Oslo and Akershus University of Applied Sciences, Oslo, Norway

METABOLIC SYNDROME

What is Metabolic Syndrome?

Metabolic syndrome (MetS) is a cluster of metabolic risk factors for cardiovascular disease (CVD) and type 2 diabetes mellitus (T2D). These risk factors include abdominal obesity, dyslipidemia, hypertension, and hyperglycemia (Alberti et al., 2009). The impact of MetS on public health is profound through the increased risk of morbidity and mortality (Alberti et al., 2005). MetS has been recognized as a major risk factor for several additional diseases such as common cancers (Bhandari et al., 2014; Esposito et al., 2012), and is associated with a doubling of CVD-risk (Cornier et al., 2008) and a fivefold increased risk for incident T2D (Cornier et al., 2008). Lately, MetS has been associated with nonalcoholic fatty liver disease (NAFLD) and with liver manifestations of steatosis, fibrosis and cirrhosis although, the mechanisms by which this occurs are not fully understood (Asrih and Jornayvaz, 2015). Inflammation is present in both MetS and NAFLD and insulin resistance seems to be a key factor that links MetS and NAFLD, promoting inflammation and endoplasmic reticulum stress (Asrih and Jornayvaz, 2015).

The clustering of different metabolic abnormalities in MetS has been known for several decades under different names such as Syndrome X, The Deadly Quartet, and The Insulin Resistance Syndrome (Kaur, 2014). Over the years, different definitions and diagnostic criteria have been proposed by various expert groups and organizations (Alberti et al., 2009) such as the National Cholesterol Education Program Adult Treatment Panel III (ATP III) (Expert Panel on Detection, 2001) and the International Diabetes Federation (IDF; Alberti et al., 2006). To standardize reporting in epidemiological and clinical research, the definitions have been harmonized in a joint interim statement (JIS; Alberti et al., 2009). Here a single set of cut points is used for all the components in the MetS, except for waist circumference where population- and country-specific definitions are given.

According to the JIS, MetS is diagnosed if any three of five risk factors are present: elevated waist circumference, elevated triglycerides, reduced HDL-cholesterol, elevated blood pressure, and elevated fasting glucose (Alberti et al., 2009). For waist circumference, different thresholds are recommended in different populations and ethnic groups. For people of European origin, the recommended cut points are ≥94 cm in men and ≥80 cm in women. However, higher thresholds (men ≥102 cm, women ≥88 cm) have been used in United States, Canada and Europe. Further, lower thresholds are used in Asia and among ethnic Central and South Americans (men ≥90 cm, women ≥80 cm) and among Middle East, Mediterranean, and Sub-Saharan Africans (men ≥94 cm, women ≥80 cm; Alberti et al., 2009). The other criteria used to diagnose MetS include triglycerides ≥150 mg/dL (1.7 mmol/L), fasting glucose ≥100 mg/dL (5.6 mmol/l), systolic blood pressure ≥130 and/or diastolic blood pressure ≥85 mm Hg. For HDL-cholesterol there are gender specific criteria: men <40 mg/dL (1.0 mmol/L) and women <50 mg/dL (1.3 mmol/L; Alberti et al., 2009). Drug treatment for elevated triglyceride, fasting glucose, HDL-cholesterol or antihypertensive drug treatment in a patient with history of hypertension is considered to be an alternate indicator (Alberti et al., 2009).

Fish and Fish Oil in Health and Disease Prevention. http://dx.doi.org/10.1016/B978-0-12-802844-5.00014-2

Prevalence and Incidence of Metabolic Syndrome

The prevalence of MetS varies by gender and ethnicity but is highly dependent on the definition(s) used (Beltran-Sanchez et al., 2013; Cornier et al., 2008). Prevalence seems to increase with age (Cho et al., 2011) and may range from 8% (Zaribaf et al., 2014) in young populations and up to 70% in elderly populations (Pasalic et al., 2011). In women, parity and an increasing number of children has been associated with higher rates of MetS (Cohen et al., 2006). However, lactation and especially longer duration of lactation may have favorable effects on metabolic risk profiles (Gunderson et al., 2010; Torris et al., 2013). Several studies have compared the prevalence of MetS among men and women, but the results are inconclusive. Some studies have seen a higher prevalence in men (Akter et al., 2013; Jung et al., 2011; Kouki et al., 2011), some in women (Fonseca et al., 2012; He et al., 2012), and some find no difference between men and women (Alvarez Leon et al., 2006; Hong et al., 2012; Pasalic et al., 2011). The use of different definitions of MetS may be responsible for the differences in prevalence rates, as the prevalence of MetS is higher when using the JIS definition (Athyros et al., 2010). In addition, different populations may also have real differences in the amount of abdominal fat which affects the occurrence of MetS (Alberti et al., 2009).

Nutritional Approaches and Metabolic Syndrome

A considerable amount of literature has been published on CVD and the benefits of fish consumption over the past decades (Panagiotakos et al., 2007a; Raatz et al., 2013), and there is an increased risk of CVD in populations with low or no intake of fish (Strom et al., 2012). Several studies have suggested an inverse relationship between consumption of fish and CVD, such as heart failure (Li et al., 2013), cerebrovascular disease (Chowdhury et al., 2012), ischemic stroke (Takata et al., 2013), and sudden coronary death risk (Streppel et al., 2008). The intake of fish is also linked to a decreased risk of T2D (Patel et al., 2009) and diabetes mortality (Takata et al., 2013). The benefits of fish intake are particularly associated with the consumption of fatty fish, high in n–3 fatty acids (Lee et al., 2009; Saravanan et al., 2010). Fatty fish such as salmon and mackerel are considered a valued source of n–3 fatty acids and vitamin D. Fatty fish is associated with prevention of CVD likely due to the high content of unsaturated fatty acids, especially n–3 fatty acids (Lee et al., 2009; Saravanan et al., 2010). Vitamin D may also play a role in the prevention of CVD, and has been associated with a lower risk of MetS (Fung et al., 2012). Several studies have investigated associations between fatty acids in fish, especially n–3 fatty acids, and MetS (Baik et al., 2010; Ebbesson et al., 2007; Noel et al., 2010; Pedersen et al., 2010). The evidence is however sparser when considering the health effects of lean fish, for example, cod, which also may contribute to a better cardiometabolic health.

Lifestyle habits and socioeconomic status (SES) appear to influence the prevalence of MetS across sex, age, and race/ethnicity (Cornier et al., 2008). Both dietary intake and lifestyle behaviors such as breakfast skipping (Shafiee et al., 2013) and increased eating speed (Zhu et al., 2015) may increase the risk of MetS. Positive associations have also been observed between MetS and diets high in processed foods such as refined grains, rice, potato chips, and pancakes (DiBello et al., 2009). Today lifestyle interventions remain the primary therapy for MetS and both diet and physical activity interventions are recommended in the management of the syndrome (Alberti et al., 2006). Dietary interventions may be the best way to treat MetS and specific foods such as fish, dietary fiber, and dark chocolate may have beneficial effects on MetS and therefore be important in treating the MetS (Potenza and Mechanick, 2009). Fish consumption (Tørris et al., 2014), the use of n–3 fatty acids (Potenza and Mechanick, 2009) and fish oil (Abete et al., 2011) may have a great impact in reversing the MetS.

FISH AND FISH OIL AND METABOLIC SYNDROME

Fish and Metabolic Syndrome

Fish contains a variety of different nutrients, which may have a protective role in the prevention of MetS (Lund, 2013; Potenza and Mechanick, 2009). However, few studies have investigated associations between consumption of fish and MetS. Recently a systematic review examined fish consumption and the development and prevalence of MetS (Tørris et al., 2014) suggested that fish consumption might have a protective role in MetS prevention. This protective role may however be related to sex, with men deriving benefit more from the consumption of fish than women (Tørris et al., 2014).

A Korean follow-up study investigated the effect of fish and n–3 fatty acid consumption on the incidence of MetS among Koreans (n = 3504, 40–69 years; Baik et al., 2010). MetS was defined by the ATP III definition (Grundy et al., 2005), except for waist circumference where alternative criteria were used (men ≥85 cm, women ≥80 cm;

Baik, 2009). Fish consumption was assessed through Food Frequency Questionnaires (FFQ) (<1/week, 1–4/week, 5–6/week and daily). They found that the average daily consumption of fish (40–70 g) reduced the risk of MetS compared with eating fish <1/week (OR 0.43, 95% CI 0.23–0.83). Associations were also found between components of MetS with lower triglyceride ($P < 0.01$) and elevated HDL-cholesterol ($P < 0.01$) among men. Consumption of n–3 polyunsaturated fatty acids (PUFA) was inversely associated with the risk of MetS, especially in those with a high consumption of n–3 PUFA (median 786 mg) compared to those with the lowest consumption (median 37 mg) (OR 0.53, 95% CI 0.28–0.99; Baik et al., 2010). Among women, no significant associations were observed (Baik et al., 2010).

A cross-sectional study from Finland investigated associations between consumption of selected food with the risk of MetS ($n = 1334$, 57–78 years; Kouki et al., 2011), defined by the ATP III definition (Expert Panel on Detection, 2001). Fish consumption was assessed with a four-day food record. An inverse association between consumption of fish and MetS was found for men only ($P = 0.001$; Kouki et al., 2011). Men in the highest (>59.5 g/day) and middle tertile (18.5–59.5 g/day) of fish consumption had 37% lower risk of having MetS, compared with those in the lowest tertile (<18.5 g/day; $P = 0.002$), when adjusting for age, smoking, and alcohol (Kouki et al., 2011).

A cross-sectional study from France investigated the relationship between various food groups and the frequency of insulin resistance syndrome (IRS) among men ($n = 912$, 45–64 years; Ruidavets et al., 2007) using the ATP III definition for MetS (Expert Panel on Detection, 2001). This population consisted only of men (45–64 years) who were randomly selected from three regions in France. The consumption of fish (gram/day) in this study included sea fish, river fish, and seafood, assessed with a 3-day food record. A negative association between IRS and fish consumption was found, with a 43% lower prevalence of IRS among those in the highest versus lowest tertile of fish consumption (OR 0.57, 95% CI 0.38–0.86; Ruidavets et al., 2007).

In Iran, a cross-sectional study found an association between fish consumption and MetS prevalence (Zaribaf et al., 2014). The study population consisted of 420 female nurses randomly selected from various hospitals in Iran (age = >30 years). MetS was defined according to the JIS definition and fish consumption was determined using a FFQ. The summation of fish consumption was calculated based on tertile cutpoints of energy-adjusted fish intake. They found that women in the highest tertile of fish intake were less likely to have the MetS compared with those in the lowest tertile (OR 0.35 95% CI 0.14–0.88; Zaribaf et al., 2014).

Dietary Patterns Containing Fish and Metabolic Syndrome

Several studies have investigated associations between a dietary pattern containing fish and MetS. In follow-up studies, diets containing fish, "healthy diets", and the Mediterranean diet (MedDiet) have been associated with reduced incidence of MetS (Baik et al., 2013; Di Daniele et al., 2013; Kesse-Guyot et al., 2013). Associations between a diet containing fish and MetS have also been seen in crosssectional studies investigating a Healthy Diet (Cho et al., 2011; Kim and Jo, 2011), MedDiet (Babio et al., 2009b), and a n–3 fatty acid/fish pattern (Noel et al., 2010). However, not all studies find associations between dietary pattern containing fish and MetS (Lutsey et al., 2008).

Studies evaluating dietary patterns may not give the expected result. When different healthy foods are consumed together, there may be an additive effect. These additive effects have been seen when fish was consumed with legumes, nuts, and berries (Pasalic et al., 2011), dairy products and grain (Ruidavets et al., 2007), and in dietary patterns containing fish such as a Healthy Diet (Baik et al., 2010) and the Med Diet (Di Daniele et al., 2013; Kesse-Guyot et al., 2013). When dietary patterns are examined, the effects of dietary exposure may be captured. These effects may be lost when evaluating a single nutrient or food. However, the use of dietary patterns may also hide positive effects when dietary intake is summarized into categories or patterns. Different food or food groups may also work against each other, such as when healthy food is placed in the same group as other foods. An example of the latter is when fish is placed in the same category as processed meat and mayonnaise (Akter et al., 2013). Further, the effects of higher fish consumption may be associated with a healthier lifestyle, whereas other factors may affect the results negatively. The preparation of food may affect the results, and positive health effects may diminish or vanish depending on how the meal is prepared. This has been demonstrated with fried fish in studies concerning CVD (Mozaffarian et al., 2003) and T2D (Patel et al., 2009).

Fish and Components of Metabolic Syndrome

Some studies have found associations between consumption of fish and components of MetS. In intervention studies, consumption of fish has been associated both with a decrease in waist circumference (Thorsdottir et al., 2007) and reduced blood pressure level (Erkkila et al., 2008; Ramel et al., 2010). A lower waist circumference has also been associated with a higher adherence to MedDiet, high in fish and seafood, in a large cross-sectional study of 10 European countries (Romaguera et al., 2009).

In participants with a high consumption of fish compared with those with no fish intake, a decrease in blood pressure and triglyceride and an increase in HDL-cholesterol was observed among adult Eskimos with a high consumption of omega-3 fatty acids from fish and marine mammals (Ebbesson et al., 2007). This was also observed among women in the Iranian study with a significant inverse association with high triglyceride (OR 0.11 95% CI 0.01–0.85), low HDL-cholesterol (OR 0.57; 95% CI 0.19–0.89) and elevated blood pressure (OR 0.23 95% CI 0.14–0.89) (Zaribaf et al., 2014). Improved HDL-cholesterol was also found in a randomized clinical trial (RCT) where participants with MetS were fed a Healthy Nordic diet, consisting of three meals fish per week (two fatty fish meals + one low-fat fish meal; Uusitupa et al., 2013).

In elderly populations, inverse associations between the consumption of fish and triglyceride, systolic blood pressure, and glucose (Panagiotakos et al., 2007b), and a positive association with HDL-cholesterol (Pasalic et al., 2011) were observed.

Gender Differences

In women, parity and an increasing number of children have been associated with higher rates of MetS (Cohen et al., 2006) which, in turn, may lead to problems in later pregnancy and labor. However, lactation, particularly a longer duration of lactation, may have favorable effects on metabolic risk profiles (Gunderson et al., 2010; Torris et al., 2013) due to the metabolic burden lactation imposed on the mother (Butte and King, 2005; Butte et al., 2001). Changes that occur during pregnancy (visceral fat accumulation, insulin resistance, and increased lipid levels; Einstein et al., 2008; Stuebe and Rich-Edwards, 2009) may therefore be reversed more quickly and more completely with lactation.

In the review of Tørris et al. (2014), several of the studies found associations between fish consumption and MetS only among men (Baik et al., 2010; Kouki et al., 2011; Ruidavets et al., 2007). In a prospective study from Korea (Baik et al., 2010), associations between a high consumption of fish and n–3 fatty acids and a lower risk of MetS was found among men, but not among women. Those with frequent fish consumption were more likely to be younger and better educated. The included participants consisted of men and women without MetS at baseline (52% men; Baik et al., 2010). Over the three-year follow-up period, 9.9% of men and 7.3% of women were newly identified with MetS (Baik et al., 2010). Of the crosssectional studies investigating fish consumption and MetS prevalence, associations between fish consumption and MetS were seen among men in two studies (Kouki et al., 2011; Ruidavets et al., 2007) and among women in one study (Zaribaf et al., 2014). In a Finnish study, both men and women with MetS reported a lower fish consumption than those without MetS (Kouki et al., 2011). However, significant associations were found only among men, where those in the highest tertile of fish consumption had almost half the risk of having MetS compared to those in the lowest third ($P = 0.002$) (Kouki et al., 2011). In a French study, where only men were included, they found that a high consumption of fish was associated with a lower probability of presenting with an IRS (Ruidavets et al., 2007). Further, that the risk of developing IRS was twice as high among men with fish consumption below the median value (33 g/day), versus those above median value (OR 0.51, 95% CI 0.36–0.71; Ruidavets et al., 2007). Only the Iranian study found associations among women; however, they included only women (Zaribaf et al., 2014). In this study, they found that high fish consumption was inversely associated with MetS (Zaribaf et al., 2014).

This lack of significant findings in women is surprising. The protective role of fish consumption might be related to gender, where it may seem like men benefit more from the consumption of fish than women do (Tørris et al., 2014). However, in the review of Tørris et al. (2014), none of the included studies adjusted for parity or length of lactation in women, which might have resulted in differences in the results among women. This is because prolonged lactation may be associated with a healthier metabolic profile and body composition, especially lipid levels and waist-to-hip ratios (Torris et al., 2013), though few studies have investigated these associations.

Gender differences with significant associations only in men have also been found in studies investigating associations between dietary patterns containing fish and MetS (Babio et al., 2009a; Thorsdottir et al., 2007). Although these associations have been observed in women, they were only significant among postmenopausal women (OR 0.60, 95% CI 0.40–0.86) for highest versus lowest quartile of a healthy dietary pattern containing fish (Cho et al., 2011). This may suggest that gender differences last until menopause and that premenopausal woman might have a natural protection against MetS. This may be related to the premenopausal women's higher estrogen levels, and to the ability of estrogens to decrease inflammation and reduce the glucocorticoid response (Alemany, 2012). Inflammatory responses are a common factor in MetS, and this inflammatory response appears to be supported by tissue malfunction and homeostatic imbalance (Scrivo et al., 2011). Adipokines and a number of bioactive peptides or proteins are fundamental in the pathogenesis of the MetS through their role in energy and vascular homeostasis, and immunity, and may modulate insulin sensitivity, cardiovascular homeostasis, inflammation, and fat mass (Maury and Brichard, 2010).

Fatty or Lean Fish

Fatty and lean fish differ in the amount of fat in their body tissues; still both lean and fatty fish may have a protective role in the prevention of MetS. Many studies have focused only on single components in marine nutrients, such as n–3 fatty acids (Robinson et al., 2007; Robinson and Mazurak, 2013). In an intervention study from Iceland where they investigated cod consumption, weight loss and CVD-risk factors, a reduced MetS prevalence was observed with increased intake. However, neither blood lipids nor glucose was affected by the consumption of cod. The decrease in waist circumference was greater among the cod consuming groups compared to the control group (Ramel et al., 2009). In a Spanish intervention study investigating the effect of lean fish (100 g/day of Namibian hake) on CVD-risk factors in patients with MetS, they found that seven servings of hake per week reduced both waist circumference and diastolic blood pressure (Vazquez et al., 2014). Lean fish is considered a superior source of protein which may be associated with reduction in body weight through its positive effect on satiety (Uhe et al., 1992). The proteins in fish are easily digestible and rich in essential amino acids.

Association between consumption of fish and the incidence of MetS, may be driven by the concentrations of triglyceride and HDL-cholesterol (Baik et al., 2010). A short-term intake of both lean and fatty fish has been observed to decrease triglyceride concentrations (Telle-Hansen et al., 2012). Increased HDL-cholesterol levels have also been observed after participants received fatty fish (salmon; Telle-Hansen et al., 2012). Dietary proteins regulate lipid metabolism, promote lipid excretion, and slow absorption and synthesis of lipids (El Khoury and Anderson, 2013). Proteins from fish have been shown to exert hypocholesterolemic activity in animal studies (El Khoury and Anderson, 2013). Fish protein may have multiple effects on plasma and liver lipids, however a HDL-lowering effect is observed with fish protein feeding in animal studies (Shukla et al., 2006). Nevertheless, beneficial effects on both hyperglycemia (Madani et al., 2012) and hyperlipidemia (Aadland et al., 2015) is observed. Further, improved insulin sensitivity in insulin resistant men and women was observed when consuming proteins from cod, compared to other animal proteins (Ouellet et al., 2007). Decreased blood pressure was associated with consumption of lean (Erkkila et al., 2008), and fatty fish (salmon; Ramel et al., 2010).

Fish Oil and Metabolic Syndrome

Long chain n–3 fatty acids may be beneficial in the treatment of conditions with an inflammatory component, such as MetS (Calder, 2006). The marine n–3 fatty acids eicosapentaenoic acid (EPA) and docosahexaenoic acid (DHA) are present mainly in fatty fish (Saravanan et al., 2010). Fish oil supplements are becoming increasingly popular, with several health benefits attributed to them (Saravanan et al., 2010), and the use of n–3 fatty acids is considered a valuable clinical tool for the treatment of hypertriglyceridemia (Davidson, 2006).

Consumption of fish oil, especially DHA, is favorably associated with HDL-metabolism (Yanai et al., 2015), and fish oil is a useful supplement to reduce triglyceride concentrations (Lewis et al., 2004). A reduction in triglyceride (56 %) was seen in rats given fish oil (Barrios-Ramos et al., 2012). Intervention studies have observed both reduced triglycerides and increased HDL-cholesterol ($P = 0.01$) in participants with early-stage T2D or MetS (Lee et al., 2014), as well as a reduction in triglycerides (P, 0.05) in overweight premenopausal women receiving fish oil (Dunn et al., 2014). However, the latter study was a lifestyle intervention where the women received Med Diet advice and high-intensity exercise, in addition to a daily n–3 supplementation (Dunn et al., 2014). There was an increase of HDL-cholesterol among overweight adolescent boys consuming fish oil in an intervention study investigating fish oil and CVD-risk factors (Pedersen et al., 2010). In a follow-up study where hypertriglyceridemia participants with untreated normal-high blood pressure were included, fish oil also increased HDL-cholesterol after 3 months of treatment (Cicero et al., 2010).

A decrease in systolic blood pressure was observed ($P < 0.05$) in overweight premenopausal women (Dunn et al., 2014), as well as a reduction in diastolic blood pressure in overweight participants receiving fish oil (Ramel et al., 2010). Among hypertriglyceridemia patients a decrease in blood pressure was observed after 12 months of PUFA supplementation (Cicero et al., 2010) and among overweight adolescent boys consuming fish oil for 16 weeks (Pedersen et al., 2010). A reduction was observed in waist circumference ($P < 0.001$) in overweight premenopausal women receiving fish oil (Dunn et al., 2014), and in blood glucose (26 %) in rats given fish oil (Barrios-Ramos et al., 2012).

Fish oil may be beneficial in reducing MetS, both through its modulation of lipid metabolism and its effect in reducing inflammation. The n–3 fatty acids may be more efficacious when consumed through fish rather than the equivalent amounts provided as fish oil capsules (Visioli et al., 2003). Still the benefits of fish oil have been seen at higher doses (Vannice, 2010). However, in addition to the fatty acids, fish provides quality protein, vitamins, and minerals which may independently work to reduce MetS (Vannice, 2010).

CONCLUSION

Fish consumption may prevent or improve metabolic health and play a protective role in the prevention of MetS. This protective role may be related to gender, as men may benefit more from the consumption of fish. Both fish and fish oil may be beneficial in reducing MetS through modulation of lipid metabolism and its effect in reducing inflammation. Further, both lean and fatty fish may play a protective role through its positive effect on satiety and due to the variety of different nutrients they provide. Additional research is required to further explore these associations to improve or reverse MetS and its components.

References

Aadland, E.K., Lavigne, C., Graff, I.E., Eng, O., Paquette, M., Holthe, A., Mellgren, G., Jacques, H., Liaset, B., 2015. Lean-seafood intake reduces cardiovascular lipid risk factors in healthy subjects: results from a randomized controlled trial with a crossover design. Am. J. Clin. Nutr. 102, 582–592.

Abete, I., Goyenechea, E., Zulet, M.A., Martinez, J.A., 2011. Obesity and metabolic syndrome: potential benefit from specific nutritional components. Nutr. Metab. Cardiovasc. Dis. 21 (Suppl. 2), B1–B15.

Akter, S., Nanri, A., Pham, N.M., Kurotani, K., Mizoue, T., 2013. Dietary patterns and metabolic syndrome in a Japanese working population. Nutr. Metab. (London) 10, 30.

Alberti, K.G., Eckel, R.H., Grundy, S.M., Zimmet, P.Z., Cleeman, J.I., Donato, K.A., Fruchart, J.C., James, W.P., Loria, C.M., Smith, Jr., S.C., 2009. Harmonizing the metabolic syndrome: a joint interim statement of the International Diabetes Federation Task Force on Epidemiology and Prevention; National Heart, Lung, and Blood Institute; American Heart Association; World Heart Federation; International Atherosclerosis Society; and International Association for the Study of Obesity. Circulation 120, 1640–1645.

Alberti, K.G., Zimmet, P., Shaw, J., 2005. The metabolic syndrome-a new worldwide definition. Lancet 366, 1059–1062.

Alberti, K.G., Zimmet, P., Shaw, J., 2006. Metabolic syndrome—a new world-wide definition. A Consensus Statement from the International Diabetes Federation. Diabet. Med. 23, 469–480.

Alemany, M., 2012. Do the interactions between glucocorticoids and sex hormones regulate the development of the metabolic syndrome? Front. Endocrinol. (Lausanne) 3, 27.

Alvarez Leon, E., Henriquez, P., Serra-Majem, L., 2006. Mediterranean diet and metabolic syndrome: a cross-sectional study in the Canary Islands. Public Health Nutr. 9, 1089–1098.

Asrih, M., Jornayvaz, F.R., 2015. Metabolic syndrome and nonalcoholic fatty liver disease: is insulin resistance the link? Mol. Cell Endocrinol.

Athyros, V.G., Ganotakis, E.S., Tziomalos, K., Papageorgiou, A.A., Anagnostis, P., Griva, T., Kargiotis, K., Mitsiou, E.K., Karagiannis, A., Mikhailidis, D.P., 2010. Comparison of four definitions of the metabolic syndrome in a Greek (Mediterranean) population. Curr. Med. Res. Opin. 26, 713–719.

Babio, N., Bullo, M., Basora, J., Martinez-Gonzalez, M.A., Fernandez-Ballart, J., Marquez-Sandoval F., Molina, C., Salas-Salvado, J., Nureta, P.I., 2009a. Adherence to the Mediterranean diet and risk of metabolic syndrome and its components. Nutr. Metab. Cardiovasc. Dis. 19, 563–570.

Babio, N., Bullo, M., Salas-Salvado, J., 2009b. Mediterranean diet and metabolic syndrome: the evidence. Public Health Nutr. 12, 1607–1617.

Baik, I., 2009. Optimal cutoff points of waist circumference for the criteria of abdominal obesity: comparison with the criteria of the International Diabetes Federation. Circ. J. 73, 2068–2075.

Baik, I., Abbott, R.D., Curb, J.D., Shin, C., 2010. Intake of fish and n-3 fatty acids and future risk of metabolic syndrome. J. Am. Diet Assoc. 110, 1018–1026.

Baik, I., Lee, M., Jun, N.R., Lee, J.Y., Shin, C., 2013. A healthy dietary pattern consisting of a variety of food choices is inversely associated with the development of metabolic syndrome. Nutr. Res. Pract. 7, 233–241.

Barrios-Ramos, J.P., Garduno-Siciliano, L., Loredo, M., Chamorro-Cevallos, G., Jaramillo-Flores, M.E., 2012. The effect of cocoa, soy, oats and fish oil on metabolic syndrome in rats. J. Sci. Food Agric. 92, 2349–2357.

Beltran-Sanchez, H., Harhay, M.O., Harhay, M.M., McElligott, S., 2013. Prevalence and trends of metabolic syndrome in the adult U.S. population, 1999–2010. J. Am. Coll. Cardiol. 62, 697–703.

Bhandari, R., Kelley, G.A., Hartley, T.A., Rockett, I.R., 2014. Metabolic syndrome is associated with increased breast cancer risk: a systematic review with meta-analysis. Int. J. Breast Cancer 2014, 189384.

Butte, N.F., King, J.C., 2005. Energy requirements during pregnancy and lactation. Public Health Nutr. 8, 1010–1027.

Butte, N.F., Wong, W.W., Hopkinson, J.M., 2001. Energy requirements of lactating women derived from doubly labeled water and milk energy output. J. Nutr. 131, 53–58.

Calder, P.C., 2006. n-3 polyunsaturated fatty acids, inflammation, and inflammatory diseases. Am. J. Clin. Nutr. 83, 1505S–1519S.

Cho, Y.A., Kim, J., Cho, E.R., Shin, A., 2011. Dietary patterns and the prevalence of metabolic syndrome in Korean women. Nutr. Metab. Cardiovasc. Dis. 21, 893–900.

Chowdhury, R., Stevens, S., Gorman, D., Pan, A., Warnakula, S., Chowdhury, S., Ward, H., Johnson, L., Crowe, F., Hu, F.B., Franco, O.H., 2012. Association between fish consumption, long chain omega 3 fatty acids, and risk of cerebrovascular disease: systematic review and meta-analysis. BMJ 345, e6698.

Cicero, A.F., Derosa, G., Di Gregori, V., Bove, M., Gaddi, A.V., Borghi, C., 2010. Omega 3 polyunsaturated fatty acids supplementation and blood pressure levels in hypertriglyceridemic patients with untreated normal-high blood pressure and with or without metabolic syndrome: a retrospective study. Clin. Exp. Hypertens. 32, 137–144.

Cohen, A., Pieper, C.F., Brown, A.J., Bastian, L.A., 2006. Number of children and risk of metabolic syndrome in women. J. Womens Health (Larchmt.) 15, 763–773.

Cornier, M.A., Dabelea, D., Hernandez, T.L., Lindstrom, R.C., Steig, A.J., Stob, N.R., Van Pelt, R.E., Wang, H., Eckel, R.H., 2008. The metabolic syndrome. Endocr. Rev. 29, 777–822.

Davidson, M.H., 2006. Mechanisms for the hypotriglyceridemic effect of marine omega-3 fatty acids. Am. J. Cardiol. 98, 27i–33i.

Di Daniele, N., Petramala, L., Di Renzo, L., Sarlo, F., Della Rocca, D.G., Rizzo, M., Fondacaro, V., Iacopino, L., Pepine, C.J., De Lorenzo, A., 2013. Body composition changes and cardiometabolic benefits of a balanced Italian Mediterranean Diet in obese patients with metabolic syndrome. Acta. Diabetol. 50, 409–416.

DiBello, J.R., McGarvey, S.T., Kraft, P., Goldberg, R., Campos, H., Quested, C., Laumoli, T.S., Baylin, A., 2009. Dietary patterns are associated with metabolic syndrome in adult Samoans. J. Nutr. 139, 1933–1943.

Dunn, S.L., Siu, W., Freund, J., Boutcher, S.H., 2014. The effect of a lifestyle intervention on metabolic health in young women. Diabetes Metab. Syndr. Obes. 7, 437–444.

Ebbesson, S.O., Tejero, M.E., Nobmann, E.D., Lopez-Alvarenga, J.C., Ebbesson, L., Romenesko, T., Carter, E.A., Resnick, H.E., Devereux, R.B., MacCluer, J.W., Dyke, B., Laston, S.L., Wenger, C.R., Fabsitz, R.R., Comuzzie, A.G., Howard, B.V., 2007. Fatty acid consumption and metabolic syndrome components: the GOCADAN study. J. Cardiometab. Syndr. 2, 244–249.

Einstein, F.H., Fishman, S., Muzumdar, R.H., Yang, X.M., Atzmon, G., Barzilai, N., 2008. Accretion of visceral fat and hepatic insulin resistance in pregnant rats. Am. J. Physiol. Endocrinol. Metab. 294, E451–455.

El Khoury, D., Anderson, G.H., 2013. Recent advances in dietary proteins and lipid metabolism. Curr. Opin. Lipidol. 24, 207–213.

Erkkila, A.T., Schwab, U.S., de Mello, V.D., Lappalainen, T., Mussalo, H., Lehto, S., Kemi, V., Lamberg-Allardt, C., Uusitupa, M.I., 2008. Effects of fatty and lean fish intake on blood pressure in subjects with coronary heart disease using multiple medications. Eur. J. Nutr. 47, 319–328.

Esposito, K., Chiodini, P., Colao, A., Lenzi, A., Giugliano, D., 2012. Metabolic syndrome and risk of cancer: a systematic review and meta-analysis. Diabetes Care 35, 2402–2411.

Expert Panel on Detection, E., Treatment of High Blood Cholesterol in, A., 2001. Executive Summary of The Third Report of The National Cholesterol Education Program (NCEP) Expert Panel on Detection, Evaluation, And Treatment of High Blood Cholesterol In Adults (Adult Treatment Panel III). JAMA 285, 2486–2497.

Fonseca, M.J., Gaio, R., Lopes, C., Santos, A.C., 2012. Association between dietary patterns and metabolic syndrome in a sample of Portuguese adults. Nutr. J. 11, 64.

Fung, G.J., Steffen, L.M., Zhou, X., Harnack, L., Tang, W., Lutsey, P.L., Loria, C.M., Reis, J.P., Van Horn, L.V., 2012. Vitamin D intake is inversely related to risk of developing metabolic syndrome in African American and white men and women over 20 y: the Coronary Artery Risk Development in Young Adults study. Am. J. Clin. Nutr. 96, 24–29.

Grundy, S.M., Cleeman, J.I., Daniels, S.R., Donato, K.A., Eckel, R.H., Franklin, B.A., Gordon, D.J., Krauss, R.M., Savage, P.J., Smith, Jr., S.C., Spertus, J.A., Costa, F., American Heart, A., National Heart, L., Blood, I., 2005. Diagnosis and management of the metabolic syndrome: an American Heart Association/National Heart, Lung, and Blood Institute Scientific Statement. Circulation 112, 2735–2752.

Gunderson, E.P., Jacobs, Jr., D.R., Chiang, V., Lewis, C.E., Feng, J., Quesenberry, Jr., C.P., Sidney, S., 2010. Duration of lactation and incidence of the metabolic syndrome in women of reproductive age according to gestational diabetes mellitus status: a 20-year prospective study in CARDIA (Coronary Artery Risk Development in Young Adults). Diabetes 59, 495–504.

He, Y., Li, Y., Lai, J., Wang, D., Zhang, J., Fu, P., Yang, X., Qi, L., 2012. Dietary patterns as compared with physical activity in relation to metabolic syndrome among Chinese adults. Nutr. Metab. Cardiovasc. Dis.

Hong, S., Song, Y., Lee, K.H., Lee, H.S., Lee, M., Jee, S.H., Joung, H., 2012. A fruit and dairy dietary pattern is associated with a reduced risk of metabolic syndrome. Metabolism 61, 883–890.

Jung, H.J., Han, S.N., Song, S., Paik, H.Y., Baik, H.W., Joung, H., 2011. Association between adherence to the Korean Food Guidance System and the risk of metabolic abnormalities in Koreans. Nutr. Res. Pract. 5, 560–568.

Kaur, J., 2014. A comprehensive review on metabolic syndrome. Cardiol. Res. Pract. 2014, 943162.

Kesse-Guyot, E., Ahluwalia, N., Lassale, C., Hercberg, S., Fezeu, L., Lairon, D., 2013. Adherence to Mediterranean diet reduces the risk of metabolic syndrome: a 6-year prospective study. Nutr. Metab. Cardiovasc. Dis. 23, 677–683.

Kim, J., Jo, I., 2011. Grains, vegetables, and fish dietary pattern is inversely associated with the risk of metabolic syndrome in South Korean adults. J. Am. Diet Assoc. 111, 1141–1149.

Kouki, R., Schwab, U., Hassinen, M., Komulainen, P., Heikkila, H., Lakka, T.A., Rauramaa, R., 2011. Food consumption, nutrient intake and the risk of having metabolic syndrome: the DR's EXTRA Study. Eur. J. Clin. Nutr. 65, 368–377.

Lee, J.H., O'Keefe, J.H., Lavie, C.J., Harris, W.S., 2009. Omega-3 fatty acids: cardiovascular benefits, sources and sustainability. Nat. Rev. Cardiol. 6, 753–758.

Lee, T.C., Ivester, P., Hester, A.G., Sergeant, S., Case, L.D., Morgan, T., Kouba, E.O., Chilton, F.H., 2014. The impact of polyunsaturated fatty acid-based dietary supplements on disease biomarkers in a metabolic syndrome/diabetes population. Lipids Health Dis. 13, 196.

Lewis, A., Lookinland, S., Beckstrand, R.L., Tiedeman, M.E., 2004. Treatment of hypertriglyceridemia with omega-3 fatty acids: a systematic review. J. Am. Acad. Nurse Pract. 16, 384–395.

Li, Y.H., Zhou, C.H., Pei, H.J., Zhou, X.L., Li, L.H., Wu, Y.J., Hui, R.T., 2013. Fish consumption and incidence of heart failure: a meta-analysis of prospective cohort studies. China Med. J. (England) 126, 942–948.

Lund, E.K., 2013. Health benefits of seafood; is it just the fatty acids? Food Chem. 140, 413–420.

Lutsey, P.L., Steffen, L.M., Stevens, J., 2008. Dietary intake and the development of the metabolic syndrome: the Atherosclerosis Risk in Communities study. Circulation 117, 754–761.

Madani, Z., Louchami, K., Sener, A., Malaisse, W.J., Ait Yahia, D., 2012. Dietary sardine protein lowers insulin resistance, leptin and TNF-alpha and beneficially affects adipose tissue oxidative stress in rats with fructose-induced metabolic syndrome. Int. J. Mol. Med. 29, 311–318.

Maury, E., Brichard, S.M., 2010. Adipokine dysregulation, adipose tissue inflammation and metabolic syndrome. Mol. Cell Endocrinol. 314, 1–16.

Mozaffarian, D., Lemaitre, R.N., Kuller, L.H., Burke, G.L., Tracy, R.P., Siscovick, D.S., Cardiovascular Health, S., 2003. Cardiac benefits of fish consumption may depend on the type of fish meal consumed: the Cardiovascular Health Study. Circulation 107, 1372–1377.

Noel, S.E., Newby, P.K., Ordovas, J.M., Tucker, K.L., 2010. Adherence to an (n-3) fatty acid/fish intake pattern is inversely associated with metabolic syndrome among Puerto Rican adults in the Greater Boston area. J. Nutr. 140, 1846–1854.

Ouellet, V., Marois, J., Weisnagel, S.J., Jacques, H., 2007. Dietary cod protein improves insulin sensitivity in insulin-resistant men and women: a randomized controlled trial. Diabetes Care 30, 2816–2821.

Panagiotakos, D.B., Pitsavos, C., Skoumas, Y., Stefanadis, C., 2007a. The association between food patterns and the metabolic syndrome using principal components analysis: the ATTICA Study. J. Am. Diet Assoc. 107, 979–987.

Panagiotakos, D.B., Zeimbekis, A., Boutziouka, V., Economou, M., Kourlaba, G., Toutouzas, P., Polychronopoulos, E., 2007b. Long-term fish intake is associated with better lipid profile, arterial blood pressure, and blood glucose levels in elderly people from Mediterranean islands (MEDIS epidemiological study). Med. Sci. Monit. 13, CR307–CR312.

Pasalic, D., Dodig, S., Corovic, N., Pizent, A., Jurasovic, J., Pavlovic, M., 2011. High prevalence of metabolic syndrome in an elderly Croatian population—a multicentre study. Public Health Nutr. 14, 1650–1657.

Patel, P.S., Sharp, S.J., Luben, R.N., Khaw, K.T., Bingham, S.A., Wareham, N.J., Forouhi, N.G., 2009. Association between type of dietary fish and seafood intake and the risk of incident type 2 diabetes: the European prospective investigation of cancer (EPIC)-Norfolk cohort study. Diabetes Care 32, 1857–1863.

Pedersen, M.H., Molgaard, C., Hellgren, L.I., Lauritzen, L., 2010. Effects of fish oil supplementation on markers of the metabolic syndrome. J. Pediatr. 157, 395–400, 400 e391.

Potenza, M.V., Mechanick, J.I., 2009. The metabolic syndrome: definition, global impact, and pathophysiology. Nutr. Clin. Pract. 24, 560–577.

Raatz, S.K., Silverstein, J.T., Jahns, L., Picklo, M.J., 2013. Issues of fish consumption for cardiovascular disease risk reduction. Nutrients 5, 1081–1097.

Ramel, A., Jonsdottir, M.T., Thorsdottir, I., 2009. Consumption of cod and weight loss in young overweight and obese adults on an energy reduced diet for 8-weeks. Nutr. Metab. Cardiovasc. Dis. 19, 690–696.

Ramel, A., Martinez, J.A., Kiely, M., Bandarra, N.M., Thorsdottir, I., 2010. Moderate consumption of fatty fish reduces diastolic blood pressure in overweight and obese European young adults during energy restriction. Nutrition 26, 168–174.

Robinson, L.E., Buchholz, A.C., Mazurak, V.C., 2007. Inflammation, obesity, and fatty acid metabolism: influence of n-3 polyunsaturated fatty acids on factors contributing to metabolic syndrome. Appl. Physiol. Nutr. Metab. 32, 1008–1024.

Robinson, L.E., Mazurak, V.C., 2013. N-3 polyunsaturated fatty acids: relationship to inflammation in healthy adults and adults exhibiting features of metabolic syndrome. Lipids 48, 319–332.

Romaguera, D., Norat, T., Mouw, T., May, A.M., Bamia, C., Slimani, N., Travier, N., Besson, H., Luan, J., Wareham, N., Rinaldi, S., Couto, E., Clavel-Chapelon, F., Boutron-Ruault, M.C., Cottet, V., Palli, D., Agnoli, C., Panico, S., Tumino, R., Vineis, P., Agudo, A., Rodriguez, L., Sanchez, M.J., Amiano, P., Barricarte, A., Huerta, J.M., Key, T.J., Spencer, E.A., Bueno-de-Mesquita, H.B., Buchner, F.L., Orfanos, P., Naska, A., Trichopoulou, A., Rohrmann, S., Kaaks, R., Bergmann, M., Boeing, H., Johansson, I., Hellstrom, V., Manjer, J., Wirfalt, E., Uhre Jacobsen, M., Overvad, K., Tjonneland, A., Halkjaer, J., Lund, E., Braaten, T., Engeset, D., Odysseos, A., Riboli, E., Peeters, P.H., 2009. Adherence to the Mediterranean diet is associated with lower abdominal adiposity in European men and women. J. Nutr. 139, 1728–1737.

Ruidavets, J.B., Bongard, V., Dallongeville, J., Arveiler, D., Ducimetiere, P., Perret, B., Simon, C., Amouyel, P., Ferrieres, J., 2007. High consumptions of grain, fish, dairy products and combinations of these are associated with a low prevalence of metabolic syndrome. J. Epidemiol. Commun. Health 61, 810–817.

Saravanan, P., Davidson, N.C., Schmidt, E.B., Calder, P.C., 2010. Cardiovascular effects of marine omega-3 fatty acids. Lancet 376, 540–550.

Scrivo, R., Vasile, M., Bartosiewicz, I., Valesini, G., 2011. Inflammation as "common soil" of the multifactorial diseases. Autoimmun. Rev. 10, 369–374.

Shafiee, G., Kelishadi, R., Qorbani, M., Motlagh, M.E., Taheri, M., Ardalan, G., Taslimi, M., Poursafa, P., Heshmat, R., Larijani, B., 2013. Association of breakfast intake with cardiometabolic risk factors. J. Pediatr. (Rio Janerio) 89, 575–582.

Shukla, A., Bettzieche, A., Hirche, F., Brandsch, C., Stangl, G.I., Eder, K., 2006. Dietary fish protein alters blood lipid concentrations and hepatic genes involved in cholesterol homeostasis in the rat model. Br J. Nutr. 96, 674–682.

Streppel, M.T., Ocke, M.C., Boshuizen, H.C., Kok, F.J., Kromhout, D., 2008. Long-term fish consumption and n-3 fatty acid intake in relation to (sudden) coronary heart disease death: the Zutphen study. Eur Heart J 29, 2024–2030.

Strom, M., Halldorsson, T.I., Mortensen, E.L., Torp-Pedersen, C., Olsen, S.F., 2012. Fish, n-3 fatty acids, and cardiovascular diseases in women of reproductive age: a prospective study in a large national cohort. Hypertension 59, 36–43.

Stuebe, A.M., Rich-Edwards, J.W., 2009. The reset hypothesis: lactation and maternal metabolism. Am. J. Perinatol. 26, 81–88.

Takata, Y., Zhang, X., Li, H., Gao, Y.T., Yang, G., Gao, J., Cai, H., Xiang, Y.B., Zheng, W., Shu, X.O., 2013. Fish intake and risks of total and cause-specific mortality in 2 population-based cohort studies of 134,296 men and women. Am. J. Epidemiol. 178, 46–57.

Telle-Hansen, V.H., Larsen, L.N., Hostmark, A.T., Molin, M., Dahl, L., Almendingen, K., Ulven, S.M., 2012. Daily intake of cod or salmon for 2 weeks decreases the 18:1n-9/18:0 ratio and serum triacylglycerols in healthy subjects. Lipids 47, 151–160.

Thorsdottir, I., Tomasson, H., Gunnarsdottir, I., Gisladottir, E., Kiely, M., Parra, M.D., Bandarra, N.M., Schaafsma, G., Martinez, J.A., 2007. Randomized trial of weight-loss-diets for young adults varying in fish and fish oil content. Int. J. Obes. (London) 31, 1560–1566.

Torris, C., Thune, I., Emaus, A., Finstad, S.E., Bye, A., Furberg, A.S., Barrett, E., Jasienska, G., Ellison, P., Hjartaker, A., 2013. Duration of lactation, maternal metabolic profile, and body composition in the Norwegian EBBA I-study. Breastfeed Med. 8, 8–15.

Tørris, C., Molin, M., Cvancarova Småstuen, M., 2014. Fish consumption and its possible preventive role on the development and prevalence of metabolic syndrome - a systematic review. Diabetol.ogy Metabol.ic Syndrome 6, 112.

Uhe, A.M., Collier, G.R., O'Dea, K., 1992. A comparison of the effects of beef, chicken and fish protein on satiety and amino acid profiles in lean male subjects. J. Nutr. 122, 467–472.

Uusitupa, M., Hermansen, K., Savolainen, M.J., Schwab, U., Kolehmainen, M., Brader, L., Mortensen, L.S., Cloetens, L., Johansson-Persson, A., Onning, G., Landin-Olsson, M., Herzig, K.H., Hukkanen, J., Rosqvist, F., Iggman, D., Paananen, J., Pulkki, K.J., Siloaho, M., Dragsted, L.,

Barri, T., Overvad, K., Bach Knudsen, K.E., Hedemann, M.S., Arner, P., Dahlman, I., Borge, G.I., Baardseth, P., Ulven, S.M., Gunnarsdottir, I., Jonsdottir, S., Thorsdottir, I., Oresic, M., Poutanen, K.S., Riserus, U., Akesson, B., 2013. Effects of an isocaloric healthy Nordic diet on insulin sensitivity, lipid profile and inflammation markers in metabolic syndrome - a randomized study (SYSDIET). J. Intern. Med. 274, 52–66.

Vannice, G.K., 2010. n-3s from fish and the risk of metabolic syndrome. J. Am. Diet Assoc. 110, 1014–1017.

Vazquez, C., Botella-Carretero, J.I., Corella, D., Fiol, M., Lage, M., Lurbe, E., Richart, C., Fernandez-Real, J.M., Fuentes, F., Ordonez, A., de Cos, A.I., Salas-Salvado, J., Burguera, B., Estruch, R., Ros, E., Pastor, O., Casanueva, F.F., Investigators, W.-C.S., 2014. White fish reduces cardiovascular risk factors in patients with metabolic syndrome: the WISH-CARE study, a multicenter randomized clinical trial. Nutr. Metab. Cardiovasc. Dis. 24, 328–335.

Visioli, F., Rise, P., Barassi, M.C., Marangoni, F., Galli, C., 2003. Dietary intake of fish vs. formulations leads to higher plasma concentrations of n-3 fatty acids. Lipids 38, 415–418.

Yanai, H., Katsuyama, H., Hamasaki, H., Abe, S., Tada, N., Sako, A., 2015. Effects of dietary fat intake on HDL metabolism. J. Clin. Med. Res. 7, 145–149.

Zaribaf, F., Falahi, E., Barak, F., Heidari, M., Keshteli, A.H., Yazdannik, A., Esmaillzadeh, A., 2014. Fish consumption is inversely associated with the metabolic syndrome. Eur. J. Clin. Nutr. 68, 474–480.

Zhu, B., Haruyama, Y., Muto, T., Yamazaki, T., 2015. Association between eating speed and metabolic syndrome in a three-year population-based cohort study. J. Epidemiol. 25, 332–336.

CHAPTER

15

Dietary and Supplemental Long-Chain N3 Fatty Acids and Incident Type 2 Diabetes

L.M. Steffen, B.T. Steffen***

*Division of Epidemiology and Community Health, University of Minnesota School of Public Health, Minneapolis, Minnesota, United States; **Department of Laboratory Medicine and Pathology, University of Minnesota, Minneapolis, Minnesota, United States

INTRODUCTION

The prevalence of type 2 diabetes (T2D) has more than doubled over the past 30 years (CDC, 2013). A host of research has described the relations between dietary intake and risk of developing T2D. Numerous studies have shown the beneficial effects of n–3 fatty acids, both dietary intake of fatty fish and seafood, as well as long chain n–3 fatty acid supplement use on coronary heart disease (CHD) and some risk factors for cardiovascular disease (CVD), and markers of atherosclerosis and thrombosis (DeCaterina, 2011; Mozafarrian and Wu, 2011). N–3 fatty acids are known for their anti-inflammatory properties and antiarrhythmic and antiatherogenic effects. Some studies have also reported lower blood pressure and heart rate and improved insulin sensitivity with n–3 fatty acid intake. Therefore, we would expect that n–3 fatty acids would also be beneficially related to T2D. However, results from individual studies of fish and n–3 fatty acid intakes relative to T2D are inconsistent. Therefore, five meta-analyses including up to 26 epidemiologic observational studies were conducted that examined the relations of dietary intakes of fish and/or n–3 fatty acids with risk of developing T2D in adults living in Asia, Europe, or the United States (Wallin et al., 2012; Wu et al., 2012; Xun and He, 2012; Zheng et al., 2012; Zhou et al., 2012).

In this chapter, we discuss the results and interpretation of the individual and meta-analytic studies. Long chain n–3 fatty acids are defined as the sum of eicosapentaenoic acid (EPA) and docosahexaenoic acid (DHA) fatty acids.

INTERVENTION STUDIES

There have been no intervention studies conducted in humans testing the effectiveness of dietary intake of fish or n–3 supplement use on reducing the risk of developing T2D.

OBSERVATIONAL STUDIES

Numerous epidemiologic observational, mainly prospective studies have been conducted about the relations of dietary intakes of fish and long chain n–3 fatty acids with risk of developing T2D; however study findings have been inconsistent (Table 15.1). Participants enrolled in these prospective studies were adults aged 18–98 years, generally healthy men and women, and were of Caucasian, African American, or Asian race although mostly Caucasian. Twelve prospective studies showed no relation, while a significant and positive relation between fish intake and incident T2D was observed in four prospective studies (Table 15.1). Findings from 11 prospective studies about the

Fish and Fish Oil in Health and Disease Prevention. http://dx.doi.org/10.1016/B978-0-12-802844-5.00015-4

TABLE 15.1 Individual Studies Included in Each of the Five Meta-analysis Conducted About Dietary Intakes of Fish and Long Chain n–3 Fatty Acids Relative to Incident Type 2 Diabetes (T2D)

Author, year published	Study population	Geographic location	Hazard ratio (95% C.I)[a]	Xun	Wallin	Zhou	Wu	Zheng
Fish intake								
Montonen et al. (2005)	Finnish Mobile Clinic Health Exam Survey	Finland	1.08 (0.80, 1.45)	X	X			
Vang et al. (2008)	Seventh Day Adventist	United States	1.12 (0.88, 1.44)		X		X	
Kaushik et al. (2009)	Nurses Health Study	United States	1.29 (1.05, 1.58)	X	X	X	X	X
Kaushik et al. (2009)	Nurses Health Study 2	United States	1.32 (1.00, 1.75)	X	X	X	X	X
Kaushik et al. (2009)	Health Professionals Follow-up Study	United States	1.16 (0.96, 1.41)	X	X	X	X	X
Patel et al. (2009)	EPIC_Norfolk	United Kingdom	0.81 (0.60, 1.11)	X	X		X	X
van Woudenbergh et al. (2009)	Rotterdam Study	Netherlands	1.32 (1.02, 1.70)	X	X	X	X	X
Krishnan et al. (2010)	Black Women's Health Study	United States	0.89 (0.64, 1.24)			X		
Brostow et al. (2011)	Singapore Health Study	Singapore	1.06 (0.91, 1.23)		X		X	X
Djousse et al. (2011a)	Women's Health Study	United States	1.49 (1.30, 1.70)	X	X	X	X	X
Djousse et al. (2011b)	Coronary Heart Study	United States	1.07 (0.35, 3.29)	X	X	X	X	X
Nanri et al. (2011)	JPHC-Men	Japan	0.73 (0.54, 1.00)	X	X		X	X
Nanri et al. (2011)	JPHC-Women	Japan	1.01 (0.69, 1.49)	X	X		X	X
Villegas et al. (2011)	Shanghai Women's Health Study	Shanghai	0.89 (0.78, 1.01)	X	X	X	X	X
Villegas et al. (2011)	Shanghai Men's Health Study	Shanghai	0.94 (0.75, 1.18)	X	X	X	X	X
He, unpublished	CARDIA	United States	0.99 (0.52, 1.88)	X				
Total number of studies				**12**	**13**	**9**	**13**	**11**
Dietary n–3 fatty acids[b]								
Meyer et al. (2001)	Iowa Women's Health Study	United States	1.20 (1.03, 1.39)	X	X	X	X	X
van Dam et al. (2002)	Health Professional Followup Study	United States	0.90 (0.75, 1.07)			X		
Song et al. (2004)	Nurses Health Study	United States	1.10 (0.93, 1.30)			X		
Hodge et al. (2007)	Melbourne Collaborative Cohort Study	Australia	0.74 (0.50, 1.11)		X		X	X
van Woudenbergh et al. (2009)	Rotterdam Study	Netherlands	1.05 (0.80, 1.38)	X	X		X	X
Kaushik et al. (2009)	Nurses Health Study	United States	1.23 (1.11, 1.37)	X	X	X	X	X
Kaushik et al. (2009)	Nurses Health Study 2	United States	1.25 (1.10, 1.42)	X	X	X	X	X
Kaushik et al. (2009)	Health Professional Followup Study	United States	1.12 (0.98, 1.28)	X	X	X	X	X
Patel et al. (2010)	EPIC_Norfolk	United Kingdom	0.57 (0.32, 1.05)		X		X	
Brostow et al. (2011)	Singapore Health Study	Singapore	0.78 (0.65, 0.94)	X	X	X	X	X
Djousse et al. (2011a)	Women's Health Study	United States	1.44 (1.25, 1.65)	X	X	X	X	X

TABLE 15.1 Individual Studies Included in Each of the Five Meta-analysis Conducted About Dietary Intakes of Fish and Long Chain n–3 Fatty Acids Relative to Incident Type 2 Diabetes (T2D) (*cont.*)

Author, year published	Study population	Geographic location	Hazard ratio (95% C.I)[a]	Xun	Wallin	Zhou	Wu	Zheng
Djousse et al. (2011a,b)	Cardiovascular Heart Study(CHS)	United States	1.04 (0.67, 1.60)	X	X	X	X	X
Kroger et al. (2011)	EPIC_Potsdam	Germany	1.29 (0.95, 1.75)		X		X	X
Nanri et al. (2011)	JPHC-Men	Japan	0.79 (0.59, 1.05)				X	
Nanri et al. (2011)	JPHC-Women	Japan	0.93 (0.67, 1.29)				X	
Villegas et al. (2011)	Shanghai Women's Health Study	Shanghai	0.84 (0.74, 0.95)	X	X	X	X	X
Villegas et al. (2011)	Shanghai Men's Health Study	Shanghai	0.89 (0.70, 1.13)	X	X	X	X	X
Total no. of studies				**10**	**13**	**11**	**15**	**12**

[a] *The hazard ratio (HR) and 95% confidence intervals (95% C.I.) compares the highest versus lowest intake of fish or n–3 fatty acids relative to T2D.*
[b] *Dietary long chain n–3 fatty acids defined as eicosapentaenoic acid (EPA) + docosahexaenoic acid (DHA).*

relation between long chain n–3 (EPA + DHA) fatty acids and incident T2D were null; four studies observed a positive relation; and finally, two studies reported an inverse relation with T2D. Given these inconsistent findings, five meta-analyses were conducted to clarify the role of n–3 fatty acids in the development of T2D (Wallin et al., 2012; Wu et al., 2012; Xun and He, 2012; Zheng et al., 2012; Zhou et al., 2012). The individual studies included in each meta-analysis are shown in Table 15.1. A meta-analysis is a tool or method used to systematically combine results from several selected studies and draw a conclusion that has more statistical power than a single study.

Characteristics of the five meta-analytic studies are shown in Table 15.2 including the number of cohort studies examined, sample size, and number of incident T2D cases, years of follow-up, method of dietary intake and/or n–3 fatty acid biomarker assessment, and geographic location of study conduct. There were 12–18 cohort studies

TABLE 15.2 Characteristics of Five Published Meta-analyses for the Associations of Dietary Intakes of Fish and Long Chain n–3 Fatty Acids With Type 2 Diabetes (T2D)

Author, year published	No. of studies; follow-up time	Participants; no. T2D cases	Assessment of exposure	T2D study definition	Geographic location strata
Xun and He (2012)	12 cohorts; 11.4 years follow-up	*n* = 438,214 T2D cases *n* = 18,711 Age: 18–98 years	FFQ; fish and n–3 fatty acid intake	Self report or study diagnosed	Western, Asia
Wallin et al. (2012)	16 cohorts; years follow-up not reported	*n* = 527,441 T2D cases *n* = 24,082 Age: 26–98 years	FFQ; fish and n–3 fatty acid intake	Self report or study diagnosed	United States, Europe, Asia
Zhou et al. (2012)	13 cohorts; years follow-up not reported	*n* = 367,757, fish intake T2D cases *n* = 17,799 *n* = 506,665, n–3 intake T2D cases *n* = 21,866 Age: 26–78 years	FFQ; fish and n–3 fatty acid intake	Self report or study diagnosed	Did not stratify by geographic location
Wu et al. (2012)	18 cohorts; Follow-up ranged from 4.0–16.7 years	*n* = 540,184 T2D cases *n* = 25,670 Mean age: 36–75 years	FFQ; fish and n–3 fatty acid intake	Self report or study diagnosed	Western, Asia
Zheng et al. (2012)	16 cohorts and 9.9 years followup; 10 case-control studies	*n* = 515,537 T2D cases *n* = 23,226; 8727 controls and 1629 T2D cases Age: 26–79 years	FFQ; fish and n–3 fatty acid intake	Self report or study diagnosed	United States, Europe, Asia

Dietary long-chain n–3 fatty acids defined as eicosapentaenoic acid (EPA) + docosahexaenoic acid (DHA) fatty acids.
Western = USA + Europe.

TABLE 15.3 Relative Risk Estimates of Type 2 Diabetes Associated With Dietary Intakes of Fish and Long Chain n–3 Fatty Acids: Results From Five Meta-analyses

Author, year published	No. of cohorts	Fish intake (per 100 g/day) relative risk (95% C.I.)	No. of cohorts	n–3 fatty acid intake (per 250 mg/day) relative risk (95% C.I.)
Xun and He (2012)	12	0.99 (0.85, 1.16)	11	1.04 (0.92, 1.18)
Wallin et al. (2012)	13	1.01 (0.99, 1.03)	13	1.06 (0.97, 1.14)
Zhou et al. (2012)	9	1.15 (0.98, 1.35)	11	1.08 (0.96, 1.21)
Wu et al. (2012)	13	1.12 (0.94, 1.34)	16	1.04 (0.97, 1.10)
Zheng et al. (2012)	11	1.07 (0.91, 1.25)	12	1.07 (0.95, 1.20)

Dietary long-chain n–3 fatty acids defined as eicosapentaenoic acid (EPA) + docosahexaenoic acid (DHA).
95% C.I. = 95% confidence interval.

included in these meta-analyseses with over 18,000–25,000 incident cases of T2D identified from over 368,000 to over 540,000 study participants. Participants' age ranged from 18 to 98 years at baseline. Dietary intake of fish and n–3 fatty acids was assessed using a food frequency questionnaire (FFQ), although not the same FFQ. T2D was self-report or diagnosed according to the study definition. Data were stratified by geographic location.

For each meta-analysis study (Table 15.3), results of the main effects analysis were null for both intakes of fish and long-chain n–3 fatty acids, but were consistent across the five meta-analytic studies. After stratifying data by geographic location (Table 15.4), the risk of developing T2D was higher in individuals who consumed higher

TABLE 15.4 Relative Risk Estimates of Type 2 Diabetes Associated With Dietary Intakes of Fish and n–3 Long-Chain Fatty Acids According to Geographic Location: Results From Five Meta-analyses

Author, year published	No. of studies	Fish intake (per 100 gm/day) relative risk (95% C.I.)	No. of studies	n–3 fatty acid intake (per 250 mg/day) relative risk (95% C.I.)
USA				
Xun and He (2012)	9[a]	1.09 (0.94, 1.27)	—	NR
Wallin et al. (2012)	6	1.05 (1.02, 1.09)	6	1.17 (1.09, 1.26)
Zhou et al. (2012)	—	NR	—	NR
Wu et al. (2012)	8[a]	1.38 (1.13, 1.70)	—	NR
Zheng et al. (2012)	5	1.33 (1.20, 1.48)	6	1.22 (1.13, 1.33)
Europe				
Xun and He (2012)	—	NR	—	NR
Wallin et al. (2012)	3	1.03 (0.95, 1.11)	3	0.98 (0.70, 1.37)
Zhou et al. (2012)	—	NR	—	NR
Wu et al. (2012)	—	NR	—	NR
Zheng et al. (2012)	2	1.00 (0.57, 1.73)	2	1.15 (0.94, 1.41)
Asia				
Xun and He (2012)	3	0.79 (0.66, 0.96)	—	NR
Wallin et al. (2012)	5	1.00 (0.97, 1.03)	4	0.90 (0.82, 0.98)
Zhou et al. (2012)	—	NR	—	NR
Wu et al. (2012)	5	0.89 (0.81, 0.98)	—	NR
Zheng et al. (2012)	4	0.89 (0.81, 0.98)	3	0.87 (0.79, 0.96)

Dietary long chain n–3 fatty acids defined as eicosapentaenoic acid (EPA) + docosahexaenoic acid (DHA).
NR, not reported.
[a] *Data were stratified by Western countries (USA + Europe).*

versus lower fish and lived in western countries, while opposing findings were observed for Asian countries; that is, higher intake of fish was inversely related to incident T2D. Similar results were observed for long chain n–3 fatty acids.

Since the five meta-analyses were published in 2012, investigators from Finland recently examined the associations of incident T2D with intakes of dietary fish and n–3 fatty acids EPA, DHA, the combination of EPA + DHA, docosapentaenoic acid (DPA), and the combination of EPA + DHA + DPA in 2,212 Finnish men over 19.3 years of follow-up (Virtanen et al., 2014). A significantly lower risk (33%) of incident T2D was observed in men who consumed the highest amount of EPA + DHA + DPA, but not for intakes of fish, EPA, DHA, or the combination of EPA + DHA. DPA, a long chain n–3 fatty acid, structurally similar to EPA, is found in fish oil, salmon, and beef. No other published study had included DPA in their analysis.

DISCUSSION

In main effects analysis, no relation was observed between fish or n–3 fatty acid intake and risk of developing T2D. But stratification of data by geographic location resulted in differential associations between intakes of fish or n–3 fatty acid intakes and incident T2D. Risk of developing T2D was lower in individuals living in Asia compared to residents of western countries for consumption of fish (100 g/day) and n–3 fatty acids (250 mg/day) (Wallin et al., 2012; Wu et al., 2012; Xun and He, 2012; Zheng et al., 2012). This finding was unexpected. One explanation may be heterogeneity of the main effects analysis found in all meta-analytic studies. When stratified by geographic location, no heterogeneity was observed in the results for Asian countries; however, significant heterogeneity across the study results remained for the western countries. Reasons for heterogeneity of effects by region may be true biologic diversity, methodologic diversity among studies, publication bias, or chance (Wu et al., 2012).

It is important to point out the differences in fish intake between Asian and Western populations. Average intakes of EPA/DHA in many Asian populations is >1000 mg per day with average US intakes <100 mg. In addition, the type of fish consumed in each country may also explain these disparate results.

Different foods or dietary pattern consumed in each country may contribute to these diverse study results (Tanabe et al., 2013). The positive association of fish or n–3 fatty acid intakes with T2D observed in the western country studies may be due to inadequate fruit and vegetable intake and excessive red and processed meat intake, allowing greater susceptibility of polyunsaturated fatty acids to oxidation (Østerud and Elvevoll, 2011; White and Collinson, 2013). Inflammation is associated with lower fruit and vegetable intake and greater red and processed meat intake, which has been shown to promote insulin resistance, leading to the development of T2D (Vykoukal and Davies, 2011; White and Collinson, 2013). It may be that Asian populations consume more fish, greater amount and variety of vegetables, and less red and processed meat than western populations, thus, promoting greater insulin sensitivity from n–3 fatty acid intake while greater vegetable or antioxidant intake and less meat intake prevents susceptibility to lipid peroxidation. A discussion of n–3 fatty acids and inflammation is included in Chapter: Fish/Fish Oil Intake and Inflammatory Biomarkers, Endothelial Function.

Other explanations for these opposing study findings by geographic location include; (1) diverse cooking methods (deep-fried, pan-fried, steamed, or baked), and (2) different availability of types of fish such as fresh (including fresh frozen), canned, or commercially breaded fish – all of which have varying fatty acid composition. For example, some commercially breaded fish purchased in the United States has the same fatty acid content as red meat. Last, diet assessment methodology may not capture true dietary intake. In United States studies measuring plasma fatty acid biomarkers, n–3 fatty acids have not associated with higher risk of incident T2D (Wu et al., 2012). Thus, measurement error associated with self-reported dietary intake may explain study findings. In addition, diet assessment tools, that is, food frequency questionnaires, used to capture dietary intake, specifically fish intake, do not accurately capture the type of fish consumed, such as lean or fatty/oily fish or whether the fish was fresh, frozen, salted, or breaded, or method of food preparation, which influences the fatty acid composition of the fish consumed. Thus, we were unable to sort out if type of fish selected (fresh vs frozen and breaded) and consumed in the United States is related to incident diabetes.

The 2010 Dietary Guidelines for Americans recommend consuming eight ounces of fish and seafood each week, including oily fish such as salmon, trout, halibut, and herring, and seafood such as shrimp, scallops, lobster, and mussels (USDA, 2010). These guidelines could also recommend 'eating fresh fish and seafood' and avoid the breaded selections that reflect a fatty acid composition similar to red and processed meat. It would also be prudent to emphasize consuming more fruit and vegetables and less meat consumption for health promotion and disease prevention (USDA, 2010; Mozafarrian and Wu, 2011).

References

Brostow, D.P., Odegaard, A.O., Koh, W.P., Duval, S., Gross, M.D., Yuan, J.M., Pereira, M.A., 2011. Omega-3 fatty acids and incident type 2 diabetes: the Singapore Chinese Health Study. Am. J. Clin. Nutr. 94, 520–526.

Centers for Disease Control and Prevention, National Center for Health Statistics, Division of Health Interview Statistics, data from the National Health Interview Survey. Statistical analysis by the Centers for Disease Control and Prevention, National Center for Chronic, Disease Prevention and Health Promotion, Division of Diabetes Translation, 2013. http://www.cdc.gov/diabetes/statistics/prev/national/figpersons.htm

DeCaterina, R., 2011. N-3 fatty acids in cardiovascular disease. N. Engl. J. Med. 364, 2439–2450.

Djousse, L., Gaziano, J.M., Buring, J.E., Lee, I.M., 2011a. Dietary omega-3 fatty acids and fish consumption and risk of type 2 diabetes. Am. J. Clin. Nutr. 93, 143–150.

Djousse, L., Biggs, M.L., Lemaitre, R.N., King, I.B., Song, X., Ix, J.H., Mukamal, K.J., Siscovick, D.S., Mozaffarian, D., 2011b. Plasma omega-3 fatty acids and incident diabetes in older adults. Am. J. Clin. Nutr. 94, 527–533.

Hodge, A.M., English, D.R., O'Dea, K., Sinclair, A.J., Makrides, M., Gibson, R.A., Giles, G.G., 2007. Plasma phospholipid and dietary fatty acids as predictors of type 2 diabetes: interpreting the role of linoleic acid. Am. J. Clin. Nutr. 86, 189–197.

Kaushik, M., Mozaffarian, D., Spiegelman, D., Manson, J.E., Willett, W.C., Hu, F.B., 2009. Long-chain omega-3 fatty acids, fish intake, and the risk of type 2 diabetes mellitus. Am. J. Clin. Nutr. 90, 613–620.

Krishnan, S., Coogan, P.F., Boggs, D.A., Rosenberg, L., Palmer, J.R., 2010. Consumption of restaurant foods and incidence of type 2 diabetes in African American women. Am. J. Clin. Nutr. 91, 465–471.

Kroger, J., Zietemann, V., Enzenbach, C., Weikert, C., Jansen, E.H., Döring, F., Joost, H.G., Boeing, H., Schulze, M.B., 2011. Erythrocyte membrane phospholipid fatty acids, desaturase activity, and dietary fatty acids in relation to risk of type 2 diabetes in the European Prospective Investigation into Cancer and Nutrition (EPIC)-Potsdam Study. Am. J. Clin. Nutr. 93, 127–142.

Meyer, K.A., Kushi, L.H., Jacobs, Jr., D.R., Folsom, A.R., 2001. Dietary fat and incidence of type 2 diabetes in older Iowa women. Diabetes Care 24, 1528–1535.

Montonen, J., Jarvinen, R., Heliovaara, M., Reunanen, A., Aromaa, A., Knekt, P., 2005. Food consumption and the incidence of type II diabetes mellitus. Eur. J. Clin. Nutr. 59, 441–448.

Mozafarrian, D., Wu, J.H.Y., 2011. Omega-3 fatty acids and cardiovascular disease effects on risk factors, molecular pathways, and clinical events. J. Am. Coll. Cardiol. 58, 2047–2067.

Nanri, A., Mizoue, T., Noda, M., Takahashi, Y., Matsushita, Y., Poudel-Tandukar, K., Kato, M., Oba, S., Inoue, M., Tsugane, S., 2011. Fish intake and type 2 diabetes in Japanese men and women: the Japan Public Health Center–based prospective study. Am. J. Clin. Nutr. 94, 884–891.

Østerud, B., Elvevoll, E.O., 2011. Dietary omega-3 fatty acids and risk of type 2 diabetes: lack of antioxidants? Am. J. Clin. Nutr. 94, 617–618.

Patel, P.S., Sharp, S.J., Luben, R.N., Khaw, K.T., Bingham, S.A., Wareham, N.J., Forouhi, N.G., 2009. Association between type of dietary fish and seafood intake and the risk of incident type 2 diabetes: the European prospective investigation of cancer (EPIC)-Norfolk cohort study. Diabetes Care 32, 1857–1863.

Patel, P.S., Sharp, S.J., Jansen, E., Luben, R.N., Khaw, K.T., Wareham, N.J., Forouhi, N.G., 2010. Fatty acids measured in plasma and erythrocyte-membrane phospholipids and derived by food-frequency questionnaire and the risk of new-onset type 2 diabetes: a pilot study in the European Prospective Investigation into Cancer and Nutrition (EPIC)-Norfolk cohort. Am. J. Clin. Nutr. 92, 1214–1222.

Song, Y., Manson, J.E., Buring, J.E., Liu, S., 2004. A prospective study of red meat consumption and type 2 diabetes in middle-aged and elderly women: the women's health study. Diabetes Care 27, 2108–2115.

Tanabe, F.H., Drehmer, M., Neutzling, M.B., 2013. Food consumption and dietary factors involved in health and disease in Nikkeis: systematic review. Rev. Saúde Pública 47, 1–12.

United States Department of Agriculture and United States Department of Health and Human Services. Dietary Guidelines for Americans, 2010. Seven ed., Washington, DC: United States Government Printing Office.

van Dam, R.M., Willett, W.C., Rimm, E.B., Stampfer, M.J., Hu, F.B., 2002. Dietary fat and meat intake in relation to risk of type 2 diabetes in men. Diabetes Care 25, 417–424.

van Woudenbergh, G.J., van Ballegooijen, A.J., Kuijsten, A., Sijbrands, E.J., van Rooij, F.J., Geleijnse, J.M., Hofman, A., Witteman, J.C., Feskens, E.J., 2009. Eating fish and risk of type 2 diabetes: a population-based, prospective follow-up study. Diabetes Care 32, 2021–2026.

Vang, A., Singh, P.N., Lee, J.W., Haddad, E.H., Brinegar, C.H., 2008. Meats, processed meats, obesity, weight gain and occurrence of diabetes among adults: findings from Adventist Health Studies. Ann. Nutr. Metab. 52, 96–104.

Villegas, R., Xiang, Y.B., Elasy, T., Li, H.L., Yang, G., Cai, H., Ye, F., Gao, Y.T., Shyr, Y., Zheng, W., Shu, X.O., 2011. Fish, shellfish, and long-chain n-3 fatty acid consumption and risk of incident type 2 diabetes in middle-aged Chinese men and women. Am. J. Clin. Nutr. 94, 543–551.

Virtanen, J.K., Mursu, J., Voutilainen, S., Uusitupa, M., Tuomainen, T.-P., 2014. Serum omega-3 polyunsaturated fatty acids and risk of incident type 2 diabetes in men: the Kuopio Ischemic Heart Disease Risk Factor Study. Diabetes Care 37, 189–196.

Vykoukal, D., Davies, M.G., 2011. Vascular biology of metabolic syndrome. J. Vasc. Surg. 54, 819–831.

Wallin, A., Giuseppe, D.D., Orsini, N., Patel, P.S., Forouhi, P.S., Wolk, A., 2012. Fish consumption, dietary long-chain n-3 fatty acids, and risk of type 2 diabetes: systematic review and meta-analysis of prospective studies. Diabetes Care 35, 918–925.

White, D.L., Collinson, A., 2013. Red meat, dietary heme iron, and risk of type 2 diabetes: the involvement of advanced lipoxidation endproducts. Adv Nutr. 4, 403–411.

Wu, J.H.Y., Micha, R., Imamura, F., Pan, A., Biggs, M.L., Ajaz, O., Djousse, L., Hu, F.B., Mozaffarian, D., 2012. Omega-3 fatty acids and incident type 2 diabetes: a systematic review and meta-analysis. Brit. J. Nutr. 107, S214–S227.

Xun, P., He, K., 2012. Fish consumption and incidence of diabetes. Diabetes Care 35, 930–938.

Zheng, J.S., Huang, T., Yang, J., Fu, Y.-Q., Li, D., 2012. Marine n-3 polyunsaturated fatty acids are inversely associated with risk of type 2 diabetes in Asians: a systematic review and meta-analysis. Plos One 7, e44525.

Zhou, Y., Tian, C., Jia, C., 2012. Association of fish and n-3 fatty acid intake with the risk of type 2 diabetes: a meta-analysis of prospective studies. Brit. J. Nutr. 108, 408–417.

CHAPTER

16

Seafood Consumption and Fasting Leptin and Ghrelin in Overweight and Obese

B.E. Birgisdottir, I. Thorsdottir***

*Unit for Nutrition Research, Faculty of Food Science and Nutrition, University of Iceland, Reykjavik; Landspitali University Hospital, Reykjavík, Iceland; **School of Health Sciences, University of Iceland, Háskóli Íslands, Iceland

Overweight and obesity are defined as body weight above the ideal body weight evidently related to health and well-being. A body weight that is too high in relation to height is associated with higher proportion of adipose tissue in the body and a number of diseases. The prevalence of overweight and obesity in the world has doubled over the last 25 years. In 2014, 39% of adults over 18 years were overweight. The prevalence is still increasing in many wealthy countries and, with increased standards of living, the trend has reached less affluent countries as well (WHO, 2016, web reference). Efforts to treat overweight and obesity include factors such as restriction of energy intake, increased physical activity, and other life style programs, as well as surgical methods. A better understanding of the underlying causes is still needed. Two hormones, leptin and ghrelin, call for special attention in this regard as their production and secretion are associated with satiety and hunger and their levels in blood vary with body weight and adipose tissue (Woods and D'Alessio, 2008).

ROLE AND PRODUCTION OF LEPTIN AND GHRELIN

The main role of leptin, also called the satiety hormone, is to mediate satiety and reduce appetite by way of a circulating signal. It also gives an adaptive response to starvation (Ahima et al., 1996; Friedman, 2009) and it has been hypothesized that the primary role of leptin may be to signal starvation that is, through low leptin levels and, as such, aid to avoid depletion of fat stores, and support survival when food is scarce. Leptin is therefore both a satiety mediator to prevent overeating and a player to support the body's energy storage. In opposition to leptin, ghrelin (also named lenomorelin) has been called the hunger hormone (Dickson et al., 2011) as it regulates appetite and is important in regulating the distribution and rate of energy use in the body (Burger and Berner, 2014). Receptors for ghrelin and leptin are found on the same cells in the brain (Perello et al., 2012). The main production of leptin is in the adipocytes of white adipose tissue. It is also produced in brown adipose tissue, fundic glands of the stomach fundus, and gastric chief cells (Bado et al., 1998) as well as in mammary epithelial cells, bone marrow, placenta, ovaries, and skeletal muscles (Margetic et al., 2002). The production of ghrelin, a peptide hormone, is in ghrelinergic cells in the gastrointestinal tract and it is mainly secreted from cells in the stomach (Inui et al., 2004; Sakata and Sakai, 2010).

CONDITIONS AFFECTING BLOOD LEVELS OF LEPTIN AND GHRELIN

In healthy individuals, leptin and ghrelin levels in blood are affected by many conditions. Large fat mass produces disproportionally more leptin than a smaller fat mass. Leptin is found both in free form and bound to proteins in the blood (Lonnqvist et al., 1995; Madej, 1998; Sinha et al., 1996b). Gender affects leptin levels as these are higher in women compared to men, and concurrently correlate negatively with testosterone levels and positively with

Fish and Fish Oil in Health and Disease Prevention. http://dx.doi.org/10.1016/B978-0-12-802844-5.00016-6

estrogen levels (Ahima & Flier, 2000). This is in line with the proportional higher fat percentage of women's body weight compared to men. However, there are also variations in leptin levels in blood which are not associated with adipose tissues and the amount or proportion of body fat mass. Exercise and training, for example, have been found to reduce leptin levels (de Salles et al., 2010; Hickey et al., 1996; Hickey et al., 1997) which stimulates food intake after the increased usage of energy during exercise and training periods. Measurements of leptin have shown higher blood levels from midnight to early morning which may be associated with rest and therefore lower appetite during the night's sleep (Sinha et al., 1996a). However, the everyday pulse of leptin levels in blood can be changed by serving meals at different time points, as well as through timing of waking hours and sleep (Schoeller et al., 1997). Fasting leptin levels decrease after a short-term fasting of 24–72 h, although no changes in fat mass can be seen (Chan et al., 2003; Kolaczynski et al., 1996a; Kolaczynski et al., 1996b). Fasting blood leptin levels are higher in obese individuals, as compared to normal weight individuals, a condition that should lead to more satiety and less food intake (Caro et al., 1996). The lack of stretching of stomach cells controls the secretion of ghrelin when the stomach is empty, and when the stomach cells are stretched, secretion stops (Dickson et al., 2011). In normal weight individuals, the levels of ghrelin in plasma change in the period from midnight to dawn when there is an increase in the ghrelin concentration. However, the circadian rhythm of ghrelin release has been shown to be altered by exposure to, for example, light at night (Fonken and Nelson, 2014).

Shorter duration of sleep leads to hormonal changes which may increase food intake and lead to obesity (Cappuccio et al., 2008). The high ghrelin levels may be the reason for more intake dependent on ghrelin-mediated hunger. Increasing levels of ghrelin and decreasing levels of leptin over a period of short sleep or disturbed sleep duration both mediate increased hunger and may lead to more food intake, a constantly positive energy balance, surplus energy storage, and finally obesity (Cappuccio et al., 2008). In a recent study fragmented sleep, shown by increased number of waking episodes, predicted less weight reduction in women who participated in a weight-loss programs (Sawamoto et al., 2014). Anorexia nervosa leads to higher ghrelin concentrations (Misra and Klibanski, 2014) than found in normal weight individuals (Germain et al., 2007). Opposite to leptin, fasting ghrelin levels are lower in obese individuals than in normal weight individuals (Cummings et al., 2002) and it has been suggested that there might be a flaw in the circadian rhythm in obese individuals leading to these differences (Yildiz et al., 2004). Obese children 11–15 years old also show significantly lower ghrelin concentrations and higher leptin levels than overweight and normal weight children (Rambhojan et al., 2015).

FASTING LEPTIN AND GHRELIN LEVELS IN OVERWEIGHT AND OBESE PARTICIPANTS AFTER DIFFERENT TYPES OF SEAFOOD DIETS AND WEIGHT LOSS

The roles of leptin and ghrelin in healthy subjects and their interesting association to obesity call for studies on the effects of different diets and weight change on the blood levels of leptin and ghrelin. Seafood has constituents of special interest. Both the long chain (LC) n–3 fatty acids as well as fish proteins, especially the amino acid taurine, have been suggested to support weight loss in energy restricted diets (Buckley and Howe, 2010). A randomized controlled dietary intervention trial, SEAFOODplus Young, was performed at our unit in Iceland, Unit for Nutrition Research at School of Health Sciences, University of Iceland and Landspitali University Hospital, together with colleagues from Ireland and Spain at the School of Food and Nutritional Sciences, University College Cork, and the Department of Physiology and Nutrition, University of Navarra, Pamplona, respectively.

In total, 324 overweight and obese young adults were recruited into the study (138 men and 186 women, aged 20–40 years, BMI 27.5–32.5). Of these 278 or 86% completed an 8 week intervention. The participants were asked to follow an individually tailored energy restricted diet, lowering calculated individual energy needs by 30%, giving a total daily intake close to 1500 kcal on average (ie, 500–800 kcal less energy daily). The primary objective was to investigate the effect of fish and seafood on health and disease in young, overweight, or obese Europeans. The participants were randomly assigned to one of four different diets with varying seafood content. A control diet contained no seafood but included six placebo capsules per day with no long chain (LC) omega-3 (n–3) fatty acids (Diet 1). Diet 2 provided 150 g lean fish (cod) three times a week and gave 0.26 g/day of eicosapentaenoic acid (EPA) and docosahexaenoic acid (DHA). Diet 3 provided 150 g fatty fish (salmon) three times a week providing 2.1 g/day of EPA and DHA, and Diet 4 was similar to Diet 1, but included six oil capsules per day giving 1.3 g/day of EPA and DHA. The energy distribution of all the diets was similar with total fat contributing 30% of total energy, carbohydrates 50%, protein 20%, and dietary fiber was 20–25 g. At baseline just before the start of the intervention period, information on lifestyle factors was collected, and participants were instructed not to change their physical activity level during the 8 week intervention period. Physical activity level was taken into account when total energy expenditure was estimated. Detailed information on the intervention has been published (Thorsdottir et al., 2007).

Blood samples were collected after an overnight fast at baseline and after the 8 week intervention. The results of the energy restriction for all the diets showed lower body weight, by on average roughly 5 kg or 6%. Leptin concentration in plasma was lower by ~10 ng/mL while plasma ghrelin concentration increased by ~50 pg/mL (Ramel et al., 2009). Many other health indicators changed over the course of the SEAFOODplus Young intervention, including changes towards a healthier blood lipid profile (Gunnarsdottir et al., 2008), lower insulin and insulin resistance (Ramel et al., 2008), lower blood pressure (Ramel et al., 2010b) and lower measured inflammatory markers (Ramel et al., 2010a) as well as reduced oxidative stress (Parra et al., 2007). Compliance to the diets was verified through two types of measurements to check the reported intake (Birgisdottir et al., 2008; Thorsdottir et al., 2009) and with biochemical measures. LC n–3 fatty acids in erythrocyte phospholipids changed in good agreement with the amount of LC n–3 fatty acids found in the different diets (Bandarra et al., 2007). Some of the health improvement markers were found to be increased in the seafood containing diets (Diets 2–4) compared to the control (Diet 1), such as weight loss, improved blood lipid profile, and lower oxidative stress. Remarkably, this was true for all the seafood diets, the lean fish (Diet 2) as well as the salmon and the diet including LC n–3 fatty acid capsules (Diets 3 and 4). However, gender apparently plays a role as the main outcome, weight loss, was only significant in men when gender was part of the model. Furthermore, it was tested whether seafood could protect loss of bone during weight loss, but no differences were observed between the four diets (Lucey et al., 2008).

Weight loss after all diet treatments was on average 6.5 kg for men and just above 4 kg for women, resulting in weight loss of 6.7% and 5.1% for men and women, respectively. Levels of fasting leptin decreased more among women, or about 13 ng/mL on average, than men who showed on average a decrease of about 6 ng/mL, after the 8 weeks of energy restriction. Fasting baseline leptin levels seemed to provide a very small, but significant, indication of the weight loss outcome (Ramel et al., 2010) but a recent systematic review does not support this finding (Strohacker et al., 2014).

Separate statistical models were constructed for men and women to predict endpoint for leptin due to the difference in leptin levels by gender. Leptin levels in men were 23% lower after the diet including salmon compared to the control. A smaller effect (ie, a 20% reduction in leptin concentration) was seen after the EPA and DHA capsule diet when compared to control. The difference in leptin levels between those who received salmon in their diet and control was no longer statistically significant after including weight loss in the model. In women, no significant difference in leptin levels was found between the four diet groups which is in accordance with no difference in weight loss between the four diets among women. There was an approximate 10% reduction in leptin concentration was seen with each kg in body weight loss among women.

About 6% higher endpoint ghrelin levels were observed among participants receiving EPA and DHA capsules compared to controls. When adjusted for gender, EPA and DHA capsule intake increased ghrelin only in women, not in men. When including weight loss in the model, the association with gender was still evident, but the effect of the diet including EPA and DHA capsules, was no longer statistically significant. Fasting insulin was reduced during the 8 week intervention. It was associated with increased endpoint ghrelin level and reduced endpoint leptin in men and women. A 14% reduction of was observed after the diet including EPA and DHA capsules compared to control, even after inclusion of weight loss in the model. The significant insulin reduction after Diet 3 which included salmon, observed in a linear model did not remain after the inclusion of weight loss in the model.

Even though the consumption of lean fish (cod) did affect several of the health outcomes positively as compared to controls, (eg, weight loss, decreased antioxidative stress, triglycerides), it did not seem to affect the circulating hormones leptin, ghrelin, or insulin more than the diet without any seafood (control). However, the 8 week intervention including salmon or fish oil decreased concentration of leptin and insulin and increased concentration of ghrelin in blood. As the study found no effect of lean fish consumption on the concentration of hormones, the principal bioactive components of seafood might be the LC n–3 fatty acids as the difference could not be explained by other factors. For example, the vitamin D intake was kept at the same level in all four diets and the energy intake was similar (Thorsdottir et al., 2007). Even though Diet 2, including lean fish, gave 0.26 g/day of EPA and DHA, it is only a small fraction of the amount of EPA and DHA in the diets with salmon and with capsules including EPA and DHA. This seems to support that increased weight loss and modification of circulating hormones by the salmon or fish oil diets as compared to control was mediated through the LC n–3 fatty acids, but the increased weight loss observed with the lean seafood diet compared to control, was mediated through another constituent found in lean fish and not through affecting the hormones levels. Therefore, the effect of the two fatty seafood diets on leptin and ghrelin may be more complex than through the weight loss alone.

ADDITIONAL ASPECTS

Studies in vitro and in animals have shown effects of LC n–3 fatty acids, EPA, and DHA on lowering leptin levels. In vitro EPA and DHA have been shown to reduce the expression of leptin and both plasma leptin and mRNA expression have been found to be lowered by LC n–3 fatty acid supplementation in rats (Ukropec et al., 2003). This effect has not been so definite in humans. A double-blinded, randomized trial in males with no energy restriction found that supplementation with 5 g of LC n–3 fatty acids per day did not affect plasma leptin concentration. However, the authors suggested that lower plasma concentrations do not automatically have to follow altered leptin expression (Reseland et al., 2001). The effect of salmon consumption on circulating leptin in men in the SEAFOODplus Young intervention seems to have been mediated by the greater weight loss following the salmon diet. The association between n–3 fatty acids and ghrelin needs to be studied further. Only a few studies have investigated the long-term effects of diet composition on fasting ghrelin. As an example, fat restriction only does not give the same effect on ghrelin levels as the increase induced by dietary energy restriction (Weigle et al., 2003). Furthermore, several weeks of high protein intake increases ghrelin concentrations (Weigle et al., 2005). Insulin is a key factor in acute studies investigating the response of ghrelin to changes in macronutrient composition of meals (Blom et al., 2005; Tannous dit El Khoury et al., 2006; Teff et al., 2004). The SEAFOODplus Young study showed that in the EPA and DHA group, the concentration of ghrelin was higher compared to controls in women but no effect was seen in males, either for EPA and DHA or in the salmon group. When including weight loss in the model for women, the significant effects of EPA and DHA disappeared indicating that in this group higher ghrelin concentrations are to some degree a consequence of weight loss rather than the higher LC n–3 fatty acid consumption. However, as ghrelin is an orexigenic hormone, women would be put at higher risk of increased food intake with higher ghrelin concentrations which seems contrary to studies finding increase in fat oxidation after intake of fish oil (Couet et al., 1997) and others indicating that n–3 fatty acids have positive effect on weight loss (Kunesova et al., 2006; Thorsdottir et al., 2009). Interestingly, in the SEAFOODplus Young study (Thorsdottir et al., 2009) the significant association between intake of EPA and DHA and weight loss was only found in men, not women (Kunesova et al., 2006). The study also found hunger sensations to decrease, not to increase, with intake of n–3 fatty acid after single meals (Parra et al., 2008) and postprandial satiety seemed tempered by intake of LC n–3 fatty acids during weight loss among the participants. Whether LC n–3 fatty acids improves compliance to nutritional treatment in overweight and obesity, as well as in weight loss maintenance, needs to be studied further (Parra et al., 2008). However, the calculated energy intake was similar between the four intervention diets indicating that the real effect on energy intake was not large.

As shown above, more weight loss was seen following all the seafood including diets when compared to the control diet in men, also the lean fish diet. As the lean fish diet included LC n–3 fatty acids as well, but in a smaller amount than the other two seafood diets, it might indicate that for some outcomes only a small amount of LC n–3 fatty acids are needed or that another lean fish constituent has an effect. A smaller study ($n = 32$ overweight or obese subjects) including a fish-based diet versus a control diet for an 8 week period, showed a larger reduction in leptin concentrations after the fish-based diet (ie, from 38 ng/mL to 24 ng/mL versus 38 to 34 ng/mL in the control diet; Abete et al., 2008). Some studies have shown an opposite effect of n–6 fatty acids. A study on diabetic/obese mice found a four-week diet including fish oil and taurine decreased fat accumulation and leptin levels when compared to a 4-week diet including soy bean oil (Mikami et al., 2012). A study in mice fed different diets for 16 weeks found that n–6 (linoleic acid) promotes weight gain compared to the control group (Alvheim et al., 2014). The SEAFOODplus Young intervention found that regular consumption of EPA and DHA decreased fasting insulin by 14.4% independent of weight loss. According to the statistical model this change is equivalent to a weight loss of ~4 kg (Ramel et al., 2009). Studies have found insulin to be an important regulator of both leptin and ghrelin levels as it was found to decrease ghrelin and increase leptin dose-dependently in human studies using hyperinsulinemic–euglycemic clamps (Boden et al., 1997; Saad et al., 2002). Similar results, although reversed, were found in the SEAFOODplus Young study as reductions of fasting insulin during the eight weeks were significantly associated with increased ghrelin and reduced leptin concentrations. Other studies investigating the effect of energy intake and weight loss on circulating leptin and ghrelin levels are in line with the findings from the SEAFOODplus Young study (Ariyasu et al., 2001; Cummings et al., 2001; Kolaczynski et al., 1996a; Romon et al., 2006; Weigle et al., 1997). However, the decrease in body weight of 5 kg or 6% on average, was not in direct correlation with changes of circulating hormones of a 6% increase for ghrelin and a 35% decrease for leptin. In our investigation the most consistent predictor of hormonal changes seemed to be weight loss. It has been hypothesized that leptin resistance develops in obesity making the receptors less prone to receive the leptin message and therefore accumulate at a higher level (Myers et al., 2008; Oswal & Yeo, 2010). This has been compared to resistance of insulin in type 2 diabetes, such that the elevated hormone level fails to control hunger and modulate weight (Myers et al., 2008). Similar resistance has been seen in rats given access to palatable, energy dense food (Wang et al., 2001) while the effect is reversed when the animals are put back on a low energy diet (Enriori et al., 2007). As leptin levels signal that there is enough energy stored (Banks et al., 2006) leptin resistance might be a normal part of human physiology even indicating a survival advantage (Myers et al., 2008) or an evolutionary advantage (Obici & Rossetti, 2003).

CONCLUSION

Fatty fish and LC n–3 fatty acids are important in the discussion about potential benefit of specific foods and nutrients in treatment of overweight and obese individuals and may improve insulin and leptin levels and improve weight loss (Abete et al., 2011). More long term trials are needed to discern the effect and mechanism behind the potential benefit of LC n–3 fatty acid supplementation indicated in human intervention trials. These should be combined with energy restricted diets and/or exercise (Buckley and Howe, 2010). Other aspects should also be explored such as potential interaction between the intestinal microflora and leptin and ghrelin levels (Clarke et al., 2014). In our 8 week intervention the consumption of fatty seafood (salmon group or EPA and DHA oil capsules) modulated the fasting levels of insulin, ghrelin and leptin. The effects were specific for gender but were most consistently explained by weight loss. However, as consumption of lean fish had several similar effects on health indicators as the fatty seafood diets, but did not affect the circulating hormones in comparison to the control group, there seems to be two different ways of achieving weight loss, with or without the effect on leptin and ghrelin. Therefore, the potential effects on leptin and ghrelin of EPA and DHA might be more complex than through the weight loss alone.

References

Abete, I., Parra, D., Crujeiras, A.B., Goyenechea, E., Martinez, J.A., 2008. Specific insulin sensitivity and leptin responses to a nutritional treatment of obesity via a combination of energy restriction and fatty fish intake. J. Hum. Nutr. Diet 21 (6), 591–600.

Abete, I., Goyenechea, E., Zulet, M.A., Martinez, J.A., 2011. Obesity and metabolic syndrome: potential benefit from specific nutritional components. Nutr. Metab. Cardiovasc. Dis. 21 (Suppl. 2), B1–B15.

Ahima, R.S., Flier, J.S., 2000. Leptin. Annu. Rev. Physiol. 62, 413–437.

Ahima, R.S., Prabakaran, D., Mantzoros, C., Qu, D., Lowell, B., Maratos-Flier, E., Flier, J.S., 1996. Role of leptin in the neuroendocrine response to fasting. Nature 382 (6588), 250–252.

Alvheim, A. R., Torstensen, B. E., Lin, Y. H., Lillefosse, H. H., Lock, E. J., Madsen, L., Malde, M. K., 2014. Dietary linoleic acid elevates the endocannabinoids 2-AG and anandamide and promotes weight gain in mice fed a low fat diet. Lipids, 49 (1); pp. 59–69.

Ariyasu, H., Takaya, K., Tagami, T., Ogawa, Y., Hosoda, K., Akamizu, T., Nakao, K., 2001. Stomach is a major source of circulating ghrelin, and feeding state determines plasma ghrelin-like immunoreactivity levels in humans. J. Clin. Endocrinol. Metab. 86 (10), pp. 4753–4758.

Bado, A., Levasseur, S., Attoub, S., Kermorgant, S., Laigneau, J.P., Bortoluzzi, M.N., Lewin, M.J., 1998. The stomach is a source of leptin. Nature, 394 (6695), pp. 790–793.

Bandarra, N.M., Monteiro, M., Martinez, J.A., Kiely, M., Thorsdottir, I., 2007. Erythrocyte membrane fatty acid incorporation as a marker of fish diet in young overweight Europeans. J. Aquatic Food Prod. Technol. 16 (4), 3–11.

Banks, W.A., Farr, S.A., Morley, J.E., 2006. The effects of high fat diets on the blood-brain barrier transport of leptin: failure or adaptation? Physiol. Behav. 88 (3), 244–248.

Birgisdottir, B.E., Kiely, M., Martinez, J.A., Thorsdottir, I., 2008. Validity of a food frequency questionnaire to assess intake of seafood in adults in three European countries. Food Control 19 (7), 648–653.

Blom, W.A., Stafleu, A., de Graaf, C., Kok, F.J., Schaafsma, G., Hendriks, H.F., 2005. Ghrelin response to carbohydrate-enriched breakfast is related to insulin. Am. J. Clin. Nutr. 81 (2), 367–375.

Boden, G., Chen, X., Kolaczynski, J.W., Polansky, M., 1997. Effects of prolonged hyperinsulinemia on serum leptin in normal human subjects. J. Clin. Invest. 100 (5), 1107–1113.

Buckley, J.D., Howe, P.R., 2010. Long-chain omega-3 polyunsaturated fatty acids may be beneficial for reducing obesity-a review. Nutrients 2 (12), 1212–1230.

Burger, K.S., Berner, L.A., 2014. A functional neuroimaging review of obesity, appetitive hormones and ingestive behavior. Physiol. Behav. 136, 121–127.

Cappuccio, F.P., Taggart, F.M., Kandala, N.B., Currie, A., Peile, E., Stranges, S., Miller, M.A., 2008. Meta-analysis of short sleep duration and obesity in children and adults. Sleep 31 (5), 619–626.

Caro, J.F., Sinha, M.K., Kolaczynski, J.W., Zhang, P.L., Considine, R.V., 1996. Leptin: the tale of an obesity gene. Diabetes 45 (11), 1455–1462.

Chan, J.L., Heist, K., DePaoli, A.M., Veldhuis, J.D., Mantzoros, C.S., 2003. The role of falling leptin levels in the neuroendocrine and metabolic adaptation to short-term starvation in healthy men. J. Clin. Invest. 111 (9), 1409–1421.

Clarke, G., Stilling, R.M., Kennedy, P.J., Stanton, C., Cryan, J.F., Dinan, T.G., 2014. Minireview: gut microbiota: the neglected endocrine organ. Mol. Endocrinol. 28 (8), 1221–1238.

Couet, C., Delarue, J., Ritz, P., Antoine, J.M., Lamisse, F., 1997. Effect of dietary fish oil on body fat mass and basal fat oxidation in healthy adults. Int. J. Obes. Relat. Metab. Disord. 21 (8), 637–643.

Cummings, D.E., Purnell, J.Q., Frayo, R.S., Schmidova, K., Wisse, B.E., Weigle, D.S., 2001. A preprandial rise in plasma ghrelin levels suggests a role in meal initiation in humans. Diabetes 50 (8), 1714–1719.

Cummings, D.E., Weigle, D.S., Frayo, R.S., Breen, P.A., Ma, M.K., Dellinger, E.P., Purnell, J.Q., 2002. Plasma ghrelin levels after diet-induced weight loss or gastric bypass surgery. N. Engl. J. Med. 346 (21), 1623–1630.

de Salles, B.F., Simao, R., Fleck, S.J., Dias, I., Kraemer-Aguiar, L.G., Bouskela, E., 2010. Effects of resistance training on cytokines. Int. J. Sports. Med. 31 (7), 441–450.

Dickson, S.L., Egecioglu, E., Landgren, S., Skibicka, K.P., Engel, J.A., Jerlhag, E., 2011. The role of the central ghrelin system in reward from food and chemical drugs. Mol. Cell. Endocrinol. 340 (1), 80–87.

Enriori, P. J., Evans, A. E., Sinnayah, P., Jobst, E. E., Tonelli-Lemos, L., Billes, S. K., Cowley, M. A., 2007. Diet-induced obesity causes severe but reversible leptin resistance in arcuate melanocortin neurons. Cell Metab. 5 (3), pp. 181—194.

Fonken, L.K., Nelson, R.J., 2014. The effects of light at night on circadian clocks and metabolism. Endocr. Rev. 35 (4), 648–670.

Friedman, J.M., 2009. Leptin at 14 y of age: an ongoing story. Am. J. Clin. Nutr. 89 (3), 973S–979S.

Germain, N., Galusca, B., Le Roux, C. W., Bossu, C., Ghatei, M. A., Lang, F., Estour, B., 2007. Constitutional thinness and lean anorexia nervosa display opposite concentrations of peptide YY, glucagon-like peptide 1, ghrelin, and leptin. Am. J. Clin. Nutr. 85 (4), pp. 967–971.

Gunnarsdottir, I., Tomasson, H., Kiely, M., Martinez, J.A., Bandarra, N.M., Morais, M.G., Thorsdottir, I., 2008. Inclusion of fish or fish oil in weight-loss diets for young adults: effects on blood lipids. Int. J. Obes. (London) 32 (7), 1105–1112.

Hickey, M. S., Considine, R. V., Israel, R. G., Mahar, T. L., McCammon, M. R., Tyndall, G. L., Caro, J. F., 1996. Leptin is related to body fat content in male distance runners. Am J Physiol. 271 (5 Pt 1), pp. E938–E940.

Hickey, M. S., Houmard, J. A., Considine, R. V., Tyndall, G. L., Midgette, J. B., Gavigan, K. E., Caro, J. F., 1997. Gender-dependent effects of exercise training on serum leptin levels in humans. Am. J. Physiol. 272 (4 Pt 1), pp. E562-E566.

Inui, A., Asakawa, A., Bowers, C.Y., Mantovani, G., Laviano, A., Meguid, M.M., Fujimiya, M., 2004. Ghrelin, appetite, and gastric motility: the emerging role of the stomach as an endocrine organ. FASEB J. 18 (3), 439–456.

Kolaczynski, J. W., Considine, R. V., Ohannesian, J., Marco, C., Opentanova, I., Nyce, M. R., Caro, J. F., 1996. Responses of leptin to short-term fasting and refeeding in humans: a link with ketogenesis but not ketones themselves. Diabetes, 45 (11), pp. 1511–1515.

Kolaczynski, J.W., Ohannesian, J.P., Considine, R.V., Marco, C.C., Caro, J.F., 1996b. Response of leptin to short-term and prolonged overfeeding in humans. J. Clin. Endocrinol. Metab. 81 (11), 4162–4165.

Kunesova, M., Braunerova, R., Hlavaty, P., Tvrzicka, E., Stankova, B., Skrha, J., Svacina, S. 2006. The influence of n-3 polyunsaturated fatty acids and very low calorie diet during a short-term weight reducing regimen on weight loss and serum fatty acid composition in severely obese women. Physiol. Res. 55 (1), pp. 63–72.

Lonnqvist, F., Arner, P., Nordfors, L., Schalling, M., 1995. Overexpression of the obese (ob) gene in adipose tissue of human obese subjects. Nat. Med. 1 (9), 950–953.

Lucey, A.J., Paschos, G.K., Cashman, K.D., Martinez, J.A., Thorsdottir, I., Kiely, M., 2008. Influence of moderate energy restriction and seafood consumption on bone turnover in overweight young adults. Am. J. Clin. Nutr. 87 (4), 1045–1052.

Madej, T., 1998. Considerations in the use of lipid-based drug products. J. Intraven. Nurs. 21 (6), 326.

Margetic, S., Gazzola, C., Pegg, G.G., Hill, R.A., 2002. Leptin: a review of its peripheral actions and interactions. Int. J. Obes. Relat. Metab. Disord. 26 (11), 1407–1433.

Mikami, N., Hosokawa, M., Miyashita, K., 2012. Dietary combination of fish oil and taurine decreases fat accumulation and ameliorates blood glucose levels in Type 2 diabetic/obese KK-A(y) Mice. J. Food Sci. 77 (6), H114–H120.

Misra, M., Klibanski, A., 2014. Endocrine consequences of anorexia nervosa. Lancet Diabetes Endocrinol. 2 (7), 581–592.

Myers, M.G., Cowley, M.A., Munzberg, H., 2008. Mechanisms of leptin action and leptin resistance. Annu. Rev. Physiol. 70, 537–556.

Obici, S., Rossetti, L., 2003. Minireview: nutrient sensing and the regulation of insulin action and energy balance. Endocrinology 144 (12), 5172–5178.

Oswal, A., Yeo, G., 2010. Leptin and the control of body weight: a review of its diverse central targets, signaling mechanisms, and role in the pathogenesis of obesity. Obesity (Silver Spring) 18 (2), 221–229.

Parra, D., Bandarra, N.M., Kiely, M., Thorsdottir, I., Martinez, J.A., 2007. Impact of fish intake on oxidative stress when included into a moderate energy-restricted program to treat obesity. Eur. J. Nutr. 46 (8), 460–467.

Parra, D., Ramel, A., Bandarra, N., Kiely, M., Martinez, J.A., Thorsdottir, I., 2008. A diet rich in long chain omega-3 fatty acids modulates satiety in overweight and obese volunteers during weight loss. Appetite 51 (3), 676–680.

Perello, M., Scott, M. M., Sakata, I., Lee, C. E., Chuang, J. C., Osborne-Lawrence, S., Zigman, J. M., 2012. Functional implications of limited leptin receptor and ghrelin receptor coexpression in the brain. J Comp Neurol. 520 (2), pp. 281–294.

Rambhojan, C., Bouaziz-Amar, E., Larifla, L., Deloumeaux, J., Clepier, J., Plumasseau, J., Foucan, L., 2015. Ghrelin, adipokines, metabolic factors in relation with weight status in school-children and results of a 1-year lifestyle intervention program. Nutr. Metab. (London), 12, 43.

Ramel, A., Martinez, A., Kiely, M., Morais, G., Bandarra, N.M., Thorsdottir, I., 2008. Beneficial effects of long-chain n-3 fatty acids included in an energy-restricted diet on insulin resistance in overweight and obese European young adults. Diabetologia 51 (7), 1261–1268.

Ramel, A., Parra, D., Martinez, J.A., Kiely, M., Thorsdottir, I., 2009. Effects of seafood consumption and weight loss on fasting leptin and ghrelin concentrations in overweight and obese European young adults. Eur. J. Nutr. 48 (2), 107–114.

Ramel, A., Arnarson, A., Parra, D., Kiely, M., Bandarra, N.M., Martinez, J.A., Thorsdottir, I., 2010. Gender difference in the prediction of weight loss by leptin among overweight adults. Ann. Nutr. Metab. 56 (3), 190–197.

Ramel, A., Martinez, J.A., Kiely, M., Bandarra, N.M., Thorsdottir, I., 2010a. Effects of weight loss and seafood consumption on inflammation parameters in young, overweight and obese European men and women during 8 weeks of energy restriction. Eur. J. Clin. Nutr. 64 (9), 987–993.

Ramel, A., Martinez, J.A., Kiely, M., Bandarra, N.M., Thorsdottir, I., 2010b. Moderate consumption of fatty fish reduces diastolic blood pressure in overweight and obese European young adults during energy restriction. Nutrition 26 (2), 168–174.

Reseland, J. E., Haugen, F., Hollung, K., Solvoll, K., Halvorsen, B., Brude, I. R., Drevon, C. A., 2001. Reduction of leptin gene expression by dietary polyunsaturated fatty acids. J. Lipid Res. 42 (5), pp. 743–750.

Romon, M., Gomila, S., Hincker, P., Soudan, B., Dallongeville, J., 2006. Influence of weight loss on plasma ghrelin responses to high-fat and high-carbohydrate test meals in obese women. J. Clin. Endocrinol. Metab. 91 (3), 1034–1041.

Saad, M.F., Bernaba, B., Hwu, C.M., Jinagouda, S., Fahmi, S., Kogosov, E., Boyadjian, R., 2002. Insulin regulates plasma ghrelin concentration. J. Clin. Endocrinol. Metab. 87 (8), 3997–4000.

Sakata, I., Sakai, T., 2010. Ghrelin cells in the gastrointestinal tract. Int. J. Pept.

Sawamoto, R., Nozaki, T., Furukawa, T., Tanahashi, T., Morita, C., Hata, T., Sudo, N., 2014. Higher sleep fragmentation predicts a lower magnitude of weight loss in overweight and obese women participating in a weight-loss intervention. Nutr. Diabetes 4.

Schoeller, D.A., Cella, L.K., Sinha, M.K., Caro, J.F., 1997. Entrainment of the diurnal rhythm of plasma leptin to meal timing. J. Clin. Invest. 100 (7), 1882–1887.

Sinha, M. K., Ohannesian, J. P., Heiman, M. L., Kriauciunas, A., Stephens, T. W., Magosin, S., Caro, J. F., 1996. Nocturnal rise of leptin in lean, obese, and non-insulin-dependent diabetes mellitus subjects. J. Clin. Invest. 97 (5), pp. 1344–1347.

Sinha, M. K., Opentanova, I., Ohannesian, J. P., Kolaczynski, J. W., Heiman, M. L., Hale, J., Caro, J. F., 1996. Evidence of free and bound leptin in human circulation. Studies in lean and obese subjects and during short-term fasting. J. Clin. Invest. 98 (6), 1277–1282.

Strohacker, K., McCaffery, J.M., MacLean, P.S., Wing, R.R., 2014. Adaptations of leptin, ghrelin or insulin during weight loss as predictors of weight regain: a review of current literature. Int. J. Obes. (London) 38 (3), 388–396.

Tannous dit El Khoury, D., Obeid, O., Azar, S.T., Hwalla, N., 2006. Variations in postprandial ghrelin status following ingestion of high-carbohydrate, high-fat, and high-protein meals in males. Ann. Nutr. Metab. 50 (3), 260–269.

Teff, K. L., Elliott, S. S., Tschop, M., Kieffer, T. J., Rader, D., Heiman, M., Havel, P. J., 2004. Dietary fructose reduces circulating insulin and leptin, attenuates postprandial suppression of ghrelin, and increases triglycerides in women. J. Clin. Endocrinol. Metab. 89 (6), pp. 2963–2972.

Thorsdottir, I., Tomasson, H., Gunnarsdottir, I., Gisladottir, E., Kiely, M., Parra, M. D., Martinez, J. A., 2007. Randomized trial of weight-loss-diets for young adults varying in fish and fish oil content. Int. J. Obes. (London), 31 (10), pp. 1560–1566.

Thorsdottir, I., Birgisdottir, B., Kiely, M., Martinez, J., Bandarra, N., 2009. Fish consumption among young overweight European adults and compliance to varying seafood content in four weight loss intervention diets. Public Health Nutr. 12 (5), 592–598.

Ukropec, J., Reseland, J. E., Gasperikova, D., Demcakova, E., Madsen, L., Berge, R. K., Sebokova, E., 2003. The hypotriglyceridemic effect of dietary n-3 FA is associated with increased beta-oxidation and reduced leptin expression. Lipids, 38 (10), pp. 1023–1029.

Wang, J., Obici, S., Morgan, K., Barzilai, N., Feng, Z., Rossetti, L., 2001. Overfeeding rapidly induces leptin and insulin resistance. Diabetes 50 (12), 2786–2791.

Weigle, D.S., Duell, P.B., Connor, W.E., Steiner, R.A., Soules, M.R., Kuijper, J.L., 1997. Effect of fasting, refeeding, and dietary fat restriction on plasma leptin levels. J. Clin. Endocrinol. Metabol. 82 (2), 561–565.

Weigle, D. S., Cummings, D. E., Newby, P. D., Breen, P. A., Frayo, R. S., Matthys, C. C., Purnell, J. Q., 2003. Roles of leptin and ghrelin in the loss of body weight caused by a low fat, high carbohydrate diet. J. Clin. Endocrinol. Metab. 88 (4), pp. 1577–1586.

Weigle, D.S., Breen, P.A., Matthys, C.C., Callahan, H.S., Meeuws, K.E., Burden, V.R., Purnell, J.Q., 2005. A high-protein diet induces sustained reductions in appetite, ad libitum caloric intake, and body weight despite compensatory changes in diurnal plasma leptin and ghrelin concentrations. Am. J. Clin. Nutr. 82 (1), 41–48.

World Health Organization (WHO), 2016. http://www.who.int/mediacentre/factsheets/fs311/en/

Woods, S.C., D'Alessio, D.A., 2008. Central control of body weight and appetite. J. Clin. Endocrinol. Metab. 93 (11 Suppl. 1), S37–S50.

Yildiz, B.O., Suchard, M.A., Wong, M.L., McCann, S.M., Licinio, J., 2004. Alterations in the dynamics of circulating ghrelin, adiponectin, and leptin in human obesity. Proc. Natl. Acad. Sci. USA 101 (28), 10434–10439.

CHAPTER

17

Fish/Fish Oil Intake and Inflammatory Biomarkers, Endothelial Function

B.T. Steffen, L.M. Steffen***

*Department of Laboratory Medicine and Pathology, University of Minnesota, Minneapolis, Minnesota, United States; **Division of Epidemiology and Community Health, University of Minnesota School of Public Health, Minneapolis, Minnesota, United States

OVERVIEW

Evidence that the fish oil fatty acids EPA and DHA have health benefits, protect against disease development, or slow/reverse disease progression has been presented in previous chapters, yet it must be acknowledged that the mechanisms by which EPA and DHA may exert their effects remain controversial. Habitual dietary intake of fish and high plasma levels of fish oil fatty acids have been shown to reduce cardiac arrhythmias (Billman et al., 1994; Jacobsen et al., 1997; Mozaffarian et al., 2004) and favorably influence cholesterol profiles (lower triglycerides and modestly increase HDL) and lower blood pressure (Iketani et al., 2013; Geleijnse et al., 2002). Apart from these, EPA and DHA suppress certain biological phenomena that promote disease states—specifically, inflammation and endothelial activation.

Inflammation and endothelial activation (ie, endothelial dysfunction) represent two separate, but related, processes for initiating and maintaining the immune response necessary for homeostasis, repairing damaged tissue, as well as fighting pathogens and infection. Often characterized by redness, swelling, and soreness, inflammation increases blood flow and permeability of blood vessels in order to deliver plasma exudates as well as leukocytes and other immune cells to the inflamed tissue. Also facilitating the movement of these cells in to tissue, endothelial activation results in the expression of proteins and adhesion molecules on the endothelial surface of vessels which then bind to immune cells, slowing them in a process called 'leukocyte rolling' and mediating their transport across the endothelial membrane. Though acute inflammation is critical in host defense, *chronic* inflammation and endothelial activation have been found to contribute to disease development including atherosclerosis and cardiovascular disease. Furthermore, their chronic activity has been found to contribute to peripheral insulin resistance and type II diabetes. Though specific pathophysiologies and origins of diseases are beyond the scope of the present chapter, it must be recognized that there is an inflammatory component to certain disease states that may be prevented, diminished, or reversed with fish oil fatty acid intake. The remaining sections will present the current evidence from the scientific literature that fish oil fatty acids reduce inflammation and endothelial activation.

EPA Competes with Arachidonic Acid

One of the first antiinflammatory mechanisms hypothesized for fish oil fatty acids related to their competition with arachidonic acid and its metabolism to the inflammatory eicosanoids. To understand this paradigm, it must first be recognized that a cell membrane is a phospholipid bilayer composed of a complex of fatty acids, proteins, glycoproteins, carbohydrates, and free cholesterol. Fatty acids within the cell membrane serve a multitude of functions—among them, they are substrates for intracellular enzymes and signal transduction pathways that mediate inflammation (as well as having a host of other functions).

Fish and Fish Oil in Health and Disease Prevention. http://dx.doi.org/10.1016/B978-0-12-802844-5.00017-8

Importantly, it has been found that the fatty acid composition of immune cell membranes may influence inflammation in either direction. In the case of the omega-6 fatty acid, arachidonic acid, is a critical intermediary of inflammation through its production of inflammatory mediators via the arachidonate 5-lipoxygenase (ALOX-5) enzyme, cyclooxygenase, and cytochrome P450 enzymes (Bagga et al., 2003). Arachidonic acid-derived mediators such as the 4-series leukotrienes and 2-series prostaglandins are instrumental in initiating and maintaining the inflammatory response, inducing vascular permeability, and immune cell chemotaxis in target tissues (Figs. 17.1 and 17.2).

Similar to omega-6 arachidonic acid, omega-3 EPA is metabolized to inflammatory mediators by ALOX-5 activity; however, those derived from EPA, the 5-series leukotrienes and 3-series prostaglandins among them, are less inflammatory—specifically, these eicosanoids are less potent in inducing chemotaxis and proinflammatory cytokine production in immune cells as compared to AA-derived counterparts (Goldman et al., 1983; Lee et al., 1984; Bagga et al., 2003). Although EPA-derived eicosanoids are less inflammatory than those generated from AA (Barham et al., 2000), it is unlikely that this proposed antiinflammatory mechanism of EPA represents the sole effect that accounts for the antiinflammatory influence of fish oil fatty acids.

EPA/DHA Suppress the Inflammatory Nuclear Factor-κB Pathway

The nuclear factor-κB (NF-κB) pathway is one of the most prominent and well-studied pathways involved in acute inflammatory response, inflammatory cytokine synthesis, endothelial activation, and has also been shown to be involved in disease development. At a cellular level, an inflammatory stimulus caused by interleukin 1 (IL-1), tumor necrosis factor alpha (TNF-α), or bacterial-associated lipopolysacharide activates the NF-κB transcription factor through the phosphorylation and subsequent degradation of a bound inhibitory element, IκB. Following its dissociation with IkB, NF-κB is free to enter the nucleus and initiate transcription of dozens of inflammatory and endothelial activation-related genes—among the most well-known: IL-1α, IL-1β, IL-1 receptor antagonist, IL-6, IL-8, IL-10, IL-12, TNF-α, ICAM-1, P-selectin, and VCAM-1.

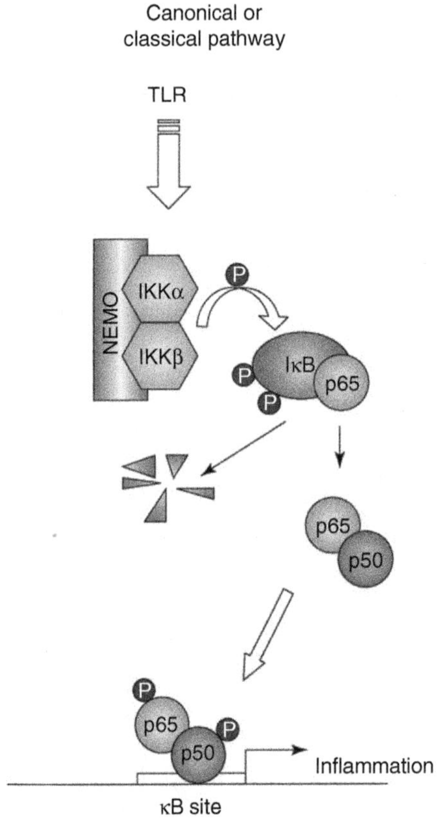

FIGURE 17.1 **Classical NF-κB pathway.** Activation by TNF-α or toll-like receptors result in ubiquitination and degradation of the IκB inhibitory element, phosphorylation, activation of the p65/p50 transcription factor, and ultimately in inflammatory gene expression. *Source: Illustration of AA versus EPA cascade producing alternative.*

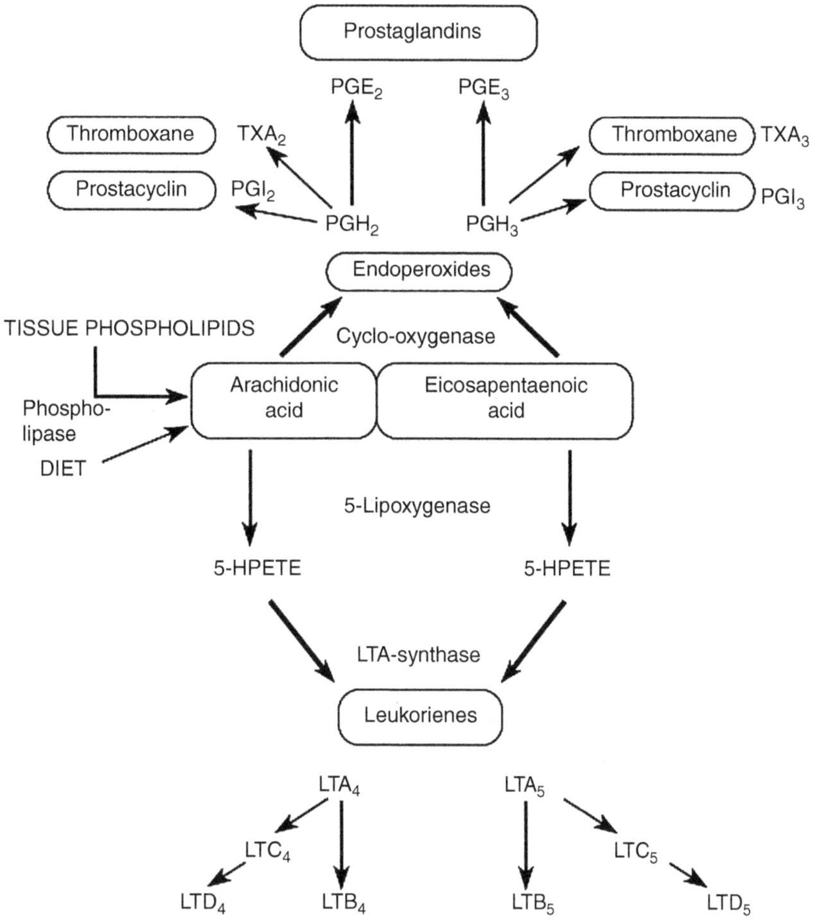

FIGURE 17.2 **Differential metabolism of fatty acids.** The omega-3 eicosapentaenoic acid (EPA) and omega-6 arachidonic acid (AA) metabolize in to different eicosanoids (leukotrienes, prostaglandins, etc.) which have distinct implications for inducing inflammation. *Source: illustration of IkB-NFkB-transcription.*

Evidence that the marine n–3 fatty acids reduce NF-κB activity has been found in cell culture and animal models, as well as in human studies. Direct exposure of EPA and DHA to cultured macrophages, neutrophils, and other differentiated immune cells has been found to reduce expression of inflammatory cytokines (De Caterina et al., 1994; Khalfoun et al., 1997; Chu et al., 1999) and has been shown to occur with a concomitant reduction in IκB phosphorylation or reduced NF-κB activity (Lo et al., 1999; Lee et al., 2001; Novak et al., 2003; Zhao et al., 2004; Mullen et al., 2010). However, as direct exposure of moderate to high concentrations of EPA and DHA to cells in a culture dish does not capture the in vivo situation, animal studies have therefore been conducted to better determine whether fish oil affects immune cell function. Though there are a number of methods to examine the effect of EPA and DHA on inflammation in a living system, a common study design involves a group of *experimental* rodents fed high intakes of EPA and DHA compared to *control* animals fed standard rodent chow. After an allotted period of time, blood is collected from both sets of animals and immune cells can then be harvested and isolated. Isolated immune cells are then 'challenged' often with lipopolysaccharide, to induce a classical acute immune response characterized by upregulation of inflammatory cytokine genes, inflammatory protein expression, and their release—all of which can be assessed to evaluate the amplitude of the immune response. Similar to results using cell culture models, immune cells from animals fed higher levels of EPA and DHA were shown to generate lower levels of inflammatory cytokine and inflammatory gene expression (Renier et al., 1993; Chandrasekar and Fernandes, 1994; Robinson et al., 1996; Calder 2013), as well as showing lower NF-κB activity (Xi et al., 2001). Though both cell culture and animal models have shown that EPA and DHA suppress the inflammatory response in immune cells, it remains unclear whether this is through direct interaction. Intermediaries have been suggested—activation of peroxisome proliferator-activated receptor γ (Kliewer et al., 1997; Huang et al., 2011; Li et al., 2005) and the G-protein receptor 120 (Oh et al., 2010) are likely modes of EPA/DHA-directed suppression of the NFkB pathway. Cell culture models have shown that n–3 fatty acids inhibit

TNF-activated, proinflammatory pathways and this inhibition was dependent on functional GPR120. Using a gene knockout approach in mice revealed that high intake of n–3 fatty acids reduced inflammation, but only in animals with functional GPR 120 protein (Oh et al., 2010). Whether GPR120 mediates an antiinflammatory effect in humans has yet to be determined.

EPA and DHA Promote the Resolution of Inflammation

Two critical aspects of the inflammatory response are its locality and duration, both of which must be limited lest inflammation expands to adjacent tissue and/or continues over a longer time frame, damaging healthy tissue, and promoting pathological events. Historically, both its confinement and inflammatory resolution were considered passive processes that were resolved once the underlying infection and cellular debris were cleared, injured tissue had healed, or tissue homeostasis restored. However, in the year 2000 a proresolving metabolite of EPA was discovered (Serhan et al., 2000; Serhan et al., 2002). EPA-derived resolvin E1 represents one of the first Specialized Proresolving Mediators (SPMs) [though AA-derived lipoxin could be argued as the first proresolution lipid mediators identified in 1984 (Serhan et al., 1984)]. SPMs are a class of compounds shown to mediate the 'resolution' phase, or endpoint, of an inflammatory response but they also suppress inflammation at crucial junctures in the inflammatory response. Proresolving lipid mediators represent another potential mechanism that contributes to the antiinflammatory effects of fish oil fatty acids.

SPMs are a growing family of lipid mediators composed of dozens of subclasses including resolvins, protectins, and maresins—notably, as EPA and DHA are structurally distinct, they generate different lipid mediators. The E-series resolvins (RvE1, RvE2, RvE3, etc.) are metabolic products of EPA while the D-series resolvins (RvD1–RvD6) and protectins (PD1, PDX) are generated from DHA (Serhan et al., 2000; Serhan et al., 2004). The resolvins and protectins are found in white blood cells as well as various tissues—among them, lymph nodes, spleen, and lungs (Colas et al., 2014). Although individual metabolites have unique tissue-specific functions that also depend on the stage of the inflammatory response, many of their effects have been shown to overlap. Among these effects, resolvins and protectins have been shown to reduce: (1) chemotaxis and transendothelial migration; (2) cell adhesion molecule expression on leukocytes and endothelial cells; (3) neutrophil recruitment and activation; (4) proinflammatory cytokine and chemokine activity (Arita et al., 2005; Schwab et al., 2007; Serhan et al., 2015). In contrast to the resolvins and protectins, the maresins (macrophage mediators in resolving inflammation) have so far been found to be expressed in macrophages alone. Maresins show many of the same functions, but also have been shown to promote phagocytosis of apoptotic neutrophils and macrophages, and the exodus of leukocytes from tissue—effectively stimulating the removal of cells and cellular debris from the site of inflammation.

Lipoprotein-Associated Phospholipase A_2

The lipoprotein-associated phospholipase A_2 (Lp-PLA$_2$) enzyme is considered as a marker of vascular inflammation and has been shown to be an independent risk factor for cardiovascular disease. Given the inflammatory component of Lp-PLA$_2$, it has been hypothesized that n–3 fish oil fatty acids may reduce its expression and/or enzymatic activity. Observation studies showed that EPA and DHA levels inversely associate with Lp-PLA$_2$ concentrations (Schmidt et al., 2008; Steffen et al., 2013); however, results from dietary intervention studies of EPA or DHA supplementation have been inconclusive. No effect of EPA + DHA on Lp-PLA$_2$ mass has been reported by one study (Pedersen et al., 2009; Nelson et al., 2011), while EPA has been shown to reduce Lp-PLA$_2$ levels by a modest 6% in another study (Schaefer et al., 2010). Two clinical trials examining fish oil in conjunction with lipid lowering statin treatment (Davidson et al., 2009; Maki et al., 2011) demonstrated that their combination lowered Lp-PLA$_2$ mass to a greater extent than placebo + statin treatment. The origin of the inconsistency found in studies of Lp-PLA$_2$ is unknown but is discussed later.

Responders and Non-Responders?

Despite years of research in to the n–3 fatty acids and their potential effects, there remains a controversy in both research and clinical communities as to whether they provide a tangible health benefit for all individuals. In the context of inflammation, some studies, including metaanalyses, have demonstrated a significant antiinflammatory effect while others show EPA/DHA have little to no effect on inflammatory markers. A hypothesis has been put forth to explain the inconsistent findings—that there is a responder/non-responder phenomenon among study populations. With intake of certain macronutrients, supplements, and even pharmaceutical therapies, variable responses from one person to another are not uncommon. In the case of n–3 fatty acids, it has been found that some individuals respond well, showing the noncontroversial effects of fish oil including lower triglycerides and modestly higher HDL, while other individuals remain unaffected.

Unsurprisingly, genetic differences among individuals have been suggested as the primary mechanism that account for differences in fish oil responsiveness. Recent studies have shown that variation in multiple genes including phospholipase A_2 (Tremblay et al., 2015) arachidonate 5-lipoxygenase (Armstrong et al., 2012), ATP citrate lyase (*ACLYI*), and acetyl-CoA carboxylase α (Bouchard-Mercier et al., 2013) partially account for variation in differential responses to fish oil supplementation. Though the above research focused on the triglyceride-lowering effect of fish oil, further studies may reveal additional genes that account for the variability in the antiinflammatory effect of fish oils. Apart from specific genes that influence this responder–nonresponder phenomenon, individuals respond differently to n–3 supplementation vis-à-vis how quickly they are incorporated in to plasma fractions (Johnson et al., 2012) and cell membranes. For example, 'responders' are characterized by quick incorporation of n–3 fatty acids in to cell membranes and plasma subfractions. This in turn would be expected to negatively influence downstream inflammatory pathways. However, it appears that nonresponders 'catch-up' within a subsequent 6-month period (Johnson et al., 2012). Ultimately, this responder–nonresponder paradigm has implications for: (1) modifying expectations for individuals or patients that begin fish oil supplementation and (2) examining the effects of the fish oil fatty acids in a study population, and whether a longer time frame is possible to ensure all individuals have the opportunity to incorporate n–3 fatty acids in to plasma and cell membranes.

SUMMARY

The concept that marine n–3 fatty acids, EPA and DHA, suppress inflammatory and endothelial activation pathways has been hypothesized for over three decades. EPA and DHA have been shown to reduce inflammatory and endothelial activation responses by directly antagonizing major inflammatory signaling mediators such as NF-kB, competing with arachidonic acid for ALOX-5 activity to produce less inflammatory eicosanoids, and by metabolizing in to powerful SPMs, including the resolvins and protectins to actively resolve inflammation. Though their clinical value remains controversial, research continues to further elucidate the precise mechanisms of the putative health benefits of the marine n–3 fatty acids.

References

Arita, M., Bianchini, F., Aliberti, J., Sher, A., Chiang, N., Hong, S., Yang, R., Petasis, N.A., Serhan, C.N., 2005. Stereochemical assignment, antiinflammatory properties, and receptor for the omega-3 lipid mediator resolvin E1. J. Exp. Med. 201, 713–722.

Armstrong, P., Kelley, D.S., Newman, J.W., Staggers, Sr., F.E., Hartiala, J., Allayee, H., Stephensen, C.B., 2012. Arachidonate 5-lipoxygenase gene variants affect response to fish oil supplementation by healthy African Americans. J. Nutr. 142 (8), 1417–1428.

Bagga, D., Wang, L., Farias-Eisner, R., Glaspy, J.A., Reddy, S.T., 2003. Differential effects of prostaglandin derived from omega-6 and omega-3 polyunsaturated fatty acids on COX-2 expression and IL-6 secretion. Proc. Natl. Acad. Sci. 100, 1751–1756.

Barham, J.B., Edens, M.B., Fonteh, A.N., Johnson, M.M., Easter, L., Chilton, F.H., 2000. Addition of eicosapentaenoic acid to gamma-linolenic acid-supplemented diets prevents serum arachidonic acid accumulation in humans. J. Nutr. 130, 1925–1931.

Billman, G.E., Hallaq, H., Leaf, A., 1994. Prevention of ischemia-induced arrhythmias by n-3 fatty acids. Proc. Natl. Acad. Sci. 91, 4427–4430.

Bouchard-Mercier, A., Rudkowska, I., Lemieux, S., Couture, P., Vohl, M.C., 2013. Polymorphisms, de novo lipogenesis, and plasma triglyceride response following fish oil supplementation. J. Lipid Res. 54, 2866–2873.

Calder, P.C., 2013. Omega-3 polyunsaturated fatty acids and inflammatory processes: nutrition or pharmacology? Br. J. Clin. Pharmacol. 75, 645–662.

Chandrasekar, B., Fernandes, G., 1994. Decreased pro-inflammatory cytokines and increased antioxidant enzyme gene expression by omega-3 lipids in murine lupus nephritis. Biochem. Biophys. Res. Commun. 200, 893–898.

Chu, A.J., Walton, M.A., Prasad, J.K., Seto, A., 1999. Blockade by polyunsaturated n-3 fatty acids of endotoxin-induced monocytic tissue factor activation is mediated by the depressed receptor expression in THP-1 cells. J. Surg. Res. 87, 217–224.

Colas, R.A., Shinohara, M., Dalli, J., Chiang, N., Serhan, C.N., 2014. Identification and signature profiles for pro-resolving and inflammatory lipid mediators in human tissue. Am. J. Physiol. Cell Physiol. 307, C39–C54.

Davidson, M.H., Maki, K.C., Bays, H., Carter, R., Ballantyne, C.M., 2009. Effects of prescription omega-3-acid ethyl esters on lipoprotein particle concentrations, apolipoproteins AI and CIII, and lipoprotein-associated phospholipase A(2) mass in statin-treated subjects with hypertriglyceridemia. J. Clin. Lipidol. 3, 332–340.

De Caterina, R., Cybulsky, M.I., Clinton, S.K., Gimbrone, Jr., M.A., Libby, P., 1994. The omega-3 fatty acid docosahexaenoate reduces cytokine-induced expression of proatherogenic and proinflammatory proteins in human endothelial cells. Arterioscler. Thromb. 14, 1829–1836.

Geleijnse, J.M., Giltay, E.J., Grobbee, D.E., Donders, A.R., Kok, F.J., 2002. Blood pressure response to fish oil supplementation: metaregression analysis of randomized trials. J. Hypertens. 20, 1493–1499.

Goldman, D.W., Pickett, W.C., Goetzl, E.J., 1983. Human neutrophil chemotactic and degranulating activities of leukotriene B5 (LTB5) derived from eicosapentaenoic acid. Biochem. Biophys. Res. Commun. 117, 282–288.

Huang, F., Wei, H., Luo, H., Jiang, S., Peng, J., 2011. EPA inhibits the inhibitor of κBα (IκBα)/NF-κB/muscle RING finger 1 pathway in C2C12 myotubes in a PPARγ-dependent manner. Br. J. Nutr. 105, 348–356.

Iketani, T., Takazawa, K., Yamashina, A., 2013. Effect of eicosapentaenoic acid on central systolic blood pressure. Prostagland. Leukot. Essen. Fatty Acid. 88, 191–195.

Jacobsen, A.N., Du, X.J., Dart, A.M., Woodcock, E.A., 1997. Ins-(1,4.5)-P and arrhythmogenic responses during myocardial reperfusion. Am. J. Physiol. 273, H1119–H1125.

Johnson, M., Månsson, J.E., Ostlund, S., Fransson, G., Areskoug, B., Hjalmarsson, K., Landgren, M., Kadesjö, B., Gillberg, C., 2012. Fatty acids in ADHD: plasma profiles in a placebo-controlled study of Omega 3/6 fatty acids in children and adolescents. Atten. Defic. Hyperact. Disord. 4, 199–204.

Khalfoun, B., Thibault, F., Watier, H., Bardos, P., Lebranchu, Y., 1997. Docosahexaenoic and eicosapentaenoic acids inhibit in vitro human endothelial cell production of interleukin-6. Adv. Exp. Med. Biol. 400B, 589–597.

Kliewer, S.A., Sundseth, S.S., Jones, S.A., Brown, P.J., Wisely, G.B., Koble, C.S., Devchand, P., Wahli, W., Willson, T.M., Lenhard, J.M., Lehmann, J.M., 1997. Fatty acids and eicosanoids regulate gene expression through direct interactions with peroxisome proliferator-activated receptors a and g. Proc. Natl. Acad. Sci. 94, 4318–4323.

Lee, T.H., Menica-Huerta, J.M., Shih, C., Corey, E.J., Lewis, R.A., Austen, K.F., 1984. Characterization and biologic properties of 5,12-dihydroxy derivatives of eicosapentaenoic acid, including leukotriene B5 and the double lipoxygenase product. J. Biol. Chem. 259, 2383–2389.

Lee, J.Y., Sohn, K.H., Rhee, S.H., Hwang, D., 2001. Saturated fatty acids, but not unsaturated fatty acids, induce the expression of cyclooxygenase-2 mediated through Toll-like receptor 4. J. Biol. Chem. 276, 16683–16689.

Li, H., Ruan, X.Z., Powis, S.H., Fernando, R., Mon, W.Y., Wheeler, D.C., Moorhead, J.F., Varghese, Z., 2005. EPA and DHA reduce LPS-induced inflammation responses in HK-2 cells: evidence for a PPAR-gamma-dependent mechanism. Kidney Int. 67, 867–874.

Lo, C.J., Chiu, K.C., Fu, M., Lo, R., Helton, S., 1999. Fish oil decreases macrophage tumor necrosis factor gene transcription by altering the NF kappa B activity. J. Surg. Res. 82, 216–221.

Maki, K.C., Bays, H.E., Dicklin, M.R., Johnson, S.L., Shabbout, M., 2011. Effects of prescription omega-3-acid ethyl esters, coadministered with atorvastatin, on circulating levels of lipoprotein particles, apolipoprotein CIII, and lipoprotein-associated phospholipase A2 mass in men and women with mixed dyslipidemia. J. Clin. Lipidol. 5, 483–492.

Mozaffarian, D., Psaty, B., Rimm, E.B., Lemaitre, R.N., Burke, G.L., Lyles, M.F., Lefkowitz, D., Siscovick, D.S., 2004. Fish intake and risk of incident atrial fibrillation. Circulation 110, 368–373.

Mullen, A., Loscher, C.E., Roche, H.M., 2010. Anti-inflammatory effects of EPA and DHA are dependent upon time and dose-response elements associated with LPS stimulation in THP-1-derived macrophages. J. Nutr. Biochem. 21, 444–450.

Nelson, T.L., Hokanson, J.E., Hickey, M.S., 2011. Omega-3 fatty acids and lipoprotein associated phospholipase A(2) in healthy older adult males and females. Eur. J. Nutr. 50, 185–193.

Novak, T.E., Babcock, T.A., Jho, D.H., Helton, W.S., Espat, N.J., 2003. NF-kappa B inhibition by omega-3 fatty acids modulates LPS-stimulated macrophage TNF-alpha transcription. Am. J. Physiol. Lung Cell Mol. Physiol. 284, L84–L89.

Oh, D.Y., Talukdar, S., Bae, E.J., Imamura, T., Morinaga, H., Fan, W., Li, P., Lu, W.J., Watkins, S.M., Olefsky, J.M., 2010. GPR120 is an omega-3 fatty acid receptor mediating potent anti-inflammatory and insulin-sensitizing effects. Cell 142, 687–698.

Pedersen, M.W., Koenig, W., Christensen, J.H., Schmidt, E.B., 2009. The effect of marine omega-3 fatty acids in different doses on plasma concentrations of Lp-PLA2 in healthy adults. Eur. J. Nutr. 48, 1–5.

Renier, G., Skamene, E., DeSanctis, J., Radzioch, D., 1993. Dietary n-3 polyunsaturated fatty acids prevent the development of atherosclerotic lesions in mice. Modulation of macrophage secretory activities. Arterioscler. Thromb. 13, 1515–1524.

Robinson, D.R., Urakaze, M., Huang, R., Taki, H., Sugiyama, E., Knoell, C.T., Xu, L., Yeh, E.T., Auron, P.E., 1996. Dietary marine lipids suppress continuous expression of interleukin-1 beta gene transcription. Lipids 31 (Suppl.), S23–S31.

Schaefer, E.J., Asztalos, I.B., Gleason, J.A., 2010. Effects of eicosapentaenoic acid, docosahexaenoic acid, and olive oil on cardiovascular disease risk factors. Circulation 122, A20007.

Schmidt, E.B., Koenig, W., Khuseyinova, N., Christensen, J.H., 2008. Lipoprotein-associated phospholipase A2 concentrations in plasma are associated with the extent of coronary artery disease and correlate to adipose tissue levels of marine omega-3 fatty acids. Atherosclerosis 196, 420–424.

Schwab, J.M., Chiang, N., Arita, M., Serhan, C.N., 2007. Resolvin E1 and protectin D1 activate inflammation-resolution programmes. Nature 447, 869–874.

Serhan, C.N., Hamberg, M., Samuelsson, B., 1984. Lipoxins: novel series of biologically active compounds formed from arachidonic acid in human leukocytes. Proc. Natl. Acad. Sci. USA. 81, 5335–5339.

Serhan, C.N., Clish, C.B., Brannon, J., Colgan, S.P., Chiang, N., Gronert, K., 2000. Novel functional sets of lipid-derived mediators with antiinflammatory actions generated from omega-3 fatty acids via cyclooxygenase 2-nonsteroidal antiinflammatory drugs and transcellular processing. J. Exp. Med. 192, 1197–1204.

Serhan, C.N., Hong, S., Gronert, K., Colgan, S.P., Devchand, P.R., Mirick, G., Moussignac, R.L., 2002. Resolvins: a family of bioactive products of omega-3 fatty acid transformation circuits initiated by aspirin treatment that counter proinflammation signals. J. Exp. Med. 196, 1025–1037.

Serhan, C.N., Gotlinger, K., Hong, S., Arita, M., 2004. Protectins and maresins: new pro-resolving families of mediators in acute inflammation and resolution bioactive metabolome. Prostagland. Other Lipid Mediat. 73, 155–172.

Serhan, C.N., Dalli, J., Colas, R.A., Winkler, J.W., Chiang, N., 2015. Protectins and maresins: new pro-resolving families of mediators in acute inflammation and resolution bioactive metabolome. Biochim. Biophys. Acta 1851, 397–413.

Steffen, B.T., Steffen, L.M., Liang, S., Tracy, R., Jenny, N.S., Tsai, M.Y., 2013. n-3 and n-6 Fatty acids are independently associated with lipoprotein-associated phospholipase A2 in the Multi-Ethnic Study of Atherosclerosis. Br. J. Nutr. 110, 1664–1671.

Tremblay, B.L., Cormier, H., Rudkowska, I., Lemieux, S., Couture, P., Vohl, M.C., 2015. Association between polymorphisms in phospholipase A2 genes and the plasma triglyceride response to an n-3 PUFA supplementation: a clinical trial. Lipids Health Dis. 14, 12.

Xi, S., Cohen, D., Barve, S., Chen, L.H., 2001. Fish oil suppressed cytokines and nuclear factor kB induced by murine AIDS virus infection. Nutr. Res. 21, 865–878.

Zhao, Y., Joshi-Barve, S., Barve, S., Chen, L.H., 2004. Eicosapentaenoic acid prevents LPS-induced TNF-alpha expression by preventing NF-kappaB activation. J. Am. Coll. Nutr. 23, 71–78.

CHAPTER

18

Omega-3 Fatty Acids and Risk for Cardiovascular Disease

W.S. Harris, C. von Schacky***

*Department of Internal Medicine, Sanford School of Medicine, University of South Dakota, Sioux Falls, South Dakota; OmegaQuant Analytics, LLC, Sioux Falls, South Dakota, United States; **Preventive Cardiology, Medical Clinic I, Ludwig Maximilians-University, Munich; Omegametrix, Martinsried, Germany

INTRODUCTION

During the last 40 years, there have been numerous epidemiologic, observational, experimental, and randomized controlled trials (RCTs) examining the effects of the marine n–3 FAs on coronary heart disease (CHD) risk. The reader is referred to several comprehensive reviews (De Caterina, 2011; Flock et al., 2013a; Harris et al., 2013; Kromhout et al., 2012; Lavie et al., 2009; Mozaffarian and Wu, 2011; Saravanan et al., 2010). Regarding ALA, there are some data suggesting it also may have CHD benefits (Fleming and Kris-Etherton, 2014), but whether they are completely independent of their conversion to EPA + DHA is not clear. The evidence relating to the marine n–3 fatty acids and CHD risk from RCTs and epidemiological investigations will be considered below.

RANDOMIZED TRIALS

The 11 major RCTs with n–3 FAs that examine effects on clinical CHD endpoints are summarized in Table 18.1. Among these trials, four would be considered positive, six as neutral, and one as negative. Such heterogeneity invites metaanalyses (Harris, 2013), with no less than five being published in 2012 alone (Delgado-Lista et al., 2012; Kotwal et al., 2012; Kwak et al., 2012; Rizos et al., 2012; Trikalinos et al., 2012) and one in 2014 (Chowdhury et al., 2014).

The most influential metaanalysis of omega-3 fatty acids and CVD to date was published in September 2012 in JAMA (Rizos et al., 2012). These authors included 20 randomized controlled studies that primarily used omega-3 capsules whether placebo-controlled or open label. They also included the two dietary advice studies (Burr et al., 2003; Burr et al., 1989). This was an improvement on an earlier metaanalysis that did not include the four major nonplacebo controlled trials (Burr et al., 2003; Burr et al., 1989; Marchioli et al., 2002; Yokoyama et al., 2007). Nevertheless, Rizos and coworkers concluded that there was no statistically significant effect of omega-3 supplements on risk for cardiovascular disease. The primary reason why they reached this "no effect" conclusion was because they inflated the critical value for significance to 0.006 instead of the standard 0.05. Another "no effect" meta-analysis has been criticized for discrepancies between data published in the original articles, and the data reported in the metaanalysis (Kwak et al., 2012; von Schacky, 2013). However, other metaanalyses were not criticized for such issues like the one by Kotwal and coworkers or Chowdhury and coworkers, which also came to a "no effect" conclusion, putting meta-analyses with a positive conclusion into a minority position (Delgado-Lista et al., 2012). Clearly, science is not a democratic process. However, it might be more productive to seek reasons for failures of the original trials to show an effect than it is to criticize their metaanalyses.

Fish and Fish Oil in Health and Disease Prevention. http://dx.doi.org/10.1016/B978-0-12-802844-5.00018-X

TABLE 18.1 The 11 Largest (>2000 Participants) n–3 Fatty Acid Randomized Controlled Trials Assessing Cardiovascular Outcomes

Trial, year	Population	Intervention	Duration, years	Primary endpoint(s)	No. of events	RR (95% CI)
Primary prevention of CHD						
Risk and prevention (Roncaglioni et al., 2013)	12,513 patients at increased risk for CHD but without MI	850 mg/day EPA+DHA versus placebo (olive oil)	5	Death, nonfatal MI or stroke, CVD death or hospitalization for CVD cause	1478	0.98 (0.88–1.08)
Secondary prevention of CHD						
DART (Burr et al., 1989)	2,033 men with recent MI (mean ~ 1.5 months)	2 servings/week fatty fish or fish oil capsules (XX mg/day) versus usual care (open label)	2	CHD death or nonfatal MI CHD death	224 194	0.84 (0.66–1.07) 0.71 (0.54–0.93)
GISSI-prevenzione (Marchioli et al., 2002)	11,324 men with recent MI (≤3 months)	882 mg/day EPA+DHA versus usual care (open label)	3.5	Death, nonfatal MI, and nonfatal stroke CVD death, nonfatal MI, and nonfatal stroke	1513 1187	0.85 (0.74–0.98) 0.80 (0.68–0.94)
OMEGA (Rauch et al., 2010)	3804 patients with recent MI (≤2 week)	840 mg/day EPA+DHA versus placebo (olive oil)	1	Sudden deaths or sudden cardiac arrest followed by successful resuscitation but death with 3 weeks	57	0.95 (0.56–1.60)
Alpha–omega (Kromhout et al., 2010)	4837 patients with history of MI (median 3.7 years)	376 mg/day EPA+DHA versus placebo margarine and ALA (1.9 g/day) groups combined ("omega-3 versus non-omega-3")	3.4	Major cardiovascular events (fatal and nonfatal CVD events plus coronary revascularization)	675	1.01 (0.87–1.17) 0.95 (0.68–1.32)
SU.FOL.OM3 (Galan et al., 2010)	2501 patients with recent coronary or cerebral ischemic event (median 101 days)	600 mg/day EPA + DHA versus placebo (not defined)	4.7	Major cardiovascular events (nonfatal MI, stroke, or CVD death)	157	1.08 (0.79–1.47)
Mixed populations						
DART 2 * (Burr et al., 2003)	3114 men receiving treatment for self-reported angina	2 servings/week fatty fish or fish oil capsules (XX mg/day) versus other dietary advice	3–9	Total mortality Cardiac deaths Sudden deaths	525 319 120	1.15 (0.96-1.36) 1.26 (1.00–1.58) 1.54 (1.06–2.23)
JELIS (Yokoyama et al., 2007)	18,645 patients with total cholesterol ≥6.5 mmol/L (with and without CHD history) on statins	1.8 g/day EPA versus usual care (open label)	4.6	Major coronary event (combined sudden cardiac death, fatal and nonfatal MI, unstable angina pectoris, coronary revascularization)	586	0.81 (0.69–0.95)
GISSI-HF (Investigators, 2008)	6975 patients with heart failure	840 mg/day EPA+DHA versus placebo (olive oil)	3.9	Total mortality Total mortality or hospitalization for CVD	1969 4034	0.91 (0·83–0.99) 0.92 (0.85–0.99)
ORIGIN (Bosch et al., 2012)	12,536 patients with diabetes, IGT, or IFG, most with CVD	840 mg/day EPA+DHA versus placebo (olive oil)	6.2	CVD death	1055	1.01 (0.93–1.10)
AREDS2 (Bonds et al., 2014)	4203 patients at risk for macular degeneration and no CVD events in last 12 months	1000 mg/day EPA+DHA versus placebo (not specified)	4.8	CVD mortality (sudden death; death due to MI, heart failure, or stroke) plus CVD morbidity (MI; stroke; unstable angina; coronary and carotid revascularization; hospitalized CHF; resuscitated cardiac arrest).	370	0.95 (0.78–1.17)

CHD, coronary heart disease; *CV*, cardiovascular; *DART*, Diet and Reinfarction Trial; *HDL*, high density lipoprotein; *HDL-C*, HDL cholesterol; *IFG*, impaired fasting glucose; *IGT*, impaired glucose tolerance; *IHD*, ischemic heart disease; *LDL*, low density lipoprotein; *LDL-C*, LDL cholesterol; *MI*, myocardial infarction; *NR*, not reported; *ORIGIN*, outcome reduction with initial glargine intervention; *RCT*, randomized control trial; *SU.FOL.OM3*, Supplementation en Folates et Omega-3.

Why have fish oils been apparently less effective in the more recent studies than in the earlier ones? There are several possible explanations that have been discussed by several authors (Harris, 2013; James et al., 2014; von Schacky, 2015; Wu and Mozaffarian, 2014):

- The heightened awareness of the benefits of fish and fish oils may have increased background utilization of these fatty acids (placebo-treated patients can easily take off-study fish oil pills 'just in case') and reduced the tissue deficiency to the point where additional (at least 1 g) omega-3 fatty acid intakes had nothing to improve upon.
- The average RCT included in Rizos' metaanalyses tracked the effects of about 1 g of EPA + DHA in medically well-treated patients with a history of CHD (or at high risk for it) who were in their early 60s and who were treated for a median of only 2 years. In this context it is not at all surprising that adding a small amount of fish oil on top of a multi-drug regimen and following patients for only a few years did not reduce event rates. These studies did not examine the effects of decades of increased omega-3 intake on CVD risk in the typical consumer.
- Very few patients in the real world are actually "on optimal medical therapy" since noncompliance rates are around 50% within a year of getting a prescription (Frishman, 2007) and even less after 2 years (Jackevicius et al., 2002). So, the findings of research trials cannot always be extrapolated to the real world.
- In addition, 84% of the subjects in the Rizos' metaanalyses were taking ethyl esters. It is now clear that taking ethyl esters on an empty stomach (as opposed to with a meal) results in very poor absorption (Davidson et al., 2012). So, the true dose may have been even smaller than the average of 1 g that characterized these studies.
- The omega-3 status of patients was never used as an inclusion criterion in any of these studies, so individuals already at cardio protective levels would have been included along with patients with very low levels, and all were given the same dose of omega-3. Obviously, the inclusion of all patients regardless of omega-3 blood levels would dilute any anticipated benefit.
- To make matters worse, interindividual variability of uptake of EPA + DHA into blood fatty acid components (plasma or erythrocytes) varies by up to a factor of 13 (eg, Flock et al., 2013b; Kohler et al., 2010). This cannot be explained by issues in compliance since the same phenomenon was observed in a single-dose "metabolic cage" trial in humans (Kohler et al., 2015).
- Combined, the effects of the interindividual variability just discussed and the recruiting irrespective of baseline values of EPA + DHA, resulted in a large overlap between levels in placebo and verum groups in terms of levels of EPA + DHA which indeed has been observed (Muhlhausler et al., 2014).
- Finally, in considering why fish oils did not work in several large trials one must include the possibility that they simply do not reduce risk for CHD, but this flies in the face of so many other lines of evidence (outlined in this volume) as to strain credulity.

Unfortunately, using the same trial design, and continued use of a fixed dose 1 g of EPA + DHA per day in RCTs [like VITAL (Manson et al., 2012) and ASCEND (Clinicaltrials.gov, NCT00135226)] will likely continue to produce the same results as summarized by Rizos. Unfortunately, these trials were designed long before the results of these more recent studies were published; one can only hope that those designing future RCTs with EPA + DHA will learn from previous experience. In that regard, two on-going RCTs are of particular interest as they are using much higher doses. The Reduction of Cardiovascular Events with EPA—Intervention Trial (REDUCE-IT; ClinicalTrials.gov identifier: NCT01492361)—is evaluating supplementation with 4 g/day of EPA ethyl esters (icosapent ethyl) in 8000 patients at high risk for CHD, who are on a background of statins. Another trial, a Phase III, double-blind, long-term outcomes study to asses Statin Residual Risk Reduction with Epanova in High Cardiovascular Risk Patients with Hypertriglyceridemia (STRENGTH, Clinicaltrial.gov identifier NCT02104817) will test supplementation with 4 g of EPA + DHA given in a free fatty acid form in a similar population. The results of both REDUCE-IT and STRENGTH are expected to be available between 2017 and 2019. However, as discussed in more detail elsewhere (von Schacky, 2015), trials recruiting participants based on low levels of EPA + DHA, integrating the current knowledge on bioavailability, and using variable dosing to achieve a separation between verum and placebo groups will not only be a more efficient trial design, but will also generate clearer results as to the effects of marine omega-3 fatty acids. Based on known unpublished data, the same is to be expected for other fatty acids.

Another aspect that merits consideration is the safety of EPA + DHA. Based on large amounts of data analyzed, both the American Food and Drug Administration (FDA) and the European Food Safety Authority (EFSA) consider EPA + DHA as safe (FDA up to 3 g, EFSA up to 5 g per day). Therefore, within the dose range mentioned, RCT's will not contribute to resolving the question of the relation of benefit versus risk of EPA + DHA, because there is no risk to start with. This is in stark contrast to RCT's with pharmaceutical compounds that primarily aim to establish the balance of risk and benefit. An extreme position would be to refuse the need for RCT's with safe compounds. However, in the case of a safe compound, RCT's with clinical endpoints, especially with the methodologic shortcomings discussed above, should not be the ultimate evidence to rely upon.

EPIDEMIOLOGY

While prospective cohort studies also have significant limitations, the relations between nutrient intakes (or, better, nutrient biomarker levels) and disease outcomes should be considered complimentary and equally important as RCT data [see Discussion in (Harris et al., 2009a)]. There have been at least 16 cohort studies that have used dietary estimates of EPA + DHA intake as the exposure marker for CHD endpoints, and 13 studies that have used circulating EPA + DHA levels. These have been included in a major meta-analysis that examined all fatty acids, not just the omega-3's (Chowdhury et al., 2014). In this analysis, higher intakes of long chain n–3 FAs were associated with a 13% (95% CI, 3%–22%) reduction in CHD events, and this class of FAs was the only one linked to a lower risk of adverse events (Table 18.2). Also consistent with this, higher circulating levels of these two n–3 FA (and levels of docosapentaenoic acid, DPA) were significantly associated with reduced risk for CHD events. This indicates that, in the long run and in more 'natural' settings outside of clinical trials, n–3 FAs are consistently and directly associated with better cardiac health.

MECHANISMS OF ACTION OF N–3 FATTY ACIDS

Detailed reviews of n–3 FAs mechanisms of action at both the cellular and the systemic level have been recently published (Harris et al., 2008; Jump et al., 2012; Mozaffarian and Wu, 2011). Unlike drugs that typically inhibit or activate a specific enzyme or receptor, n–3 FAs alter biology in a more global and fundamental manner and can affect many molecular pathways. The n–3 FAs are incorporated as structural components into the phospholipids of the cell membrane, and therefore increase membrane (especially lipid raft) fluidity. This incorporation can nonspecifically impact cellular function by altering the activity of membrane-associated receptors, ion channels, transporters, and enzymes. In addition, n–3 FAs serve as natural substrates for cyclooxygenases, lipoxygenases, and cytochrome P450 monooxygenases (Arnold et al., 2010; Serhan and Petasis, 2011; Shearer and Newman, 2009; Wada et al., 2007) and thereby generate hundreds of molecular species, including prostaglandins, leukotrienes, epoxides, resolvins, protectins, and maresins.

TABLE 18.2 Relative Risk (RR) for Coronary Outcomes in Prospective Cohort Studies of Dietary Fatty Acid Intake and of Circulating Fatty Acid Composition

Fatty acid intake	**Studies, *n***	**RR (95% CI)**
Saturated total	20	1.03 (0.98–1.07)
Monounsaturated total	9	1.00 (0.91–1.10)
18:3n-3	7	0.99 (0.86–1.14)
20:5n–3, 22:5n–3, and/or 22:6n–3	16	**0.87 (0.78–0.97)**
n–6 total	8	0.98 (0.90–1.06)
Trans total	5	**1.16 (1.06–1.27)**
Blood fatty acid composition		
18:3n–3	8	0.93 (0.83–1.03)
20:5n–3	13	**0.78 (0.65–0.94)**
22:5n–3	4	**0.64 (0.47–0.89)**
22:6n–3	13	**0.79 (0.67–0.93)**
20:5n–3 + 22:6n–3	13	**0.75 (0.62–0.89)**
18:2n–6	10	0.99 (0.77–1.28)
20:4n–6	10	**0.83 (0.74–0.92)**

From Chowdhury et al., 2014.

These molecules produce favorable changes in a wide range of cellular activities important to cardiovascular function (eg, vasodilation and vasoconstriction, cellular adhesion process, inflammatory responses, and platelet aggregation). Additionally, n–3 FAs [or eicosanoids (20-carbon metabolites) and docosanoids (22-carbon metabolites)] produced from them serve as ligands for nuclear transcription factors that control genes such as peroxisome proliferator-activated receptors α and γ which, when activated, regulate expression of genes for FA uptake and metabolism (Jump, 2011). Together, and in ways not precisely understood, these basic mechanisms influence several factors important in the development of CHD (Harris et al., 2008) including reductions in serum triglyceride levels (Balk et al., 2006), blood pressure (Geleijnse et al., 2002), platelet aggregation (Violi et al., 2010), heart rate (Mozaffarian et al., 2005), susceptibility to ventricular fibrillation in some settings (Rauch and Senges, 2012), and plaque vulnerability (Cawood et al., 2010; Thies et al., 2003) along with improvements in endothelial function (Pase et al., 2011). There appear to be no effects on atrial fibrillation (Mariani et al., 2013) even for patients in the postcardiac surgery setting (Mozaffarian et al., 2012).

CONCLUSION

The long-chain marine n–3 fatty acids are clearly cardio protective when incorporated into dietary patterns for decades. The failure of many recent RCTs is that they do not demonstrate a benefit in the short term; low dose trials in patients receiving modern background therapy and should not be interpreted as indicating that n–3 fatty acids "are not cardio protective." Consumption of at least 250 mg of EPA + DHA per day and between 5% and 10% of energy as linoleic acid (Harris et al., 2009b) appears to be the optimal combination for reducing risk for CHD.

ACKNOWLEDGMENT

Conflict of Interest Statement

William S. Harris, PhD, is the owner of OmegaQuant Analytics, LLC, and a scientific advisor to Aker Biomarine. Clemens von Schacky, MD, is the owner of Omegametrix.

References

Arnold, C., Markovic, M., Blossey, K., Wallukat, G., Fischer, R., Dechend, R., Konkel, A., von, S.C., Luft, F.C., Muller, D.N., Rothe, M., Schunck, W.H., 2010. Arachidonic acid-metabolizing cytochrome P450 enzymes are targets of {omega}-3 fatty acids. J. Biol. Chem. 285, 32720–32733.

Balk, E.M., Lichtenstein, A.H., Chung, M., Kupelnick, B., Chew, P., Lau, J., 2006. Effects of omega-3 fatty acids on serum markers of cardiovascular disease risk: a systematic review. Atherosclerosis 189, 19–30.

Bonds, D.E., Harrington, M., Worrall, B.B., Bertoni, A.G., Eaton, C.B., Hsia, J., Robinson, J., Clemons, T.E., Fine, L.J., Chew, E.Y., 2014. Effect of long-chain omega-3 fatty acids and lutein + zeaxanthin supplements on cardiovascular outcomes: results of the Age-Related Eye Disease Study 2 (AREDS2) randomized clinical trial. JAMA Intern. Med. 174, 763–771.

Bosch, J., Gerstein, H.C., Dagenais, G.R., Diaz, R., Dyal, L., Jung, H., Maggiono, A.P., Probstfield, J., Ramachandran, A., Riddle, M.C., Ryden, L.E., Yusuf, S., 2012. N-3 fatty acids and cardiovascular outcomes in patients with dysglycemia. N. Eng. J. Med. 367, 309–318.

Burr, M.L., Fehily, A.M., Gilbert, J.F., Rogers, S., Holliday, R.M., Sweetnam, P.M., Elwood, P.C., Deadman, N.M., 1989. Effects of changes in fat, fish, and fibre intakes on death and myocardial reinfarction: diet and reinfarction trial (DART). Lancet 2, 757–761.

Burr, M.L., Ashfield-Watt, P.A., Dunstan, F.D., Fehily, A.M., Breay, P., Ashton, T., Zotos, P.C., Haboubi, N.A., Elwood, P.C., 2003. Lack of benefit of dietary advice to men with angina: results of a controlled trial. Eur. J. Clin. Nutr. 57, 193–200.

Cawood, A.L., Ding, R., Napper, F.L., Young, R.H., Williams, J.A., Ward, M.J., Gudmundsen, O., Vige, R., Payne, S.P., Ye, S., Shearman, C.P., Gallagher, P.J., Grimble, R.F., Calder, P.C., 2010. Eicosapentaenoic acid (EPA) from highly concentrated n-3 fatty acid ethyl esters is incorporated into advanced atherosclerotic plaques and higher plaque EPA is associated with decreased plaque inflammation and increased stability. Atherosclerosis 212, 252–259.

Chowdhury, R., Warnakula, S., Kunutsor, S., Crowe, F., Ward, H.A., Johnson, L., Franco, O.H., Butterworth, A.S., Forouhi, N.G., Thompson, S.G., Khaw, K.T., Mozaffarian, D., Danesh, J., Di Angelantonio, E., 2014. Association of dietary, circulating, and supplement fatty acids with coronary risk: a systematic review and meta-analysis. Ann. Intern. Med. 160, 398–406.

Davidson, M.H., Johnson, J., Rooney, M.W., Kyle, M.L., Kling, D.F., 2012. A novel omega-3 free fatty acid formulation has dramatically improved bioavailability during a low-fat diet compared with omega-3-acid ethyl esters: The ECLIPSE (Epanova compared to Lovaza in a pharmacokinetic single-dose evaluation) study. J. Clin. Lipidol. 6, 573–584.

De Caterina, R., 2011. n-3 fatty acids in cardiovascular disease. N. Engl. J. Med. 364, 2439–2450.

Delgado-Lista, J., Perez-Martinez, P., Lopez-Miranda, J., Perez-Jimenez, F., 2012. Long chain omega-3 fatty acids and cardiovascular disease: a systematic review. Br. J. Nutr. 107 (Suppl. 2), S201–S213.

Fleming, J.A., Kris-Etherton, P.M., 2014. The evidence for alpha-linolenic acid and cardiovascular disease benefits: comparisons with eicosapentaenoic acid and docosahexaenoic acid. Adv. Nutr 5, 863s–876s.

Flock, M.R., Harris, W.S., Kris-Etherton, P.M., 2013a. Long-chain omega-3 fatty acids: time to establish a dietary reference intake. Nutr. Rev. 71, 692–707.

Flock, M.R., Skulas-Ray, A.C., Harris, W.S., Etherton, T.D., Fleming, J.A., Kris-Etherton, P.M., 2013b. Determinants of erythrocyte omega-3 fatty acid content in response to fish oil supplementation: a dose-response randomized controlled trial. J. Am. Heart Assoc. 2, e000513.

Frishman, W.H., 2007. Importance of medication adherence in cardiovascular disease and the value of once-daily treatment regimens. Cardiol. Rev. 15, 257–263.

Galan, P., Kesse-Guyot, E., Czernichow, S., Briancon, S., Blacher, J., Hercberg, S., 2010. Effects of B vitamins and omega 3 fatty acids on cardiovascular diseases: a randomised placebo controlled trial. BMJ 341, c6273.

Geleijnse, J.M., Giltay, E.J., Grobbee, D.E., Donders, A.R., Kok, F.J., 2002. Blood pressure response to fish oil supplementation: metaregression analysis of randomized trials. J. Hypertens. 20, 1493–1499.

Harris, W.S., 2013. Are n-3 fatty acids still cardioprotective? Curr. Opin. Clin. Nutr. Metab. Care 16, 141–149.

Harris, W.S., Miller, M., Tighe, A.P., Davidson, M.H., Schaefer, E.J., 2008. Omega-3 fatty acids and coronary heart disease risk: clinical and mechanistic perspectives. Atherosclerosis 197, 12–24.

Harris, W.S., Mozaffarian, D., Lefevre, M., Toner, C.D., Colombo, J., Cunnane, S.C., Holden, J.M., Klurfeld, D.M., Morris, M.C., Whelan, J., 2009a. Towards establishing dietary reference intakes for eicosapentaenoic and docosahexaenoic acids. J. Nutr. 139, 804S–819S.

Harris, W.S., Mozaffarian, D., Rimm, E.B., Kris-Etherton, P.M., Rudel, L.L., Appel, L.J., Engler, M.M., Engler, M.B., Sacks, F.M., 2009b. Omega-6 fatty acids and risk for cardiovascular disease: a science advisory from the American heart association nutrition committee. Circulation 119, 902–907.

Harris, W.S., Dayspring, T.D., Moran, T.J., 2013. Omega-3 fatty acids and cardiovascular disease: new developments and applications. Postgrad. Med. 125, 100–113.

Investigators, G.-H., 2008. Effect of n-3 polyunsaturated fatty acids in patients with chronic heart failure (the GISSI-HF trial): a randomised, double-blind, placebo-controlled trial. Lancet 372, 1223–1230.

Jackevicius, C.A., Mamdani, M., Tu, J.V., 2002. Adherence with statin therapy in elderly patients with and without acute coronary syndromes. JAMA 288, 462–467.

James, M.J., Sullivan, T.R., Metcalf, R.G., Cleland, L.G., 2014. Pitfalls in the use of randomised controlled trials for fish oil studies with cardiac patients. Br. J. Nutr. 112, 812–820.

Jump, D.B., 2011. Fatty acid regulation of hepatic lipid metabolism. Curr. Opin. Clin. Nutr. Metab. Care 14, 115–120.

Jump, D.B., Depner, C.M., Tripathy, S., 2012. Omega-3 fatty acid supplementation and cardiovascular disease. J. Lipid. Res. 53, 2525–2545.

Kohler, A., Bittner, D., Low, A., von Schacky, C., 2010. Effects of a convenience drink fortified with n-3 fatty acids on the n-3 index. Br. J. Nutr. 104, 729–736.

Kohler, A., Sarkkinen, E., Tapola, N., Niskanen, T., Bruheim, I., 2015. Bioavailability of fatty acids from krill oil, krill meal and fish oil in healthy subjects—a randomized, single-dose, cross-over trial. Lipids Health Dis. 14, 19.

Kotwal, S., Jun, M., Sullivan, D., Perkovic, V., Neal, B., 2012. Omega 3 Fatty acids and cardiovascular outcomes: systematic review and meta-analysis. Circ. Cardiovasc. Qual. Outcomes 5, 808–818.

Kromhout, D., Giltay, E.J., Geleijnse, J.M., 2010. n-3 fatty acids and cardiovascular events after myocardial infarction. N. Engl. J. Med. 363, 2015–2026.

Kromhout, D., Yasuda, S., Geleijnse, J.M., Shimokawa, H., 2012. Fish oil and omega-3 fatty acids in cardiovascular disease: do they really work? Eur. Heart J. 33, 436–443.

Kwak, S.M., Myung, S.K., Lee, Y.J., Seo, H.G., 2012. Efficacy of omega-3 fatty acid supplements (eicosapentaenoic acid and docosahexaenoic acid) in the secondary prevention of cardiovascular disease: a meta-analysis of randomized, double-blind, placebo-controlled trials. Arch. Intern. Med. 172, 686–694.

Lavie, C.J., Milani, R.V., Mehra, M.R., Ventura, H.O., 2009. Omega-3 polyunsaturated fatty acids and cardiovascular diseases. J. Am. Coll. Cardiol. 54, 585–594.

Manson, J.E., Bassuk, S.S., Lee, I.M., Cook, N.R., Albert, M.A., Gordon, D., Zaharris, E., Macfadyen, J.G., Danielson, E., Lin, J., Zhang, S.M., Buring, J.E., 2012. The VITamin D and OmegA-3 TriaL (VITAL): rationale and design of a large randomized controlled trial of vitamin D and marine omega-3 fatty acid supplements for the primary prevention of cancer and cardiovascular disease. Contemp. Clin. Trials 33, 159–171.

Marchioli, R., Barzi, F., Bomba, E., Chieffo, C., Di Gregorio, D., Di Mascio, R., Franzosi, M.G., Geraci, E., Levantesi, G., Maggioni, A.P., Mantini, L., Marfisi, R.M., Mastrogiuseppe, G., Mininni, N., Nicolosi, G.L., Santini, M., Schweiger, C., Tavazzi, L., Tognoni, G., Tucci, C., Valagussa, F., 2002. Early protection against sudden death by n-3 polyunsaturated fatty acids after myocardial infarction: time-course analysis of the results of the Gruppo Italiano per lo Studio della Sopravvivenza nell'Infarto Miocardico (GISSI)-Prevenzione. Circulation 105, 1897–1903.

Mariani, J., Doval, H.C., Nul, D., Varini, S., Grancelli, H., Ferrante, D., Tognoni, G., Macchia, A., 2013. N-3 polyunsaturated Fatty acids to prevent atrial fibrillation: updated systematic review and meta-analysis of randomized controlled trials. J. Am. Heart Assoc. 2, e005033.

Mozaffarian, D., Wu, J.H.Y., 2011. Omega-3 fatty acids and cardiovascular disease: effects on risk factors, molecular pathways and clinical events. J. Am. Coll. Cardiol. 58, 2047–2067.

Mozaffarian, D., Geelen, A., Brouwer, I.A., Geleijnse, J.M., Zock, P.L., Katan, M.B., 2005. Effect of fish oil on heart rate in humans: a meta-analysis of randomized controlled trials. Circulation 112, 1945–1952.

Mozaffarian, D., Marchioli, R., Macchia, A., Silletta, M.G., Ferrazzi, P., Gardner, T.J., Latini, R., Libby, P., Lombardi, F., O'Gara, P.T., Page, R.L., Tavazzi, L., Tognoni, G., 2012. Fish oil and postoperative atrial fibrillation: the Omega-3 Fatty Acids for Prevention of Post-operative Atrial Fibrillation (OPERA) randomized trial. JAMA 308, 2001–2011.

Muhlhausler, B.S., Gibson, R.A., Yelland, L.N., Makrides, M., 2014. Heterogeneity in cord blood DHA concentration: towards an explanation. Prostagland. Leukotr. Essen. Fatty Acid. 91, 135–140.

Pase, M.P., Grima, N.A., Sarris, J., 2011. Do long-chain n-3 fatty acids reduce arterial stiffness? A meta-analysis of randomised controlled trials. Br. J. Nutr. 106, 974–980.

Rauch, B., Senges, J., 2012. The effects of supplementation with omega-3 polyunsaturated fatty acids on cardiac rhythm: anti-arrhythmic, pro-arrhythmic, both or neither? Front Physiol. 3, 1–9.

Rauch, B., Schiele, R., Schneider, S., Diller, F., Victor, N., Gohlke, H., Gottwik, M., Steinbeck, G., Del, C.U., Sack, R., Worth, H., Katus, H., Spitzer, W., Sabin, G., Senges, J., 2010. OMEGA, a randomized, placebo-controlled trial to test the effect of highly purified omega-3 fatty acids on top of modern guideline-adjusted therapy after myocardial infarction. Circulation 122, 2152–2159.

Rizos, E.C., Ntzani, E.E., Bika, E., Kostapanos, M.S., Elisaf, M.S., 2012. Association between omega-3 fatty acid supplementation and risk of major cardiovascular disease events: a systematic review and meta-analysis. JAMA 308, 1024–1033.
Roncaglioni, M.C., Tombesi, M., Silletta, M.G., 2013. n-3 fatty acids in patients with cardiac risk factors. New England J. Med. 369, 781–782.
Saravanan, P., Davidson, N.C., Schmidt, E.B., Calder, P.C., 2010. Cardiovascular effects of marine omega-3 fatty acids. Lancet 376, 540–550.
Serhan, C.N., Petasis, N.A., 2011. Resolvins and protectins in inflammation resolution. Chem. Rev. 111, 5922–5943.
Shearer, G.C., Newman, J.W., 2009. Impact of circulating esterified eicosanoids and other oxylipins on endothelial function. Curr. Atheroscler. Rep. 11, 403–410.
Thies, F., Garry, J.M., Yaqoob, P., Rerkasem, K., Williams, J., Shearman, C.P., Gallagher, P.J., Calder, P.C., Grimble, R.F., 2003. Association of n-3 polyunsaturated fatty acids with stability of atherosclerotic plaques: a randomised controlled trial. Lancet 361, 477–485.
Trikalinos, T.A., Lee, J., Moorthy, D., Yu, W.W., Lau, J., Lichtenstein, A.H., Chung, M., 2012. Effects of eicosapentaenoic acid and docosahexaenoic acid on mortality across diverse settings: systematic review and meta-analysis of randomized trials and prospective cohorts. Rockville, MD.
Violi, F., Pignatelli, P., Basili, S., 2010. Nutrition, supplements, and vitamins in platelet function and bleeding. Circulation 121, 1033–1044.
von Schacky, C., 2013. Meta-analysing randomised controlled trials with omega-3 fatty acids in cardiovascular disease. Evid. Based Med. 18, e33.
von Schacky, C., 2015. Omega-3 fatty acids in cardiovascular disease—an uphill battle. Prostagland. Leukotr. Essen. Fatty Acid. 92, 41–47.
Wada, M., Delong, C.J., Hong, Y.H., Rieke, C.J., Song, I., Sidhu, R.S., Yuan, C., Warnock, M., Schmaier, A.H., Yokoyama, C., Smyth, E.M., Wilson, S.J., FitzGerald, G.A., Garavito, R.M., Sui, D.X., Regan, J.W., Smith, W.L., 2007. Enzymes and receptors of prostaglandin pathways with arachidonic acid-derived versus eicosapentaenoic acid-derived substrates and products. J Biol. Chem. 282, 22254–22266.
Wu, J.H., Mozaffarian, D., 2014. omega-3 fatty acids, atherosclerosis progression and cardiovascular outcomes in recent trials: new pieces in a complex puzzle. Heart 100, 530–533.
Yokoyama, M., Origasa, H., Matsuzaki, M., Matsuzawa, Y., Saito, Y., Ishikawa, Y., Oikawa, S., Sasaki, J., Hishida, H., Itakura, H., Kita, T., Kitabatake, A., Nakaya, N., Sakata, T., Shimada, K., Shirato, K., 2007. Effects of eicosapentaenoic acid on major coronary events in hypercholesterolaemic patients (JELIS): a randomised open-label, blinded endpoint analysis. Lancet 369, 1090–1098.

CHAPTER

19

Salmon and Vascular Risk in Young Healthy Subjects

*J. Lara**, *M. Lean***

*Department of Applied Sciences, Faculty of Health and Life Sciences, Northumbria University, Newcastle upon Tyne, United Kingdom;
**School of Medicine, University of Glasgow, Glasgow Royal Infirmary, Glasgow, Scotland

FISH AND SEAFOOD IN HEALTH AND HUMAN NUTRITION

Fish and seafood have been an important component of diverse and nutritious diets worldwide since ancient times. Their contribution to good health and human nutrition is well documented and has become a research topic of growing interest. These foods represent important sources of high-quality protein, healthy lipids [particularly polyunsaturated fatty acids (PUFA)], vitamin D and selenium. Fish and seafood are a central element to most dietary guidelines, often recommending the consumption of at least two portions of fish per week, including one portion of oil-rich fish. Fish and seafood are also an important element of healthy dietary patterns such as the Mediterranean (Bach-Faig et al., 2011) and the Japanese (Nakamura et al., 2002) diets, as well as of dietary recommendations (Scottish-Government, 2008). Fish and seafood are included in other dietary indices such the DASH diet, the Programme National Nutrition Santé Guideline Score, and are a common element of a posteriori defined dietary patterns positively associated with health.

A range of health benefits have been associated with fish consumption, particularly through the intake of PUFA from oil-rich species such as salmon, sardines, fresh tuna, and mackerel, among others. Fish consumption is acknowledged as an important component of a cardio protective diet (Mozaffarian et al., 2011). Significant epidemiological evidence consistently suggests an association between habitual fish consumption and lower risk for coronary heart disease (CHD), ischemic stroke and mortality among generally healthy populations (Chowdhury et al., 2012; Leung Yinko et al., 2014; Mozaffarian et al., 2011). This evidence has encouraged the design and implementation of controlled studies on the effect of fish consumption as well as fish oils.

In 1989, the report of the innovative diet and reinfarction trial (DART, Burr et al., 1989) reported that advice to increase fatty fish intake among 2033 men who have recovered from myocardial infarction (MI), was associated with 29% reduction in all-cause mortality after 2 years, independent of confounding factors.

The world supply of oil-rich fish is insufficient to meet recommended intakes. Fish farming is a potential solution, and farmed salmon is now widely available and affordable. In this chapter we will focus on the health aspects of salmon consumption, particularly on its impact on vascular risk factors among healthy subjects.

SALMON AS FOOD

Salmon is the common name for several species of fish (family Salmonidae) found in the North Atlantic (genus *Salmo*) and Pacific Ocean (genus *Oncorhynchus*). The life cycle of wild salmon is extraordinary; salmon are born in fresh water; then migrate to the ocean to mature, and return to fresh water to reproduce. However, populations

Fish and Fish Oil in Health and Disease Prevention. http://dx.doi.org/10.1016/B978-0-12-802844-5.00019-1

of several species are restricted to fresh water through their lives. Many species of salmon have been introduced into nonnative environments such as the Great lakes of North America and the Patagonia in South America. Salmon are also intensively produced in farms in many parts of the world such as in Scandinavia, Chile, Canada, and the United States and in the Scottish sea-lochs around the North-West coast, Wester Isles, Shetland, and Orkney.

Salmon has been the most frequently consumed seafood product in United States for most of the past decade (SeafoodHealthFacts.org, 2015). Recent market analysis has shown that farmed salmon is now considered affordable, and one of United Kingdom's most popular dishes. It features on 53% of restaurants menus, second only to grilled chicken at 60%. Likewise, retail sales for the years 2008–09 indicate that on a value basis, salmon is United Kingdom's best-selling fish outperforming all traditional favorites.

Raw Atlantic salmon contains approximately 13 g of fat per 100 g of fish; of these, 3.9 g are PUFAs [0.6 g eicosapentaenoic acid (EPA), and 1.3 g docosahexaenoic acid (DHA)].

MARKERS OF VASCULAR RISK

With cardiovascular disease being one of the major causes of death (Murray et al., 2015), there is value in identifying objectively assessed outcomes measures and biomarkers to be used as surrogate endpoints in population studies and for use in other settings (eg, community-based intervention studies). There is great interest in identifying and developing novel biomarkers of cardiovascular risk and guidelines and benchmarks have been proposed (Morrow and de Lemos, 2007). In addition to being capable of predicting health risks (van Holten et al., 2013), such biomarkers would be expected to change with interventions (Lara et al., 2015). In this chapter we review and discuss the evidence on the effects consuming salmon on such biomarkers.

EXPERIMENTAL STUDIES: SALMON AND VASCULAR RISK FACTORS

In 2007, our group reported the results of a clinical trial testing the effect of consuming 125 g of salmon every day for a four-week period on vascular risk factors, among young healthy subjects (Lara et al., 2007). That study was an initial 'proof-of-concept' trial, and used a high dose which could not be sustained in a realistic setting. Since then other experimental studies testing the efficacy of consuming salmon on vascular risk factors have been published, using more achievable consumption levels.

To evaluate the evidence on the topic, we undertook a systematic review of the literature targeting clinical trials using salmon as food. In June 2015, PUBMED was searched from inception. The search strategy involved combining words from the following concepts: (1) salmon, fish diet; (2) clinical trials; and (3) vascular risk factors.

The search identified eleven publications reporting seven studies that met our inclusion criteria (Table 19.1). Two studies originated from United Kingdom, two from China, and one study from Norway, United States, and a collaborative study from Iceland/Spain/Ireland. Sample size in the studies ranged from 25 to 324, and interventions ranged from 4 to 16 weeks. The frequencies for consuming salmon ranged from twice a week to daily consumption, and the portion size of salmon to be consumed on a given day ranged from 80 to 150 g. All studies identified in our search provided the fish to be consumed during the intervention. One study involved men only, two studies involved women only, while the four studies included mixed sex samples. Two studies involved healthy subjects, two studies involved subjects with hyperlipidemia, one study on overweight/obese, one study on pregnant women, and one study on CHD patients. Different vascular risk factors (blood lipids, inflammatory factors, and hemostasis) were evaluated in these studies.

BLOOD LIPIDS

Six out of the seven studies identified were meta-analysed using random effects models to evaluate the effects of consuming salmon on blood lipids. Forest plots presented these results are shown in Fig. 19.1. This analysis excluded the study from Norway because such study evaluated the dose response of salmon with different concentrations of n–3 fatty acids and did not include a comparative control arm. Overall, consuming salmon resulted in significant

TABLE 19.1 Characteristics of Interventions Included in Systematic Review of Salmon Eating on Vascular Risk Factors

Author/year	Sample population	Mean or range age (years)	Mean BMI (kg/m^2)	Participants health status	Baseline sample size (sex % female)	Intervention length (dose and frequency of consumption)	Control
(Seierstad et al., 2005)	Norway	63	26–29	CHD patients	60 (13)	6 weeks of differently fed salmon (80 g of salmon, herring or pompano 5 times/week)	No control
(Lara et al., 2007)	UK	28	23	Healthy	48 (66)	4 weeks (125 g/day of salmon daily)	Follow-up period with no fish
(Rajaram et al., 2009)	USA	23–65 (range)	24.8	Healthy	25 (44)	4 weeks (113 g of salmon 2 times/week)	No fish diet
(Zhang et al., 2010)	China	50	26	Hyperlip-idemia	92 (0)	8 weeks (100 g of salmon 5 times/week)	100 g of pork, chicken or beef 5 times/week Or 100 g of hairtail or freshwater carp 5 times/week
(Zhang et al., 2012)	China	35–70 (range)	26–28	Hyper-triglyceri-demia	126 (100)	8 weeks (80 g of salmon, herring or pompano 5 times/week)	80 g of pork, chicken, beef, or lean fish five times/week
(García-Rodríguez et al., 2012)	UK	18–40 (range)	–	Pregnancy (19 week gestation)	123 (100)	From week 19 of pregnancy until delivery (150 g of salmon 2 times/week)	Habitual diet
(Gunnarsdottir et al., 2008) (Paulo et al., 2008; Ramel et al., 2010)	Iceland/Spain/Ireland	20–40 (range)	30	Over-weight and obese	324 (57)	8 weeks (150 g of salmon or Cod or six fish oil capsules 3 times/week)	Sunflower oil six capsules 3 times/week

decreases in triglycerides (−0.16 mmol/L) and increases in HDL cholesterol (0.08 mmol/L) concentrations. These changes although statistically significant, are of moderate size. Contrasting with these results, the evidence available indicates that consuming salmon does not affect the concentrations of total or LDL cholesterol.

Among these studies, only our study (Lara et al., 2007) reported VLDL cholesterol, with salmon significantly reducing VLDL by 0.05 mmol/L. Available evidence indicates that VLDL have significant predictive power for (Eckel, 2014; Prenner et al., 2014).

BLOOD PRESSURE

Some of these studies report that consuming salmon improved other vascular risk factors such as blood pressure. Our group (Lara et al., 2007) reported significant reductions in systolic (mean −5 mmHg) and diastolic (−3 mmHg) blood pressure after consuming 125 g of salmon daily for 4 weeks. In addition, a recent publication from the SEAFOOD plus YOUNG study (www.seafoodplus.org; Ramel et al., 2010) reported that consuming 150g of salmon three times per week for 8 weeks decreased diastolic blood pressure (DBP). These authors reported that the endpoint DBP was significantly lower with salmon intake compared with consuming cod (DBP −2.9 mmHg, $P = 0.022$); they also reported that similar reductions on DBP were observed after consuming six fish oil capsules 3 times per week for 8 weeks (Ramel et al., 2010).

(a) **Triglycerides**

Study or Subgroup	Experimental Mean	SD	Total	Control Mean	SD	Total	Weight	Mean Difference IV, Random, 95% CI
Garcia-Rodriguez et al., 2012	1.41	3.937	62	1.5	3.1241	61	0.6%	−0.09 [−1.34, 1.16]
Gunnarsdottir et aL., 2008	0.92	0.52	80	1.03	0.59	80	34.4%	−0.11 [−0.28, 0.06]
Lara et al., 2007	0.82	0.35	48	0.97	0.37	41	45.2%	−0.15 [−0.30, 0.00]
Rajaram et al., 2009	1	0.55	25	1.12	0.55	25	11.0%	−0.12 [−0.42, 0.18]
Zhang et al., 2010	2.08	1.1649	32	2.76	2.4906	30	1.1%	−0.68 [−1.66, 0.30]
Zhang et al., 2012	1.75	0.6223	32	2.23	0.8485	32	7.7%	−0.48 [−0.84, 0.12]
Total (95% CI)			**279**			**269**	**100.0%**	**−0.16 [−0.26, −0.06]**

Heterogeneity: Tau^2 = 0.00; Chi^2 = 4.46, df = 5 (P = 0.49); I^2 = 0%
Test for overall effect: Z = 3.17 (P = 0.002)

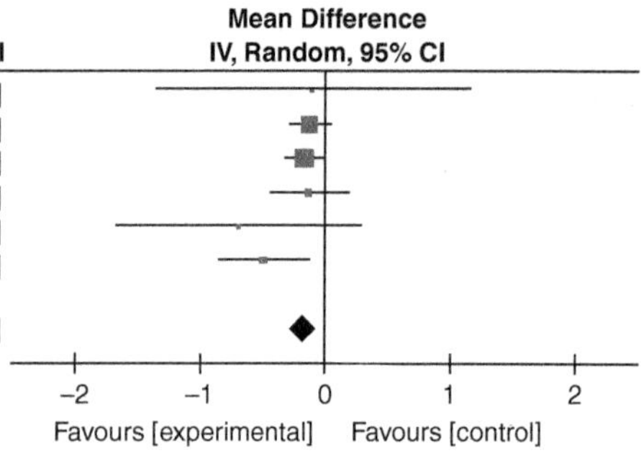

(b) **HDL cholesterol**

Study or Subgroup	Experimental Mean	SD	Total	Control Mean	SD	Total	Weight	Mean Difference IV, Random, 95% CI
Garcia-Rodriguez et al., 2012	1.8	3.937	62	1.7	3.1241	61	0.3%	0.10 [−1.15, 1.35]
Gunnarsdottir et aL., 2008	1.31	0.44	80	1.35	0.36	80	21.9%	−0.04 [−0.16, 0.08]
Lara et al., 2007	1.42	0.34	48	1.33	0.28	41	20.9%	0.09 [−0.04, 0.22]
Rajaram et al., 2009	1.23	0.25	25	1.19	0.25	25	18.8%	0.04 [−0.10, 0.18]
Zhang et al., 2010	1.21	0.416	32	1.09	0.1339	30	16.4%	0.12 [−0.03, 0.27]
Zhang et al., 2012	1.34	0.2263	32	1.16	0.2828	32	21.7%	0.18 [0.05, 0.31]
Total (95% CI)			**279**			**269**	**100.0%**	**0.08 [0.01, 0.15]**

Heterogeneity: Tau^2 = 0.00; Chi^2 = 6.60, df = 5 (P = 0.25); I^2 = 24%
Test for overall effect: Z = 2.14 (P = 0.03)

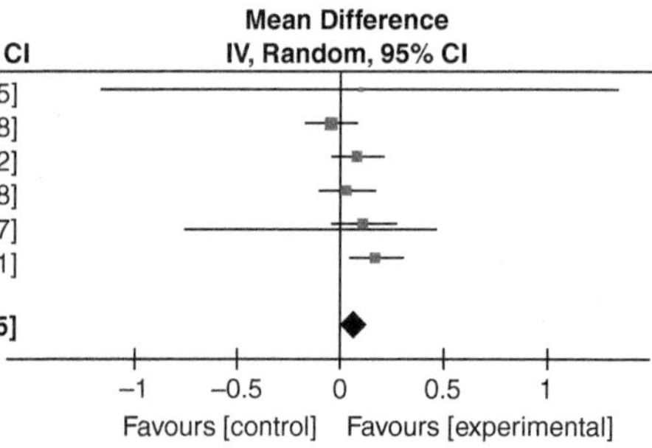

(c) **Total cholesterol**

Study or Subgroup	Experimental Mean	SD	Total	Control Mean	SD	Total	Weight	Mean Difference IV, Random, 95% CI
Garcia-Rodriguez et al., 2012	5.4	7.874	62	5.7	5.4672	61	4.0%	−0.30 [−2.69, 2.09]
Gunnarsdottir et aL., 2008	4.69	0.88	80	5.82	0.87	80	20.2%	−1.13 [−1.40, −0.86]
Lara et al., 2007	4.33	0.85	48	4.37	0.71	41	19.7%	−0.04 [−0.36, 0.28]
Rajaram et al., 2009	5.33	0.9	25	5.14	0.9	25	17.9%	0.19 [−0.31, 0.69]
Zhang et al., 2010	5.16	0.527	32	5.13	0.7499	30	19.7%	0.03 [−0.29, 0.35]
Zhang et al., 2012	5.23	0.7354	32	5.26	1.0748	32	18.5%	−0.03 [−0.48, 0.42]
Total (95% CI)			**279**			**269**	**100.0%**	**−0.21 [−0.74, 0.32]**

Heterogeneity: Tau^2 = 0.34; Chi^2 = 46.99, df = 5 (P < 0.00001); I^2 = 89%
Test for overall effect: Z = 0.79 (P = 0.43)

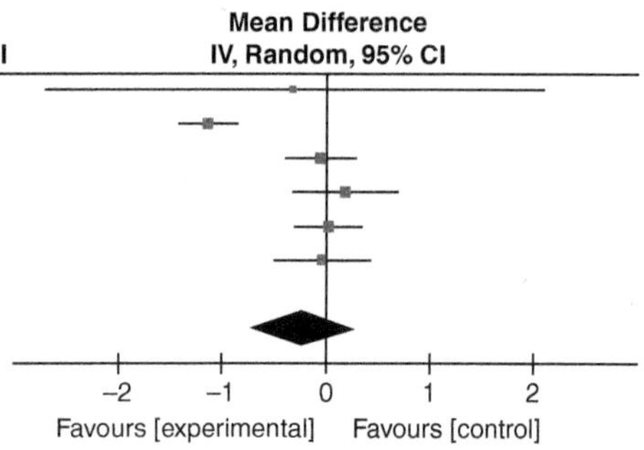

(d) **LDL cholesterol**

Study or Subgroup	Experimental Mean	SD	Total	Control Mean	SD	Total	Weight	Mean Difference IV, Random, 95% CI
Garcia-Rodriguez et al., 2012	2.9	6.2992	62	3.3	5.4672	61	0.5%	−0.40 [−2.48,1.68]
Gunnarsdottir et aL., 2008	2.86	0.8	80	3	0.74	80	35.8%	−0.14 [−0.38, 0.10]
Lara et al., 2007	2.31	0.74	48	2.48	0.64	41	24.9%	−0.17 [−0.46, 0.12]
Rajaram et al., 2009	3.2	0.75	25	3.06	0.15	25	22.7%	0.14 [−0.16, 0.44]
Zhang et al., 2010	3.58	1.47	32	3.54	0.9909	30	5.3%	0.04 [−0.58, 0.66]
Zhang et al., 2012	3.58	0.7354	32	3.72	1.0182	32	10.8%	−0.14 [−0.58, 0.30]
Total (95% CI)			**279**			**269**	**100.0%**	**−0.08 [−0.22, 0.07]**

Heterogeneity: Tau^2 = 0.00; Chi^2 = 2.99, df = 5 (P = 0.70); I^2 = 0%
Test for overall effect: Z = 1.03 (P = 0.30)

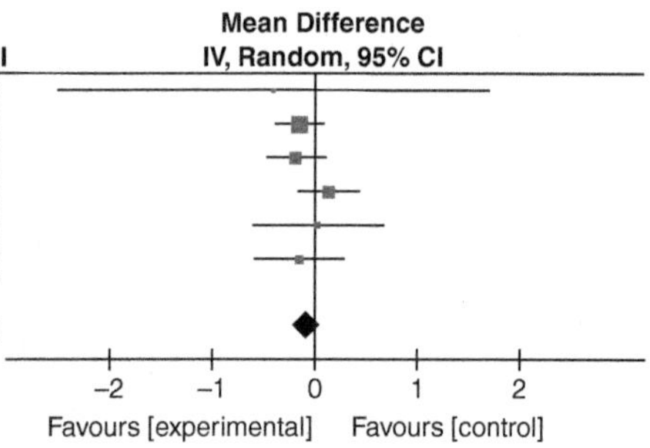

FIGURE 19.1 **Trials reporting the effects of consuming salmon on several vascular risk factors.**

INTERCELLULAR ADHESION MOLECULES (ICAM VCAM)

Intercellular adhesion molecule 1 (ICAM) and vascular cell adhesion molecule 1 (VCAM) are members of the adhesion molecule superfamily, to which monocytes and lymphocytes can bind. These inflammatory cells move through the endothelium and release cytokines and enzymes, important components in the progression of atherosclerosis.

Three studies (Lara et al., 2007; Paulo et al., 2008; Zhang et al., 2012) reported the impact of Salmon consumption on ICAM, while only two (Paulo et al., 2008; Zhang et al., 2012) reported VCAM. No significant effect of salmon intervention was detected on these biomarkers in any of these trials.

INFLAMMATION MARKERS

C reactive protein. C reactive protein (CRP), a protein synthesized by the liver, is a sensitive marker of inflammation. CRP concentration has continuous associations with the risk of coronary heart disease, ischemic stroke, and vascular mortality (Kaptoge et al., 2010).

Three studies reported the effects of consuming salmon, either 125 g of salmon daily for 4 weeks (Lara et al., 2007) among healthy participants or 80 g of salmon 5 times a week for 8 weeks among individuals with hyperlipidemia (Zhang et al., 2012; Zhang et al., 2010), on CRP. None of these reported a significant effect of intervention on CRP after eating salmon.

Interleukin 6. Interleukin 6 (IL-6) is a pro-inflammatory cytokine. Elevated long term IL-6 levels are associated with CHD risk about as strongly as are some of the other major established risk factors (Danesh et al., 2008).

In the present literature review, three studies reported effects of interventions on IL-6 (García-Rodríguez et al., 2012; Zhang et al., 2012; Zhang et al., 2010). These studies found that 80 g of salmon five times a week for 8 weeks reduced IL-6 significantly by 0.03 ng/dL ($P < 0.01$) in dyslipidemic Chinese men and women (Zhang et al., 2012; Zhang et al., 2010); however 150 g of salmon 2 times a week for 16 weeks (intervention started at 19 weeks of pregnancy) did not affect IL-6 in pregnant British women (García-Rodríguez et al., 2012).

Tumor Necrosis Factors Alpha

Tumor necrosis factor—alpha (TNFα) is a cytokine that has a wide variety of functions. Recent evidence indicates that higher concentrations of TNFα are associated with 10–25% higher risk of nonfatal myocardial infarction or CHD death.

In the present review, only one study reported the effects of salmon intake on TNFα (Zhang et al., 2012), reporting that eating 80 g of salmon 5 times a week for 8 weeks, lowered TNFα by 1.26 ng/L among Chinese hyperlipidemic women.

OTHER VASCULAR RISK FACTORS

Other vascular risk factors evaluated in the reviewed studies included:

Fibrinogen

Plasma fibrinogen is involved in hemostasis and blood viscosity and elevated concentrations are associated with increased cardiovascular disease risk (Danesh et al., 2005); to our knowledge only our group has evaluated the effects of daily salmon consumption (125g/day for 4 weeks) on plasma fibrinogen levels among healthy individuals. We observed no significant changes in response to salmon intake (Lara et al., 2007).

Adiponectin

Serum adiponectin, a cytokine with cardiovascular protective actions (Parker-Duffen and Walsh, 2014) has been reported in two studies supplementing salmon. While one study (Lara et al., 2007) reported no changes after 4 weeks of daily salmon consumption (125 g/day), a second study (Zhang et al., 2012) reported that 8 weeks of salmon consumption (80 g 5 times per week) raised adiponectin concentrations by 0.72 μg/mL in Chinese women.

Apolipoproteins

Three studies have reported the effect of consuming salmon on circulating concentrations of apolipoproteins. Results showed that neither 113 g of salmon 2 times a week for 4 weeks in healthy individuals (Rajaram et al., 2009), nor 80 g of salmon 5 times a week for 8 weeks among hyperlipidemic Chinese men and women (Zhang et al., 2012; Zhang et al., 2010), affected Apo A1 or Apo B.

INCREASING OMEGA-3 3 PUFA CONCENTRATIONS IN SALMON

Some studies have evaluated the effect of feeding salmon with different types of diet in order to modify their omega-3 (n–3) PUFA content for human consumption. In a recent 6-week intervention study (Seierstad et al., 2005), significant reductions of serum triglycerides (−0.50 mmol/L), VCAM (−56 ng/mL), and IL-6 (−1.49 ng/mL) were reported in CHD patients consuming 700 g/week of salmon fed with a fish oil-based diet, thus having a greater content of n–3 fatty acids (30.2% weight) than in volunteers fed with salmon fillets containing intermediate (20.5% weight) and lower (11.7%) concentrations of n–3 PUFAs. These findings highlight the possibility of adapting salmon farming practices to provide food with enhanced cardio protective properties. A lower intake of salmon with increased n–3 fatty acids concentrations might then be able to improve health outcomes.

HEALTH RISKS OF CONSUMING OIL-RICH FISH

There has been concern about the potential health risks associated with consuming fish, particularly farmed fish, and the levels of environmental contaminants such as mercury (mainly in wild sea fish), PCBs, DDT, dioxins, and lead in their flesh and fat (Hites et al., 2004). Farmed fish are also often exposed to regular treatment with pesticides, for example to control sea lice infestations. Currently, long term data on the cardiovascular risk or benefit from regular consumption of farmed salmon are not available. Recent analysis of the mortality of Finnish fishermen and their wives, who have a high consumption of contaminated fish (Turunen et al., 2008) showed a lower risk for mortality from all cause (−22%), ischemic heart disease (−27%), and malignant neoplasms (−33%) than the general population. These results are in broad accordance with the reduced mortality rates of Dutch fish consumers (Kromhout et al., 1985). There is therefore a general agreement that the health benefits of fish intake exceed the potential risks, but additional data would be welcomed (Mozaffarian and Rimm, 2006; Tuomisto et al., 2004).

CONCLUDING REMARKS

The available evidence on the effects of eating salmon, and specifically farmed salmon, on vascular risk factors supports the view that consuming this type of fish has positive effects on well-established vascular risk factors such as blood pressure, triglycerides, and HDL-cholesterol. There are at least no adverse effects on other risk factors. Among the mechanisms behind the lowering effects of n–3 fatty acids on triglycerides is a decreased hepatic fatty acid output as a result of both increased fatty acid oxidation and a decreased lipogenesis (Shearer et al., 2012).

In relation with improving HDL-cholesterol concentrations after salmon, some evidence indicate that HDL-cholesterol increases are likely due to specific increases in the cardio protective HDL-2 sub-fraction as reported previously (Lara et al., 2007; Lindgren et al., 1991). Furthermore, some evidence suggest that fish consumption may increase the levels of HDL-cholesterol not only through mechanism involving n–3 fatty acids, but also possibly through effects exerted by fish proteins on lipid metabolism as previously reported in studies on rabbits (Bergeron et al., 1992) and rats (Wergedahl et al., 2004). Reduction in the activity of acyl-CoA:cholesterol acyltransferase activity which plays an important role in VLDL secretion and cholesteryl ester accumulation, has been associated with reductions in total cholesterol and increases in HDL-cholesterol in rats fed a fish protein hydrolysate (Wergedahl et al., 2004).

These results are very similar to those obtained from taking "fish oil" supplements, so at least some of the benefits of salmon consumption probably derive from their content of n–3 fatty acids. There is also benefit from replacing high saturated fatty acid-containing foods such as meat products which might tend to raise LDL cholesterol. Studies focusing on fish as food offer real-life examples of the benefits of eating fish such as salmon. Most of these studies have reported good compliance with fish interventions by showing significant increases of EPA and DHA in blood.

There are already good commercial opportunities for farmed fish. Current fish consumption is low in most countries, and people are often reluctant to eat it more frequently, so social marketing is needed to increase consumptions. Improved feeding of farmed salmon to generate a more potent cardio protective effect from less frequent consumption offers an important public health approach.

References

Bach-Faig, A., Berry, E.M., Lairon, D., Reguant, J., Trichopoulou, A., Dernini, S., Medina, F.X., Battino, M., Belahsen, R., Miranda, G., Serra-Majem, L., Mediterranean Diet Foundation Expert, G., 2011. Mediterranean diet pyramid today. Science and cultural updates. Public Health Nutr. 14, 2274–2284.

Bergeron, N., Deshaies, Y., Jacques, H., 1992. Dietary fish protein modulates high density lipoprotein cholesterol and lipoprotein lipase activity in rabbits. J. Nutr. 122, 1731–1737.

Burr, M.L., Fehily, A.M., Gilbert, J.F., Rogers, S., Holliday, R.M., Sweetnam, P.M., Elwood, P.C., Deadman, N.M., 1989. Effects of changes in fat, fish, and fibre intakes on death and myocardial reinfarction: diet and reinfarction trial (DART). Lancet 2, 757–761.

Chowdhury, R., Stevens, S., Gorman, D., Pan, A., Warnakula, S., Chowdhury, S., Ward, H., Johnson, L., Crowe, F., Hu, F.B., Franco, O.H., 2012. Association between fish consumption, long chain omega 3 fatty acids, and risk of cerebrovascular disease: systematic review and meta-analysis. BMJ, 345.

Danesh, J., Kaptoge, S., Mann, A.G., Sarwar, N., Wood, A., Angleman, S.B., Wensley, F., Higgins, J.P., Lennon, L., Eiriksdottir, G., Rumley, A., Whincup, P.H., Lowe, G.D., Gudnason, V., 2008. Long-term interleukin-6 levels and subsequent risk of coronary heart disease: two new prospective studies and a systematic review. PLoS Med. 5, e78.

Danesh, J., Lewington, S., Thompson, S.G., Lowe, G.D., Collins, R., Kostis, J.B., Wilson, A.C., Folsom, A.R., Wu, K., Benderly, M., Goldbourt, U., Willeit, J., Kiechl, S., Yarnell, J.W., Sweetnam, P.M., Elwood, P.C., Cushman, M., Psaty, B.M., Tracy, R.P., Tybjaerg-Hansen, A., Haverkate, F., de Maat, M.P., Fowkes, F.G., Lee, A.J., Smith, F.B., Salomaa, V., Harald, K., Rasi, R., Vahtera, E., Jousilahti, P., Pekkanen, J., D'Agostino, R., Kannel, W.B., Wilson, P.W., Tofler, G., Arocha-Pinango, C.L., Rodriguez-Larralde, A., Nagy, E., Mijares, M., Espinosa, R., Rodriquez-Roa, E., Ryder, E., Diez-Ewald, M.P., Campos, G., Fernandez, V., Torres, E., Marchioli, R., Valagussa, F., Rosengren, A., Wilhelmsen, L., Lappas, G., Eriksson, H., Cremer, P., Nagel, D., Curb, J.D., Rodriguez, B., Yano, K., Salonen, J.T., Nyyssonen, K., Tuomainen, T.P., Hedblad, B., Lind, P., Loewel, H., Koenig, W., Meade, T.W., Cooper, J.A., De Stavola, B., Knottenbelt, C., Miller, G.J., Cooper, J.A., Bauer, K.A., Rosenberg, R.D., Sato, S., Kitamura, A., Naito, Y., Palosuo, T., Ducimetiere, P., Amouyel, P., Arveiler, D., Evans, A.E., Ferrieres, J., Juhan-Vague, I., Bingham, A., Schulte, H., Assmann, G., Cantin, B., Lamarche, B., Despres, J.P., Dagenais, G.R., Tunstall-Pedoe, H., Woodward, M., Ben-Shlomo, Y., Davey Smith, G., Palmieri, V., Yeh, J.L., Rudnicka, A., Ridker, P., Rodeghiero, F., Tosetto, A., Shepherd, J., Ford, I., Robertson, M., Brunner, E., Shipley, M., Feskens, E.J., Kromhout, D., Dickinson, A., Ireland, B., Juzwishin, K., Kaptoge, S., Lewington, S., Memon, A., Sarwar, N., Walker, M., Wheeler, J., White, I., Wood, A., 2005. Plasma fibrinogen level and the risk of major cardiovascular diseases and nonvascular mortality: an individual participant meta-analysis. JAMA 294, 1799–1809.

Eckel, R.H., 2014. What is it about very low density lipoproteins (VLDL) and cardiovascular disease in patients with type 2 diabetes mellitus: is it the triglycerides or the cholesterol? Atherosclerosis 237, 138–139.

García-Rodríguez, C.E., Olza, J., Aguilera, C.M., Mesa, M.D., Miles, E.A., Noakes, P.S., Vlachava, M., Kremmyda, L.-S., Diaper, N.D., Godfrey, K.M., Calder, P.C., Gil, A., 2012. Plasma inflammatory and vascular homeostasis biomarkers increase during human pregnancy but are not affected by oily fish intake. J. Nutr. 142, 1191–1196.

Gunnarsdottir, I., Tomasson, H., Kiely, M., Martinez, J.A., Bandarra, N.M., Morais, M.G., Thorsdottir, I., 2008. Inclusion of fish or fish oil in weight-loss diets for young adults: effects on blood lipids. Int. J. Obes. 32, 1105–1112.

Hites, R.A., Foran, J.A., Carpenter, D.O., Hamilton, M.C., Knuth, B.A., Schwager, S.J., 2004. Global assessment of organic contaminants in farmed salmon. Science 303, 226–229.

Kaptoge, S., Di Angelantonio, E., Lowe, G., Pepys, M.B., Thompson, S.G., Collins, R., Danesh, J., 2010. C-reactive protein concentration and risk of coronary heart disease, stroke, and mortality: an individual participant meta-analysis. Lancet 375, 132–140.

Kromhout, D., Bosschieter, E.B., de Lezenne Coulander, C., 1985. The inverse relation between fish consumption and 20-year mortality from coronary heart disease. N. Engl. J. Med. 312, 1205–1209.

Lara, J.J., Economou, M., Wallace, A.M., Rumley, A., Lowe, G., Slater, C., Caslake, M., Sattar, N., Lean, M.E.J., 2007. Benefits of salmon eating on traditional and novel vascular risk factors in young, non-obese healthy subjects. Atherosclerosis 193, 213–221.

Lara, J., Cooper, R., Nissan, J., Ginty, A.T., Khaw, K.T., Deary, I.J., Lord, J.M., Kuh, D., Mathers, J.C., 2015. A proposed panel of biomarkers of healthy ageing. BMC Med. 13, 222.

Leung Yinko, S.S.L., Stark, K.D., Thanassoulis, G., Pilote, L., 2014. Fish consumption and acute coronary syndrome: a meta-analysis. Am. J. Med. 127, 848.e842–857.e842.

Lindgren, F.T., Adamson, G.L., Shore, V.G., Nelson, G.J., Schmidt, P.C., 1991. Effect of a salmon diet on the distribution of plasma lipoproteins and apolipoproteins in normolipidemic adult men. Lipids 26, 97–101.

Morrow, D.A., de Lemos, J.A., 2007. Benchmarks for the assessment of novel cardiovascular biomarkers. Circulation 115, 949–952.

Mozaffarian, D., Appel, L.J., Van Horn, L., 2011. Components of a cardioprotective diet: new insights. Circulation 123, 2870–2891.

Mozaffarian, D., Rimm, E.B., 2006. Fish intake, contaminants, and human health: evaluating the risks and the benefits. JAMA 296, 1885–1899.

Murray, C.J., Barber, R.M., Foreman, K.J., Ozgoren, A.A., Abd-Allah, F., Abera, S.F., Aboyans, V., Abraham, J.P., Abubakar, I., Abu-Raddad, L.J., Abu-Rmeileh, N.M., Achoki, T., Ackerman, I.N., Ademi, Z., Adou, A.K., Adsuar, J.C., Afshin, A., Agardh, E.E., Alam, S.S., Alasfoor, D., Albittar, M.I., Alegretti, M.A., Alemu, Z.A., Alfonso-Cristancho, R., Alhabib, S., Ali, R., Alla, F., Allebeck, P., Almazroa, M.A., Alsharif, U., Alvarez, E., Alvis-Guzman, N., Amare, A.T., Ameh, E.A., Amini, H., Ammar, W., Anderson, H.R., Anderson, B.O., Antonio, C.A., Anwari, P., Arnlov, J., Arsenijevic, V.S., Artaman, A., Asghar, R.J., Assadi, R., Atkins, L.S., Avila, M.A., Awuah, B., Bachman, V.F., Badawi, A., Bahit, M.C., Balakrishnan, K., Banerjee, A., Barker-Collo, S.L., Barquera, S., Barregard, L., Barrero, L.H., Basu, A., Basu, S., Basulaiman, M.O., Beardsley, J., Bedi, N., Beghi, E., Bekele, T., Bell, M.L., Benjet, C., Bennett, D.A., Bensenor, I.M., Benzian, H., Bernabe, E., Bertozzi-Villa, A., Beyene, T.J., Bhala, N., Bhalla, A., Bhutta, Z.A., Bienhoff, K., Bikbov, B., Biryukov, S., Blore, J.D., Blosser, C.D., Blyth, F.M., Bohensky, M.A., Bolliger, I.W., Basara, B.B., Bornstein, N.M., Bose, D., Boufous, S., Bourne, R.R., Boyers, L.N., Brainin, M., Brayne, C.E., Brazinova, A., Breitborde, N.J., Brenner, H., Briggs, A.D., Brooks, P.M., Brown, J.C., Brugha, T.S., Buchbinder, R., Buckle, G.C., Budke, C.M., Bulchis, A., Bulloch, A.G., Campos-Nonato, I.R., Carabin, H., Carapetis, J.R., Cardenas, R., Carpenter, D.O., Caso, V., Castaneda-Orjuela, C.A., Castro, R.E., Catala-Lopez, F., Cavalleri, F., Cavlin, A., Chadha, V.K., Chang, J.C., Charlson, F.J., Chen, H., Chen, W., Chiang, P.P., Chimed-Ochir, O., Chowdhury, R., Christensen, H., Christophi, C.A., Cirillo, M., Coates, M.M., Coffeng, L.E., Coggeshall, M.S., Colistro, V., Colquhoun, S.M., Cooke, G.S., Cooper, C., Cooper, L.T., Coppola, L.M., Cortinovis, M., Criqui, M.H., Crump, J.A., Cuevas-Nasu, L., Danawi, H., Dandona, L.,

Dandona, R., Dansereau, E., Dargan, P.I., Davey, G., Davis, A., Davitoiu, D.V., Dayama, A., De Leo, D., Degenhardt, L., Del Pozo-Cruz, B., Dellavalle, R.P., Deribe, K., Derrett, S., Jarlais, D.C., Dessalegn, M., Dharmaratne, S.D., Dherani, M.K., Diaz-Torne, C., Dicker, D., Ding, E.L., Dokova, K., Dorsey, E.R., Driscoll, T.R., Duan, L., Duber, H.C., Ebel, B.E., Edmond, K.M., Elshrek, Y.M., Endres, M., Ermakov, S.P., Erskine, H.E., Eshrati, B., Esteghamati, A., Estep, K., Faraon, E.J., Farzadfar, F., Fay, D.F., Feigin, V.L., Felson, D.T., Fereshtehnejad, S.M., Fernandes, J.G., Ferrari, A.J., Fitzmaurice, C., Flaxman, A.D., Fleming, T.D., Foigt, N., Forouzanfar, M.H., Fowkes, F.G., Paleo, U.F., Franklin, R.C., Furst, T., Gabbe, B., Gaffikin, L., Gankpe, F.G., Geleijnse, J.M., Gessner, B.D., Gething, P., Gibney, K.B., Giroud, M., Giussani, G., Dantes, H.G., Gona, P., Gonzalez-Medina, D., Gosselin, R.A., Gotay, C.C., Goto, A., Gouda, H.N., Graetz, N., Gugnani, H.C., Gupta, R., Gupta, R., Gutierrez, R.A., Haagsma, J., Hafezi-Nejad, N., Hagan, H., Halasa, Y.A., Hamadeh, R.R., Hamavid, H., Hammami, M., Hancock, J., Hankey, G.J., Hansen, G.M., Hao, Y., Harb, H.L., Haro, J.M., Havmoeller, R., Hay, S.I., Hay, R.J., Heredia-Pi, I.B., Heuton, K.R., Heydarpour, P., Higashi, H., Hijar, M., Hoek, H.W., Hoffman, H.J., Hosgood, H.D., Hossain, M., Hotez, P.J., Hoy, D.G., Hsairi, M., Hu, G., Huang, C., Huang, J.J., Husseini, A., Huynh, C., Iannarone, M.L., Iburg, K.M., Innos, K., Inoue, M., Islami, F., Jacobsen, K.H., Jarvis, D.L., Jassal, S.K., Jee, S.H., Jeemon, P., Jensen, P.N., Jha, V., Jiang, G., Jiang, Y., Jonas, J.B., Juel, K., Kan, H., Karch, A., Karema, C.K., Karimkhani, C., Karthikeyan, G., Kassebaum, N.J., Kaul, A., Kawakami, N., Kazanjan, K., Kemp, A.H., Kengne, A.P., Keren, A., Khader, Y.S., Khalifa, S.E., Khan, E.A., Khan, G., Khang, Y.H., Kieling, C., Kim, D., Kim, S., Kim, Y., Kinfu, Y., Kinge, J.M., Kivipelto, M., Knibbs, L.D., Knudsen, A.K., Kokubo, Y., Kosen, S., Krishnaswami, S., Defo, B.K., Bicer, B.K., Kuipers, E.J., Kulkarni, C., Kulkarni, V.S., Kumar, G.A., Kyu, H.H., Lai, T., Lalloo, R., Lallukka, T., Lam, H., Lan, Q., Lansingh, V.C., Larsson, A., Lawrynowicz, A.E., Leasher, J.L., Leigh, J., Leung, R., Levitz, C.E., Li, B., Li, Y., Li, Y., Lim, S.S., Lind, M., Lipshultz, S.E., Liu, S., Liu, Y., Lloyd, B.K., Lofgren, K.T., Logroscino, G., Looker, K.J., Lortet-Tieulent, J., Lotufo, P.A., Lozano, R., Lucas, R.M., Lunevicius, R., Lyons, R.A., Ma, S., Macintyre, M.F., Mackay, M.T., Majdan, M., Malekzadeh, R., Marcenes, W., Margolis, D.J., Margono, C., Marzan, M.B., Masci, J.R., Mashal, M.T., Matzopoulos, R., Mayosi, B.M., Mazorodze, T.T., McGill, N.W., McGrath, J.J., McKee, M., McLain, A., Meaney, P.A., Medina, C., Mehndiratta, M.M., Mekonnen, W., Melaku, Y.A., Meltzer, M., Memish, Z.A., Mensah, G.A., Meretoja, A., Mhimbira, F.A., Micha, R., Miller, T.R., Mills, E.J., Mitchell, P.B., Mock, C.N., Ibrahim, N.M., Mohammad, K.A., Mokdad, A.H., Mola, G.L., Monasta, L., Hernandez, J.C., Montico, M., Montine, T.J., Mooney, M.D., Moore, A.R., Moradi-Lakeh, M., Moran, A.E., Mori, R., Moschandreas, J., Moturi, W.N., Moyer, M.L., Mozaffarian, D., Msemburi, W.T., Mueller, U.O., Mukaigawara, M., Mullany, E.C., Murdoch, M.E., Murray, J., Murthy, K.S., Naghavi, M., Naheed, A., Naidoo, K.S., Naldi, L., Nand, D., Nangia, V., Narayan, K.M., Nejjari, C., Neupane, S.P., Newton, C.R., Ng, M., Ngalesoni, F.N., Nguyen, G., Nisar, M.I., Nolte, S., Norheim, O.F., Norman, R.E., Norrving, B., Nyakarahuka, L., Oh, I.H., Ohkubo, T., Ohno, S.L., Olusanya, B.O., Opio, J.N., Ortblad, K., Ortiz, A., Pain, A.W., Pandian, J.D., Panelo, C.I., Papachristou, C., Park, E.K., Park, J.H., Patten, S.B., Patton, G.C., Paul, V.K., Pavlin, B.I., Pearce, N., Pereira, D.M., Perez-Padilla, R., Perez-Ruiz, F., Perico, N., Pervaiz, A., Pesudovs, K., Peterson, C.B., Petzold, M., Phillips, M.R., Phillips, B.K., Phillips, D.E., Piel, F.B., Plass, D., Poenaru, D., Polinder, S., Pope, D., Popova, S., Poulton, R.G., Pourmalek, F., Prabhakaran, D., Prasad, N.M., Pullan, R.L., Qato, D.M., Quistberg, D.A., Rafay, A., Rahimi, K., Rahman, S.U., Raju, M., Rana, S.M., Razavi, H., Reddy, K.S., Refaat, A., Remuzzi, G., Resnikoff, S., Ribeiro, A.L., Richardson, L., Richardus, J.H., Roberts, D.A., Rojas-Rueda, D., Ronfani, L., Roth, G.A., Rothenbacher, D., Rothstein, D.H., Rowley, J.T., Roy, N., Ruhago, G.M., Saeedi, M.Y., Saha, S., Sahraian, M.A., Sampson, U.K., Sanabria, J.R., Sandar, L., Santos, I.S., Satpathy, M., Sawhney, M., Scarborough, P., Schneider, I.J., Schottker, B., Schumacher, A.E., Schwebel, D.C., Scott, J.G., Seedat, S., Sepanlou, S.G., Serina, P.T., Servan-Mori, E.E., Shackelford, K.A., Shaheen, A., Shahraz, S., Levy, T.S., Shangguan, S., She, J., Sheikhbahaei, S., Shi, P., Shibuya, K., Shinohara, Y., Shiri, R., Shishani, K., Shiue, I., Shrime, M.G., Sigfusdottir, I.D., Silberberg, D.H., Simard, E.P., Sindi, S., Singh, A., Singh, J.A., Singh, L., Skirbekk, V., Slepak, E.L., Sliwa, K., Soneji, S., Soreide, K., Soshnikov, S., Sposato, L.A., Sreeramareddy, C.T., Stanaway, J.D., Stathopoulou, V., Stein, D.J., Stein, M.B., Steiner, C., Steiner, T.J., Stevens, A., Stewart, A., Stovner, L.J., Stroumpoulis, K., Sunguya, B.F., Swaminathan, S., Swaroop, M., Sykes, B.L., Tabb, K.M., Takahashi, K., Tandon, N., Tanne, D., Tanner, M., Tavakkoli, M., Taylor, H.R., Ao, B.J., Tediosi, F., Temesgen, A.M., Templin, T., Ten Have, M., Tenkorang, E.Y., Terkawi, A.S., Thomson, B., Thorne-Lyman, A.L., Thrift, A.G., Thurston, G.D., Tillmann, T., Tonelli, M., Topouzis, F., Toyoshima, H., Traebert, J., Tran, B.X., Trillini, M., Truelsen, T., Tsilimbaris, M., Tuzcu, E.M., Uchendu, U.S., Ukwaja, K.N., Undurraga, E.A., Uzun, S.B., Van Brakel, W.H., Van De Vijver, S., van Gool, C.H., Van Os, J., Vasankari, T.J., Venketasubramanian, N., Violante, F.S., Vlassov, V.V., Vollset, S.E., Wagner, G.R., Wagner, J., Waller, S.G., Wan, X., Wang, H., Wang, J., Wang, L., Warouw, T.S., Weichenthal, S., Weiderpass, E., Weintraub, R.G., Wenzhi, W., Werdecker, A., Westerman, R., Whiteford, H.A., Wilkinson, J.D., Williams, T.N., Wolfe, C.D., Wolock, T.M., Woolf, A.D., Wulf, S., Wurtz, B., Xu, G., Yan, L.L., Yano, Y., Ye, P., Yentur, G.K., Yip, P., Yonemoto, N., Yoon, S.J., Younis, M.Z., Yu, C., Zaki, M.E., Zhao, Y., Zheng, Y., Zonies, D., Zou, X., Salomon, J.A., Lopez, A.D., Vos, T., 2015. Global, regional, and national disability-adjusted life years (DALYs) for 306 diseases and injuries and healthy life expectancy (HALE) for 188 countries, 1990-2013: quantifying the epidemiological transition. Lancet 386, 2145–2191.

Nakamura, K., Nashimoto, M., Okuda, Y., Ota, T., Yamamoto, M., 2002. Fish as a major source of vitamin D in the Japanese diet. Nutrition 18, 415–416.

Parker-Duffen, J.L., Walsh, K., 2014. Cardiometabolic effects of adiponectin. Best. Pract. Res. Clin. Endocrinol. Metab. 28, 81–91.

Paulo, M.C., Andrade, A.M., Andrade, M.L., Morais, M.G., Kiely, M., Parra, D., Martinéz, J.A., Thorsdottir, I., Bandarra, N.M., 2008. Influence of n-3 polyunsaturated fatty acids on soluble cellular adhesion molecules as biomarkers of cardiovascular risk in young healthy subjects. Nutr. Metabol. Cardiovascular Dis. 18, 664–670.

Prenner, S.B., Mulvey, C.K., Ferguson, J.F., Rickels, M.R., Bhatt, A.B., Reilly, M.P., 2014. Very low density lipoprotein cholesterol associates with coronary artery calcification in type 2 diabetes beyond circulating levels of triglycerides. Atherosclerosis 236, 244–250.

Rajaram, S., Haddad, E.H., Mejia, A., Sabaté, J., 2009. Walnuts and fatty fish influence different serum lipid fractions in normal to mildly hyperlipidemic individuals: a randomized controlled study. Am. J. Clin. Nutr. 89, 1657S–1663S.

Ramel, A., Martinez, J.A., Kiely, M., Bandarra, N.M., Thorsdottir, I., 2010. Moderate consumption of fatty fish reduces diastolic blood pressure in overweight and obese European young adults during energy restriction. Nutrition 26, 168–174.

Scottish-Government, 2008. Healthy eating, active living: an action plan to improve diet, increase physical activity and tackle obesity (2008–11).

SeafoodHealthFacts.org, 2015. Seafood Health Facts.

Seierstad, S.L., Seljeflot, I., Johansen, O., Hansen, R., Haugen, M., Rosenlund, G., Frøyland, L., Arnesen, H., 2005. Dietary intake of differently fed salmon; the influence on markers of human atherosclerosis. Eu. J. Clin. Investig. 35, 52–59.

Shearer, G.C., Savinova, O.V., Harris, W.S., 2012. Fish oil—how does it reduce plasma triglycerides? BBA– Mol. Cell Biol. Lipids 1821, 843–851.

Tuomisto, J.T., Tuomisto, J., Tainio, M., Niittynen, M., Verkasalo, P., Vartiainen, T., Kiviranta, H., Pekkanen, J., 2004. Risk-benefit analysis of eating farmed salmon. Science 305, 476–477.

Turunen, A.W., Verkasalo, P.K., Kiviranta, H., Pukkala, E., Jula, A., Männistö, S., Räsänen, R., Marniemi, J., Vartiainen, T., 2008. Mortality in a cohort with high fish consumption. Int. J. Epidemiol. 37, 1008–1017.

van Holten, T.C., Waanders, L.F., de Groot, P.G., Vissers, J., Hoefer, I.E., Pasterkamp, G., Prins, M.W., Roest, M., 2013. Circulating biomarkers for predicting cardiovascular disease risk; a systematic review and comprehensive overview of meta-analyses. PLoS One 8, e62080.

Wergedahl, H., Liaset, B., Gudbrandsen, O.A., Lied, E., Espe, M., Muna, Z., Mork, S., Berge, R.K., 2004. Fish protein hydrolysate reduces plasma total cholesterol, increases the proportion of HDL cholesterol, and lowers acyl-CoA:cholesterol acyltransferase activity in liver of Zucker rats. J. Nutr. 134, 1320–1327.

Zhang, J., Wang, C., Li, L., Man, Q., Meng, L., Song, P., Froyland, L., Du, Z.Y., 2012. Dietary inclusion of salmon, herring and pompano as oily fish reduces CVD risk markers in dyslipidaemic middle-aged and elderly Chinese women. Br. J. Nutr. 108, 1455–1465.

Zhang, J., Wang, C., Li, L., Man, Q., Song, P., Meng, L., Du, Z.-Y., Frøyland, L., 2010. Inclusion of Atlantic salmon in the Chinese diet reduces cardiovascular disease risk markers in dyslipidemic adult men. Nutr. Res. 30, 447–454.

CHAPTER

20

Fish and Fish Oil for Cardiovascular Disease in Diabetes

R. Ward, K. Hintze

Department of Nutrition, Dietetics and Food Sciences, Utah State University, Logan, Utah, United States

INTRODUCTION

As of the year 2015, 28 million people, or 9.3% of the American population, are estimated to have diabetes (Nathan, 2015). This figure includes both diagnosed and undiagnosed cases. More striking, perhaps, is that roughly 80 million Americans, which is more than 1 in 3 adults, are estimated to have prediabetes based on measures of fasting glucose and/or hemoglobin A_{1C} (Hb_{A1c}) levels. Recent cost estimates for diabetes in the United States in the year 2012 were 176 billion dollars for medical expenditures and 69 billion dollars for disability, lost productivity, and early death (CDC, 2014). Worldwide, there are estimated to be approximately 382 million cases of diabetes (IDF, 2013), and 80% live in low and middle income countries. More troublesome, by 2035 there may be as many as 592 million cases of diabetes worldwide (IDF, 2013).

Diabetes is a disease characterized by high blood glucose and involves both problems with insulin secretion and insulin action in target tissues. Four general types of diabetes are recognized and include type 1, or insulin-dependent diabetes, type 2, or noninsulin-dependent diabetes, gestational diabetes, and specific types of diabetes due to other causes (American Diabetes Association, 2015). Type 1 diabetes accounts for roughly 5% of the total, and onset occurs rapidly when the beta cells of the pancreas, which synthesize the hormone insulin, are killed by the body's immune system. Individuals with type 1 diabetes cannot produce sufficient insulin to control blood glucose and require exogenous delivery via pump or injection. While type 1 diabetes can occur at any age, it is most commonly diagnosed in teenagers. Type 2 diabetes (T2DM) accounts for 90%–95% of US cases, and usually develops more slowly and later in life than type 1. The development of T2DM is initiated by the inability of insulin to induce proper glucose uptake in tissues such as liver, muscles and adipose, and may involve either altered insulin secretion or insulin sensitivity in target tissues, or both. Due to its slow onset, T2DM may go undiagnosed for years and cause damage to host tissues via effects of hyperglycemia. Gestational diabetes occurs during pregnancy when some women become resistant to insulin and blood glucose levels rise due to the increased metabolic demand of pregnancy. The prevalence is between 3–8% and it is increasing across the world (Zhou et al., 2012a). Gestational diabetes affects the long term health of the child, and mothers are at an increased risk of developing T2DM later in life (IDF, 2013). Diabetes due to other causes includes monogenic diabetes syndromes, drug- or chemical-induced diabetes among other causes (American Diabetes Association, 2015).

The purpose of this chapter is to summarize the effects of fish and fish oil consumption on the development and management of cardiovascular disease in diabetes as reported in the scientific literature. Individuals with diabetes are at increased mortality and morbidity risk due to dysregulation of lipoprotein, lipid, and glucose metabolism, as well as elevated platelet aggregation, arrhythmia, and dysfunction of the endothelium (Seshasai et al., 2011). Prior to the presentation of results from human trials with fish and fish oil, basic information on diabetes will be presented, including information on the etiology, complications and the dyslipidemia common in diabetics. A brief review of evidence of the effects of fish and fish oil intake in diabetes will be presented from ecological studies and preclinical models.

Fish and Fish Oil in Health and Disease Prevention. http://dx.doi.org/10.1016/B978-0-12-802844-5.00020-8

ETIOLOGY

T2DM is a disease of carbohydrate and fat metabolism, and is characterized by high fasting glucose. T2DM is strongly associated with obesity and with a sedentary lifestyle (Zimmet et al., 2001). After meals, carbohydrates are digested and absorbed into the blood stream. To facilitate uptake into tissues and to control the increase in blood glucose, the beta cells of the pancreas secrete insulin. In T2DM, individuals may be unable to produce sufficient insulin for blood sugar control, or the tissues which use insulin to facilitate glucose uptake become insensitive to it. As the body becomes insensitive to insulin, fasting blood glucose rises from what is considered normal (≤100 mg/dL). When fasting blood sugar is between 100 and 120 mg/dL an individual is considered prediabetic. Close to half of subjects with prediabetes will progress to diabetes in 5–10 years (Zimmet et al., 2001).

As subjects become resistant to insulin, the first detectable metabolic defect in healthy, young subjects is impaired glucose transport into muscles and reduced glycogen synthesis (Petersen et al., 2012). Meanwhile, the continued high plasma glucose is compensated for by increased insulin secretion (Taylor, 2013). As insulin resistance develops, adipose tissues become nonresponsive and fail to cease lipolysis and release of free fatty acids. Increased plasma FFA and increased insulin drives hepatic triglyceride synthesis (Gaggini et al., 2013). Interestingly, increased intrahepatic triglyceride content (IHTC) has recently been tied to the metabolic consequences of obesity, including insulin resistance (Fabbrini et al., 2009). Furthermore, increased IHTC is associated with hepatic insulin resistance leading to continued liver production and secretion of both glucose and VLDL (Kotronen et al., 2008).

DYSLIPIDEMIA

The leading cause of mortality in diabetics is cardiovascular disease (CVD; Gadi and Samaha, 2007). Close to 65% of diabetes-related mortality is attributed to stroke and heart disease (Chehade et al., 2013). T2DM is associated with a dyslipidemia that includes elevated plasma triglycerides, low–high density lipoprotein (HDL) cholesterol, and small dense low density lipoprotein (LDL) cholesterol. However, although high LDL cholesterol is a known risk factor for CVD, the presence of T2DM is associated with a risk of death from CVD which is independent of LDL (Almdal et al., 2004). Interestingly, the lipoprotein pattern which is common in T2DM is present before a subject is categorized as diabetic (Gadi and Samaha, 2007), and is associated with insulin resistance, but not hyperglycemia (Haffner et al., 1990). In order to control diabetic dyslipidemia both pharmacological and dietary approaches are used. Pharmacological approaches include use of 3-hydroxy-3-methylglutaryl CoA reductase inhibitors (ie, statins), fibrates and niacin (Montori et al., 2000).

The pathogenesis associated with diabetic dyslipidemia was reviewed by Chehade et al. (2013), and begins with insulin resistance. As insulin resistance develops, adipocytes continue to release free fatty acids which are taken up by the liver. With the increased availability of fatty acids, liver triglyceride production increases as does assembly and release of very low density lipoprotein (VLDL). In the blood, VLDL triglyceride can be exchanged for cholesteryl ester with HDL via cholesteryl ester transfer protein (CETP). The resulting VLDL is reduced in triglyceride content, and more cholesterol-rich (and atherogenic), while the HDL is more triglyceride-rich. The triglycerides in the triglyceride-rich HDL are then hydrolyzed by either hepatic or lipoprotein lipase, resulting in a cholesterol-poor HDL particle. Apo A-I can dissociate from this particle and be removed by the kidney, which reduces the HDL available for reverse cholesterol transport. In addition, it has been suggested that less apo A-I may be produced in diabetes due to insulin resistance (Mooradian et al., 2004) and inflammatory cytokines (Haas and Mooradian, 2010).

A problematic aspect of the small dense LDL particles is that they are more slowly cleared from circulation and are more likely to become oxidized (Gadi and Samaha, 2007). Exchange of lipids between LDL and VLDL is partially responsible for the production of the small dense LDL associated with diabetes (Gadi and Samaha, 2007). After the cholesteryl ester in LDL is exchanged for triglycerides with VLDL, the triglyceride can be removed by hepatic lipase and/or lipoprotein lipase, which results in the small dense LDL (Chehade et al., 2013). While the LDL cholesterol levels in individuals with diabetes do not differ substantially from those without diabetes, the particle number is increased as are other characteristics such as glycosylation and oxidation state (Chehade et al., 2013).

DIABETIC COMPLICATIONS

Long term complications of diabetes include damage to the eyes (retinopathy), damage to the kidneys (nephropathy), as well as nerve damage (neuropathy; Nathan, 1993). Between the years 2005–08, nearly 33% of adults over 40 years of age with diabetes had retinopathy or advanced retinopathy (CDC, 2014). In addition, 44% of all new cases of kidney failure reported in 2011 were due to diabetes. Diabetes is a serious risk factor for CVD and diabetics are at a two- to four-fold higher risk of developing CVD (Preis et al., 2009). While rates of CVD mortality have been decreasing in the general population, rates are increasing in women with diabetes (Mooradian, 2009). Furthermore, diabetes is an independent risk factor for CVD and amplifies other well known risk factors such as hypertension, hypercholesterolemia, and smoking (Mooradian, 2009). In addition, diabetes has been associated with an increased risk of several forms of cancer (Harding et al., 2015). Diabetes increases the risk of cancers of the liver, pancreas, and endometrium by at least twofold, and cancers of the colon, rectum, bladder, and breast between 1.2- and 1.5-fold (Giovannucci et al., 2010). Evidence for the role of diabetes in cancers such as kidney and non-Hodgkin lymphoma is inconclusive, whereas diabetic men are less frequently diagnosed with prostate cancer.

FISH OIL AND DIABETES, PRECLINICAL MODELS

Evidence from the animal model literature indicates long-chain omega-3 (n–3) polyunsaturated fatty acid (PUFA) has beneficial effects on metabolism as related to diabetes, by reducing obesity, inflammation, hyperinsulemia, and increasing glucose tolerance. The majority of these studies have used high fat diets, typically >35% of energy from fat, in conjunction with obesity-prone mice or rats to induce adiposity, and the resulting metabolic sequelae including hyperinsulemia and glucose intolerance. In an early study, Storlien et al. (1987), found that replacing 6% of dietary linoleic acid with fish oil prevented insulin resistance in rats fed high fat diets. Using the high fat feeding, C57BL/6 mouse obesity model, Ruzickova et al. (2004), reported that increasing the long chain n-3 PUFA concentration of the diet from 1–12% (weight to weight basis) decreased adiposity and improved markers of glucose and lipid metabolism. When compared to high fat diets with lard as the fat source, Jelinek et al. (2013) observed that C57BL/6 mice had improved glucose tolerance when 25% of the lard was replaced with fish oil. Similarly, Kalupahana et al. (2010) reported increased glucose tolerance in C57BL/6 mice fed high fat diets when 17% of the lard was exchanged with eicosapentaenoic acid (EPA) ethyl ester. Using a similar model, Rossmeisl et al. (2009) replaced 1.5% of lipids in a corn oil-based, high fat diet with four different docosahexaenoic acid (DHA) derivatives. Of the derivatives tested, ethyl docosahexaenoate had the strongest metabolic effects; mice on this dietary treatment had impressive reductions in circulating triglycerides, nonesterified fatty acids, cholesterol, weight gain, adiposity, and had increased glucose tolerance.

Several studies have investigated the influence of increased long chain n–3 PUFA on diabetes specific parameters using the transgenic fat-1 mouse. The fat-1 mouse carries a n–3 fatty acid desaturase enzyme from *Caenorhabditis elegans* and is able to convert omega-6 (n–6) to n–3 fatty acids thereby increasing the overall organismal n–3/n–6 ratio (Kang et al., 2004). Several investigators have compared phenotypes between fat-1 mice and wild type controls and have reported that by endogenously increasing n–3 fatty acids with the fat-1 gene, glucose tolerance is improved (Li et al., 2014; Smith et al., 2010; White et al., 2010). Moreover, the fat-1 gene confers protection against beta cell damage from ER stress (Wang et al., 2015) and streptozotocin (Hwang et al., 2015) suggesting a protective role of long chain n–3 PUFA for type 1 diabetes.

Taken together, the animal model data suggests a protective effect of long chain n–3 PUFA for both type 1 and 2 diabetes. However, translating these preclinical results to human populations is problematic. The diet induced obesity models used to induce metabolic disturbances are extreme in fat content and protective effects of long chain n–3 PUFA are typically only observed when fed at levels not relevant to most human diets. Moreover, it is difficult to translate the findings from the fat-1 transgenic model to human populations as these mice have altered fatty acid metabolism due to their functional n–3 fatty acid desaturase transgene.

FISH OIL AND DIABETES, ECOLOGICAL EVIDENCE

There has been interest in the possible benefits of fish oil against diabetes since the 1960s when a low incidence was reported among the Inuit in Greenland (Friedberg et al., 1998). The traditional Inuit diet is high in marine n–3 fatty acids, and among those consuming the traditional diet there was little metabolic or cardiovascular disease (Dyerberg et al., 1975). In follow-up studies from the Dutch and Finnish cohorts of the Seven Countries Study, fish intake was inversely related with a 2 h glucose level (Feskens et al., 1991; Feskens et al., 1995). An ecological study that covered 41 countries in 5 continents reported that in countries with high obesity rates, incidence of T2DM was reduced in those 20–44 year olds consuming more seafood and fish (2.5 ± 1.8% versus 0.9 ± 0.7%; $p = 0.007$). In the 45–64 year old cohort, the incidence was 11.0 ± 3.9% versus 6.2 ± 4.1%; $p = 0.041$ (Nkondjock and Receveur, 2003). In an epidemiological study from Japan that involved around 55,000 men and women from 45 to 75 years who were diabetes free at baseline, total fish/seafood intake was associated with a lower odds ratio of developing T2DM at a 5 year follow-up (0.73, 95% CI; 0.54–1.00) (Nanri, 2013). However, this association was attenuated after adjustment for PUFA and vitamin D intake.

PROSPECTIVE COHORT STUDIES ON FISH OIL, LONG CHAIN n–3 FATTY ACIDS AND DIABETES RISK

Prior to discussing the effects of fish and fish oil on CVD in individuals with diabetes, it is of interest to address whether these dietary constituents affect the development of diabetes. Interestingly, there do not appear to be any published metaanalyses of prospective cohort studies investigating the effects of fish or long chain n–3 consumption on diabetes incidence prior to 2012, a year in which at least five were published (Muley et al., 2014; Wallin et al., 2012; Wu et al., 2012; Xun and He, 2012; Zhang et al., 2013; Zheng et al., 2012; Zhou et al., 2012b). While these analyses used a core of the same studies, the approaches were different and each contributes unique information to the field. The individual study details are presented in Table 20.1, along with the relevant findings. Across all studies there was agreement that fish and long chain n–3 intake is not clearly associated with either the incidence or prevention of T2DM. However, subgroup analysis of the individual studies suggests quite different responses in Asian and Western populations. A more detailed description of two studies is provided later.

Wu et al. (2012) conducted a metaanalysis of prospective cohort studies evaluating the role of n–3 intake on the development of T2DM. The analysis included 18 cohorts with 540,184 individuals and 25,670 cases of incident diabetes. Using 13 studies, the association of fish and/or seafood intake and incident T2DM was determined, and the results indicated there was no effect. The relative risk (RR) per intake of 100g/day fish was 1.12 (95% CI: 0.94–1.34). In addition, the RR of EPA + DHA intake, measured in 16 cohorts, was 1.04 per 250 mg/day (95% CI 0.97–1.10). In

TABLE 20.1 Metaanalyses of Prospective Cohort Studies on Fish and Fish Oil Intake and Type 2 Diabetes Incidence

Study	Cohorts	Subjects	T2DM	Major findings
Xun and He (2012)	12	438,241	18,711	12 Studies with fish, 9 with long chain–3 PUFA. RR not different for increasing levels of fish or long chain n–3 PUFA intake. Lower RR in studies from Asia.
Wallin et al. (2012)	16	527,441	24,082	Heterogeneity between study results precluded combining all studies. Sensitivity analyses indicated geographical variability among study results. No publication bias.
Wu et al. (2012)	18	540,184	25,670	Heterogeneity despite high quality of studies. RR was lower in Asian studies with little heterogeneity, higher in North American/European studies with high heterogeneity. Colinearity across study location, BMI and study duration.
Zhou et al. (2012b)	13	526,271	25,283	'Leave one out' analysis used to reduce heterogeneity. Resulting RR indicated weak positive association with fish and long chain n–3 PUFA on T2DM incidence.
Zheng et al. (2012)	24	545,275	24,509	Subgroup analysis found heterogeneity explained by geographical location, with fish and FO protective in Asian populations and detrimental in Western populations. Subjects with T2DM had lower tissue concentrations of ALA.
Zhang et al. (2013)	13	549,955	NR	No effect of fish/seafood or long chain n–3 PUFA and T2DM risk. Protective effect of oily fish with each 80 g/day increase reducing risk by 20%.
Muley et al. (2014)	16	765,070	NR	Confirmed previous findings that long chain n–3 PUFA increase risk of T2DM in Americans, but reduce risk in Asians.

RR, relative risk; *ALA*, alpha linolenic acid; *BMI*, body mass index; *NR*, not reported.

five cohorts, circulating levels of EPA + DHA were not associated with incident diabetes as the RR was 0.94 per 3% of total fatty acids in the biomarker (95% CI: 0.75–1.17).

Using Begg's test for publication bias the authors determined there was no publication bias for either fish/seafood intake, nor for EPA + DHA intake. However, there was significant heterogeneity between the results from the cohorts included in the analysis despite the fact that studies were judged to mostly have high quality scores (ie, ≥4). Similar to other metaanalyses (Table 20.1), this work found that studies conducted in Asia showed EPA + DHA consumption was associated with a lower incidence of T2DM (per 250 mg/day, RR = 0.95, 95% CI: 0.91–0.99) whereas those from North America/Europe EPA + DHA consumption was associated with a higher incidence of T2DM (RR = 1.12, 95% CI: 1.05–1.20). Additionally, there was little heterogeneity in the Asian studies ($I^2 = 14.7\%$) yet significant heterogeneity in the North/American studies ($I^2 = 67.5\%$). Due to the nature of the studies in the different geographical regions, there was collinearity across study location, average BMI and study duration, and a lack of statistical power to ascertain the independent contribution of these variables. Based on the results of the analysis, the authors concluded that EPA + DHA and fish/seafood intake appear to not have a substantial negative or positive effects on the development of T2DM in moderately overweight, but otherwise healthy people.

Zheng et al. (2012) also conducted a meta analysis on the effects of marine n–3 PUFA on T2DM, but included a supplementary analysis of tissue levels of these fatty acids (Zheng et al., 2012). This analysis included 24 studies with 545,275 subjects, of which 24,509 had T2DM. Overall, there was no effect of fish, marine n–3 PUFA or alpha-linolenic acid on the RR of diabetes when the entire study population was evaluated. However, subgroup analysis found that for Asian populations, the summary RR for high versus. low consumption was 0.89 (95% CI: 0.81–0.98) and 0.87 (95% CI: 0.70–0.96) for fish and marine n–3 PUFA, respectively. Conversely, for Western populations, fish and marine n–3 PUFA were associated with a higher risk of T2DM, as the RR was 1.20 (95% CI: 1.0–1.44) and 1.16 (95% CI: 1.04–1.28), respectively. Across all studies, subjects with T2DM had significantly lower standard mean difference (SMD) tissue concentrations of alpha-linolenic acid (SMD: −0.48; 95% CI: −0.86 to −0.11), whereas there were no differences in long-chain n–3 PUFA. However, when stratified by study location, the SMD for DHA in Asian countries was −1.43 (95% CI: −1.75 to −1.12) whereas that of the Western countries was 0.16 (95% CI: −0.05 to 0.37). For total n–3 PUFA, the SMD was −1.41 (95% CI: −2.23 to −0.59) for Asian countries and 0.18 (95% CI: 0.08– 0.28). The authors suggested that factors such as genetics and gene–diet interactions may explain some of the apparent heterogeneity in the findings.

RANDOMIZED, CONTROLLED TRIALS WITH LONG-CHAIN OMEGA-3 FATTY ACIDS AND CARDIOVASCULAR DISEASE IN DIABETICS

There have been a number of metaanalyses of clinical trials that were conducted to test the hypothesis that intake of fish and fish oil may affect biomarkers of cardiovascular disease risk in diabetics (Table 20.2). However, none of the metaanalyses identified trials that measured primary outcomes of fatal myocardial infarction, sudden cardiac death, or coronary revascularization procedures (Hartweg et al., 2008). Therefore, these metaanalyses have focused on CVD biomarkers, or secondary outcomes from randomized clinical trials such as effects of fish and fish oil on triglycerides, cholesterol, lipoproteins, Hb_{A1C}, concentrations, and blood glucose control in diabetic populations.

The focus of a metaanalysis by Friedberg et al. (1998) was glycemic control, but several CVD risk factors were analyzed as well. Their analysis included studies with more than five diabetic subjects (both type 1 and type 2) that included glycemic and lipid endpoints as affected by fish oil supplementation. Collectively, 26 studies were identified that met the inclusion criteria, and changes in serum triglycerides, total cholesterol, LDL cholesterol, HDL cholesterol, Hb_{A1c}, and fasting glucose were determined. The analysis included 12 studies with 185 type 1 diabetics, and 14 studies with 240 type 2 diabetics. The average fish oil dose given to subjects was 2.7 g of EPA and 1.6 g DHA per day, and study durations ranged from 2 to 36 weeks. The combined and weighted results indicated there was a significant effect of the fish oil treatment on triglycerides, which were reduced by roughly 30%. In addition, there was a modest, but significant increase in LDL cholesterol of 5%. When the analysis was restricted to subjects with T2DM, the effects on both triglycerides and LDL cholesterol remained significant and of the same magnitude. In type 1 diabetics, there was significant effect of FO supplementation on fasting glucose which was reduced by ~16% and increases in both total (~4%) and HDL cholesterol (11%). The FO treatment did not affect LDL cholesterol in type 1 diabetics, but the effect on triglycerides was still significant with an approximate 25% decline.

In 2000, Montori et al. (2000) conducted a systematic review of randomized, placebo-controlled trials in which fish oil administration was the sole intervention in individuals with T2DM. This analysis was also published as a Cochrane Database Systematic Review and included 18 trials and 823 subjects that were published before Sep. 1998. FO supplementation ranged from 3 to 18 g/day and lasted on average 12 weeks (Hartweg et al., 2008). The main

TABLE 20.2 Metaanalyses of Randomized Clinical Trials on Fish and Fish Oil Intake and Biomarkers of CVD Risk in Subjects with T2DM

Study	Trials	Subjects	Length	Focus	Major findings
Friedberg et al. (1998)	26	425	2–36 weeks	Glycemic control/ CVD risk factors	In combined studies, long chain n–3 PUFA reduced triglycerides by 30%, with a slight increase in LDL cholesterol (5%). n-3 PUFA reduced fasting glucose in type 1 diabetes.
Montori et al. (2000)	18	823	2–24 weeks	Effects of n–3 HUFA on CVD factors	Long-chain n–3 PUFA significantly lowered triglycerides and raised LDL cholesterol. Effects were most pronounced in subjects with hypertriglyceridemia and with highest doses.
Balk et al. (2006)	21	NR	4–52 weeks	CVD risk factors	Long-chain n–3 PUFA consumption reduced triglycerides according to dose.
Hartweg et al. (2007b)	23	1,075	Average 8.9 weeks	Lipoproteins and other CVD risk factors	Triglycerides were reduced by ~25%, VLDL cholesterol by 36%, VLDL triglyceride reduced by 40%. LDL cholesterol increased by 6%.
Hartweg et al. (2007a)	12	847	Average 8.5 weeks	Hematological and thrombogenic factors	Long chain n–3 PUFA reduced diastolic pressure by 1.8 mmHg, and increased factor VII by 24%.
Hartweg et al. (2009)	24	1,633	2–36 weeks	Lipid, glycemic and hematological risk factors in T2DM	Long chain n–3 PUFA reduced triglycerides by 7% and increased LDL cholesterol by 3%. Plasma fibrinogen reduced by 10% and platelet aggregation.

NR, not reported.

parameters studied were glycemic control and lipid profiles. Similar to the Friedberg analysis, there was a significant effect of FO on lowering triglycerides (−0.56 mmol/L; 95% CI: −0.71 to −0.41) and in raising LDL cholesterol (0.21 mmol/L; 95% CI: 0.02–0.41). FO supplementation did not affect total cholesterol, HDL cholesterol, fasting glucose or Hb_{A1c}. Interestingly, the effect of FO in lowering triglycerides and in raising LDL cholesterol was greatest in those trials in which subjects had more pronounced hypertriglyceridemia and in which larger doses of fish oil were used.

In discussing their work, the authors made some valuable observations with respect to study design and the challenges of pooling data from numerous studies. Eleven of the studies included in the metaanalyses were crossover designed and only four of them included washout periods, which is problematic as fish oil fatty acids are incorporated into tissue membranes and may have effects that outlast the study duration. To check if design affected the results the analysis was run with all the pooled data and with only the parallel data, and the main findings were the same. Another concern that the authors raised was with respect to Hb_{A1c} which is thought to reflect blood sugar levels over a period of roughly 12 weeks. Therefore, it is not a valid measurement in studies of shorter duration.

Balk et al. (2006) conducted a systematic review on n–3 fatty acid consumption and serum markers of cardiovascular risk. While the inclusion of studies in this review was not restricted to those containing subjects with diabetes, many of the studies included in the analysis did. The authors restricted the analysis to studies with <6 g/day of n–3 fatty acid intake and to studies >4 weeks in duration. The main findings of these analyses, with respect to the topic of this chapter, is that fish oil consumption was associated with a decrease in triglycerides and that the effect was dose-dependent and influenced by baseline triglyceride levels.

Hartweg and coworkers, performed a metaanalysis of randomized, controlled clinical trials focused on the effects of long-chain n–3 PUFA consumption on lipoproteins and other CVD markers in subjects with T2DM (Hartweg et al., 2007b; Hartweg et al., 2008) and a second metaanalysis on the n–3, long-chain PUFA consumption on hematological and thrombogenic factors in subjects with T2DM (Hartweg et al., 2007a). The studies included in the first analysis ranged from 1966 to Dec. of 2006. Collectively, 23 studies were included in the analysis incorporating 1075 subjects and an average duration of 8.9 weeks. The variables investigated were total cholesterol, HDL, LDL, and VLDL, and subfractions, lipid ratios, apolipoproteins, and cholesterol particle sizes. According to the results, long chain n-3 PUFA intake resulted in statistically significant changes in four outcomes. First, triglyceride levels were reduced by approximately 25% (mean 0.45 mmol/L; 95% CI: −0.58 to −0.32; $p < 0.00001$). VLDL cholesterol was reduced by 36%

(0.07 mmol/L; 95% CI: −0.13 to 0.00; $p = 0.04$). VLDL triglyceride was reduced by ~40% (0.44 mmol/L; 95% CI: −0.83 to −0.05; $p = 0.03$). Similar to the previous meta-analyses, LDL cholesterol was increased by ~6% (0.11 mmol/L; 95% CI: 0.00 to 0.22; $p = 0.05$). There were no differences in plasma cholesterol, HDL-2, HDL-3, HDL-TG, LDL-TG, and the LDL: HDL ratio or concentration of apolipoproteins.

Another metaanalysis conducted by Hartweg et al. (2007a) on hematological and thrombogenic factors was also published in 2007, and included 847 subjects in 12 trials. The parameters measured included plasma fibrinogen, heart rate, blood pressure, and factor VII. The results of the analysis indicated that n–3 PUFA treatment significantly reduced diastolic pressure by 1.8 mm Hg (95% CI: 0.0–3.6, $p = 0.05$), and increased factor VII by 24% (95% CI: 7.2–42.6), $p = 0.006$). The average dose of n–3 PUFA used was 4.3 g/day (range 0.9 to 10g/day) and the average treatment duration was 8.5 weeks. In discussing the limitations of the analysis, the authors point out that the trials included in the analysis were small (average ~40 participants). Nonetheless, the reduction in diastolic blood pressure is consistent with other metaanalyses on the effect of fish oil on blood pressure in normal and hypertensive individuals (Geleijnse et al., 2002). Furthermore, although the change is small, it may have a meaningful effect in reducing CVD (Cook et al., 1995).

In 2009 Hartweg et al. (2009) published a follow-up metaanalysis on the effects of n–3 supplementation on an expanded set of markers of CVD. In the updated study, 24 trials were included that were conducted between 1966 and 2008 and included 1533 subjects. The mean intake of n–3 fatty acids was 2.4 g/day. Similar to previous metaanalyses, the results indicated long chain n–3 fatty acids decreased triglycerides by 7% (mean −0.17 mmol/L; 95% CI: −0.23 to −0.11) compared to controls. While this change was statistically significant ($p < 0.00001$) there was also significant heterogeneity in the results of the studies included ($p < 0.00001$). LDL cholesterol was significantly increased 3% (mean 0.08 mmol/L; 95% CI: 0.02–0.13; $p = 0.006$). Several other indices of dyslipidemia (total cholesterol, HDL, VLDL, ratio of small dense LDL to total, ApoB and ApoA1) were evaluated and were not changed as a function of long chain n–3 supplementation. The metaanalysis also included evaluation of inflammatory markers and vascular and thrombogenic factors. Of these, plasma fibrinogen was significantly reduced by 10% (mean −0.96; 95% CI: −1.76 to −0.15), as were ADP platelet aggregation to ADP (22% reduction; mean −10.3%; CI: −12.34 to −8.26) and platelet aggregation to collagen (21% reduction; mean −10.55%; 95% CI; −12.3% to −8.8%).

To further explore the effects of long chain n–3 supplementation on triglycerides and LDL, the authors performed a subgroup analysis to explore the effects of baseline triglyceride levels, dose of n−3 intake and study duration. In two studies that included 72 hypertriglyceridemic subjects at baseline, the long chain n−3 supplementation did not cause a significant reduction in triglycerides ($p = 0.13$), but did in the 22 studies with 1530 subjects who were not hypertriglyceridemic ($p < 0.00001$). In the same set of 72 hypertriglyceridemic subjects at baseline in 2 studies, the long chain n−3 did not significantly increase LDL cholesterol, whereas it was increased in the 1032 subjects who had triglycerides <0.40 mmol/L at baseline ($p < 0.007$).

The subgroup analysis indicated there was a dose−response relationship with long chain n−3 supplementation and triglycerides. In studies where more than 2 g/day of EPA + DHA were given (15 studies with 513 subjects), the reduction in triglycerides was −0.53 mmol/L (95% CI: −0.67 to −0.39), whereas it was −0.11 mmol/L (95% CI; −018 to −0.04) in eight trials with 656 subjects. In 856 subjects in 14 trials, high doses of long chain omega-3 fatty acids increased LDL cholesterol by 0.09 mmol/L (95% CI; 0.02 mmol/L to 0.16 mmol/L; $p = 0.01$) whereas the increase was not significant in subjects that consumed lower doses.

Study trial duration had a significant effect on both the triglyceride and LDL cholesterol response to n–3 supplementation. In trials longer than 2 months (10 trials with 685 subjects) triglycerides were reduced by −0.58 mmol/L (95% CI: −0.73 to −0.44, $p < 0.00001$) compared to −0.10 mmol/L (95% CI −0.17 to -0.03 mmol/L, $p < .004$) in 12 trials with 484 subjects. The weighted mean difference in LDL cholesterol was the same in trials of both longer and shorter duration. One caveat in interpretation of the subgroup analysis is that most of the trials of longer duration also used higher doses of n–3 supplementation. Thus, the authors caution it is difficult to evaluate which factor caused the different response.

EFFECTS OF FISH AND FISH OIL ON MORTALITY IN SUBJECTS WITH T2DM

While the metaanalyses covered in the previous section did not identify enough studies to determine effects of fish and fish oil on primary outcomes, such as mortality, Jeppesen et al. (2013) reviewed prospective cohort studies and more recent analyses where mortality was measured. In a prospective cohort study with female nurses, Hu et al. (2003) examined the relationship between fish and long chain n–3 intake and all-cause mortality in subjects who were CHD-free at baseline. The study followed 5103 nurses from 1980 to 1996, a period in which there were 468 total deaths. In those who consumed fish five or more times per week, the RR of mortality was 0.48 (95% CI: 0.29–0.80) compared to those who consumed fish less than one time per month. The multivariate analysis used included adjustment for numerous potential confounding factors such as energy intake, BMI, smoking, alcohol intake, aspirin use, *trans* fat intake, and dietary fiber.

In 2008, a 4-year follow-up study on 6975 subjects from the Gruppo Italiano per lo Studio della Soppravvienza nell'Insufficienza Cardiaca (GISSI) was published with effects of fish oil supplementation on mortality in subjects with heart failure (Tavazzi et al., 2008). In a subgroup analysis of diabetics (n = 1283), approximately 1 g of fish oil (850–882 mg EPA + DHA ethyl esters in 1:1.2 ratio) per day was associated with a hazard ratio (HR) for all-cause mortality or admission to the hospital for cardiovascular reasons of 0.89 (95% CI: 0.80–0.99) compared to an undefined placebo.

Studies with fish and long chain n–3 fatty acids in diabetics that were not included in the metaanalyses covered in the previous sections are shown in Table 20.3, and a few reported on mortality. For example, in the Alpha–Omega trial, subjects with a previous myocardial infarction (MI) consumed a margarine that was formulated to deliver either 223 mg/day EPA + 149 mg/day DHA and/or 1.9g/day ALA, or a placebo margarine (Kromhout et al., 2011). Subjects consumed the margarine for 40 months. In a subgroup analysis of 1014 subjects with T2DM, there was no effect on all-cause mortality. In 2012 the results of the ORIGIN Trial were published which included 12,536 T2DM subjects with a history of MI (Origin Trial Investigators, 2012). Subjects were given 465 mg/day EPA + 375 mg/day DHA or olive oil as a placebo and followed for over 6 years. Similar to the Alpha–Omega Trial, there was no effect of fish oil supplementation on mortality. In discussing the inconsistency of results between the GISSI, Alpha–Omega and ORIGIN trials, Jeppesen pointed out the GISSI trial summed both all-cause mortality and hospitalization and thus was not a true measure of mortality (Jeppesen et al., 2013). A second prospective cohort study supporting a role for long chain n–3 PUFA in preventing mortality was conducted by Strand et al. (2013). In a subgroup of this study, 317 subjects with T2DM were followed for 4.8 years (Table 20.3). Those in the highest tertile of long chain n–3 consumption had significantly fewer fatal MIs, as in tertile #2 HR was 0.39 (95% CI: 0.13–1.15), tertile #3 0.22 (0.06–0.81) p = 0.02 for trend. Interestingly, in nondiabetics, the highest tertile of long chain n–3 intake was associated with a significantly greater chance of a fatal MI, 4.79 (1.05–21.9).

Collectively, the results of these studies do not paint a clear picture on the effectiveness of fish or long chain n–3 fatty acids in reducing all-cause mortality in subjects with diabetes. However, two large clinical trials are currently underway and should soon contribute valuable information. A Study of Cardiovascular Events iN Diabetes (ASCEND) is currently ongoing and will finish in 2017 (NCT00135226, www.clinicaltrials.gov). The study population is both type 1 and type 2 diabetics > 40 years of age. The treatments are 100 mg of aspirin daily, and/or 1 g n–3 fatty acids. The endpoints are serious vascular events, including death, in subjects without occlusive arterial disease at baseline. The Vitamin D and Omega-3 Trial (VITAL) started in 2010 and the final data collection will be in 2017 (NCT01169259, www.clinicaltrials.gov). This is a randomized trial with 24,874 subjects that is investigating the effects of vitamin D and fish oil on cancer, heart disease, and stroke. The number of subjects with diabetes and the type are unclear, but at least one ancillary study includes endpoints specific to diabetes suggesting there will be enough subjects for such a subgroup analysis.

EFFECT OF FISH AND FISH OIL ON CARDIOVASCULAR DISEASE IN SUBJECTS WITH DIABETES

There are several prospective cohort studies that have investigated the role of fish and long chain n–3 PUFA in the prevention of heart disease. For example, in a subset of nurses with T2DM from the Nurses' Health Study who were cardiovascular disease free at baseline, there were 362 incident cases of CHD (141 deaths and 221 nonfatal MIs) over 16 years (Hu et al., 2003). When subjects in the lowest quintile of fish consumption (≤1 serving/month) were compared to those consuming more fish, the RR of CHD incidence was 0.70 (95% CI, 0.48–1.03) for consuming fish one to three times per month, 0.60 (0.42–0.85) for once per week, 0.64 (0.42–0.99) for two to four times per week, and 0.36 (0.20–0.66) for five or more times per week. Although the authors did not have a direct measure of glycemic control in the subjects, adjustments for insulin use and hypoglycemic medications did not change the results. In a prospective cohort study of postmenopausal women with coronary artery disease, increased fish intake was associated with reduced disease progression over a 3-year period, as measured by coronary artery diameter using quantitative coronary angiography (Erkkila et al., 2004). Increased long chain n–3 intake has also been associated with fewer MI events in a separate prospective cohort study with T2DM (Strand et al., 2013, Table 20.3). Using a multivariate model, the investigators found that increasing tertiles of fish consumption were associated with reduced hazard

TABLE 20.3 Relevant Studies Investigating Effects of Fish and Fish Oil in Type 2 Diabetics Published Since 2009

Study	Treatment	Length and type	Participants	Major findings
RANDOMIZED CLINICAL TRAILS				
Rizza et al. (2009)	2000 mg EPA + DHA versus olive oil	12 weeks parallel	50 offspring of subjects with T2DM, average age 31 years, average BMI 26	Decreased triglycerides, decreased TNFα, increased flow-mediated dilation of brachial artery compared with controls
JELIS (2009)	1800 mg/day EPA	4.6 years	Subanalysis of 4,565 subjects with impaired glucose metabolism in study with 18,645 subjects	EPA supplementation reduced coronary artery disease incidence by 22% in impaired glucose metabolism subjects
Stirban et al. (2010)	920 mg EPA + 760 mg DHA versus olive oil	6 weeks crossover	32 subjects with T2DM, average age 57 years, average BMI 31	Increased postprandial flow-mediated dilation of brachial artery compared with controls
Alpha Omega 2011	223 mg/day EPA + 149 mg/day DHA and/or 1.9 g/day ALA in margarine versus control margarine	40 months parallel	1014 T2DM subjects with previous MI, average age 70 years, average BMI 29	EPA + DHA + ALA group experienced less ventricular arrhythmia and few fatal myocardial infarctions
Sasaki 2012	1800 mg/day EPA versus control	6 months parallel	28 subjects with T2DM, average age 67 years, average BMI	EPA reduced LDL cholesterol and prolonged the duration of reactive hyperemia, an improvement in vascular function
Origin Trial Investiga-tors (2012)	465 mg EPA + 375 mg DHA versus olive oil	6.2 years parallel	12,536 subjects with T2DM	No significant difference in primary mortality, no effect on rates of major vascular events, triglycerides significantly lowered
Miller et al. (2013)	2.3 g/day EPA + 1.2 g/day DHA as ethyl esters versus corn oil	6 weeks crossover	29 subjects with T2DM, average age 67, average BMI 31.6	n–3 PUFA significantly reduced urinary N-acetyl β-d-glucosaminidase excretion
Ogawa et al. (2013)	250 mg/day EPA + 170 mg/day DHA in liquid enteral diet versus control liquid diet	3 months parallel	26 bedridden, T2DM subjects on enteral nutrition, average age 80.4, average BMI 20.1	Significant decline in fasting glucose, Hb_{A1c} and apoB
Spencer et al. (2013)	4 g/day n–3 ethyl esters versus corn oil	12 weeks parallel	34 subjects, 23 with impaired glucose tolerance, average BMI 33, average age 50	Fish oil reduced adipose MCP-1 and macrophages, but not in muscle. Effect was greatest in subjects with most macrophages. Fish oil increased adipose capillary area. No effect on insulin sensitivity
Kondo et al. (2014)	≥3.0 g/day n–3 PUFA from fish versus control diet	4 weeks crossover	23 postmenopausal women with T2DM	Fish-based intervention improved peak blood flow, duration of hyperemia, and flow debt replacement
Lee et al. (2014)	3.6 g/day EPA + 2.4 g/day DHA versus corn oil and borage oil	8 weeks parallel	59 subjects with early-stage T2DM or metabolic syndrome	Fish oil reduced serum triglycerides, Hb_{A1c}, and increased HDL cholesterol
PROSPECTIVE COHORT AND CROSSSECTIONAL STUDIES				
Strand et al. (2013)	Intake of fish and long chain n–3 fatty acids in tertiles	4.8 years	317 subjects with T2DM, average age 63 years, average BMI 28.4	Highest tertile of long chain n–3 intake had fewest MIs and fewest fatal MIs
Kim et al. (2015)	Crosssectional analysis		356 female subjects with T2DM, average age 55.5 years, average BMI 24.2	Fish and shellfish intake negatively associated with triglycerides and pulse wave velocity. Long chain n–3 PUFA negatively associated with triglycerides, systolic blood pressure, diastolic blood pressure, and pulse wave velocity

BMI, body mass index; *TNFα*, tumor necrosis factor; *ALA*, alpha linolenic acid; *MCP-1*, monocyte chemotactic protein; *MI*, myocardial infarction.

ratios for MI of 0.48 (95% CI: 0.22–1.06) for the second tertile and 0.38 (0.17–0.83) for the third (p for trend = 0.01; Strand et al., 2013).

The Japan EPA Lipid Intervention Study (JELIS) was a large clinical trial investigating the effects of EPA supplementation on coronary artery disease (Table 20.3). In 2008, a subgroup analysis of subjects with impaired glucose metabolism was published that included subjects with T2DM and others with a fasting glucose ≥110 mg/dL (Oikawa et al., 2009). The treatment was 1800 mg/day of purified EPA and the subjects were followed for an average of 4.6 years. The analysis indicated that subjects with impaired glucose metabolism had a higher hazard ratio for developing CAD. However, EPA treatment resulted in a 22% decrease in CAD incidence (p = 0.048) in those with impaired glucose metabolism. EPA supplementation increased blood EPA levels from 2.9 mol% in controls to 5.3 mol% in subjects given EPA. According to the authors, this indicates that EPA was effective, despite the fact that the control population had a relatively high fish intake.

In the other clinical trials in which cardiovascular disease was measured (Table 20.3) the results are not consistent. In the secondary analysis of Alpha–Omega trial that focused on subjects with T2DM with a previous MI, supplementation with long-chain n–3 PUFA did not affect fatal MI occurrence. However, supplementation of EPA–DHA–ALA resulted in less ventricular arrhythmia-related events (HR 0.16; 95% CI 0.04, 0.69) compared to placebo (Kromhout et al., 2011). In the ORIGIN trial, supplementation with long-chain n–3 PUFA in diabetic subjects with a history of MI did not affect the primary endpoint (death) or rates of major vascular events (Origin Trial Investigators, 2012).

EFFECTS OF FISH AND FISH OIL ON ENDOTHELIAL FUNCTION IN DIABETICS

Several recent studies have investigated the effects of long chain n–3 fatty acids on aspects of endothelial function (Table 20.3). Rizza et al. (2009) conducted a double-blind, placebo-controlled trial with offspring of subjects with T2DM. Subjects consumed 2000 mg of an EPA + DHA mix or olive oil for 12 weeks. In addition to metabolic metrics endothelial function was measured using flow-mediated dilation (FMD). Compared to baseline, subjects consuming the fish oil had significant improvement in FMD (9.1 ± 5.8% versus 11.7 ± 4.4%, p = 0.02), as well as significantly decreased serum triglyceride and TNFα levels. Furthermore, regression analysis indicated that reduction in TNFα was predictive of the increase in FMD. From the results, the authors concluded that fish oil supplementation improved metabolic heath in a population susceptible to diabetes and vascular complications.

Other groups have also reported positive effects of long chain n–3 supplementation on endothelial function. Based on the fact that individuals with T2DM have increased endothelial dysfunction (Calles-Escandon and Cipolla, 2001) and that this predisposes them for development of CVD (Guerci et al., 2001), Stirban and coworkers investigated whether long chain n–3 PUFA supplementation might improve postprandial endothelial function (Stirban et al., 2010). In a randomized, placebo-controlled, double-blind trial, 34 subjects with T2DM, but no history of CVD, were given 2 g/day purified EPA/DHA or olive oil for 6 weeks (Table 20.3). Subsequently, subjects consumed a high fat meal and parameters of both macrovascular and microvascular function were followed over 6 h. The area under the curve (AUC) for both postprandial flow-mediated dilation (FMD; macrovascular function) and reactive hyperemia (RH; microvascular function) were significantly lower after long chain n–3 supplementation indicating improved vascular function. These results provide support for the fact that long chain n–3 fatty acids are vasoprotective in subjects with T2DM.

Two other randomized controlled trials from Japan have investigated long chain n–3 fatty acids and endothelial function (Kondo et al., 2014; Sasaki et al., 2012; Table 20.3). In one study, 28 statin-treated subjects with T2DM were randomized into control and treatment groups and given either 1800 mg/day EPA + statin or a statin alone for 6 months. Vascular function was measured via the duration of reactive hyperemia (DRH) which is measured with plethysmogaphy as the time necessary for forearm blood flow to return to baseline after reactive hyperemia is induced (Sasaki et al., 2012). EPA treatment led to significant lowering of both LDL-C, and non HDL-C. In addition, EPA, but not the satin alone, prolonged DRH, and thus improved vascular function. Kondo et al. (2014), investigated the effects of a fish-based intervention on endothelial function in postmenopausal women with T2DM. Twenty-three women were randomized and fed control and fish-based diets for 4 weeks, and endothelial function was measured at the end of each diet period with peak forearm blood flow. To increase fish consumption, subjects were instructed to consume at least 3.0 g/day of marine PUFA from fish, and no washout period was described between the crossover arms. DRH was measured as was flow debt replacement (FDR). The fish-based diet improved peak flow by 63.7%, DRH by 27.9% and FDR by 70.7%. In 2015, a cross-sectional analysis of Korean women with T2DM was conducted to investigate the relationship between fish consumption and endothelial function (Kim et al., 2015). The study involved 356 females with an average age of 56 years and BMI of 24.2 kg/m^2 (Table 20.3). After controlling for factors such as age, BMI and disease severity, the results indicated that long chain n–3 PUFA was negatively associated with triglycerides, and both systolic and diastolic blood pressure. Additionally, the study measured pulse wave velocity (PWV), a measure of arterial stiffness. Using multiple logistic regression analysis, the authors found a significant inverse relationship between marine PUFA intake and triglycerides between those consuming higher than average PUFA versus lower than average. In addition, marine PUFA intake was negatively associated with PWV, indicating better endothelial function.

EFFECT OF FISH AND FISH OIL ON METABOLIC AND CARDIOVASCULAR RISK FACTORS IN DIABETES

Several new studies have been published since the last metaanalysis of randomized trials conducted on CVD risk factors with diabetics (Table 20.3). Ogawa et al. (2013) investigated the effects of fish oil supplementation on bedridden subjects receiving enteral nutrition. The study population was composed of 26 subjects with T2DM with an average age of 80 years and BMI of 20.1 kg/m^2. For 3 months, half of the subjects received 250 mg/day EPA + 170 mg/day DHA in their liquid diet. Compared to the control diet, the long chain n–3 PUFA supplemented diet resulted in lower fasting glucose, Hb_{A1c}, remnant-like particles and apoB. Spencer et al. (2013) fed a high dose (4 g/day) of long chain n–3 ethyl esters or corn oil to subjects with an average BMI of 33 kg/m^2 and age of 50 years. Subjects consumed the supplements for 12 weeks and then biopsies of adipose and muscle tissue were collected. Fish oil reduced plasma monocyte chemotactic protein-1 (MCP-1), but not other cytokines. This was associated with a decrease in adipose macrophages, adipose MCP-1, and an increase in adipose capillaries. The treatments did not affect insulin sensitivity or plasma adiponectin. Lastly, Lee et al. (2014) investigated the effects of a large dose of fish oil on metabolic parameters. Fifty-nine subjects with early-stage T2DM or metabolic syndrome were randomized into three groups and provided with either corn oil, borage oil, or fish oil. The fish oil group consumed 3.6 g/day EPA and 2.4 g/day DHA and the intervention lasted for 8 weeks. There was no difference from baseline in the corn oil group, but fish oil supplementation significantly decreased triglycerides (~17%), increased HDL-cholesterol (~7%), and decreased HbA1c (~3%).

CONCLUSION

Despite compelling evidence from ecological and preclinical studies, human prospective cohort and randomized clinical trials have not clearly and consistently supported a role for fish and long chain n–3 fatty acids in the prevention of diabetes incidence or the development of CVD in diabetics. Data from prospective cohort studies indicates that fish and fish oil consumption may be protective against the development of T2DM in Asian populations, but not in Western ones. Several recent studies have supported a role for fish and fish oil in the promotion of endothelial function. Metaanalyses of randomized trials published before 2010 indicate a clear triglyceride lowering effect for both fish and fish oil that is dependent on dose, yet those analyses were not able to address primary protection against CVD incidence and mortality. More recent studies have had mixed results with respect to CVD incidence and mortality. At least two large trials are currently underway that should contribute more information on the possible protective effects of fish and fish oil against CVD in diabetes.

References

Almdal, T., Scharling, H., Jensen, J.S., Vestergaard, H., 2004. The independent effect of type 2 diabetes mellitus on ischemic heart disease, stroke, and death: a population-based study of 13,000 men and women with 20 years of follow-up. Arch. Intern. Med. 164, 1422–1426.

American Diabetes Association, 2015. Standards of medical care in diabetes, Diabetes Care. 38.

Balk, E.M., Lichtenstein, A.H., Chung, M., Kupelnick, B., Chew, P., Lau, J., 2006. Effects of omega-3 fatty acids on serum markers of cardiovascular disease risk: a systematic review. Atherosclerosis 189, 19–30.

Calles-Escandon, J., Cipolla, M., 2001. Diabetes and endothelial dysfunction: a clinical perspective. Endocr. Rev. 22, 36–52.

CDC, 2014. National Diabetes Statistics Report: Estimates of Diabetes and Its Burgen in the United States. US Department of Health and Human Services, Atlanta, GA.

Chehade, J.M., Gladysz, M., Mooradian, A.D., 2013. Dyslipidemia in type 2 diabetes: prevalence, pathophysiology, and management. Drugs 73, 327–339.

Cook, N.R., Cohen, J., Hebert, P.R., Taylor, J.O., Hennekens, C.H., 1995. Implications of small reductions in diastolic blood pressure for primary prevention. Arch. Intern. Med. 155, 701–709.

Dyerberg, J., Bang, H.O., Hjorne, N., 1975. Fatty acid composition of the plasma lipids in Greenland Eskimos. Am. J. Clin. Nutr. 28, 958–966.

Erkkila, A.T., Lichtenstein, A.H., Mozaffarian, D., Herrington, D.M., 2004. Fish intake is associated with a reduced progression of coronary artery atherosclerosis in postmenopausal women with coronary artery disease. Am. J. Clin. Nutr. 80, 626–632.

Fabbrini, E., Magkos, F., Mohammed, B.S., Pietka, T., Abumrad, N.A., Patterson, B.W., Okunade, A., Klein, S., 2009. Intrahepatic fat, not visceral fat, is linked with metabolic complications of obesity. Proc. Natl. Acad. Sci. USA 106, 15430–15435.

Feskens, E.J., Bowles, C.H., Kromhout, D., 1991. Inverse association between fish intake and risk of glucose intolerance in normoglycemic elderly men and women. Diabetes Care 14, 935–941.

Feskens, E.J., Virtanen, S.M., Rasanen, L., Tuomilehto, J., Stengard, J., Pekkanen, J., Nissinen, A., Kromhout, D., 1995. Dietary factors determining diabetes and impaired glucose tolerance. A 20-year follow-up of the Finnish and Dutch cohorts of the Seven Countries Study. Diabetes Care 18, 1104–1112.

Friedberg, C.E., Janssen, M.J., Heine, R.J., Grobbee, D.E., 1998. Fish oil and glycemic control in diabetes. A meta-analysis. Diabetes Care 21, 494–500.

Gadi, R., Samaha, F.F., 2007. Dyslipidemia in type 2 diabetes mellitus. Curr. Diab. Rep. 7, 228–234.

Gaggini, M., Morelli, M., Buzzigoli, E., DeFronzo, R.A., Bugianesi, E., Gastaldelli, A., 2013. Non-alcoholic fatty liver disease (NAFLD) and its connection with insulin resistance, dyslipidemia, atherosclerosis and coronary heart disease. Nutrients 5, 1544–1560.

Geleijnse, J.M., Giltay, E.J., Grobbee, D.E., Donders, A.R., Kok, F.J., 2002. Blood pressure response to fish oil supplementation: metaregression analysis of randomized trials. J. Hypertens. 20, 1493–1499.

Giovannucci, E., Harlan, D.M., Archer, M.C., Bergenstal, R.M., Gapstur, S.M., Habel, L.A., Pollak, M., Regensteiner, J.G., Yee, D., 2010. Diabetes and cancer: a consensus report. CA Cancer J. Clin. 60, 207–221.

Guerci, B., Kearney-Schwartz, A., Bohme, P., Zannad, F., Drouin, P., 2001. Endothelial dysfunction and type 2 diabetes. Part 1: physiology and methods for exploring the endothelial function. Diabetes Metab. 27, 425–434.

Haas, M.J., Mooradian, A.D., 2010. Regulation of high-density lipoprotein by inflammatory cytokines: establishing links between immune dysfunction and cardiovascular disease. Diabetes Metab. Res. Rev. 26, 90–99.

Haffner, S.M., Stern, M.P., Hazuda, H.P., Mitchell, B.D., Patterson, J.K., 1990. Cardiovascular risk factors in confirmed prediabetic individuals. Does the clock for coronary heart disease start ticking before the onset of clinical diabetes? JAMA 263, 2893–2898.

Harding, J.L., Shaw, J.E., Peeters, A., Cartensen, B., Magliano, D.J., 2015. Cancer risk among people with type 1 and type 2 diabetes: disentangling true associations, detection bias, and reverse causation. Diabetes Care 2015; 38: pp. 264–270. (Diabetes Care 38, 734-735.)

Hartweg, J., Farmer, A.J., Holman, R.R., Neil, H.A., 2007a. Meta-analysis of the effects of n-3 polyunsaturated fatty acids on haematological and thrombogenic factors in type 2 diabetes. Diabetologia 50, 250–258.

Hartweg, J., Farmer, A.J., Perera, R., Holman, R.R., Neil, H.A., 2007b. Meta-analysis of the effects of n-3 polyunsaturated fatty acids on lipoproteins and other emerging lipid cardiovascular risk markers in patients with type 2 diabetes. Diabetologia 50, 1593–1602.

Hartweg, J., Perera, R., Montori, V., Dinneen, S., Neil, H.A., Farmer, A., 2008. Omega-3 polyunsaturated fatty acids (PUFA) for type 2 diabetes mellitus. Cochrane Database Syst. Rev. 1, 1–38, CD003205.

Hartweg, J., Farmer, A.J., Holman, R.R., Neil, A., 2009. Potential impact of omega-3 treatment on cardiovascular disease in type 2 diabetes. Curr. Opin. Lipidol. 20, 30–38.

Hu, F.B., Cho, E., Rexrode, K.M., Albert, C.M., Manson, J.E., 2003. Fish and long-chain omega-3 fatty acid intake and risk of coronary heart disease and total mortality in diabetic women. Circulation 107, 1852–1857.

Hwang, W.M., Bak, D.H., Kim, D.H., Hong, J.Y., Han, S.Y., Park, K.Y., Lim, K., Lim, D.M., 2015. Attenuation of streptozotocin-induced pancreatic beta cell death in transgenic fat-1 mice via autophagy activation. Endocrinol. Metab. (Seoul) 30, 569–575.

IDF, 2013. IDF Diabetes Atlas, sixth edn. International Diabetes Federation, Brussels, Belgium.

Jelinek, D., Castillo, J.J., Arora, S.L., Richardson, L.M., Garver, W.S., 2013. A high-fat diet supplemented with fish oil improves metabolic features associated with type 2 diabetes. Nutrition 29, 1159–1165.

Jeppesen, C., Schiller, K., Schulze, M.B., 2013. Omega-3 and omega-6 fatty acids and type 2 diabetes. Curr. Diab. Rep. 13, 279–288.

Kalupahana, N.S., Claycombe, K., Newman, S.J., Stewart, T., Siriwardhana, N., Matthan, N., Lichtenstein, A.H., Moustaid-Moussa, N., 2010. Eicosapentaenoic acid prevents and reverses insulin resistance in high-fat diet-induced obese mice via modulation of adipose tissue inflammation. J. Nutr. 140, 1915–1922.

Kang, J.X., Wang, J., Wu, L., Kang, Z.B., 2004. Transgenic mice: fat-1 mice convert n-6 to n-3 fatty acids. Nature 427, 504.

Kim, H., Park, S., Yang, H., Choi, Y.J., Huh, K.B., Chang, N., 2015. Association between fish and shellfish, and omega-3 PUFAs intake and CVD risk factors in middle-aged female patients with type 2 diabetes. Nutr. Res. Pract. 9, 496–502.

Kondo, K., Morino, K., Nishio, Y., Kondo, M., Nakao, K., Nakagawa, F., Ishikado, A., Sekine, O., Yoshizaki, T., Kashiwagi, A., Ugi, S., Maegawa, H., 2014. A fish-based diet intervention improves endothelial function in postmenopausal women with type 2 diabetes mellitus: a randomized crossover trial. Metabolism 63, 930–940.

Kotronen, A., Seppala-Lindroos, A., Bergholm, R., Yki-Jarvinen, H., 2008. Tissue specificity of insulin resistance in humans: fat in the liver rather than muscle is associated with features of the metabolic syndrome. Diabetologia 51, 130–138.

Kromhout, D., Geleijnse, J.M., de Goede, J., Oude Griep, L.M., Mulder, B.J., de Boer, M.J., Deckers, J.W., Boersma, E., Zock, P.L., Giltay, E.J., 2011. n-3 fatty acids, ventricular arrhythmia-related events, and fatal myocardial infarction in postmyocardial infarction patients with diabetes. Diabetes Care 34, 2515–2520.

Lee, T.C., Ivester, P., Hester, A.G., Sergeant, S., Case, L.D., Morgan, T., Kouba, E.O., Chilton, F.H., 2014. The impact of polyunsaturated fatty acid-based dietary supplements on disease biomarkers in a metabolic syndrome/diabetes population. Lipids Health Dis. 13, 196.

Li, J., Li, F.R., Wei, D., Jia, W., Kang, J.X., Stefanovic-Racic, M., Dai, Y., Zhao, A.Z., 2014. Endogenous omega-3 polyunsaturated fatty acid production confers resistance to obesity, dyslipidemia, and diabetes in mice. Mol. Endocrinol. 28, 1316–1328.

Miller, 3rd, E.R., Juraschek, S.P., Anderson, C.A., Guallar, E., Henoch-Ryugo, K., Charleston, J., Turban, S., Bennett, M.R., Appel, L.J., 2013. The effects of n-3 long-chain polyunsaturated fatty acid supplementation on biomarkers of kidney injury in adults with diabetes: results of the GO-FISH trial. Diab. Care. 36, 1462–1469.

Montori, V.M., Farmer, A., Wollan, P.C., Dinneen, S.F., 2000. Fish oil supplementation in type 2 diabetes: a quantitative systematic review. Diabetes Care 23, 1407–1415.

Mooradian, A.D., 2009. Dyslipidemia in type 2 diabetes mellitus. Nat. Clin. Pract. Endocrinol. Metab. 5, 150–159.

Mooradian, A.D., Haas, M.J., Wong, N.C., 2004. Transcriptional control of apolipoprotein A-I gene expression in diabetes. Diabetes 53, 513–520.
Muley, A., Muley, P., Shah, M., 2014. ALA, fatty fish or marine n-3 fatty acids for preventing DM?: a systematic review and meta-analysis. Curr. Diabetes Rev. 10, 158–165.
Nanri, A., 2013. Nutritional epidemiology of type 2 diabetes and depressive symptoms. J. Epidemiol. 23, 243–250.
Nathan, D.M., 1993. Long-term complications of diabetes mellitus. New England J. Med. 328, 1676–1685.
Nathan, D.M., 2015. Diabetes: advances in diagnosis and treatment. Jama 314, 1052–1062.
Nkondjock, A., Receveur, O., 2003. Fish-seafood consumption, obesity, and risk of type 2 diabetes: an ecological study. Diabetes Metab. 29, 635–642.
Ogawa, S., Abe, T., Nako, K., Okamura, M., Senda, M., Sakamoto, T., Ito, S., 2013. Eicosapentaenoic acid improves glycemic control in elderly bedridden patients with type 2 diabetes. Tohoku J. Exp. Med. 231, 63–74.
Oikawa, S., Yokoyama, M., Origasa, H., Matsuzaki, M., Matsuzawa, Y., Saito, Y., Ishikawa, Y., Sasaki, J., Hishida, H., Itakura, H., Kita, T., Kitabatake, A., Nakaya, N., Sakata, T., Shimada, K., Shirato, K., 2009. Suppressive effect of EPA on the incidence of coronary events in hypercholesterolemia with impaired glucose metabolism: Sub-analysis of the Japan EPA Lipid Intervention Study (JELIS). Atherosclerosis 206, 535–539.
Origin Trial Investigators, 2012. n–3 fatty acids and cardiovascular outcomes in patients with dysglycemia, New England J. Med., 367 pp. 309–318.
Petersen, K.F., Dufour, S., Morino, K., Yoo, P.S., Cline, G.W., Shulman, G.I., 2012. Reversal of muscle insulin resistance by weight reduction in young, lean, insulin-resistant offspring of parents with type 2 diabetes. Proc. Natl. Acad. Sci. USA 109, 8236–8240.
Preis, S.R., Hwang, S.J., Coady, S., Pencina, M.J., D'Agostino, Sr., R.B., Savage, P.J., Levy, D., Fox, C.S., 2009. Trends in all-cause and cardiovascular disease mortality among women and men with and without diabetes mellitus in the Framingham Heart Study, 1950 to 2005. Circulation 119, 1728–1735.
Rizza, S., Tesauro, M., Cardillo, C., Galli, A., Iantorno, M., Gigli, F., Sbraccia, P., Federici, M., Quon, M.J., Lauro, D., 2009. Fish oil supplementation improves endothelial function in normoglycemic offspring of patients with type 2 diabetes. Atherosclerosis 206, 569–574.
Rossmeisl, M., Jelenik, T., Jilkova, Z., Slamova, K., Kus, V., Hensler, M., Medrikova, D., Povysil, C., Flachs, P., Mohamed-Ali, V., Bryhn, M., Berge, K., Holmeide, A.K., Kopecky, J., 2009. Prevention and reversal of obesity and glucose intolerance in mice by DHA derivatives. Obesity (Silver Spring) 17, 1023–1031.
Ruzickova, J., Rossmeisl, M., Prazak, T., Flachs, P., Sponarova, J., Veck, M., Tvrzicka, E., Bryhn, M., Kopecky, J., 2004. Omega-3 PUFA of marine origin limit diet-induced obesity in mice by reducing cellularity of adipose tissue. Lipids 39, 1177–1185.
Sasaki, J., Miwa, T., Odawara, M., 2012. Administration of highly purified eicosapentaenoic acid to statin-treated diabetic patients further improves vascular function. Endocr. J. 59, 297–304.
Seshasai, S.R., Kaptoge, S., Thompson, A., Di Angelantonio, E., Gao, P., Sarwar, N., Whincup, P.H., Mukamal, K.J., Gillum, R.F., Holme, I., Njolstad, I., Fletcher, A., Nilsson, P., Lewington, S., Collins, R., Gudnason, V., Thompson, S.G., Sattar, N., Selvin, E., Hu, F.B., Danesh, J., 2011. Diabetes mellitus, fasting glucose, and risk of cause-specific death. New England J. Med. 364, 829–841.
Smith, B.K., Holloway, G.P., Reza-Lopez, S., Jeram, S.M., Kang, J.X., Ma, D.W., 2010. A decreased n-6/n-3 ratio in the fat-1 mouse is associated with improved glucose tolerance. Appl. Physiol. Nutr. Metab. 35, 699–706.
Spencer, M., Finlin, B.S., Unal, R., Zhu, B., Morris, A.J., Shipp, L.R., Lee, J., Walton, R.G., Adu, A., Erfani, R., Campbell, M., McGehee, Jr., R.E., Peterson, C.A., Kern, P.A., 2013. Omega-3 fatty acids reduce adipose tissue macrophages in human subjects with insulin resistance. Diabetes 62, 1709–1717.
Stirban, A., Nandrean, S., Gotting, C., Tamler, R., Pop, A., Negrean, M., Gawlowski, T., Stratmann, B., Tschoepe, D., 2010. Effects of n-3 fatty acids on macro- and microvascular function in subjects with type 2 diabetes mellitus. Am. J. Clin. Nutr. 91, 808–813.
Storlien, L.H., Kraegen, E.W., Chisholm, D.J., Ford, G.L., Bruce, D.G., Pascoe, W.S., 1987. Fish oil prevents insulin resistance induced by high-fat feeding in rats. Science 237, 885–888.
Strand, E., Pedersen, E.R., Svingen, G.F., Schartum-Hansen, H., Rebnord, E.W., Bjorndal, B., Seifert, R., Bohov, P., Meyer, K., Hiltunen, J.K., Nordrehaug, J.E., Nilsen, D.W., Berge, R.K., Nygard, O., 2013. Dietary intake of n-3 long-chain polyunsaturated fatty acids and risk of myocardial infarction in coronary artery disease patients with or without diabetes mellitus: a prospective cohort study. BMC Med. 11, 216.
Tavazzi, L., Maggioni, A.P., Marchioli, R., Barlera, S., Franzosi, M.G., Latini, R., Lucci, D., Nicolosi, G.L., Porcu, M., Tognoni, G., 2008. Effect of n-3 polyunsaturated fatty acids in patients with chronic heart failure (the GISSI-HF trial): a randomised, double-blind, placebo-controlled trial. Lancet 372, 1223–1230.
Taylor, R., 2013. Type 2 diabetes: etiology and reversibility. Diabetes Care 36, 1047–1055.
Wallin, A., Di Giuseppe, D., Orsini, N., Patel, P.S., Forouhi, N.G., Wolk, A., 2012. Fish consumption, dietary long-chain n-3 fatty acids, and risk of type 2 diabetes: systematic review and meta-analysis of prospective studies. Diabetes Care 35, 918–929.
Wang, J., Song, M.Y., Bae, U.J., Lim, J.M., Kwon, K.S., Park, B.H., 2015. n-3 Polyunsaturated fatty acids protect against pancreatic beta-cell damage due to ER stress and prevent diabetes development. Mol. Nutr. Food Res. 59, 1791–1802.
White, P.J., Arita, M., Taguchi, R., Kang, J.X., Marette, A., 2010. Transgenic restoration of long-chain n-3 fatty acids in insulin target tissues improves resolution capacity and alleviates obesity-linked inflammation and insulin resistance in high-fat-fed mice. Diabetes 59, 3066–3073.
Wu, J.H., Micha, R., Imamura, F., Pan, A., Biggs, M.L., Ajaz, O., Djousse, L., Hu, F.B., Mozaffarian, D., 2012. Omega-3 fatty acids and incident type 2 diabetes: a systematic review and meta-analysis. Br. J. Nutr. 2 (Suppl. 107), S214–227.
Xun, P., He, K., 2012. Fish Consumption and Incidence of Diabetes: meta-analysis of data from 438,000 individuals in 12 independent prospective cohorts with an average 11-year follow-up. Diabetes Care 35, 930–938.
Zhang, M., Picard-Deland, E., Marette, A., 2013. Fish and marine omega-3 polyunsatured Fatty Acid consumption and incidence of type 2 diabetes: a systematic review and meta-analysis. Int. J. Endocrinol. 2013, 501015.
Zheng, J.S., Huang, T., Yang, J., Fu, Y.Q., Li, D., 2012. Marine N-3 polyunsaturated fatty acids are inversely associated with risk of type 2 diabetes in Asians: a systematic review and meta-analysis. PLoS ONE 7, e44525.
Zhou, S.J., Yelland, L., McPhee, A.J., Quinlivan, J., Gibson, R.A., Makrides, M., 2012a. Fish-oil supplementation in pregnancy does not reduce the risk of gestational diabetes or preeclampsia. Am. J. Clin. Nutr. 95, 1378–1384.
Zhou, Y., Tian, C., Jia, C., 2012b. Association of fish and n-3 fatty acid intake with the risk of type 2 diabetes: a meta-analysis of prospective studies. Br J. Nutr. 108, 408–417.
Zimmet, P., Alberti, K.G., Shaw, J., 2001. Global and societal implications of the diabetes epidemic. Nature 414, 782–787.

C H A P T E R

21

Fish Consumption and Heart Rate Variability

A.L. Hansen, B. Grung***

*Department of Clinical Psychology, University of Bergen, Bergen; Centre for Research and Education in Forensic Psychiatry, Haukeland University Hospital, Bergen, Norway; **Department of Chemistry, University of Bergen, Bergen, Norway

INTRODUCTION

Fish contains many different key nutrients important for growth and development as well as maintenance of good health and well-being across the lifespan. Lean fish, for instance pike, pollock, and cod, is a good source of iodine, which is important for brain development and cognitive abilities (Alexander et al., 2007; Gordon et al., 2009). Fatty fish like salmon, herring, halibut, and mackerel are rich sources of vitamin D and the marine omega-3 fatty acids, eicosapentaenoic acid (EPA, 20:5n-3) and docosahexaenoic acid (DHA, 22:6n-3; Alexander et al., 2007). These key nutrients are especially important for brain development (McCann and Ames, 2008; Nyaradi et al., 2004) and prevention of both coronary heart diseases (Mozaffarian and Rimm, 2006) and mental health problems (Lansdowne and Provost, 1998; Appleton et al., 2007). Fatty fish seems to be more important with regard to prevention of cardiovascular heart diseases than lean fish (Mozaffarian and Rimm, 2006). However, consumption of lean fish has also been shown to reduce blood pressure in patients with coronary heart disease (Erkkilä et al., 2008). Fish and seafood in general is a unique source of key nutrients like selenium, vitamin B_{12}, and high quality proteins (Alexander et al., 2007). Thus, fish consumption as whole food has been shown to possess beneficial effects on health. The health status of an individual can of course be categorized in many different ways, and in this chapter we will argue for the use of *heart rate variability* (HRV) as a particularly useful measure.

Both dietary self-report studies and fish intervention studies have shown a positive relationship between fish consumption and improved HRV (eg, Mozaffarian et al., 2008; Hansen et al., 2014a,b). The present chapter will start with some background information concerning HRV and then we will review research focusing on the relationship between fish consumption and HRV. Finally, possible underlying mechanisms involved in the beneficial effects and implications for further research are discussed.

HEART RATE VARIABILITY

In humans, the autonomic nervous system (ANS) regulates and controls bodily functions without conscious involvement. Actions such as respiration, digestion, and sexual arousal are examples of bodily functions governed by the ANS. A very important bodily function controlled by the ANS is the beating of the heart. The heart rate is of course an important measure of the health status of an individual, but HRV is an equally important and interesting characteristic. The HRV is a measure of the time period between each successive heartbeat. This is also referred to as the inter-beat intervals (IBI), and it is expressed in milliseconds. The ANS is divided into two parts or systems with different functions. These are the sympathetic and parasympathetic nervous systems. Changes in the heart rate and its variability are mainly determined by these two subsystems' input to the sinoatrial node (the cardiac pacemaker)

Fish and Fish Oil in Health and Disease Prevention. http://dx.doi.org/10.1016/B978-0-12-802844-5.00021-X

of the heart. When an organism experiences lack of control (eg, stress) or perception of a threatening stimulus, the sympathetic nervous system swings into action and mobilizes energy to a fight-or-flight response. This system secretes neurotransmitters such as norepinephrine (noradrenaline) and adrenaline which causes the heart rate to speed up. This shortens the time period between successive heart beats. The complementary part of the ANS is the parasympathetic nervous system. It is dominant when the organism is at rest conditions and in a homeostatic balance, and is thus often referred to as responsible for the rest-and-digest responses of the organism. The tenth cranial nerve is the *vagus* nerve, and it plays an important role in the parasympathetic control of the heart. The parasympathetic nervous system is mediated by acetylcholine via the vagus nerve, and due to this neurotransmitter the parasympathetic component of the ANS affects the heart rate much faster (milliseconds instead of seconds) and causes longer inter-beat intervals compared to the sympathetic component (Thayer et al. 2010, Hugdahl, 2001; Malik, 1996). By stimulation of the sympathetic and parasympathetic or the vagal influence simultaneously, the effect of vagal influence is shown to be dominant (Levy, 1990). Thus, the parasympathetic branch of the ANS has greater influence on the heart rate than the sympathetic. As argued by Porges et al. (1996) vagal activity can be described as a brake. The vagal brake keeps the heart rate slow by increasing the vagal output and inhibiting the sympathetic influences. On the other hand, upon release of the vagal brake, vagal inhibition on the sinoatrial node is reduced and sympathetic influences increase the heart rate.

In healthy humans (and other organisms) the relationship between the sympathetic and parasympathetic nervous systems is usually reciprocally and negatively connected. This is referred to as *coupled reciprocal* modes, and increased activity in one mode is thus associated with decreased activity in the other. However, the activity of the two modes might also be *coupled nonreciprocal*. The two modes are then positively correlated, so increased activity in one mode causes increased activity in the other. Finally, the modes may be *uncoupled*, so that activity changes in the two modes are uncorrelated (Berntson et al., 1991). These different patterns in sympathetic and parasympathetic activity may be caused by vulnerability to pathologic events (Thayer et al., 2010; Eckberg, 1997). They may also be caused by different kinds of physiological interventions. When cold water is splashed in ones face (the 'diving reflex'), a parallel reduction in sympathetic and vagal activity is caused: a coupled nonreciprocal change (Malliani, 1999; Eckberg, 1997). The patterns may also be caused by individual differences in responses to stress and thresholds for activation of the two ANS divisions, as shown by uncoupled modes (Berntson et al., 1997). However, HRV is regarded as a measure of the continuous interplay between the two different modes of the ANS on the heart (Appelhans and Luecken, 2006), and higher HRV is associated with higher adaptabilities and flexibilities (Porges, 1992). Thus, HRV is regarded as an important index of parasympathetic activity, which has shown to be an important biomarker of both physical and mental health (Thayer et al., 2010).

HRV AS AN INDEX OF HEALTH

HRV's role in relation to physical health, such as cardiovascular diseases has been widely investigated, and low HRV has been shown to be a major risk factor for morbidity and mortality (Thayer and Lane, 2007). However, the neurovisceral integration model, linking underlying physiological structures (eg, central nervous system structures, peripheral end organs, and the cardiovascular system) and psychological functions (eg, cognitive and affective processes), illuminates HRV as an index of both emotion- and self-regulation as well (Thayer and Lane, 2000). Numerous studies have demonstrated that there is a link between HRV and performance on so called executive function tasks (Thayer et al., 2009 for an overview). Executive functioning is associated with activation in the prefrontal cortex and these underlying cognitive mechanisms are essential for planning, reasoning, decision making, and impulsive control (Shimamura, 2000). The neurovisceral integration model describes the central autonomic network, a functional unit within the central nervous system, and how different structural components within the central autonomic network (eg, prefrontal cortex and brain stem regions involved in control of visceral responses) are reciprocally interconnected. Moreover, the model emphasizes how the central autonomic network is related to the preganglionic sympathetic and parasympathetic neurons and how these neurons supply the heart through stellate ganglia and vagus nerve (Thayer and Lane, 2000; Thayer et al., 2009). As also demonstrated by Porges (1992), cardiac vagal tone has shown to be related to cognitive processes such as attentional control, an important cognitive component in self-regulation. HRV is therefore an important index of mental states and self-regulation (Thayer and Lane, 2000).

Low HRV has been associated with a number of psychiatric conditions and emotional health problems such as anxiety (Chalmers et al., 2014), depression (Kemp et al., 2010), and schizophrenia (Bar et al., 2008). Notably, subjects with severe psychiatric and emotional problems, usually on a mix of different kinds of medications, have shown to have a shorter life expectancy compared to normal, healthy subjects (Nome and Holsten, 2012). This shorter life expectancy may be related to many different risk factors associated with cardiovascular diseases such as side effects of medication, low physical activity, smoking, and poor diet. Thus, emotional problems are highly related to cardiovascular diseases (Newcomer and Hennekens, 2007). Since HRV is an important index of physical and mental health, it can be used as an objective outcome measure in clinical use and when evaluating the effect of various intervention studies, for example, fish diet or fish oil supplement intervention studies. The fact that HRV measurements are noninvasive and fairly simple to conduct are also attractive features of the method.

MEASURING HEART RATE VARIABILITY

HRV can easily be measured by different kinds of noninvasive assessment systems (eg, the Actiheart system, ambulatory monitoring systems, exercise watches). Thus, dependent on software or systems, the heart activity is measured by electrocardiography (ECG) or impedance cardiography (ICG) recordings (Thayer et al., 2010). Electrodes are placed on the body surface and several waveforms can be identified. Each waveform corresponds to different components of heart beats (eg, P-wave, QRS-complex, and T-wave). However, inter-beat-intervals (IBI) are usually defined as the temporal distance between R-spikes, which corresponds with the heart's ventricular contractions. Note, that IBIs are often labeled as normal-to-normal (NN) intervals (Appelhans and Luecken, 2006).

DESCRIBING HEART RATE VARIABILITY

In order to describe HRV, numerous different assessment methods and techniques have been developed. In 1996, the Task Force of the European Society of Cardiology and the North American Society of Pacing and Electrophysiology compiled a report, and Berntson and coworkers argued in 1997 that this was an important step towards standardization of the field. The most common approaches used to calculate the HRV have been the time domain and the frequency domain methods, but nonlinear analysis methods have also been suggested.

The time domain approach is the easier way to calculate the HRV. Two major groups of methods exist. The first group consists of methods that deal with standard deviations of the IBI. *SDNN* calculates the standard deviation of all IBI. The IBI is often referred to as N-N intervals—thus the name SDNN. The 'N' itself stands for 'normal'. Sometimes, an average IBI is calculated for a 5 min period. The standard deviation of these averages, recorded over a 24 h period, is referred to as *SDANN*. The second group of time domain measures deals with differences between successive IBI. The most frequently reported variable of this type is the root mean square of successive differences (*RMSSD*), which reflects the vagal modulation of the sinoatrial node during normal circumstances (Stein and Kleiger, 1999; Malik, 1996).

The frequency domain approach is mathematically more complex, but provides a more sophisticated measure. This is particularly true for the parasympathetic activity. Three main frequency bands are defined. These are the high frequency band (HF; 0.15–0.4 Hz), the low frequency band (LF; 0.04–0.15 Hz), and the very low frequency (VLF; 0.0033–0.04 Hz). However, the most reported frequency bands are the HF and the LF, because they are easier to interpret than the VLF (Thayer et al., 2010, Malik, 1996; Stein and Kleiger, 1999).

There is abundant evidence showing that the HF power is a pure measure of parasympathetic activity (see for instance Malik, 1996; Stein and Kleiger, 1999, Thayer et al., 2010). The HF power also reflects the respiration mediated HRV (Stein and Kleiger, 1999). However, there are discrepancies in the literature when it comes to the LF power. It has been argued that the LF power is a direct measure of the sympathetic nervous system (Malliani et al., 1991). Others have argued that it is a measure of both the sympathetic and the parasympathetic nervous systems (Stein and Kleiger, 1999). Others again have claimed that there is no clear evidence for any relationship between LF power and sympathetic activity (Eckberg, 1997), and even a clear positive relationship between LF power and HF power has been reported (Wang et al., 2005). This may seem confusing, but it is important to note that there is no disagreement in the literature with regards to the HF power which predominantly measures the variability in heart rate induced by respiration. The correlation between HF power and time domain measures such as RMSSD is shown to be very high (about 0.90; Friedman et al., 2002).

The three main frequency components are usually measured as absolute values of power (in units of squared milliseconds; Malik, 1996). The absolute values of spectral components correlate with the variance corresponding to the total power (Malliani, 1999). However, the LF and HF components can also be measured as normalized units (nu). Task Force of The European Society, 1996 described these normalized units to "*represent the relative value of each power component in portion to the total power minus the VLF power*". Thus, these normalized units are regarded as a measure of the changes in sympathetic and parasympathetic tone. The normalized LF and HF units may also be expressed as

LF = LF/(LF + HF) and HF = HF/(LF + HF) or the ratio of absolute LF to absolute HF power (LF/HF; Eckberg, 1997). The LF/HF ratio which has been regarded as the sympatovagal balance has therefore been reported by many researchers (Appelhans and Luecken, 2006). However, due to the lack of evidence linking the LF power to sympathetic activity, the construct of the sympathovagal balance has been questioned and criticized (Eckberg, 1997).

The most popular nonlinear method is the use of Poincaré plots (Woo et al., 1992; Brennan et al., 2001). This is a two dimensional plot in which the previous RR interval is plotted against the current. Each point in the plot thus represents two successive beats. It has been shown that it is possible to separate healthy and unhealthy individuals based on the shape of the resulting plots.

Some more advanced methods make use of the concept of entropy. Entropy, originally a term from thermodynamics, is a measure of the amount of disorder or uncertainty in a system. In information science, entropy is used to denote the amount of information in a message. The HRV data can be regarded as time series data, and approximate entropy can be calculated, describing the degree of regularity in the data. Fleisher et al. (1993) reported using approximate entropy for heart rate data, and Goldberger et al. (1994) used approximate entropy for HRV data. An extension of approximate entropy, referred to as sample entropy, was developed by Richman and Moorman (2000). More recently (Isler and Kuntalp, 2007), wavelet entropy measures have also been used to discriminate healthy individuals from patients suffering from congestive heart failure. A detailed description of the various entropy related methods is beyond the scope of this chapter.

CHANGES IN HRV PARAMETERS INDUCED BY FISH CONSUMPTION AND POSSIBLE MECHANISMS INVOLVED

Mozaffarian et al. (2008) investigated the relationship between self-reported habitual fish intake as well as omega-3 consumption and different measures of HRV. This was a population-based study focusing on older adults. The results revealed that consumption of tuna or other fish was positively linked with greater parasympathetic activity (eg, RMSSD and HF), which indicates beneficial health effects. Moreover, their results indicated that fish consumption was associated with lower (normalized) LF power, interpreted as enhanced vagal activity and parasympathetic predominance. They also found a relationship between dietary EPA + DHA and higher RMSSD and HF, but lower LF power (and LF/HF ratio).

Another study, a short-term fish intervention study of 8 weeks (Erkkilä et al., 2008), compared the effects of *lean* and *fatty fish* interventions on different parameters (eg, fatty acid composition of serum lipids, vitamin D status, and HRV) in subjects with coronary heart disease. The amount of fish was 100–150 g/meal 4 times per week. The lean fish meal consisted of fish species like pike, pike-perch, perch, pollock, or cod, while the fatty fish meals consisted of salmon, rainbow trout, herring, or whitefish. The results from this study indicated higher blood levels of EPA + DHA in the fatty fish group, but the study did not report any relationship between EPA + DHA and blood pressure. Thus, in the fatty fish group there was no reduction on blood pressure. However, systolic and diastolic blood pressure decreased in the lean fish group. Surprisingly, vitamin D status and the HRV did not change significantly in any of the fish groups. As they argued, the lack of association between fish consumption and HRV could be due to the short intervention period.

A long term fatty fish intervention study of six months (salmon, herring or halibut three times per week) in Norwegian inmates demonstrated significant increase in HF power and a significant decrease in LF/HF ratio (Hansen et al., 2010). Thus, the results from this intervention study were in line with the results of Mozaffarian et al. (2008). However, due to the disagreement concerning the LF power, one should interpret the LF/HF ratio results with caution. Moreover, the results from this study showed that fish consumption caused an increase in vitamin D status (Hansen et al., 2010). Not surprisingly, overall this group of participants with restricted access to normal daylight had very low vitamin D status at pretest measures. However, one important limitation with this Norwegian study was the low sample size (n = 15). Thus, a larger follow-up study was conducted among American forensic inpatients (n = 95), who also had restricted access to daylight due to their imprisonment. The participants were randomly assigned into two groups, a fish group or a control group. The fish group was served Atlantic salmon (150–200 g) three times per week and the control group was served an alternative meal, for example, chicken, pork, or beef during the same period. Importantly, the results from this latter study demonstrated a clear causal relationship between fatty fish consumption and increased HF power (Hansen et al., 2014a) as well as increased RMSSD (Hansen et al., 2014b). Thus, again the results from Mozaffarian et al. (2008) selfreport study were supported, suggesting that fish consumption results in higher HRV. High HRV is generally considered to be an indicator of good cardiovascular health (Thayer and Lane, 2007).

The LF power results from the United States project were less convincing. However, the results from a small subsample of participants using different kinds of medications throughout the fish intervention period had a larger reduction in LF power compared to those participants not on medication (Grung et al., 2015). The results also showed that participants in the fish group using many different drugs responded differently during the recovery phase (resting HRV after a mild cognitive stress procedure), as they had a much higher RMSSD compared to the rest of the participants. This study, an exploratory study using multivariate analysis to detect the effects of fatty fish consumption and different types of medication known to influence the HRV (eg, antidepressant and heart medication) raises several important questions and hypotheses which remain to be investigated. Since psychiatric inpatients are known to have lower life expectancy (cf. Nome and Holsten, 2012), often related to sudden death caused by cardiovascular diseases (Colton and Manderscheid, 2006), one important question is; will increased fatty fish consumption increase life expectancy in patients with severe mental health problems? This may be possible as fatty fish seems to positively influence HRV, an important risk factor for mortality and morbidity caused by cardiovascular diseases. There is also the fact that a meal of fatty fish replaces another meal: one which may be composed of less healthy ingredients. This replacement effect makes the health benefit of regular fish meals more efficient than nutrient supplements. The close relationship between mental health and HRV leads one to expect that fish interventions may boost the effects of standard health care interventions, both medical and psychological. However, very few randomized experimental fish intervention studies have been conducted to test this hypothesis.

HRV recordings are usually conducted over shorter periods of time. Often only a baseline HRV measure of 5–10 min is registered in a sitting or supine position. However, HRV is sensitive to different environmental conditions including mental and physical challenges, and can therefore be regarded as a biomarker of stress (Thayer et al., 2012). Exploring the HRV *reactivity* to different kinds of conditions as part of a fish or fish oil intervention experiment is particularly interesting. These various conditions may include resting, exposure to a stress situation, followed by resting recovery. This may add important and differentiated information with regard to the sympathetic and parasympathetic influence on the heart under various conditions (cf. the disagreement concerning the LF power, and LF/HF ratio). Interestingly, a study done by Macartney et al. (2014) investigating fish oil supplementation for 8 weeks in healthy, physically fit males demonstrated that fish oil caused a reduction in mean heart rate during maximal exercise and improved heart rate during recovery. However, the heart rate during supine rest condition was not affected by fish oil supplementation. The control/placebo (olive oil) group did not show any changes in heart rate or other outcome measures from pre- to posttest.

In the study by Grung et al. (2015) the focus was on how each individual's HRV changed during the intervention. Based on this study, one may speculate whether people with complex mental health problems may have better effects of fish interventions/increased fish consumption compared to subjects without mental health problems. A metaanalysis (Mozaffarian et al., 2005) investigating the effect of fish oil on heart rate in humans revealed that fish oil supplementation caused a greater heart rate reduction in populations with higher heart rate at baseline (≥ 69 bpm) compared to populations with lower heart rate (<69 bpm) at baseline. Moreover, this metaanalysis also showed that longer intervention periods (≥ 12 weeks) had better effects than shorter intervention periods (<12 weeks). However, regular dietary fish consumption is associated with reduced risk of cardiac mortality, and an omega-3 index of < 5% is associated with an elevated risk of cardiac diseases (Macartney et al., 2014). Thus, fish consumption will likely have health promotion and disease prevention effects in healthy subjects.

As there is a relationship between HRV and executive functioning, fish intervention may also improve and strengthen these underlying mechanisms involved in selfregulation. Notably, a direct relationship between fatty fish consumption and executive functioning has been found (Dangour et al., 2009). However, more research is needed in order to find out whether these changes are mediated by the HRV.

To our knowledge only few fish intervention studies focusing on the effect on HRV have been performed. Most studies focusing on this topic have been based on self-report. By using the words "fish intervention" and "heart rate variability" a search in Web of Science resulted in 16 hits (May, 2015). However, only five of them were *fish intervention studies* and the remaining 11 studies were based on *fish oil/omega-3 supplements*. Numerous studies have actually focused on omega-3 supplements instead of fish consumption. This has also been due to practical reasons, since supplement studies are easier to conduct than fish intervention studies. Supplement studies also have other advantages because they can be carried out as double blind trials. Blinded food intervention studies are still impossible.

Moreover, most of the human studies investigating the relationship between fish consumption and HRV have used noninvasive assessment methods. Little is known about the precise nutrients and the real mechanisms responsible for the beneficial effects of fish consumption such as specific key nutrients (eg, omega-3, vitamin D), their interaction with each other, and their interaction with underlying human biology. HRV may just be one of many biological components affected by fish consumption. Based on the evidence related to omega-3 supplementation and HRV (Mozaffarian et al., 2005; Christensen et al., 2001), one may also assume that the beneficial effects of fatty fish consumption could be due to the high level of omega-3.

Even if the real mechanisms underlying the relationship between fish consumption or supplement use and health benefit are still not established, animal models have been very useful in gaining a deeper understanding of possible mechanisms involved. Interestingly, Minami et al. (1997) investigated the effects of DHA on acetylcholine in rats and found that dietary DHA supplementation significantly increased the level of acetylcholine. In line with these observations Nishimura et al. (2000) found that EPA administration in diabetic rats decreased cardiac noradrenaline concentration. There is also a relationship between omega-3 (EPA and or DHA) and serotonin, which is very important for the regulation of HRV (Hibbeln et al., 2006). Thus, there is abundant evidence that the beneficial effects of fatty fish consumption may be caused by the omega-3 content. A metaanalysis (Xin et al., 2013) also revealed that there was a significant relationship between omega-3 supplementation and HF power. However, no significant relationships were found between fish oil and time domain measures (eg, RMSSD). Nor was any relationship between LF power and fish oil consumption detected, but the LF/HF ratio was marginally influenced by fish oil supplements. Thus, even if the RMSSD correlates highly with the HF power (Friedman et al., 2002) these results illustrate the importance of investigating different HRV parameters in relation to fish consumption.

Not all studies indicate that the beneficial effects of fish consumption are related to omega-3. For instance, Schiepers et al. (2010) found a relationship between fish consumption and physical well-being, but no relationship between well-being and fatty acids were found. In the Hansen et al. (2014a) study both the DHA and the EPA increased significantly in the fish group. In addition to improvement in HRV parameters the participants in the fish group also showed improvement on other outcome variables such as sleep and anxiety (Hansen et al., 2014a, 2014b). However, there was no relationship between omega-3, neither DHA nor EPA, and any of the other outcome variables. Notably, vitamin D correlated positively with both HRV and sleep. Vitamin D is linked to the regulation of serotonin (Stumpf and Privette, 1989), which is involved in the regulation of other physiological functions such as energy balance and sleep (Praschak-Rieder et al., 2008). Also, since fatty fish is a rich source of tryptophan, an essential amino acid that is converted to serotonin in the brain (Halson, 2008), there is reason to speculate whether some of the beneficial effects of fish consumption are related to stimulation of serotonin caused by tryptophan. However, fish is a rich source of many different nutrients, and the beneficial effects in humans may be related to many different mechanisms and interactions.

IMPLICATIONS FOR CLINICAL PRACTICE, HEALTH PROMOTION AND DISEASE PREVENTION

To date, most of the knowledge concerning fish consumption and HRV is acquired through studies focusing on the elderly, patients with coronary heart diseases, or mental health problems. Based on the research presented, fish interventions may have important clinical implications. In many hospitals and psychiatric institutions fresh fish is rarely served. However, the economic and health implications of regular fish consumption may be substantial for patients in institutions and hospitals, but regular fish consumption in healthy subjects may have significant health promotion and disease prevention effects.

SUMMARY AND CONCLUDING COMMENTS

Very few randomized controlled fish intervention studies have been performed due to expense, complexity, and possibly ethical concerns. Studies of self-reporting of habitual fish intake may therefore be more ethical. However, experimental fish intervention studies will overcome limitations related to self report studies such as lack of accuracy concerning frequency, amount and type of fish consumed. Moreover, in many countries, fish constitutes a minor part of the diet, and the balance of omega-6 and omega-3 fatty acids in the diet has shifted in favor of omega-6 fatty acids. This is particularly true in many Western countries. Thus, people with low fish and seafood intake are at risk for inadequate intake of key nutrients suggested to have important roles for physical and mental health across the lifespan. As the world's population is rapidly increasing, more efficient utilization of the earth's resources becomes increasingly important as well. Replacing meat with fish provides exactly that.

References

Alexander, J., Frøyland, L., Hemre, G.I., Jacobsen, B.K., Lund, E., Meltzer, H.M., Skåre, J.U., 2007. A comprehensive assessment of fish and other seafood in the Norwegian diet. Report from Norwegian Scientific Committee for Food Safety. ISBN 978-82-8082-207-9. http://www.vkm.no/dav/d94dff429b.pdf

Appelhans, B.M., Luecken, L.J., 2006. Heart rate variability as an index of regulated emotional responding. Rev. General Psychol. 10, 229–240.

Appleton, K., Woodside, J.V., Yarnell, J.W.G., Arveiler, D., Haas, B., Amouyel, P., Montaye, M., Ferrières, J., Ruidavets, J.B., Ducimetiere, P., Bingham, A., Evans, A, 2007. Depressed mood and dietary fish intake: direct relationship or indirect relationship as a result of diet and lifestyle. J. Affective Disorder. 104, 217–223.

Bar, K.J., Wernich, K., Boettger, S., Cordes, J., Boettger, M.K., Loffler, S., Kornischka, J., Agelink, M.-W., 2008. Relationship between cardiovagal modulation and psychotic state in patients with paranoid schizophrenia. Psychiatr. Res. 157, 255–257.

Berntson, G.G., Cacioppo, J.T., Quigley, K.S., 1991. Autonomic determinism: the modes of autonomic control, the doctrine of autonomic scape, and the laws of autonomic constraint. Psychological Rev. 98, 459–487.

Berntson, G.G., Bigger, J.T., Eckberg, D.L., Grossman, P., Kaufmann, P.G., Malik, M., Nagaraja, H.N., Porges, S., 1997. Heart rate variability: origins, methods, and interpretive caveats. Psychophysiology 34, 623–647.

Brennan, M., Palaniswami, M., Kamen, P., 2001. Do existing measures of poincaré plot geometry reflect nonlinear features of heart rate variability? IEEE Trans. Biomed. Eng. 48, 1342–1347.

Chalmers, J., Quintana, D.S., Abbott, M.J.-A., Kemp, A.H., 2014. Anxiety disorders are associated with reduced heart rate variability: a meta-analysis. Frontier. Psychiatr. 5, 10.3389.

Christensen, J.H., Skou, H.A., Madsen, T., Tørring, I., Smidt, E.B., 2001. Heart rate variability and n-3 polynsaturated fatty acids in patients with diabetes mellitus. J. Intern. Med. 249, 545–552.

Colton, C.W., Manderscheid, R.W., 2006. Congruencies in increased mortality rates, years of potential life lost, and causes of death among public mental health clients in eight states. Prevention Chronic Disease 3, A42, URL: http://www.cdc.gov/pcd/issues/2006/apr/05_0180.htm

Dangour, A.D., Allen, E., Elbourne, D., Fletcher, A., Richards, M., Uauy, R., 2009. Fish consumption and cognitive function among older people in the UK: baseline data from the OPAL study. J. Nutr. Health Aging 13, 198–202.

Eckberg, D.L., 1997. Sympathovagal balance—a critical appraisal. Circulation 96, 3224–3232.

Erkkilä, A., Schwab, U.S., De Mello, V.D.E., Lappalainen, T., Mussalo, H., Lehto, S., Kemi, V., Lamberg-Allardt, C., Uustupa, M.I.J., 2008. Effects of fatty and lean fish intake on blood pressure in subjects with coronary heart disease using multiple medications. Eur. J. Nutr. 47, 319–328.

Fleisher, L.A., Pincus, S.M., Rosenbaum, S.H., 1993. Approximate entropy of heart rate as correlate of postoperative ventricular dysfunction. Anesthesiology 78, 683–692.

Friedman, B.H., Allen, M.T., Christe, I.C., Santucci, A.K., 2002. Validity concerns of common heart-rate variability indices: addressing quantification issues in time- and frequency-domain measures of HRV. IEEE Eng. Med. Biol. 21, 35–40.

Goldberger, A.L., Mietus, J.E., Rigney, D.R., Wood, M.L., Fortney, S.M., 1994. Effects of head-down bed rest on complex heart rate variability: response to LBNP testing. J. Appl.Physiol. 77, 2863–2869.

Gordon, R.C., Rose, M.C., Skeaff, S.A., Gray, A.R., Morgan, K.M.D., Ruffman, T., 2009. Iodine supplementation improves cognition in mildly iodine-deficient children. Am. J. Clin. Nutr. 90, 1264–1271.

Grung, B., Hansen, A.L., Berg, M., Møen-Knudseth, M.P., Olson, G., Thornton, D., Dahl, L., Thayer, J.F., 2015. Exploratory multivariate analysis of the effect of fatty fish consumption and medicinal use on heart rate and heart rate variability data. Frontier. Psychol., 00135.

Halson, S., 2008. Nutrition, sleep and recovery. Eur. J. Sport Sci. 8, 119–126.

Hansen, A.L., Dahl, L., Bakke, L., Frøyland, L., Thayer, J.F., 2010. Fish consumption and heart rate variability. preliminary results. J. Psychophysiol. 24, 41–47.

Hansen, A.L., Dahl, L., Olson, G., Thornton, D., Graff, I.E., Frøyland, L., Thayer, J.F., Pallesen, S., 2014a. Fish consumption, sleep, daily functioning and heart rate variability. J. Clin. Sleep Med. 10, 567–575.

Hansen, A.L., Olson, G., Dahl, L., Thornton, D., Grung, B., Graff, I.E., Frøyland, L., Thayer, J.F., 2014b. Reduced anxiety in forensic inpatients after a long-term intervention with Atlantic salmon. Nutrients 6, 5392–5404.

Hibbeln, J.R., Ferguson, T.A., Blasbalg, T.L., 2006. Omega-3 fatty acid deficiencies in neurodevelopment, aggression, and autonomic dysregulation: opportunities for intervention. Int. Rev. Psychiatr. 18, 107–118.

Hugdahl, K, 2001. Psychophysiology. The Mind-Body Perspective. Harvard University Press.

Isler, Y., Kuntalp, M., 2007. Combining classical HRV indices with wavelet entropy measures improves to performance in diagnosing congestive heart failure. Computer. Biol. Med. 37, 1502–1510.

Kemp, A.H., Quintana, D.S., Gray, M.A., Felmingham, K.L., Brown, K., Gatt, J.M., 2010. Impact of depression and antidepressant treatment on heart rate variability: a review and metaanalysis. Biol. Psychiatr. 67, 1067–1074, 2010.

Lansdowne, A.T.G., Provost, S.C., 1998. Vitamin D3 enhances mood in healthy subjects during winter. Psychopharmacology 135, 319–323.

Levy, M.N., 1990. Autonomic interactions in cardiac control. Annal. NY Acad. Sci. 601, 209–221.

Macartney, M.J., Hingley, L., Brown, M.A., Peoples, G.E., McLennan, P.L., 2014. Intrinsic heart rate recovery after dynamic exercise is improved with an increased omega-3 index in healthy males. Br. J. Nutr. 112, 1984–1992.

Malik, M., 1996. Task force of the European society of cardiology and the North American society of pacing and electrophysiology. Eur. Heart J. 17, 354–381.

Malliani, A., Pagani, M., Lombardi, F., Cerutti, S., 1991. Cardiovascular neural regulation explored in the frequency domain. Circulation 84, 482–492.

Malliani, A., 1999. The pattern of sympathovagal balance explored in the frequency domain. News Physiol. Sci. 14, 111–117.

McCann, J.C., Ames, B.N., 2008. Is there convincing biological or behavioural evidence linking vitamin D deficiency to brain dysfunction. FASEB J. 22, 982–1001.

Minami, M., Kimura, S., Endo, T., Hamaue, N., Hirafuji, M., Togashi, H., Matsumoto, M., Yoshioka, M., Saito, H., Watanabe, S., Kobayashi, T., Okuyama, H., 1997. Dietary docosahexaenoic acid increases cerebral acetylcholine levels and improves passive avoidance performance in stroke-prone spontaneously hypertensive rats. Pharmacol. Biochem. Behavior 58, 1123–1129.

Mozaffarian, D., Geelen, A., Brouwer, I.A., Geleijnse, J.M., Zock, P.L., Katan, M.B., 2005. Effectof fish oil on heart rate in humans. A metaanalysis of randomized controlled trials. Circulation 112, 1945–1952.

Mozaffarian, D., Rimm, E.B., 2006. Fish intake, contaminants, and human health. JAMA 296, 1895–1899.

Mozaffarian, D., Stein, P.K., Prineas, R.J., Siscovick, D.S., 2008. Dietary fish ω-3 fatty acid consumption and heart rate variability in US adults. Circulation 117, 1130–1137.

Newcomer, J.W., Hennekens, C.H., 2007. Severe mental illness and risk of cardiovascular disease. JAMA J. Med. Assoc. 298, 1794–1796.

Nishimura, M., Nanbu, A., Komori, T., Ohtsuka, K., Takahashi, H., Yoshimura, M., 2000. Eicosapentaenoic acid stimulates nitric oxide production and decreases cardiac noradrenaline. Clin. Experiment. Pharmacol. Physiol. 27, 618–624.

Nome, S., Holsten, F., 2012. Changes in mortality after first psychiatric admission: a 20-year prospective longitudinal clinical study. Nordic J. Psychiatr. 66, 97–106.

Nyaradi, A., Li, J., Hickling, S., Foster, J., Oddy, W.H., 2004. The role of nutrition in children's neurocognitive development, from pregnancy through childhood. Frontiers Human Neurosci. 7.

Porges, S.W., 1992. Autonomic regulation and attention. In: Campbell, B.A., Hayne, H., Richardson, R. (Eds.), Attention and Information Processing in Infants and Adults. Erlbaum, Hillside, NJ, pp. 201–223.

Porges, S.W., Doussard-Roosevelt, J.A., Portales, A.L., Greenspan, S.I., 1996. Infant regulation of the vagal "brake" predicts child behavior problems: a psychobiological model of social. Develop. Psychobiol. 29, 697–712.

Praschak-Rieder, N., Willeit, M., Wilson, A.A., Houle, S., Meyer, J.H., 2008. Seasonal variation in human brain serotonin transporter binding. Archive. General Psychiatr. 65, 1072–1078.

Richman, J.S., Moorman, J.R., 2000. Physiological time-series analysis using approximate entropy and sample entropy. Am. J. Physiol. Heart Circulator. Physiol. 278, H2039–H2049.

Schiepers, O.J.G., de Groot, R.H.M., Jolles, J., van Boxtel, M.P.J., 2010. Fish consumption, not fatty acid status, is related to quality of life in a healthy population. Prostagland. leukotr. Essent. Fatty Acid. 83, 31–35.

Shimamura, A.P., 2000. The role of the prefrontal cortex in dynamic filtering. Psychobiology 28, 207–218.

Stein, P.K., Kleiger, R.E., 1999. Insights from the study of heart rate variability. Annual Rev. Med. 50, 249–261.

Stumpf, W.E., Privette, T.H., 1989. Light, vitamin D and psychiatry: Role of 1,25-dihydroxyvitamin D3 (soltriol) in etiology and therapy of seasonal affective disorder and other mental processes. Psychopharmacology 97, 285–294.

Task Force of The European Society of Cardiology and The North American Society of Pacing and Electrophysiology, 1996. Heart rate variability. Standards of measurement, physiological interpretation, and clinical use. Eur. Heart J. 17, 354–381.

Thayer, J.F., Lane, R.D., 2000. A model of neurovisceral integration in emotion regulation and dysregulation. J. Affective Disorder. 61, 201–216.

Thayer, J.F., Lane, R.D., 2007. The role of vagal function in the risk for cardiovascular disease and mortality. Biol. Psychol. 74, 224–242.

Thayer, J.F., Hansen, A.L., Saus, E.R., Johnsen, B.H., 2009. Heart rate variability, prefrontal neural function, and cognitive performance: the neurovisceral integration perspective. Annal. Behavioural Med. 37, 141–153.

Thayer, J.F., Hansen, A.L., Johnsen, B.H., 2010. The noninvasive assessment of autonomic influences on the heart using impedance cardiography and heart rate variability. In: Steptoe, A. (Ed.), Handbook of Behavioural Medicine - Methods and applications. Springer, London, UK, pp. 723–740.

Thayer, J.F., Åhs, F., Fredrikson, M., Sollers, J.J., Wager, R.D., 2012. A metaanalysis of heart rate variability and neuroimagine studies: Implications for heart rate variability as a maker of stress and health. Neurosci. Biobehavioral Rev. 36, 747–756.

Wang, X., Thayer, J.F., Treiber, F., Snieder, H., 2005. Ethnic differences and heritability of heart rate variability in African- and European American youth. Am. J. Cardiol. 96, 1166–1172.

Woo, M.A., Stevenson, W.G., Moser, D.K., Trelease, R.B., Harper, R.H., 1992. Patterns of beat-to-beat heart rate variability in advanced heart failure. Am. Heart J. 123, 704–710.

Xin, W., Wei, W., Li, X.-Y., 2013. Short-term effects of fish-oil supplementation on heart rate variability in humans: a metaanalysis of randomized controlled trials. Am. J. Clin. Nutr. 97, 926–935.

CHAPTER

22

Fish and Fish Oil and Lipoprotein Particle Number and Size

A. Erkkilä, M. Lankinen

Institute of Public Health and Clinical Nutrition, University of Eastern Finland, Kuopio, Finland

INTRODUCTION

In this review, we will discuss the effect of fish and fish oil on serum lipoprotein particles. First, we present how the lipoprotein particle size and number measurements are done and discuss how they are relevant in dietary studies. In the second part, we review the human studies evaluating the effects of fish and fish oils on very low density lipoprotein (VLDL), low density lipoprotein (LDL) and high density lipoprotein (HDL) particle numbers and sizes.

LIPOPROTEIN PARTICLES

Lipoproteins are complex aggregates of lipids and proteins, which are able to transport lipids throughout the circulation. Lipoproteins are synthesized in both the liver and the intestines. Lipoproteins have a spherical structure with polar lipids (phospholipids, cholesterol) on the surface and hydophobic lipids (cholesterol esters and triglycerides) in the core (Fig. 22.1). Furthermore, the protein component of lipoproteins, the apolipoproteins or apoproteins, are attached to the surface of particles, making lipoproteins more soluble and detectable for enzymes and receptors. Within the circulation, lipoproteins are in a state of constant flux, changing in composition and physical structure as the peripheral tissues take up the various components before the remnants return to the liver (Christie, 2014; Hevonoja et al., 2000).

Lipoproteins are classified into chylomicrons (CM), VLDL, LDL, and HDL based on their relative contents of protein and lipid which determine the densities of these lipoprotein classes. In addition to the density and composition, lipoproteins vary in size. The size and density of the lipoproteins affects their functions and their effects on health. The principle function for the CMs is to carry triglycerides from the intestine to the liver and other tissues, whereas VLDL particles carry endogenously synthesized triglycerides from the liver to other tissues. LDL particles are the major carriers of cholesterol in the blood, supplying it to the cells, whereas the role of HDL is to transfer cholesterol from peripheral tissues to the liver.

Classically, increased LDL concentrations are causally linked to atherosclerosis, whereas HDL is believed to have protective effects. However, this issue is more complex than initially believed. Modern genome-wide and Mendelian randomization studies have failed to show a causal link between total HDL cholesterol concentration and coronary artery disease (CAD; CADIGOGENICS Consortium et al., 2013; Haase et al., 2012), which might be related to the fact that HDL is a heterogeneous pool of subpopulations which differ in their structure and function (Kontush et al., 2013; Rye et al., 2009). It has been shown that the concentration of large HDL particles is inversely associated with cardiovascular disease while that of small HDL particles is positively associated with cardiovascular disease (Arsenault et al., 2009; Pirillo et al., 2013). Similarly, LDL cholesterol could be divided into subclasses based on the size and density of the particles and decreased size and increased density of LDL have been associated with increased coronary heart disease risk (Diffenderfer and Schaefer, 2014).

Fish and Fish Oil in Health and Disease Prevention. http://dx.doi.org/10.1016/B978-0-12-802844-5.00022-1

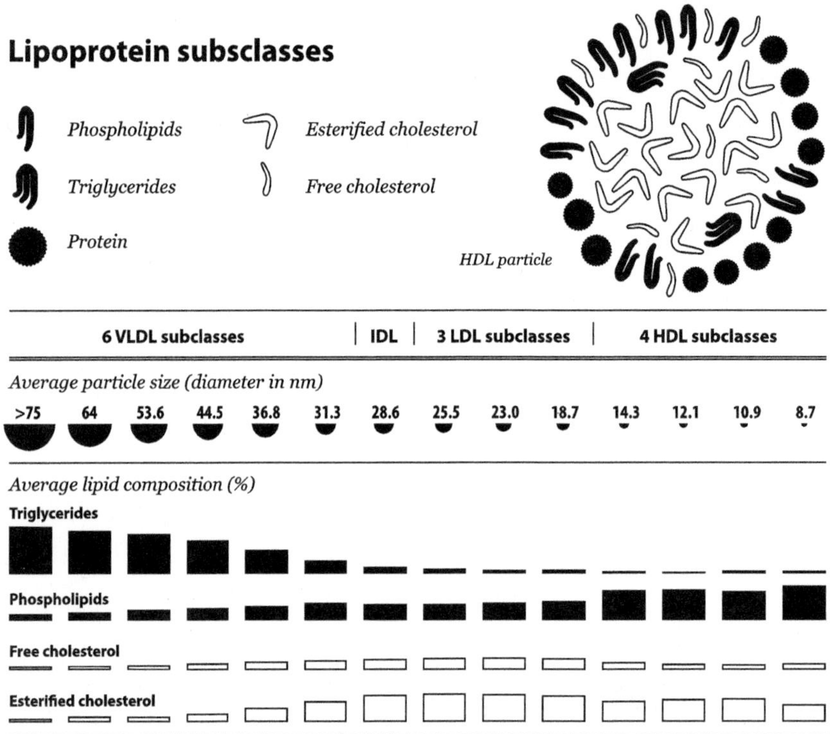

FIGURE 22.1 **HDL particle structure, composition of lipoprotein particles and their subclasses based on size (Soininen et al., 2015).** The bars depict the proportions of triglycerides, phospholipids, free cholesterol, and esterified cholesterol in lipoprotein subclasses. HDL high density lipoprotein, LDL low density lipoprotein, VLDL very low density lipoprotein. *Source: Figure courtesy of Antti J. Kangas.*

MEASUREMENTS OF LIPOPROTEIN PARTICLE SIZE AND SUBCLASSES

The particle size or density distribution of lipoproteins can be measured by a variety of laboratory methods including analytical ultracentrifugation, density ultracentrifugation by vertical auto profile, segmented gradient gel electrophoresis, tube gel electrophoresis, nuclear magnetic resonance (NMR), and ion mobility (Sninsky et al., 2013). In nutrition science, methods based on electrophoresis or NMR are commonly used. Previously, HDL particles were often separated into two subfractions (HDL_2 and HDL_3) based on particle size by precipitation. NMR is a method which is based on the principle that each compound has a unique signal in a magnetic field and it provides the opportunity to measure a broad spectrum of metabolites including numerous lipoprotein subclasses. It has been possible to classify lipoprotein particles into 14 subclasses based on their size, including six subclasses of VLDL, IDL, three subclasses of LDL and four subclasses of HDL (Fig. 22.1; Soininen et al., 2015).

DIET AND LIPOPROTEIN PARTICLE NUMBER AND SIZE

There is a long tradition of measuring how dietary changes affect serum lipids levels. However, as the traditional lipid profile does not capture all the features of serum lipids, the lipoprotein subclasses have also been measured in dietary studies. Polyunsaturated fatty acids (PUFA) relative to saturated fatty acids (SFA) have been previously shown to decrease serum total and LDL cholesterol. The newer techniques have further clarified the cardioprotective effects on these lipoproteins. Linoleic acid, which is a n–6 PUFA, was positively associated with LDL and HDL particle sizes in men in a cross-sectional setting (Choo et al., 2010). Similarly, in a follow-up of 6 years, change in serum n-6 PUFA was positively associated with LDL particle size (Mäntyselkä et al., 2014). In addition, serum total n-6 PUFAs and linoleic acid were inversely associated with triglycerides and VLDL particle concentration, particularly with large VLDL (Jelenkovic et al., 2014).

EFFECT OF FISH INTAKE ON LIPOPROTEIN PARTICLES

Controlled dietary intervention studies and one cross-sectional study reporting effects of fish consumption on lipoprotein particle size or number are listed in Table 22.1. Studies published since the year 2000 were included. The participants were either healthy adults or adults having dyslipidemias, impaired glucose metabolism or other

TABLE 22.1 Studies Reporting the Effect of Fish Consumption on Lipoprotein Particle Number and Size in Adults

Authors	Study design	Participants	Intervention	Method	Main findings
Interventions					
Beauchesne-Rondeau et al., 2003	Randomized, controlled trial, crossover	18 men with hypercholesterolemia (age 21–73 years)	1. Lean beef 2. Lean fish (69% of daily protein) 3. Poultry for 26 days (6-week washout between the diets)	HDL_2 (large) and HDL_3 (small) subfractions were separated by dextran-sulfate precipitation	HDL_2 and HDL_2/HDL_3 ↑ in lean fish diet.
Erkkilä et al., 2014	Randomized, controlled trial, parallel	33 men and women with coronary heart disease (age < 70 years)	1. Fatty fish ≥four meals per week 2. Lean fish ≥four meals per week 3. Control diet (≤one fish meal per week) for 8 weeks	NMR	HDL particle size ↑ in fatty fish diet group. No changes in VLDL particle size.
Lacaille et al., 2000	Randomized, controlled trial, crossover	11 normolipidemic men (age 19–27 years)	1. Lean fish (70%–75% of daily protein) 2. Nonfish	HDL_2 and HDL_3 subfractions were separated by dextran-sulfate precipitation	HDL_2 and HDL_2/HDL_3 ↑ in lean fish diet.
Lankinen et al., 2014	Randomized controlled trial, parallel	106 men and women with impaired glucose metabolism and features of the metabolic syndrome (age 40–70 years)	1. Fatty fish three meals per week (+wholegrain and bilberries) 2. Habitual fish consumption (+ wholegrain) 3. Control (≤one fish meal per week) for 12 weeks	NMR	Greater increase in fish consumption → large HDL particles ↑ and HDL particle size ↑. No changes in VLDL particle size.
Li et al., 2004	Parallel intervention	22 men and women (age > 40 years)	6 weeks run-in period with average diet in the US and after that National Cholesterol Education Program diet + either 1. High fish diet (lean and fatty fish 8 times per week) 2. Low fish diet (lean and fatty fish 2 times per week) for 24 weeks	NMR	Concentration of medium and small VLDL ↓ in high fish diet group, HDL particle size ↓ in low fish diet group.
Lindqvist et al., 2009	Randomized controlled trial, crossover	35 overweight men (age 35–60 years)	1. Herring diet (five meals per week) 2. Control diet for 6 weeks (12-week washout)	HDL_2 and HDL_3 subfractions were separated by dextran-sulfate precipitation	HDL_2 ↑ in herring diet.
Ouellet et al., 2008	Randomized controlled trial, crossover	19 overweight or obese insulin resistant men and women (age 40–65 years)	1. Cod protein (58–68% of daily protein) 2. Other animal protein for 4 weeks (4-week washout)	HDL_2 and HDL_3 subfractions were separated by dextran-sulfate precipitation	No changes in HDL subfractions.
Cross-sectional studies					
Bogl et al., 2013	Cross-sectional study	663 men and women (age 21–25 years)		NMR	Habitual fish consumption (fatty fish) → VLDL particle diameter ↓, HDL particle diameter ↑.

HDL, high density lipoprotein; *LDL*, low density lipoprotein; *NMR*, nuclear magnetic resonance; and *VLDL*, very low density lipoprotein.

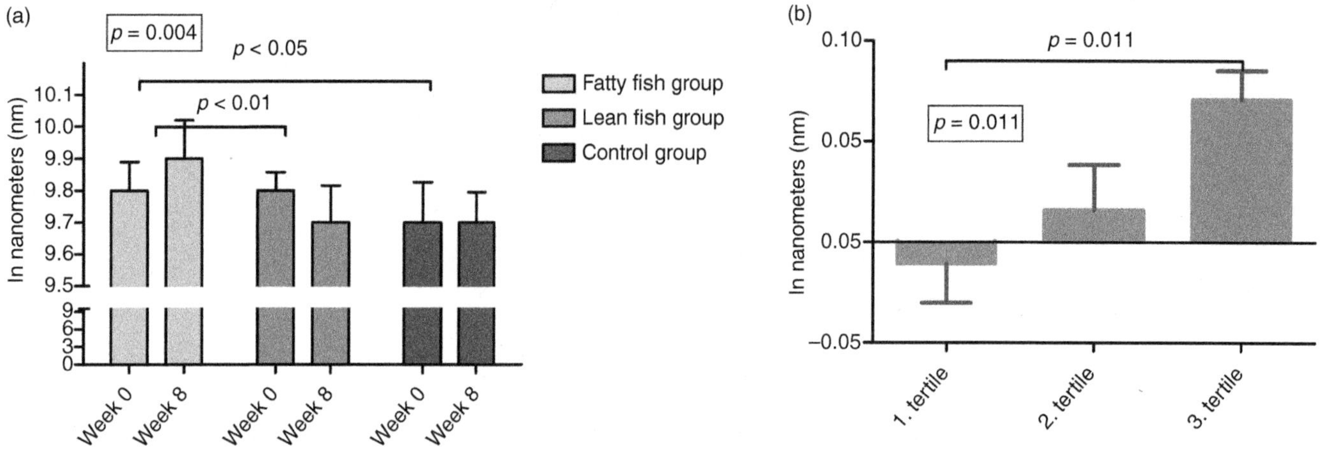

FIGURE 22.2 (a) Particle size of HDL before and after an 8-week intervention of fatty fish ($n = 11$), lean fish ($n = 12$) and control ($n = 10$) groups (Erkkilä et al., 2014). Subjects in the fish diet groups ate four fish meals per week. *P*-values are from general linear model for repeated measurements adjusted for sex and age and from Bonferroni-corrected pairwise comparisons. (b) Changes in mean diameter for HDL particles according to tertiles of changes in fish intake in the Sysdimet intervention ($n = 106$; Lankinen et al., 2014). Changes in fish intake are calculated from 4-day food records which were kept once at baseline and three times during the intervention period. *P*-values are from one-way ANOVA with Bonferroni-corrected post hoc comparisons. The daily fish consumption decreased in the first tertile (average change −40 g/day, average consumption during intervention period 26 g/day), remained nearly unchanged in the second tertile (average change +5 g/day, average intake: 28 g/day) and increased in the third tertile (average change +62 g/day, average intake 74 g/day).

features of the metabolic syndrome. One study with coronary heart disease patients is also included. It has consistently been shown that fish consumption (especially fatty fish species) increases HDL particle size when measured as average HDL particles size, as a concentration of larger HDL_2 particles, or by its ratio to smaller HDL_3 particles (Table 22.1). The changes in average size of HDL particles in two different intervention studies are shown in Fig. 22.2. In both studies, increased average HDL particle size was related to increased consumption of fatty fish (Fig. 22.2a,b), but the same was not seen after consumption of lean fish (Figure 22.2a). In some studies, increased fish consumption has also affected VLDL particle size (Table 22.2), but the results have been inconsistent, reporting decreased concentration of small and medium VLDL (Li et al., 2004), decreased average size of VLDL particles (Bogl et al., 2013) or no changes (Erkkilä et al., 2014; Lankinen et al., 2014).

FISH OILS AND LIPOPROTEIN PARTICLE NUMBER AND SIZE

Fish oils have been shown to have a serum triglyceride-lowering effect when using standard analytic methods. The studies presented in Table 22.2 describe studies that have investigated the effect of fish oils on serum lipid subclasses or lipoprotein size in controlled interventions since 2000. In addition to fish oil studies, studies supplementing EPA or DHA alone have been included. The subjects were either healthy adults or those with lipid disorders, most often elevated triglyceride concentrations. We identified 15 studies, out of which 6 used the NMR method to measure lipoprotein particle numbers and size. The doses in the studies ranged from 0.7 g/day EPA + DHA to 4 g/day of EPA or DHA.

Effect on VLDL

A consistent finding in the studies is that the size of VLDL particles was reduced after fish oil supplementation (Bays et al., 2012; Bragt and Mensink, 2012; Kelley et al., 2007; Maki et al., 2011b; Mostad et al., 2008; Neff et al., 2011). Similarly, the number of large VLDL particles was also reduced (Bays et al., 2012; Mostad et al., 2008). Furthermore, in adolescents with hypertriglyceridemia, a reduction in large VLDL particles was observed after intake of 4 g/day of fish oil for 8 weeks (Gidding et al., 2014). Smaller VLDL size was observed in users of different statins when n–3 long chain PUFA (LCPUFA) was added to the statin treatment in subjects with mixed dyslipidemias (Maki et al., 2008; Maki et al., 2011a).

Effect on LDL

The effects of fish oils on LDL particles has been more inconsistent than those reported for VLDL. While Kelley et al. (2007), Maki et al. (2011b), and Neff et al. (2011) observed increased size of LDL, Bays et al. (2012), Bragt and

TABLE 22.2 Controlled Interventions to Test the Effect of Fish Oil on Lipoprotein Particle Number and Size in Adults With or Without Lipid Abnormalities

Author	Study design	Participants	Intervention	Method	Main findings
Bays et al., 2012	Randomized, pleacebo-controlled, double-blind, parallel	229 subjects with TG 500–2000 mg/dL (age >18 years)	1. 4 g/day EPA, 2. 2 g/day EPA, 3. Placebo for for 12 weeks.	NMR	4 g EPA: ↓ VLDL size, ↓ large VLDL particle concentration, ↓ total and small LDL particle concentration and ↓ total HDL particle concentration 2 g EPA: ↓ small LDL particle concentration.
Bragt and Mensink, 2012	Randomized, placebo-controlled, double-blind, crossover	20 men and women with BMI ≥27 kg/m^2	1. Fish oil (1,7 g/day EPA and 1,2 g/day DHA) 2. 200 mg/day fenofibrate 3. Placebo (high oleic sunflower oil) for 6 weeks (2 week washout).	NMR	Compared to placebo, fish oil ↓ large VLDL particle concentration, ↑ LDL particles and ↑ large HDL particles.
Calabresi et al., 2004	Randomized, placebo-controlled, double-blind, crossover	14 subjects with familial combined hyperlipidemia	1. n–3 LCPUFA supplement (1,88 g/day EPA and 1,48 g/day DHA) 2. Placebo (corn oil) for 8 weeks.	Gradient gel electrophoresis	n–3 LCPUFA ↑ the concentrations HDL_2.
Caslake et al., 2008	Randomized, placebo-controlled, double-blind, crossover	312 subjects (age 20–70 years)	1. Fish oil (EPA+ DHA 0.7 g/day), 2. Fish oil (EPA + DHA 1.8 g/day), 3. Placebo (mixture of palm oil and soybean oil) for 8 weeks (12 week washout).	Gradient gel electrophoresis	Both doses of fish oils ↑ the proportion of HDL_2 from the total HDL.
Kelley et al., 2007	Randomized, placebo-controlled, double-blind, parallel	34 men with hypertriglyceridemia (age 39–66 years)	1. 3 g/day DHA, 2. Placebo (olive oil) for 90 days	NMR	Size and concentration of VLDL ↓, size of LDL and concentration of large LDL ↑ in DHA group. Concentration of large HDL particle ↑ and that of small HDL ↓ in DHA group.
Khandelwal et al., 2009	2 × 2 factorial, controlled, double-blind	200 Indian subjects with total cholesterol 5–8 mmol/L, BMI 18–30 kg/m^2 (age 35–55 years)	1. Control yoghurt drink and control capsules (safflower oil), 2. Control yoghurt drink and fish oil capsules (2 g/day n–3 LCPUFA), 3. Plant sterol-enriched yoghurt drink and control capsules (safflower oil) 4. Plant sterol-enriched yoghurt drink and fish oil capsules (2 g/day n–3 LCPUFA) for 4 weeks.	Gel electrophoresis	No change on LDL size in any group.
Maki et al., 2011b	Randomized, placebo-controlled, double-blind, crossover	31 subjects with primary hypercholesterolemia (age 18–79 years)	5. 4 g/day n–3 LCPUFA (EPA and DHA) 6. Placebo (corn oil) for 6 weeks.	NMR	Size and concentration of VLDL ↓ in n–3 LCPUFA group. Sizes of LDL and HDL particles ↑ and concentration of HDL particle ↓ in n–3 LCPUFA group.
Mori et al., 2000	Randomized, placebo-controlled, parallel	56 healthy men with mild hypercholesterolemia (age 20–65 years)	1. 4 g/day EPA 2. 4 g/day DHA 3. 4 g/day Placebo (olive oil) for 6 weeks.	Gradient gel electrophoresis	LDL particle size ↑ in DHA group.

(Continued)

TABLE 22.2 Controlled Interventions to Test the Effect of Fish Oil on Lipoprotein Particle Number and Size in Adults With or Without Lipid Abnormalities (*cont.*)

Author	Study design	Participants	Intervention	Method	Main findings
Mostad et al., 2008	Randomized, placebo-controlled, parallel	26 subjects with normal TG level and type 2 diabetes without insulin treatment (age 40–75 years)	1. Fish oil (1.8 g/day EPA and 3.0 g/day DHA) 2. Placebo (corn oil) for 9 weeks.	NMR	Size of VLDL ↓, concentrations of large VLDL and small HDL ↓ in fish oil group. No effect on LDL particles.
Neff et al., 2011	Randomized, placebo-controlled, double-blind, parallel	36 healthy, obese or overweight subjects (18–65 years)	1. 2 g/day algal DHA, 2. Placebo oil (mixture of corn and soybean) for 4.5 months.	NMR	Size of VLDL ↓, sizes of HDL and LDL ↑ DHA group. Concentrations of large LDL and large HDL ↑, and concentrations of small LDL and medium HDL ↓ in DHA group.
Rivellese et al., 2003	Randomized, placebo-controlled, parallel	162 subjects (age 30–65 years)	1. 3,6 g/day n-3 LCPUFA 2. Placebo (olive oil) for 90 days. The background diet was either high saturated or monounsaturated fat diet.	Gradient gel electrophoresis	LDL size was not affected by oil supplements.
de Roos et al., 2008	Randomized, placebo-controlled, double-blind, parallel	81 healthy subjects (age 50–70 years)	1. 3,5 g/day Fish oil 2. 3,5 g/day Placebo (high oleic sunflower oil) for 12 weeks	Proteomics using 2-DE gel	↑ HDL_2 particles in fish oil group.
Sanders et al., 2006	Randomized, placebo-controlled, double-blind, parallel	39 men, 40 women	1. 4 g/day algal oil (1,5 g DHA, 0,6 g DPA) 2. 4 g/day Placebo (olive oil) for 4 weeks	Iodixanol gradient centrifugation	No effect on LDL size.
Tani et al., 2013	Randomized, open-label, parallel	144 men and women with TG ≥150 mg/dL	1. 1,8 g/day EPA, 2. No placebo for 6 months.	LDL relative migration index	↑ LDL size in EPA group.
Woodman et al., 2003	Randomized, placebo-controlled, double-blind, parallel	59 men and women with diabetes and hypertension (age 40–75 years)	1. 4 g/day EPA, 2. 4 g/day DHA, 3. 4 g/day Placebo (olive oil) for 6 weeks	Gradient gel electrophoresis	↓ LDL size in EPA group, ↑ LDL size in DHA group.

BMI, body mass index; *DHA*, docosahexaenoic acid; *DPA*, docosapentaenoic acid; *EPA*, eicosapentaenoic acid; *HDL*, high density lipoprotein; *LC-PUFA*, long-chain polyunsaturated fatty acid; *LDL*, low density lipoprotein; *NMR*, nuclear magnetic resonance; *TG*, triglycerides; *VLDL*, very low density lipoprotein.

Mensink (2012), and Mostad et al. (2008) did not report significant changes in LDL particle size. Similarly, in studies that used methods other than NMR to measure LDL size the results have been mixed; two reported increased size (Mori et al., 2000; Tani et al., 2013) and three did not find an effect (Khandelwal et al., 2009; Rivellese et al., 2003; Sanders et al., 2006). There are also findings suggesting that the effects of EPA and DHA on LDL size could differ (Mori et al., 2000; Woodman et al., 2003). Two studies reported that the concentration of large LDL is increased by fish oils (Kelley et al., 2007; Neff et al., 2011). Additionally, in statin users, the size of LDL particles was increased by adding n–3 LCPUFA (Maki et al., 2008; Maki et al., 2011a).

Effect on HDL

Fish oil use was found to increase the average size of HDL particles (Maki et al., 2011b; Neff et al., 2011) or the proportion of the larger HDL_2 particles increased (Calabresi et al., 2004; Caslake et al., 2008; de Roos et al., 2008). Similar changes were observed by Kelley et al. (2007), Mostad et al. (2008) and Bragt and Mensink (2012); who reported an increase in the concentrations of large HDL or decreases in concentrations in small HDL, even though the average size of HDL particles did not significantly change.

POSTPRANDIAL LIPIDS

Only two studies have reported the postprandial effects of fish oils on lipid subclasses (Burdge et al., 2009; Kelley et al., 2007). As in fasting condition, the size of VLDL particles decreased after a test meal containing fish oil (Burdge et al., 2009) and the area under the curve for large VLDL particles decreased after consumption of a DHA containing test meal when DHA had been supplemented for 45 days (Kelley et al., 2007).

DISCUSSION AND CONCLUSIONS

The studies reviewed confirm that fish oils decrease VLDL size and the number of large VLDL particles. Fatty fish intake has not consistently been associated with VLDL particles, possibly due to lower n–3 LCPUFA intake it supplies compared to fish oil supplementation. The observed VLDL effects may reflect increased clearance of triglyceride-rich lipoprotein particles. Kinetic studies show that fish oils affect both the VLDL production and triglyceride clearance (Shearer et al., 2012). Increased levels of large VLDL particles are associated with increased risk of CAD (Freedman et al., 1998), insulin resistance (Garvey et al., 2003), and type 2 diabetes (Festa et al., 2005; Mackey et al., 2012).

These studies are inconsistent regarding LDL particle size and fish and fish oil consumption; and there seems to be a lack of change in LDL particle number. If the cascade of VLDL to IDL to LDL were more efficient, then there may be larger LDL particles. Instead, large VLDL particles result in the formation of small, dense and more atherogenic LDL particles (Millar and Packard, 1998). LDL cholesterol has been of concern as high doses of fish oils or DHA alone have been suggested to adversely affect LDL concentrations (Schwab et al. 2014). LDL cholesterol concentration may, however, be a less accurate measure of residual cardiovascular risk than the LDL particle number (Rosenson and Underberg, 2013).

Fatty fish and fish oil increase both the HDL size and the number of large HDL particles. These effects are regarded as beneficial as large HDL particle number and HDL size have been inversely associated with cardiovascular events (El Harchaoui et al., 2009; Mackey et al., 2012). The mechanism could be that the enhanced VLDL cascade delivers more surface remnants and increases the lipid transfer between LDL and HDL resulting in more larger HDL particles. Secondly, there are mixed results regarding whether fish protein, as compared to nonfish protein diets, affects HDL particles size (Beauchesne-Rondeau et al., 2003; Erkkilä et al., 2014; Ouellet et al., 2008).

The effects of fish oils or oils providing EPA and DHA have been studied more than dietary fish intake and in different populations such as those with lipid abnormalities or impaired glucose tolerance. Relatively few studies have compared the effects of EPA and DHA in regard to lipoprotein particle number and size, especially using NMR methods. Therefore, making conclusions on different dosages or types of supplements is difficult. Similarly, there are only a few studies assessing the effects of eating different types of fish on serum lipoprotein particle number and size.

To summarize, while the LDL effects seem inconsistent, intake of fish, especially fatty fish has resulted in potentially beneficial changes in HDL number and size. In addition to HDL effect, fish oils have reduced the size of VLDL particles. These results emphasize the important role of fish in cardioprotective diet.

Acknowledgment

The authors thank Antti J. Kangas, MSc, for kindly providing the Fig. 22.1.

References

Arsenault, B.J., Lemieux, I., Despres, J.P., Gagnon, P., Wareham, N.J., Stroes, E.S., Kastelein, J.J., Khaw, K.T., Boekholdt, S.M., 2009. HDL particle size and the risk of coronary heart disease in apparently healthy men and women: the EPIC-Norfolk prospective population study. Atherosclerosis 206, 276–281.

Bays, H.E., Braeckman, R.A., Ballantyne, C.M., Kastelein, J.J., Otvos, J.D., Stirtan, W.G., Soni, P.N., 2012. Icosapent ethyl, a pure EPA omega-3 fatty acid: Effects on lipoprotein particle concentration and size in patients with very high triglyceride levels (the MARINE study). J. Clin. Lipidol. 6, 565–572.

Beauchesne-Rondeau, É., Gascon, A., Bergeron, J., Jacques, H., 2003. Plasma lipids and lipoproteins in hypercholesterolemic men fed a lipid-lowering diet containing lean beef, lean fish, or poultry. Am. J. Clin. Nutr. 77, 587–593.

Bogl, L.H., Pietilainen, K.H., Rissanen, A., Kangas, A.J., Soininen, P., Rose, R.J., Ala-Korpela, M., Kaprio, J., 2013. Association between habitual dietary intake and lipoprotein subclass profile in healthy young adults. NMCD 23, 1071–1078.

Bragt, M.C., Mensink, R.P., 2012. Comparison of the effects of n-3 long chain polyunsaturated fatty acids and fenofibrate on markers of inflammation and vascular function, and on the serum lipoprotein profile in overweight and obese subjects. NMCD 22, 966–973.

Burdge, G.C., Powell, J., Dadd, T., Talbot, D., Civil, J., Calder, P.C., 2009. Acute consumption of fish oil improves postprandial VLDL profiles in healthy men aged 50-65 years. Br. J. Nutr. 102, 160–165.

Calabresi, L., Villa, B., Canavesi, M., Sirtori, C.R., James, R.W., Bernini, F., Franceschini, G., 2004. An omega-3 polyunsaturated fatty acid concentrate increases plasma high-density lipoprotein 2 cholesterol and paraoxonase levels in patients with familial combined hyperlipidemia. Metabol. Clin. Experiment. 53, 153–158.

CARDIoGRAMplusC4D Consortium, DIAGRAM Consortium, CARDIOGENICS Consortium, 2013. Large-scale association analysis identifies new risk loci for coronary artery disease. Nature genetics. 45, 25–33.

Caslake, M.J., Miles, E.A., Kofler, B.M., Lietz, G., Curtis, P., Armah, C.K., Kimber, A.C., Grew, J.P., Farrell, L., Stannard, J., Napper, F.L., Sala-Vila, A., West, A.L., Mathers, J.C., Packard, C., Williams, C.M., Calder, P.C., Minihane, A.M., 2008. Effect of sex and genotype on cardiovascular biomarker response to fish oils: the FINGEN Study. Am. J. Clin. Nutr. 88, 618–629.

Choo, J., Ueshima, H., Curb, J.D., Shin, C., Evans, R.W., El-Saed, A., Kadowaki, T., Okamura, T., Nakata, K., Otake, T., Miura, K., Abbott, R.D., Sutton-Tyrrell, K., Edmundowicz, D., Kuller, L.H., Sekikawa, A., ERA-JUMP Study Grp, 2010. Serum n-6 fatty acids and lipoprotein subclasses in middle-aged men: the population-based crosssectional ERA-JUMP Study. Am. J. Clin. Nutr. 91, 1195–1203.

Christie, W.W., 2014. The AOCS lipid library. Plasma lipoproteins. composition, structure and biochemistry. Retrieved May 2015. http://lipidlibrary.aocs.org/Lipids/lipoprot/index.htm

de Roos, B., Geelen, A., Ross, K., Rucklidge, G., Reid, M., Duncan, G., Caslake, M., Horgan, G., Brouwer, I.A., 2008. Identification of potential serum biomarkers of inflammation and lipid modulation that are altered by fish oil supplementation in healthy volunteers. Proteomics 8, 1965–1974.

Diffenderfer, M.R., Schaefer, E.J., 2014. The composition and metabolism of large and small LDL. Curr. Opin. Lipidol. 25, 221–226.

El Harchaoui, K., Arsenault, B.J., Franssen, R., Després, J., Hovingh, G.K., Stroes, E.S.G., Otvos, J.D., Wareham, N.J., Kastelein, J.J.P., Khaw, K., Boekholdt, S.M., 2009. High-density lipoprotein particle size and concentration and coronary risk. Annal. Intern. Med. 150, 84–93.

Erkkilä, A.T., Schwab, U.S., Lehto, S., de Mello, V.D., Kangas, A.J., Soininen, P., Ala-Korpela, M., Uusitupa, M.I., 2014. Effect of fatty and lean fish intake on lipoprotein subclasses in subjects with coronary heart disease: a controlled trial. J. Clin. Lipidol. 8, 126–133.

Festa, A., Williams, K., Hanley, A.J., Otvos, J.D., Goff, D.C., Wagenknecht, L.E., Haffner, S.M., 2005. Nuclear magnetic resonance lipoprotein abnormalities in prediabetic subjects in the Insulin Resistance Atherosclerosis Study. Circulation 111, 3465–3472.

Freedman, D.S., Otvos, J.D., Jeyarajah, E.J., Barboriak, J.J., Anderson, A.J., Walker, J.A., 1998. Relation of lipoprotein subclasses as measured by proton nuclear magnetic resonance spectroscopy to coronary artery disease. Arteriosclerosis Thrombosis Vascul. Biol. 18, 1046–1053.

Garvey, W.T., Kwon, S., Zheng, D., Shaughnessy, S., Wallace, P., Hutto, A., Pugh, K., Jenkins, A.J., Klein, R.L., Liao, Y., 2003. Effects of insulin resistance and type 2 diabetes on lipoprotein subclass particle size and concentration determined by nuclear magnetic resonance. Diabetes 52, 453–462.

Gidding, S.S., Prospero, C., Hossain, J., Zappalla, F., Balagopal, P., Falkner, B., Kwiterovich, P., 2014. A double-blind randomized trial of fish oil to lower triglycerides and improve cardiometabolic risk in adolescents. J. Pediatr. 165, 497–503.

Haase, C.L., Tybjaerg-Hansen, A., Qayyum, A.A., Schou, J., Nordestgaard, B.G., Frikke-Schmidt, R., 2012. LCAT, HDL cholesterol and ischemic cardiovascular disease: a Mendelian randomization study of HDL cholesterol in 54,500 individuals. J. Clin. Endocrinol. Metabol. 97, E248–E256.

Hevonoja, T., Pentikainen, M.O., Hyvonen, M.T., Kovanen, P.T., Ala-Korpela, M., 2000. Structure of low density lipoprotein (LDL) particles: basis for understanding molecular changes in modified LDL. Biochim. Biophys. Acta 1488, 189–210.

Jelenkovic, A., Bogl, L.H., Rose, R.J., Kangas, A.J., Soininen, P., Ala-Korpela, M., Kaprio, J., Silventoinen, K., 2014. Association between serum fatty acids and lipoprotein subclass profile in healthy young adults: exploring common genetic and environmental factors. Atherosclerosis 233, 394–402.

Kelley, D.S., Siegel, D., Vemuri, M., Mackey, B.E., 2007. Docosahexaenoic acid supplementation improves fasting and postprandial lipid profiles in hypertriglyceridemic men. Am. J. Clin. Nutr. 86, 324–333.

Khandelwal, S., Demonty, I., Jeemon, P., Lakshmy, R., Mukherjee, R., Gupta, R., Snehi, U., Niveditha, D., Singh, Y., van der Knaap, H.C., Passi, S.J., Prabhakaran, D., Reddy, K.S., 2009. Independent and interactive effects of plant sterols and fish oil n-3 long-chain polyunsaturated fatty acids on the plasma lipid profile of mildly hyperlipidaemic Indian adults. Br. J. Nutr. 102, 722–732.

Kontush, A., Lhomme, M., Chapman, M.J., 2013. Unraveling the complexities of the HDL lipidome. J. Lipid Res. 54, 2950–2963.

Lacaille, B., Julien, P., Deshaies, Y., Lavigne, C., Brun, L.D., Jacques, H., 2000. Responses of plasma lipoproteins and sex hormones to the consumption of lean fish incorporated in a prudent-type diet in normolipidemic men. J. Am. College Nutr. 19, 745–753.

Lankinen, M., Kolehmainen, M., Jaaskelainen, T., Paananen, J., Joukamo, L., Kangas, A.J., Soininen, P., Poutanen, K., Mykkanen, H., Gylling, H., Oresic, M., Jauhiainen, M., Ala-Korpela, M., Uusitupa, M., Schwab, U., 2014. Effects of whole grain, fish and bilberries on serum metabolic profile and lipid transfer protein activities: a randomized trial (Sysdimet). PloS One 9, e90352.

Li, Z., Lamon-Fava, S., Otvos, J., Lichtenstein, A.H., Velez-Carrasco, W., McNamara, J.R., Ordovas, J.M., Schaefer, E.J., 2004. Fish consumption shifts lipoprotein subfractions to a less atherogenic pattern in humans. J. Nutr. 134, 1724–1728.

Lindqvist, H.M., Langkilde, A.M., Undeland, I., Sandberg, A.S., 2009. Herring (*Clupea harengus*) intake influences lipoproteins but not inflammatory and oxidation markers in overweight men. Br. J. Nutr. 101, 383–390.

Mackey, R.H., Greenland, P., Goff, Jr., D.C., Lloyd-Jones, D., Sibley, C.T., Mora, S., 2012. High-density lipoprotein cholesterol and particle concentrations, carotid atherosclerosis, and coronary events: MESA (Multi-Ethnic Study of Atherosclerosis). J. Am. College Cardiol. 60, 508–516.

Maki, K.C., Bays, H.E., Dicklin, M.R., Johnson, S.L., Shabbout, M., 2011a. Effects of prescription omega-3-acid ethyl esters, coadministered with atorvastatin, on circulating levels of lipoprotein particles, apolipoprotein CIII, and lipoprotein-associated phospholipase A(2) mass in men and women with mixed dyslipidemia. J. Clin. Lipidol. 5, 483–492.

Maki, K.C., Lawless, A.L., Kelley, K.M., Dicklin, M.R., Kaden, V.N., Schild, A.L., Rains, T.M., Marshall, J.W., 2011b. Effects of prescription omega-3-acid ethyl esters on fasting lipid profile in subjects with primary hypercholesterolemia. J. Cardiovascul. Pharmacol. 57, 489–494.

Maki, K.C., McKenney, J.M., Reeves, M.S., Lubin, B.C., Dicklin, M.R., 2008. Effects of adding prescription omega-3 acid ethyl esters to simvastatin (20 mg/day) on lipids and lipoprotein particles in men and women with mixed dyslipidemia. Am. J. Cardiol. 102, 429–433.

Mäntyselkä, P., Niskanen, L., Kautiainen, H., Saltevo, J., Wurtz, P., Soininen, P., Kangas, A.J., Ala-Korpela, M., Vanhala, M., 2014. Crosssectional and longitudinal associations of circulating omega-3 and omega-6 fatty acids with lipoprotein particle concentrations and sizes: population-based cohort study with 6-year follow-up. Lipids Health Disease 13, 28.

Millar, J.S., Packard, C.J., 1998. Heterogeneity of apolipoprotein B-100-containing lipoproteins: what we have learnt from kinetic studies. Curr. Opin. Lipidol. 9, 197–202.

Mori, T.A., Burke, V., Puddey, I.B., Watts, G.F., O'Neal, D.N., Best, J.D., Beilin, L.J., 2000. Purified eicosapentaenoic and docosahexaenoic acids have differential effects on serum lipids and lipoproteins, LDL particle size, glucose, and insulin in mildly hyperlipidemic men. Am. J. Clin. Nutr. 71, 1085–1094.

Mostad, I.L., Bjerve, K.S., Lydersen, S., Grill, V., 2008. Effects of marine n-3 fatty acid supplementation on lipoprotein subclasses measured by nuclear magnetic resonance in subjects with type II diabetes. Eur. J. Clin. Nutr. 62, 419–429.

Neff, L.M., Culiner, J., Cunningham-Rundles, S., Seidman, C., Meehan, D., Maturi, J., Wittkowski, K.M., Levine, B., Breslow, J.L., 2011. Algal docosahexaenoic acid affects plasma lipoprotein particle size distribution in overweight and obese adults. J. Nutr. 141, 207–213.

Ouellet, V., Weisnagel, S.J., Marois, J., Bergeron, J., Julien, P., Gougeon, R., Tchernof, A., Holub, B.J., Jacques, H., 2008. Dietary cod protein reduces plasma C-reactive protein in insulin-resistant men and women. J. Nutr. 138, 2386–2391.

Pirillo, A., Norata, G.D., Catapano, A.L., 2013. High-density lipoprotein subfractions--what the clinicians need to know. Cardiology 124, 116–125.

Rivellese, A., Maffettone, A., Vessby, B., Uusitupa, M., Hermansen, K., Berglund, L., Louheranta, A., Meyer, B., Riccardi, G., 2003. Effects of dietary saturated, monounsaturated and n-3 fatty acids on fasting lipoproteins, LDL size and post-prandial lipid metabolism in healthy subjects. Atherosclerosis 167, 149–158.

Rosenson, R.S., Underberg, J.A., 2013. Systematic review: evaluating the effect of lipid-lowering therapy on lipoprotein and lipid values. Cardiovascul. Drugs Therapy 27, 465–479.

Rye, K.A., Bursill, C.A., Lambert, G., Tabet, F., Barter, P.J., 2009. The metabolism and anti-atherogenic properties of HDL. J. Lipid Res. 50 (Suppl.), S195–200.

Sanders, T.A., Gleason, K., Griffin, B., Miller, G.J., 2006. Influence of an algal triacylglycerol containing docosahexaenoic acid (22: 6n-3) and docosapentaenoic acid (22: 5n-6) on cardiovascular risk factors in healthy men and women. Br. J. Nutr. 95, 525–531.

Schwab, U., Lauritzen, L., Tholstrup, T., Haldorsson, T., Riserus, U., Uusitupa, M., Becker, W., 2014. Effect of the amount and type of dietary fat on cardiometabolic risk factors and risk of developing type-2 diabetes, cardiovascular disease, and cancer: a systematic review. Food Nutr. Res. 58, 25145.

Shearer, G.C., Savinova, O.V., Harris, W.S., 2012. Fish oil — How does it reduce plasma triglycerides? Biochim. Biophys. Acta 1821, 843–851.

Sninsky, J.J., Rowland, C.M., Baca, A.M., Caulfield, M.P., Superko, H.R., 2013. Classification of LDL phenotypes by 4 methods of determining lipoprotein particle size. J. Investigative Med. 61, 942–949.

Soininen, P., Kangas, A.J., Wurtz, P., Suna, T., Ala-Korpela, M., 2015. Quantitative serum nuclear magnetic resonance metabolomics in cardiovascular epidemiology and genetics circulation. Cardiovascular Genetic. 8, 192–206.

Tani, S., Nagao, K., Matsumoto, M., Hirayama, A., 2013. Highly purified eicosapentaenoic acid may increase low-density lipoprotein particle size by improving triglyceride metabolism in patients with hypertriglyceridemia. Circulation J. 77, 2349–2357.

Woodman, R.J., Mori, T.A., Burke, V., Puddey, I.B., Watts, G.F., Best, J.D., Beilin, L.J., 2003. Docosahexaenoic acid but not eicosapentaenoic acid increases LDL particle size in treated hypertensive type 2 diabetic patients. Diabetes Care 26, 253.

CHAPTER

23

Fish, Fish Oil, and Liver Cancer

S. Zheng*, T.C. Chen**

*Division of Nutrition and Food Sciences, Department of Health Sciences, California Baptist University, Riverside, California, United States; **Clinical Translational Science Institute, Boston University, Massachusetts, United States

INTRODUCTION

Liver cancer may derive from different types of liver cells that become cancerous. The most common form of liver cancer is hepatocellular carcinoma (HCC), accounting roughly for 75% of all liver cancers. Most cases of HCC are the result of hepatitis B or C infection of hepatocellular cells, the main constituent of liver tissue. The second most prevalent liver cancer is cholangiocarcinoma or bile duct cancer. It accounts for about 10–20% of all liver cancers. There are two subtypes, intrahepatic bile duct cancer that begins in the small, tube-like bile ducts within the liver and extra hepatic bile duct cancer that develops in ducts outside of the liver. The remaining cases may include angiosarcoma, also called hemangiocarcinoma, a form of fast growing cancer that begins in the blood vessels of the liver, and fibrolamellar HCC, a rare form that is relatively easier to treat than other types. There is also a secondary liver cancer, resulting from the metastasis of a primary cancer in another part of the body, such as colorectal cancer. It is also known as a liver metastasis.

Liver cancer tends to be diagnosed at a more advanced stage due to lack of specific symptoms in the early stages and because no routine and simple screening tests are available. Thus, prevention would be an important route to avoid liver cancer development. Fish oil is a rich source of omega-3 polyunsaturated fatty acids (n–3 PUFAs). In recent years, there has been considerable interest in the anticancer properties of both n–3 PUFAs and fish oil consumption. Potential health benefits related to fish oil consumption may be due to its component of n–3 PUFAs, particularly eicosapentaenoic acid (EPA), docosahexaenoic acid (DHA), and docosapentaenoic acid (DPA). Promising health benefits of fish oil have been shown in several chronic diseases as discussed in other chapters in this book, including cardiovascular disease, diabetes, rheumatoid arthritis, and other cancers, such as breast, prostate, and colorectal cancer. Fish oil may also have an impact on the development of nerve, photoreception, and reproductive systems. (Dyck et al., 2011). In this review we will focus on the beneficial effects of fish and fish oil on the prevention of HCC, the major form of liver cancer.

HEPATOCELLULAR CARCINOMA (HCC)

HCC is the fifth most common form of cancer worldwide and the third most common cause of cancer-related deaths (Raza and Sood, 2014). However, in East Asia and Sub-Saharan Africa, HCC is much more prevalent with incidence rates exceeding 20 per 100,000 persons, accounting for more than 80% of HCC cases in the world. The high prevalence is because of high rates of hepatitis B virus (HBV)-induced liver disease in these parts of the world. Fortunately, the rate has been stabilizing or decreasing due to the immunization program against HBV. However, in the United States, Canada, and Western Europe, the incidence of HCC is increasing mainly due to the increased hepatitis C viral (HCV) infection, aging, and the obesity epidemic. More than three quarters of HCC is found in patients with cirrhotic liver and therefore the disease can be considered as a complication of chronic liver diseases (Llovet et al., 2003). Epidemiologic studies have identified several risk factors associated with HCC. The major one is chronic hepatitis derived from HBV and HCV infections which constitute about 80% of HCC. The remaining 20% may come

Fish and Fish Oil in Health and Disease Prevention. http://dx.doi.org/10.1016/B978-0-12-802844-5.00023-3

from nonviral related liver cirrhosis, such as alcoholic liver disease, nonalcoholic steatohepatitis which is frequently found in people with obesity and diabetes, genetic diseases such as α1 antitrypsin deficiency, diabetes mellitus and hemochromatosis, and autoimmune hepatitis. It has also been reported that some environmental toxins, such as aflatoxin B1, may be involved in HCC development (Abrams and Marsh, 2010).

Etiology and Risk Factors for HCC

In the etiology of HCC, risk factors may include modifiable and nonmodifiable risk factors. Among modifiable risk factors, the leading risk factors for HCC include, chronic HBV and HCV infection, alcoholic cirrhosis, and non-alcoholic fatty liver disease (NAFLD).

Viral Infection

Hepatitis viruses mainly contain hepatitis A virus (HAV), HBV, and HCV. Transmission route of HAV is via ingestion of contaminated food or drinks, even in microscopic amounts, or by close or sexual contact of person-to-person. Transmission of HBV is through infectious blood, semen, and other body fluids primarily via birth from an infected mother, sexual contact with an infected person, or sharing of contaminated needles, syringes, or other injection drug equipment, needle sticks or other sharp instrument injuries. HCV is less commonly transmitted through sexual contact or infected mothers, but mainly through sharing of contaminated needles, syringes, or other injection drug equipment. HBV and HCV are the leading risk factors of viral infection for HCC (Cdc, 2014).

According to World Health Organization data, more than 5 million people in the United States and 500 million people worldwide are chronically infected with a hepatitis virus. HBV and HCV are two unrelated viruses that target the liver and replicate in hepatocytes. Chronic HBV and HCV infection has been linked to an up to 100-fold, and an up to 20-fold increase, respectively, in the risk of HCC (Fattovich et al., 2008; Yang and Roberts, 2010). HBV- and HCV-induced HCC develops in an environment of inflammation and regeneration that results from chronic liver hepatitis, fibrosis, and cirrhosis, suggesting immune-mediated mechanisms in the pathogenesis of viral HCC (Rehermann and Nascimbeni, 2005). Upon persistent virus replication, HBV- and HCV-encoded proteins alter host gene expressions and cellular phenotypes to block or alter immune responses that should resolve chronic infections (Arzumanyan et al., 2013). These changes promote growth factor independent proliferation, resistance to growth inhibition, tissue invasion and metastasis, hypoxia and angiogenesis, altered energy metabolism, and resistance to apoptosis in the face of persistent immune attack (Hanahan and Weinberg, 2011).

Alcoholic Cirrhosis Versus Nonalcoholic Fatty Liver Disease

The second leading cause of liver disease-related mortality is alcoholic liver disease (ALD), causing approximately 287,000 deaths in a 24-year-period in the United States (Paula et al., 2010). Among ALD-related mortality, alcoholic cirrhosis accounts for 40% of the cases. It has been shown that 19% of individuals who consumed on average seventy 12 oz. beers or 1.5 oz. glasses of wine per week over a period of longer than 20 years developed ALD, out of which 7% had cirrhosis (Huang et al., 2010). It is believed that there is no "safety threshold" for the effects of alcohol consumption on the liver (Donato et al., 2006). Alcoholic cirrhosis has been considered as the most probable cause for ALD-related cancer incidence, and for HCC in populations with low prevalence of HBV and HCV infection, and low exposure to aflatoxins, such as North America and Northern Europe (La Vecchia, 2007). ALD-related liver damages include acetaldehyde formation, glutathione depletion, increased intestinal permeabilization-induced lipogenesis, which therefore increases fatty acid uptake by the liver from adipose tissue, and inhibition of betaoxidation of fatty acid as a result of an increased NADH/NAD+ ratio in hepatocytes (Orman et al., 2013). Chronically, alcohol consumption also activates innate immunity, promoting secretion of proinflammatory cytokines, such as TNFα, which can lead to liver damage by recruiting lymphocytes (Kawaratani et al., 2013).

NAFLD can also lead to cirrhosis and HCC, ranging from nonalcoholic steatohepatitis (NASH) to progressive fibrosis. Sedentary lifestyles, poor eating habits, and silent progression have contributed to the NAFLD epidemic, affecting at least 25% of population in the United States (Michelotti et al., 2013). Obesity has become an independent contributor to the increased incidence of NAFLD. Due to the exponential rise of NAFLD, NASH is predicted to be the principal cause of cirrhosis and liver transplantation by 2020 (Wree et al., 2013). Nonalcoholic mechanisms that promote lipid accumulation and inflammation in the liver involve lipolysis of adipose tissue, decreased fatty acid oxidation, increased hepatic lipogenesis, and reduced secretion of very low density lipoprotein (Tilg and Moschen, 2010). Transition from NAFLD to NASH can be affected by multiple factors, including dietary cholesterol intake, endotoxemia, interference of intestinal microbiota, toll-like receptor 5 deficiencies, endoplasmic reticulum stress, and hypoadiponectinemia (Chatterjee and Mitra, 2015).

Modifiable Versus Nonmodifiable Risk Factors

Basically, the established risk factors for HCC can be classified into modifiable and nonmodifiable risk factors. The modifiable risk factors include existing latent HBV or HCV infection, alcohol consumption, smoking, dietary factors, aflatoxin, diabetes and obesity, and oral contraceptives. The nonmodifiable risk factors are gender (males have higher incidence of HCC), advanced age, and ethnicity (Blacks have significant higher HCC incidence). In addition to chronic infection with hepatitis B and C viruses and alcoholic liver disease, other modifiable risk factors have received increasing attention.

Tobacco smoking is causally associated with liver cancer (International Agency for Research on Cancer, 2004). A systematic metaanalyses of observational studies on cigarette smoking and cancer demonstrated a pooled relative risk (RR) of 1.56 on liver cancer comparing current smokers to never smokers (Gandini et al., 2008). However, no consistent synergistic interactions between smoking and HBV/HCV infection have been reported.

Some dietary factors have been reported potentially having favorable effects on liver function and liver disease, including liver cancer. The pooled RR of coffee consumption on liver cancer was 0.54 in 6 case–control studies, and 0.64 for 4 cohort investigations. Indeed, caffeine metabolism is impaired in patients with cirrhosis, who often reduce coffee intake in order to avoid discomfort side effects. The bias due to reduced coffee consumption in unhealthy subjects cannot be ignored. It is, however, unlikely that any such bias has materially influenced the findings on liver enzymes or on hepatocellular carcinoma, since the inverse associations for liver cancer were consistent across strata of cirrhosis and/or cirrhosis severity (La Vecchia, 2005). Given its effects on liver enzymes and cirrhosis and the weight of epidemiological evidence, coffee appears therefore to have a real, although moderate, effect in reducing the risk of hepatocellular carcinoma, as suggested also by limited available data on rodents (Tanaka et al., 1990). Various components of coffee have been related to such a favorable effect, including caffeine, coffee oils (kahweol and cafestol), and antioxidant substances from coffee beans (La Vecchia, 2005), but it is necessary to investigate the effect of coffee on the risk of liver cancer with or without the presence of other risk factors.

Chemopreventive Strategies of HCC

With only 13% of HCC being diagnosed at the early stage to be eligible for curative therapy, such as surgical resection or liver transplantation and the high mortality rate associated with this disease, any approaches to prevent or delay HCC initiation and progression are attractive. In this section, we describe the recent advances in the field of HCC chemoprevention.

Etiology-Specific Chemoprevention

Universal HBV vaccination has been widely implemented to reduce the incidence of new infection, and to alleviate the risk of HBV-induced HCC. In Taiwan, HCC incidence was reported to be significantly lower among children aged 6–19 years in vaccinated compared with unvaccinated birth cohorts (Chang et al., 2009).

Antiviral therapy should be considered when viral infection occurs. Based on the success rates in clinical trials, 7 drugs have been approved by the FDA for treatment of viral hepatitis: peg-interferon (IFN) α-2a, interferon α-2b, lamivudine, adefovir, tenofovir, entecavir, telbivudine, and clevudine. Antiviral therapy for patients with HBV targets on virus replication, a key risk factor for HBV associated hepatocarcinogenesis (Arzumanyan et al., 2013). Interferon and nucleotide analogues are most commonly used to treat HBV-related cirrhosis and fibrosis. IFNα therapy is recognized as the first approved treatment for chronic HBV infected patients with minimal chance to develop a drug resistant strain. It has been reported to reduce the risk of HCC in a subset of patients (~35%) with HBV-associated cirrhosis (Lai and Yuen, 2013). Compared with interferon α-2b, peg-interferon α-2a has higher efficacy and less drug resistance, with a better pharmacokinetic profile. Nucleotide analogues exhibit higher potential on the suppression of virus replication and have excellent tolerance and safety profiles for long-term treatment of HBV infection. Lamivudine, adefovir, and entecavir have shown remarkable beneficial effects in decreasing the risk of HBV-induced HCC at all stages of the disease (Liaw et al., 2004; Hosaka et al., 2013; Sung et al., 2008)

The utility of interferon-based therapy on the treatment for HCV-associated HCC have shown a marked decline in the risk of HCC. However, this decline in risk was only observed in patients who received sustained virology response (SVR; Zhang et al., 2011; Morgan et al., 2010; Morgan et al., 2013). After the crystal structures of several HCV proteins were characterized, treatment of chronic HCV infection improved significantly due to the identification of a number of potential targets for direct-acting antiviral (DAA) agents. Triple therapy combining NS3/4A protease inhibitor boceprevir or telaprevir, with pegylated IFN-α and ribavirin or with other DAAs in IFN-free regimens, showed significant SVR in 59–69% of patients with chronic HCV infection (Sarrazin et al., 2012).

Generic Chemoprevention

As the second most commonly prescribed medication for primary and secondary prevention of cardiovascular diseases, statins also have antineoplastic properties through antiproliferative, proapoptotic, antiangiogenic, immunomodulatory, and antiinfective effects (Institute for Healthcare Informatics, 2011; Demierre et al., 2005). Observational studies have shown the protective effect of statins against inflammation-driven cancers (Singh et al., 2013a), including the association between statin use and risk of incident HCC (Tsan et al., 2013; El-Serag et al., 2009; Tsan et al., 2012; Chiu et al., 2011). Besides the effect on cholesterol biosynthesis, the mechanisms of the inhibitory role of statin on 3-hydroxy-3-methylglutaryl coenzyme A (HMG-CoA) reductase include multiple pathways. This inhibition prevents posttranslational prenylation of Ras/Rho signaling, which is the key mediator of cell growth, differentiation and survival. Statins are proapoptotic, by regulating the RAF–MAPK–ERK pathway, activating caspases and decreasing the level of Bcl-2 (Marcelli et al., 1998; Wu et al., 2004). Statins also inhibit the activation of proteasome pathway through limiting the degradation of cyclin-dependent kinase inhibitors p21 and p27, therefore to inhibit tumor growth (Rao et al., 1999). In hepatocarcinogenesis, atorvastatin has been shown to block Myc phosphorylation and activation, suppressing tumor initiation and growth. However, randomized controlled trials of statins failed to demonstrate a protective effect against HCC. In a post hoc analysis of 22 randomized controlled trials and a meta-analysis of 10 studies (7 observational studies, 3 randomized controlled trials), statin users were no less likely to develop HCC than patients receiving placebo (Emberson et al., 2012; Singh et al., 2013b).

Conventional antidiabetic medications also have been demonstrated to modify the risk of cancer in patients with diabetes. Metformin and thiazolidinediones were considered to be associated with decreased risk of HCC, whereas insulin and insulin secretagogues, such as sulphonylureas, have been associated with an increased risk of HCC (Decensi et al., 2010; Chang et al., 2012). Metformin can activate AMPK signaling, which inhibits mTOR pathway (Zhou et al., 2001). It can also inhibit cell growth and promote cell death by inhibiting cyclin D1 expression and pRb phosphorylation (Chen et al., 2012). In addition, the drug can inhibit hepatocarcinogenesis by downregulating c-Myc and lipogenesis (Blandino et al., 2012). As PPARγ agonists, thiazolidinediones showed anticancer effects through inhibition of the ubiquitin–proteasome system and the ERK pathway. Thiazolidinediones also have PPARγ independent effects in preclinical models of HCC (Okumura, 2010; Wu et al., 2012a,b). Insulin and sulphonylureas can promote oncogenesis either directly or indirectly by upregulating insulin-like growth factor-1 (IGF1). The activation of IGF1 leads to abnormal stimulation of multiple cellular signaling cascades (Bowker et al., 2006).

Antiplatelet agents, such as aspirin, have been shown to have antiinflammatory and antineoplastic effects against inflammation-mediated cancers (Falk et al., 2012). In response to HBV infection, aspirin can decrease T cell-mediated chronic inflammation and decrease the risk of hepatocarcinogenesis by inhibiting the cyclooxygenase-2 enzyme (Sitia et al., 2012; Thun et al., 2012). In a large cohort study of NIH-AARP, aspirin use was associated with a 49% reduced risk of HCC, although a dose–response or duration–response relationship between aspirin use and risk modification of HCC was not observed (Sahasrabuddhe et al., 2012). However, other population-based case–control or cohort studies have not observed significant association between aspirin use and HCC risk.

Dietary Agents

Dietary agents for prevention of HCC have been under investigation. Coffee consumption has been shown to be associated with a reduced risk of HCC (Gelatti et al., 2005; Inoue et al., 2005), and of advanced fibrosis and cirrhosis, which may indirectly improve the risk of HCC (Torres and Harrison, 2013). Basically, the effect of coffee is considered dose-dependent regardless of the etiology of underlying chronic liver disease (Singh et al., 2013a). Coffee might exert its antineoplastic effects through its components, such as disterpenes, cafestol, and kahweol, which can modulate enzymes involved in carcinogen detoxification. Caffeine also has antioxidant properties (Tao et al., 2008). In a meta-analysis of 14 studies (8 cohort studies and 6 case–control studies), a 43% decline in the risk of HCC was observed in individuals who consumed coffee (Bravi et al., 2009).

Protective effects of dietary supplement on HCC have also been shown in many cohort studies. In two large cohort studies, a significantly lower risk of HCC was observed among patients in the highest quartile of dietary vitamin E intake than in the lowest quartile (Zhang et al., 2012). Similar results were demonstrated in HCC patients who consumed supplemental vitamin E in the same studies. Vitamin E is an antioxidant, which can prevent DNA damage, enhances DNA repair, promotes inactivation of carcinogenesis, and has become a first-line pharmacotherapy for patients without diabetes but with biopsy-proven NASH (Chalasani et al., 2012).

Dietary phytochemicals which possess potent antioxidant, antiinflammation or antineoplastic properties, may also decrease the risk of HCC, particularly aflatoxin-induced HCC. In chemoprevention of HCC, various biomarkers have been used for the examination of multiple agents, such as urinary aflatoxin-N7-guanine and aflatoxin-serum albumin adducts. Cruciferous vegetables, broccoli sprouts for example, might have antineoplastic effects via glucosinolates and metabolites (such as sulphoraphane) that can modulate Keap1/Nrf2 signaling and activate cytoprotective responses against oxidants (Kensler et al., 2013). Broccoli sprout extracts also showed the effects of reduced urinary excretion of sulphoraphane metabolites and aflatoxin–DNA adducts (Kensler et al., 2005). A daily consumption of oral chlorophyllin, a chlorophyll derivative, with each meal was also seen to reduce urinary aflatoxin-N7-guanine by 55% compared with placebo (Egner et al., 2001).

Curcumin, which is found in turmeric, has also been shown to have a protective effect in mouse models of aflatoxin-induced hepatocarcinogenesis (Soni et al., 1997). Although no clinical trials have been performed with curcumin in patients with HCC, curcumin has exerted proapoptotic, antiinflammatory, and antiangiogenic actions both in vitro and in vivo, and might provide protection from other cancers as well (Singh et al., 2013a). Resveratrol, a dietary polyphenol found in grapes, berries, peanuts, and red wine, also demonstrated protective effects in diethylnitrosamine-induced HCC (Bishayee and Dhir, 2009). Resveratrol can inhibit carcinogenesis by suppressing hepatic carcinogen-activating enzymes such as cytochrome P450, and by inducing oxidoreductase and glutathione S-transferase (Bishayee et al., 2010). A doubleblind placebo-controlled study showed that a daily resveratrol supplement might improve insulin sensitivity, reduce oxidative stress, and activate Akt pathway, suggesting its potent property to reduce the risk of HCC (Brasnyo et al., 2011). However, these findings were not reproduced in a more current study (Poulsen et al., 2013).

The inverse association between fish consumption and the risk of HCC has been under intensive scrutiny. In particular, dietary consumption of fish rich in n–3 PUFAs has been implicated in the reduction of HCC. The beneficial effect of n–3 PUFAs on HCC is further discussed in Section "Fish and Fish Oil" of this chapter.

Secondary Prevention

As mentioned in Section Etiology-Specific Chemoprevention, primary HCC using HBV vaccination prevention strategy has been implemented in over 150 countries with great success. Secondary prevention is defined as the prevention of tumor recurrence after hepatic resection or local ablative therapies (Colombo and Donato, 2005). In secondary prevention of HCC, multiple agents have showed effective properties. Cirrohosis and chronic HBV can induce field cancerization in the entire liver; therefore, there is a high risk of recurrence of HCC of up to 75% after surgical resection (Singh et al., 2013a). In a large cohort study of 4,569 patients who underwent curative resection of HBV-induced HCC, the treatment of nucleoside analogues significantly lowered 6-year HCC recurrence rate, and recurrence was also less frequent in statin users as well as aspirin or NSAID users (Wu et al., 2012a,b). In a case study of 216 patients with chronic HCV, the treatment of interferon and ribavirin significantly reduced the risk of HCC recurrence after 5 years, but use of statin, metformin or aspirin did not show any effects (Hsu et al., 2013). On the basis of pooled results from 7 studies, including 6 randomized controlled trials, vitamin K2 analogue has also shown a potent effect to reduce the risk of HCC at 3 years (Zhong et al., 2013).

FISH AND FISH OIL

Fish has been an important food source for humans throughout recorded history. The potential health benefits related to fish consumption are due to the presence of nutrients including: high quality protein, unsaturated essential fatty acids, minerals (calcium, iron, selenium, zinc, iodine, magnesium, potassium etc.), and water soluble (niacin, pyridoxine, and cobalamin) and fat soluble (A, D, E) vitamins in fish. The American Heart Association recommends that we eat fish at least twice a week as part of a healthy diet. Fish oil is oil derived from the tissues of oily fish, usually from the flesh or liver.

Chemistry of Fish Oil

Fish oil contains a rather large amount of saturated and unsaturated fatty acids, which are commonly linked to a glycerol backbone to form mixed triglyceride. In addition to triglyceride, fish oil contains minor amounts of phospholipids and other lipids, as well as some vitamins and minerals. An unsaturated fatty acid is a fat in which there is at least one double bond within the fatty acid chain. These long, straight-chained molecules have a series of *cis* double bonds. An unsaturated fatty acid is named depending on the position of the first double bond counting from the methyl group, n–3 for example, in which the first double bond starts from C3. The major health benefits from the consumption of fish oil are related to polyunsaturated fatty acids (PUFAs), especially n–3 PUFAs, such as *cis*-5,8,11,14,17-eicosapentaenoic acid (EPA), *cis*-4,7,10,13,16,19-docosahexaenoic acid (DHA), and docosapentaenoic acid (DPA; Arab-Tehrany et al., 2012).

Sources of n-3 Polyunsaturated Fatty Acids (n-3 PUFAs)

The fish species rich in n–3 PUFA (C20:5 EPA and C22:6 DHA) include European anchovy, striped bass, bluefish, Atlantic mackerel, Florida pompano, Atlantic herring, Pacific herring, Atlantic salmon, Chinook salmon, pink salmon, Sockeye salmon, sardines, lake trout, rainbow trout, sablefish, and tuna. According to data from the Academy of Nutrition and Dietetics, the average amount of n–3 PUFAs per meal of 227 g ranges from 1.1 to 7.5 g in these 16 species of fish. The American Heart Association dietary advisory recommends that persons with coronary heart disease should consume about one gram of fish oil daily (Kris-Etherton et al., 2002). Therefore, it appears that all these species of fish provide adequate amounts of n–3 PUFAs (1.1–7.5 g) per meal. Although α-linolenic acid (C18:3 ALA) is found in vegetable oil, its conversion to EPA and DHA in humans is low, and humans have no other means of synthesizing n-3 PUFA, so that EPA and DHA are considered essential nutrients.

Fish oil supplements are growing more popular in the global market. In the United States, fish oil supplements are usually analyzed measuring total n–3 content, EPA and DHA quantities, vitamin D and CLA (conjugated linoleic acid) amounts, methylmercury concentration, and total oxidation values.

Mechanism of Action of n-3 PUFAs

Fish oil usually contains a mix of EPA and DHA and is believed to have health benefits on cardiovascular outcomes and rheumatological conditions (De Caterina 2011; Bhangle and Kolasinski 2011). There is now emerging evidence that n–3 PUFAs may also have antitumor properties on several types of cancer, such as breast, colon and prostate cancer (Noguchi et al., 1995; Reddy 1994; Norrish et al., 1999). Knowledge of the mechanisms underlying the antineoplastic activity of n–3 PUFAs has been comprehensively reviewed (Smith, 2005; Chapkin et al., 2007; Calviello et al., 2007). The main mechanistic aspects include inhibition of COX activity, alteration of cell membrane dynamics and cell surface receptor function, increased cellular oxidative stress, and novel antiinflammatory lipid mediators derived from EPA and DHA, including resolvins, protectins and maresins, which direct fatty acid signaling via G protein-coupled receptors (Cockbain et al., 2012; Hull, 2011).

When n–3 PUFAs incorporate into cell membrane, they become a crucial component of the hydrophobic structure which affects fluidity, thickness, stability, permeability, and even domain size of the membrane. Thus, through interaction with membrane proteins, such as transporter or protein kinases, they alter various signal transduction involved in the body's biochemical activities (Simopoulos, 1986; Stubbs and Smith, 1984). The uptake of DHA by tumor cells was recently found to be related to the phosphatidylethanolamine (PE) contents in cell membrane. When DHA was conjugated with anticancer drug gemcitabine (GEM), DHA–GEM exhibited higher tumor targeting ability and enhanced therapeutic efficacy than that of GEM itself (Li et al., 2014).

Omega 3 PUFAs may mediate cell cycle arrest; probably due to control of the cell cycle regulatory cyclins and their partner kinases (Chen and Istfan, 2001; Terano et al., 1999). At least some of the beneficial effects of n–3 PUFAs are via metabolites such as prostaglandins, leukotrienes, thromboxanes, and resolvins (Vanden Heuvel, 2012). Fatty acids metabolize to prostaglandin E1 and E2 to activate protein kinase A and C leading to the phosphorylation of proteins targeted by tyrosine kinase, therefore affecting cell cycle progression.

DHA has been thought to cause cancer cell death via apoptosis (Gleissman et al., 2010; Lim et al., 2009; Wendel and Heller, 2009). Along with apoptosis, autophagy has also been indicated to play a role in the cytotoxic mechanisms of DHA in several recent reports (Jing et al., 2011; Rovito et al., 2013; Yao et al., 2014). Autophagy and apoptosis are self-destructive processes that share a key regulator ROS (reactive oxygen species), which leads to growth adaption and survival; however, excess ROS may cause irreversible cellular damage, thus provoking autophagy and/or apoptosis (Droge, 2002; Rubio et al., 2012). As a key mediator of DHA-induced cytotoxicity, ROS level and the cytotoxic effects have been shown to be abrogated by typical antioxidants (Kanno et al., 2011).

EFFECTS OF FISH OIL ON HCC

Given the reported side effects associated with chemotherapy and surgical resection, dietary intervention with n–3 PUFAs has been postulated to be an alternative way to prevent liver cancer progression and metastasis.

In Vitro Cell Culture Data

DHA has been indicated to affect cell growth through inhibiting cell cycle progression, possibly via the post-receptor signaling pathways (Bandyopadhyay et al., 1993). DHA (0–200 μM) inhibited proliferation of the human metastatic HCC cell line MHCC97L in a dose-dependent manner via targeting COX2 and other cell cycle regulations in hepatocarcinogenesis (Lee et al., 2010). A DHA and EPA treatment resulted in a dose-dependent reduction of cancer cell viability with cleavage of poly ADP ribose polymerase, caspase-3, caspase-9, and blocked β-catenin and COX2 in human HCC cell lines, therefore inhibiting HCC cell growth (Lim et al., 2009). In human HCC Bel-7402 cells, DHA induced cell apoptosis through downregulation of Bcl-2 and Bim, and upregulation of caspase-3 and Bax (Sun et al., 2013). On the other hand, excess DHA may cause cytotoxicity in human HCC cell lines. The mechanisms of the cytotoxic effects of DHA include the production of ROS. Albumin has an antioxidant property, and has been shown having protective effects against the DHA-induced cytotoxicity in three human HCC cell lines, HepG2, Hep3B, Huh7 (Kanno et al., 2011). A very recent study found EPA-induced apoptosis in HepG2 cells through ROS-Ca(2+)-JNK mitochondrial pathways (Zhang et al., 2015).

Human subjects consuming fish oil showed a significant suppression of COX2 in blood monocytes upon the stimulation in vitro with LPS, an agonist for TLR4. In a murine monocytic cell line RAW 264.7, inhibition of COX2 expression by n–3 PUFA is also mediated through the modulation of TL signaling pathways (Lee et al., 2003).

Animal Model Studies

The inhibitory effects of both EPA and DHA on growth of HCC have been demonstrated in numerous studies using animal models. EPA and DHA inhibited growth of Morris hepatocarcinoma 3924A in rats. A 50% reduction of tumor weight or volume was observed on the 19th day after transplantation for both of the n–3 PUFA groups (Calviello et al., 1998). Suppressed liver tumorigenesis was observed in fat-1 transgenic mouse model, which can endogenously produce n–3 PUFA from n–6 PUFA, with reduced plasma TNF and liver COX2 expression (Weylandt et al., 2011). EPA ameliorated steatohepatitis and development of HCC in Pten-deficient mice, based on an inhibition of MAPK activity and lowered chronic hepatic inflammation (Ishii et al., 2009). Endogenously produced n–3 PUFAs were also found to prevent liver neoplasia in a mouse hepatocarcinogenesis model via regulation on nonmammalian fat-1 gene (Griffitts et al., 2010).

Dietary fish oil suppressed a specific linoleic acid-dependent, inhibitory G protein-coupled, growth-promoting-signaling pathway in hepatoma 7288CTC in Buffalo rats (Smith et al., 2006).

Human Clinical Trials

Hanai and his colleagues (Hanai et al., 1993) evaluated 17 hepatectomized cases including 12 cases of HCC and 5 cases of metastatic liver cancer. The levels of α-linolenic acid and DHA in liver cancer tissues were found to be significantly less than those in the noncancerous reference tissues. Several studies have documented a protective effect of dietary n–3 PUFAs on the development of certain cancers (Anderson and Ma, 2009; Sasazuki et al., 2011). However, most epidemiological studies didn't consider HCV or HBV infection status. Sawada et al. (2012) found n–3 PUFAs to be associated inversely with HCC in a dose-dependent manner, and it appeared to protect against the development of HCC, even among subjects with HBV and/or HCV infection. Administration of n–3 PUFAs was reported to reduce infection rate and to improve liver function recovery in HBV-associated HCC patients after hepatectomy (Wu et al., 2012a,b). The n–3 PUFAs are also used to reduce hepatic triglyceride accumulation, while improving insulin sensitivity and reducing steatosis, and hepatic damage in patients with NAFLD (Masterton et al., 2010; Storlien et al., 1987; Levy et al., 2004). In clinical NAFLD patients studies, n–3 PUFA supplementation was demonstrated to improve ALT, AST, GGT, triglyceride, and fasting glucose concentrations (Capanni et al., 2006; Tanaka et al., 2008; Parker et al., 2012).

A metaanalysis of 11 studies (3 cohort studies, 7 retrospective case-control studies, and 1 nested case-control study) provided significant evidence that fish consumption and n–3 PUFA have inverse association with 35% reduction and 51% reduction in the risk of HCC, respectively (Gao et al., 2015). DHA has potential applications in chemotherapy. Phase III randomized controlled trials using DHA are currently underway (Hajjaji and Bougnoux, 2013). Safe and effective chemotherapeutic reagents such as DHA are needed for use against HCC, but it remains important to investigate further the cytotoxic mechanisms of DHA against HCC.

In typical American diets, the ratio of n–6 to n-3 PUFAs has been quite high. Based on evidence that such imbalance of n–6 to n–3 might be aggravating the inflammatory response and/or hindering resolution, a case study was recently carried out in the US military bases to develop ways to improve the fatty acid composition of operational rations and dining hall foods using a food-based approach (Montain, 2015). Numerous observational cohort studies and randomized controlled trials demonstrated the health effect of n–3 PUFAs in patients with cardiovascular disease or with cardiac risk factors (Roncaglioni et al., 2013; Marchioli and Levantesi, 2013). Supplementation with n–3 PUFAs has shown beneficial effects on top of modern guideline-adjusted therapy in patients after myocardial infarction (Rauch et al., 2010; Kromhout et al., 2010). However, it should be mentioned that lack of effects has also been reported in a randomized controlled trial studying a group of dysglycemia patients supplemented with one gram of n–3 fatty acids, containing 465 mg EPA and 375 mg DHA (Origin Trial investigators et al., 2012) and two metaanalyses (Rizos et al., 2012; Kwak et al., Inpress).

Synergistic Effect of Fish Oil and Vitamin D

In recent years, there has been increasing interest in the combined anticancer properties of n–3 PUFAs and vitamin D. Unlike n–3 PUFAs epidemiological studies, vitamin D studies seem to show consistent inverse correlations between its intake and the risks of certain cancers (Dyck et al., 2011). Istfan and coworkers demonstrated that the combination of 1α,25-dihydroxy vitamin D3 [1α,25(OH)2D3] and fish oil (high in n–3 PUFAs) produced significantly more inhibition of G1/S phase transition in prostate cancer cells than either treatment alone (Istfan et al., 2007). This study was the first to indicate the combined benefit of these two agents in the battle against cancer. When considering synergetic effects of fish oil with vitamin D on HCC, fish oil enhances the antiproliferative activity of 1α,25(OH)2D3 on human hepatoblastoma cells (HepG2; Chiang et al., 2009). Cod liver oil is a good source of both vitamin D and n–3 PUFAs. It could be a good option for the combined supplementation of these two molecules.

Apoptosis is an important aspect of the body's defense against tumorigenesis. As a tumor suppressor gene, p53 has been shown to be regulated by both n–3 PUFAs and vitamin D upon its phosphorylation and activation (Kim et al., 2005; Maruyama et al., 2006; Lambert et al., 2006). 1α,25(OH)2D3 represses antiapoptotic/prosurvival proteins like Bcl-2 and Bcl-X (Ylikomi et al., 2002; Diaz et al., 2000) and also suppresses p38 and COX2 expression, which have been positively associated with cancer (Nonn et al., 2006; Krishnan et al., 2007). DHA has also been shown to inactivate Bcl-2 genes (Narayanan et al., 2001). Although DHA was a p38 activator in some models (Kim et al., 2005), n–3 PUFAs exhibits inhibitory effects on COX and LOX activity and has a role in restoring apoptosis in cancerous cells (Hardman, 2002).

Angiogenesis, the formation of new blood vessels, is critical for cancer progression (Dyck et al., 2011). The n–3 PUFAs can compete with n–6 PUFAs to decrease the production of pro-angiogenic COX and LOX, thereby reducing angiogenesis (McCarty, 1996; Form and Auerbach, 1983). 1α,25(OH)2D3 also suppresses angiogenesis in prostate cancer cells by impeding endothelial cell migration and tube formation via IL8 inhibition (Bao et al., 2006).

Inflammatory environments are procarcinogenic, accompanied by elevated secretion of proinflammatory cytokines (Dyck et al., 2011). Both n–3 PUFAs and 1α,25(OH)2D3 are capable of attenuating inflammation. 1α,25(OH)2D3 downregulates IL2, IL6, IL12, and has an antiproliferative effect (Nagpa et al., 2005; Dyck et al., 2011). EPA and DHA can inhibit TNFα and IL1 (Meckling, 2007). Both n–3 PUFAs and 1α,25(OH)2D3 appear to regulate NFκB, a main regulator of inflammation, via downregulating AKT signaling and activation of p53 in various immune cells (Narayanan et al., 2001; Adorini et al., 2004; Schmitt et al., 2002).

SUMMARY AND FUTURE PROSPECTIVE STUDIES

In this chapter, we discuss the risk factors and various chemo-preventive strategies for HCC, the major form of liver cancer, with special focus on the potential benefits of fish oil, especially n–3 PUFAs. HCC affects the lives of tens of millions of people worldwide. However, only 13% were diagnosed at the early stage to be eligible for surgical resection or liver transplantation. Although pharmaceutical and biotechnology companies have spent millions to develop drugs to treat HCC, the cost of these advanced drugs is too high to be available for the majority of patients. Therefore, any low-cost approaches with lesser side-effects to prevent or delay HCC initiation and progression are desirable, such as supplementation with fish oil and n–3 PUFAs.

The beneficial effects of fish and fish oil on health were first suggested in a series of reports by two Danish physicians, Hans Olaf Bang and Jorn Dyerberg, between 1970 and 1980 (Bang et al., 1971; Bang and Dyerberg, 1972; Bang et al., 1976; Dyerberg et al., 1975; Bang et al., 1980; Dyerberg and Bang, 1980) from their studies on the Greenland Eskimos and their diet. Since then, numerous in vitro and in vivo animal studies, and human clinical trials have been conducted. In general, in vitro and in vivo animal studies all indicate the beneficial effects of n–3 PUFAs. On the contrary, some randomized clinical trials (RCT) and systemic reviews of the human studies reported either null or negative results (Origin Trial investigators et al., 2012; Rizos et al., 2012; Kwak et al., Inpress). A recent report by Fodor et al. (2014) questioned the validity of Bang and Dyerberg's initial observation and conclusion stating that Greenland's Inuit population has less cardiovascular disease due to fish and fish oil consumption.

In spite of the lack of conclusive clinical data to support the beneficial effect of fish oil on cardiovascular disease, we believe that we should not ignore the countless in vitro cell culture and in vivo animal model studies supporting the notion that fish oil and, in particular, n–3 PUFAs have positive effects on human health. The similar situation has also been found in vitamin D research. Several metaanalyses and randomized controlled trials have failed to support the beneficial effect of vitamin D supplementation on chronic diseases, such as osteoporosis and cancers. Lappe and Heaney (2012) looked into the problems that arise in the use of RCT to establish causal connection between nutrients and various clinical outcomes. They pointed out that most of the RCT studies failed to recognize that there is a sigmoid shape of nutrient intake versus endpoint effect. The effective dose varies from person to person (genetic variation) and furthermore this optimal dose range is not wide. If the patient's n–3 PUFA level was in the flat ranges of the either end of this effective dose range, supplementing the patients with a small amount of n–3 PUFAs won't show any improvement. For example, if the patient's PUFAs levels are already at the plateau range, taking more won't do any good. In other words, starting level is important in clinical trials using nutrients. In most nutritional studies, a food-frequency questionnaire is administered and the dietary intake of EPA and DHA calculated from the questionnaires (Origin Trial investigators et al., 2012) instead of the actual analysis of EPA and DHA serum levels in the study subjects at the base-line and during the course of study. Trials containing these kinds of errors are expected to generate null results. If the null data are pooled into a meta-analysis, its conclusion will inevitably be misleading and should not be used for developing nutritional policy (Lappe and Heaney, 2012).

The Nutrition Evidence Library (NEL) within the USDA's Center for Nutrition Policy and Promotion may need to pay attention to the concerns raised by Lappe and Heaney (2014).

Acknowledgments

The authors acknowledge the partial support by J W & Ida M Jameson Foundation, California Baptist University Faculty Development Micro Grant and NIH CTSA grant UL1-TR000157.

Abbreviations

ALA	α-linolenic acid
CLA	Conjugated linoleic acid
DAA	Direct-acting antiviral
DHA	Docosahexaenoic acid
DPA	Docosapentaenoic acid
EPA	Eicosapentaenoic acid
GEM	Gemcitabine
HAV	Hepatitis A virus
HBV	Hepatitis B virus
HCC	Hepatocellular carcinoma
HCV	Hepatitis C virus
HMG-CoA	3-Hydroxy-3-methylglutaryl coenzyme A
IGF-1	Insulin-like growth factor-1
IFN	Interferon
NAFLD	Nonalcoholic fatty liver disease
ALD	Alcoholic liver disease
NASH	Nonalcoholic steatohepatitis
PE	Phosphatidylethanolamine
PUFAs	Polyunsaturated fatty acids
RR	Relative risk
ROS	Reactive oxygen species
SVR	Sustained virology response
$1\alpha 25(OH)_2D_3$	1α,25-dihydroxyvitamin D_3

References

Abrams, P., Marsh, J.W., 2010. Current approach to hepatocellular carcinoma. Surg. Clin. North Am. 90, 803–816.

Adorini, L., Penna, G., Giarratana, N., Roncari, A., Amuchastegui, S., Daniel, K.C., Uskokovic, M., 2004. Dendritic cells as key targets for immunomodulation by vitamin D receptor ligands. J. Steroid Biochem. Mol. Biol. 89-90, 437–441.

Anderson, B.M., Ma, D.W., 2009. Are all n-3 polyunsaturated fatty acids created equal? Lipids Health Dis. 10, 33.

Arab-Tehrany, E., Jacquot, M., Gaiani, C., Imran, M., Desobry, S., Linder, M., 2012. Beneficial effects and oxidative stability of omega-3 long-chain polyunsaturated fatty acids. Trends Food Sci. Technol. 25, 24–33.

Arzumanyan, A., Reis, H.M., Feitelson, M.A., 2013. Pathogenic mechanisms in HBV- and HCV- associated hepatocellular carcinoma. Nat. Rev. Cancer 13, 123–135.

Bandyopadhyay, G.K., Hwang, S., Imagawa, W., Nandi, S., 1993. Role of polyunsaturated fatty acids as signal transducers: amplification of signals from growth fac-tor receptors by fatty acids in mammary epithelial cells. Prostagland. Leukotr. Essen. Fatty Acid. 48, 71–78.

Bang, H.O., Dyerberg, J., 1972. Plasma lipids and lipoproteins in Greenlandic West Coast Eskimos. Acta. Med. Scand. 192, 85–94.

Bang, H.O., Dyerberg, J., Nielsen, A.B., 1971. Plasma lipid and lipoprotein pattern in Greenlandic West-Coast Eskimos. Lancet 1, 1143–1145.

Bang, H.O., Dyerberg, J., Hjorne, N., 1976. The composition of food consumed by Greenland Eskimos. Acta Med. Scand. 200, 69–73.

Bang, H.O., Dyerberg, J., Sinclair, H.M., 1980. The composition of the Eskimo food in north western Greenland. Am. J. Clin. Nutr. 33, 2657–2661.

Bao, B.Y., Yao, J., Lee, Y.F., 2006. 1α, 25-dihydroxyvitamin D3 supresses interleukin- 8 mediated prostate cancer cell angiogenesis. Carcinogenesis 27, 1883–1893.

Bhangle, S., Kolasinski, S.L., 2011. Fish oil in rheumatic diseases. Rheum. Dis. Clin. North Am. 37, 77–84.

Bishayee, A., Dhir, N., 2009. Resveratrol-mediated chemoprevention of diethylnitrosamine-initiated hepatocarcinogenesis: inhibition of cell proliferation and induction of apoptosis. Chem. Biol. Interact. 179, 131–144.

Bishayee, A., Politis, T., Darvesh, A.S., 2010. Resveratrol in the chemoprevention and treatment of hepatocellular carcinoma. Cancer Treat Rev. 36, 43–53.

Blandino, G., Valerio, M., Cioce, M., Mori, F., Casadei, L., Pulito, C., Sacconi, A., Biagioni, F., Cortese, G., Galanti, S., Manetti, C., Citro, G., Muti, P., Strano, S., 2012. Metformin elicits anticancer effects through the sequential modulation of DICER and c-MYC. Nat. Commun. 29 (3), 865.

Bowker, S.L., Majumdar, S.R., Veugelers, P., Johnson, J.A., 2006. Increased cancer-related mortality for patients with type 2 diabetes who use sulfonylureas or insulin. Diabetes Care 29, 254–258.

Brasnyo, P., Brasnyó, P., Molnár, G.A., Mohás, M., Markó, L., Laczy, B., Cseh, J., Mikolás, E., Szijártó, I.A., Mérei, A., Halmai, R., Mészáros, L.G., Sümegi, B., Wittmann, I., 2011. Resveratrolimprovesinsulin sensitivity, reduces oxidative stress and activates the Akt pathway in type 2 diabetic patients. Br. J. Nutr. 106, 383–389.

Bravi, F., Bosetti, C., Tavani, A., La Vecchia, C., 2009. Coffee drinking and hepatocellular carcinoma: an update. Hepatology 50, 1317–1318.

Calviello, G., Palozza, P., Piccioni, E., Maggiano, N., Frattucci, A., Franceschelli, P., Bartoli, G.M., 1998. Dietary supplementation with eicosapentaenoic and docosahexaenoic acid inhibits growth of Mor-ris hepatocarcinoma 3924A in rats: effects on proliferation and apoptosis. Int. J. Cancer. 75, 699–705.

Calviello, G., Serini, S., Piccioni, E., 2007. n-3 polyunsaturated fatty acids and the prevention of colorectal cancer: molecular mechanisms involved. Curr. Med. Chem. 14, 3059–3069.

Capanni, M., Calella, F., Biagini, M.R., Genise, S., Raimondi, L., Bedogni, G., Svegliati-Baroni, G., Sofi, F., Milani, S., Abbate, R., Surrenti, C., Casini, A., 2006. Prolonged n-3 polyunsaturated fatty acid supplementation ameliorates hepatic steatosis in patients with non- alcoholic fatty liver disease: a pilot study. Aliment Pharmacol. Ther. 23, 1143–1151.

CDC, 2014. http://www.cdc.gov/hepatitis/Resources/Professionals/PDFs/ABCTable.pdf

Chalasani, N., Younossi, Z., Lavine, J.E., Diehl, A.M., Brunt, E.M., Cusi, K., Charlton, M., Sanyal, A.J., 2012. The diagnosis and management of non-alcoholic fatty liver disease: practice guideline by the American Gastroenterological Association, American Association for the Study of Liver Diseases, and American College of Gastroenterology. Gastroenterology 142, 1592–1609.

Chang, M.H., You, S.L., Chen, C.J., Liu, C.J., Lee, C.M., Lin, S.M., Chu, H.C., Wu, T.C., Yang, S.S., Kuo, H.S., Chen, D.S., 2009. Decreased incidence of hepatocellular carcinoma in hepatitis B vaccines: a 20-year follow-up study. J. Natl. Cancer Inst. 101, 1348–1355.

Chang, C.H., Lin, J.W., Wu, L.C., Lai, M.S., Chuang, L.M., 2012. Oral insulin secretagogues, insulin, and cancer risk in type 2 diabetes mellitus. J. Clin. Endocrinol. Metab. 97, E1170–E1175.

Chapkin, R.S., McMurray, D.N., Lupton, J.R., 2007. Colon cancer, fatty acids and anti-inflammatory compounds. Curr. Opin. Gastroenterol. 23, 48–54.

Chatterjee, R., Mitra, A., 2015. An overview of effective therapies and recent advances in biomarkers for chronic liver diseases and associated liver cancer. Int. Immunopharmacol. 24, 335–345.

Chen, Z.Y., Istfan, N.W., 2001. Docosahexaenoic acid, a major constituent of fish oil diets, prevents activation of cyclin-dependent kinases and S-phase entry by serum stimulation in HT-29 cells. Prostagland. Leukotr. Essen. Fatty Acid. 64, 67–73.

Chen, H.P., Shieh, J.J., Chang, C.C., Chen, T.T., Lin, J.T., Wu, M.S., Lin, J.H., Wu, C.Y., 2012. Metformin decreases hepatocellular carcinoma risk in a dose- dependent manner: population-based and in vitro studies. Gut 62, 606–615.

Chiang, K.C., Persons, K.S., Istfan, N.W., Holick, M.F., Chen, T.C., 2009. Fish oil enhances the antiproliferative effect of 1α, 25-dihydroxyvitamin D3 on liver cancer cells. Anticancer Res. 29, 3591–3596.

Chiu, H.F., Ho, S.C., Chen, C.C., Yang, C.Y., 2011. Statin use and the risk of liver cancer: a population-based case-control study. Am. J. Gastroenterol. 106, 894–898.

Cockbain, A.J., Toogood, G.J., Hull, M.A., 2012. Omega-3 polyunsaturated fatty acids for the treatment and prevention of colorectal cancer. Gut 61, 135–149.

Colombo, M., Donato, M.F., 2005. Prevention of hepatocellular carcinoma. Semin. Liver Dis. 25, 155–161.

De Caterina, R., 2011. n-3 fatty acids in cardiovascular disease. N. Engl. J. Med. 23, 2439–2450.

Decensi, A., Puntoni, M., Goodwin, P., Cazzaniga, M., Gennari, A., Bonanni, B., Gandini, S., 2010. Metformin and cancer risk in diabetic patients: a systematic review and meta-analysis. Cancer Prev. Res. 3, 1451–1461.

Demierre, M.F., Higgins, P.D., Gruber, S.B., Hawk, E., Lippman, S.M., 2005. Statins and cancer prevention. Nat. Rev. Cancer 5, 930–942.

Diaz, G.D., Paraskeva, C., Thomas, M.G., Binderup, L., Hague, A., 2000. Apoptosis is induced by the active metabolite of Vitamin D3 and its analogue EB1089 in colorectal adenoma and car-cinoma cells: possible implications for prevention and therapy. Cancer Res. 60, 2304–2312.

Donato, F., Gelatti, U., Limina, R.M., Fattovich, G., 2006. Southern Europe as an example of interaction between various environmental factors: a systematic review of the epidemiologic evidence. Oncogene 25, 3756–3770.

Droge, W., 2002. Free radicals in the physiological control of cell function. Physiol. Rev. 82, 47–95.

Dyck, M.C., Ma, D.W., Meckling, K.A., 2011. The anticancer effects of Vitamin D and omega-3 PUFAs in combination via cod-liver oil: one plus one may equal more than two. Med. Hypotheses 77, 326–332.

Dyerberg, J., Bang, H.O., 1980. All cis-5, 8, 11, 14, 17 eicosapentaenoic acid and triene prostaglandins: potential anti-thrombotic agents. Scand. J. Clin. Lab. Invest. 40, 589–593.

Dyerberg, J., Bang, H.O., Hjorne, N., 1975. Fatty acid composition of the plasma lipids in Greenland Eskimos. Am. J. Clin. Nutr. 28, 958–966.

Egner, P.A., Wang, J.B., Zhu, Y.R., Zhang, B.C., Wu, Y., Zhang, Q.N., Qian, G.S., Kuang, S.Y., Gange, S.J., Jacobson, L.P., Helzlsouer, K.J., Bailey, G.S., Groopman, J.D., Kensler, T.W., 2001. Chlorophyllin intervention reduces aflatoxin-DNA adducts in individuals at high risk for liver cancer. Proc. Natl. Acad. Sci. 98, 14601–14606.

El-Serag, H.B., Johnson, M.L., Hachem, C., Morgana, R.O., 2009. Statins are associated with a reduced risk of hepatocellular carcinoma in a large cohort of patients with diabetes. Gastroen-terology 136, 1601–1608.

Emberson, J.R., Kearney, P.M., Blackwell, L., Newman, C., Reith, C., Bhala, N., Holland, L., Peto, R., Keech, A., Collins, R., Simes, J., Baigent, C., 2012. Lack of effect of lowering LDL cholesterol on cancer: meta-analysis of individual data from 175,000 people in 27 randomised trials of statin therapy. PLoS One 7, e29849.

Falk, G.W., Buttar, N.S., Foster, N.R., Ziegler, K.L., Demars, C.J., Romero, Y., Marcon, N.E., Schnell, T., Corley, D.A., Sharma, P., Cruz-Correa, M.R., Hur, C., Fleischer, D.E., Chak, A., Devault, K.R., Weinberg, D.S., Della'Zanna, G., Richmond, E., Smyrk, T.C., Mandrekar, S.J., Limburg, P.J., Cancer Prevention Network, 2012. A combination of esomeprazole and aspirin reduces tissue concentrations of prostaglandin E(2) in patients with Barrett's esophagus. Gastroenterology 143, 917–926, e-911.

Fattovich, G., Bortolotti, F., Donato, F., 2008. Natural history of chronic hepatitis B: special emphasis on disease progression and prognostic factors. J. Hepatol. 48, 335–352.

Fodor, J.G., Helis, E., Yazdekhasti, N., Vohnout, B., 2014. "Fishing" for the origins of the "Eskimos and heart disease" story: facts or wishful thinking? Can. J. Cardiol. 30, 864–868.

Form, D.M., Auerbach, R., 1983. PGE2 and angiogenesis. Proc. Soc. Exp. Biol. Med. 172, 214–218.

Gandini, S., Botteri, E., Iodice, S., Boniol, M., Lowenfels, A.B., Maisonneuve, P., Boyle, P., 2008. Tobacco smoking and cancer: a meta-analysis. Int. J. Cancer 122, 155–164.

Gao, M., Sun, K., Guo, M., Gao, H., Liu, K., Yang, C., Li, S., Liu, N., 2015. Fish consumption and n-3 polyunsaturated fatty acids, and risk of hepatocellular carcinoma: systematic review and metaanalysis. Cancer Causes Control 26, 367–376.

Gelatti, U., Covolo, L., Franceschini, M., Pirali, F., Tagger, A., Ribero, M.L., Trevisi, P., Martelli, C., Nardi, G., Donato, F., 2005. Coffee consumption reduces the risk of hepatocellular carcinoma independently of its aetiology: a case–control study. J. Hepatol. 42, 528–534.

Gleissman, H., Yang, R., Martinod, K., Lindskog, M., Serhan, C.N., Johnsen, J.I., Kogner, P., 2010. Docosahexaenoic acid metabolome in neural tumors: identification of cytotoxic intermediates. FASEB J. 24, 906–915.

Griffitts, J., Saunders, D., Tesiram, Y.A., Reid, G.E., Salih, A., Liu, S., Lydic, T.A., Busik, J.V., Kang, J.X., Towner, R.A., 2010. Non-mammalian fat-1 gene prevents neoplasia when introduced to a mouse hepatocarcinogene-sis model: omega-3 fatty acids prevent liver neoplasia. Biochim. Biophys. Acta 1801, 1133–1144.

Hajjaji, N., Bougnoux, P., 2013. Selective sensitization of tumors to chemotherapy by marine-derived lipids: a review. Cancer Treat Rev. 39, 473–488.

Hanahan, D., Weinberg, R.A., 2011. Hallmarks of cancer: the next generation. Cell 144, 646–674.

Hanai, T., Hashimoto, T., Nishiwaki, K., Ono, M., Akamo, Y., Tanaka, M., Mizuno, I., Yura, J., 1993. Comparison of prostanoids and their precursor fatty acids in human hepatocellular carcinoma and noncancerous reference tissues. J. Surg. Res. 54, 57–60.

Hardman, W.E., 2002. Omega-3 fatty acids to augment cancer therapy. J. Nutr. 132, 3508S–3512S.

Hosaka, T., Suzuki, F., Kobayashi, M., Seko, Y., Kawamura, Y., Sezaki, H., Akuta, N., Suzuki, Y., Saitoh, S., Arase, Y., Ikeda, K., Kobayashi, M., Kumada, H., 2013. Long-term entecavir treatment reduces hepatocellular carcinoma incidence in patients with hepatitis B virus infection. Hepatology 58, 98–107.

Hsu, Y.C., Ho, H.J., Wu, M.S., Lin, J.T., Wu, C.Y., 2013. Postoperative peg-interferon plus rib-avirin is associated with reduced recurrence of hepatitis C virus-related hepatocellular carcinoma. Hepatology 58, 150–157.

Huang, Y.W., Yang, S.S., Kao, J.H., 2010. Pathogenesis and management of alcoholic liver cirrhosis: a review. Hepat. Med. Evid. Res. 2011, 1–11.

Hull, M.A., 2011. Omega-3 polyunsaturated fatty acids. Best Pract. Res. Clin. Gastroenterol. 25, 547–554.

Inoue, M., Yoshimi, I., Sobue, T., Tsugane, S., 2005. Influence of coffee drinking on subsequent risk of hepatocellular carcinoma: a prospective study in Japan. J. Natl. Cancer Inst. 97, 293–300.

Institute for Healthcare Informatics, 2011. The Use of Medicines in the United States: Review of 2010. http://www.imshealth.com/imshealth/Glob-al/Content/IMS%20Institute/Documents/IHII_UseOfMed_report%20.pdf

International Agency for Research on Cancer, 2004. Tobacco smoke, in: IARC Monograph on the Evaluation of Carcinogenic Risks to Humans, vol. 83. In: Tobacco Smoke and Involuntary Smoking, IARC, Lyon, pp. 1–1438.

Ishii, H., Horie, Y., Ohshima, S., Anezaki, Y., Kinoshita, N., Dohmen, T., Kataoka, E., Sato, W., Goto, T., Sasaki, J., Sasaki, T., Watanabe, S., Suzuki, A., Ohnishi, H., 2009. Eicosapentaenoic acid ameliorates steatohepatitis and hepatocellular carcinoma in hepatocyte-specific Pten-deficient mice. J. Hepatol. 50, 562–571.

Istfan, N.W., Person, K.S., Holick, M.F., Chen, T.C., 2007. 1α, 25-dihydroxyvitamin D and fish oil synergistically inhibit G(1)/S-phase transition in prostate cancer cells. J. Steroid Biochem. Mol. Biol. 103, 726–730.

Jing, K., Song, K.S., Shin, S., Kim, N., Jeong, S., Oh, H.R., Park, J.H., Seo, K.S., Heo, J.Y., Han, J., Park, J.I., Han, C., Wu, T., Kweon, G.R., Park, S.K., Yoon, W.H., Hwang, B.D., Lim, K., 2011. Docosahexaenoic acid induces autophagy through p53/AMPK/mTOR signaling and promotes apoptosis in human cancer cells harboring wild-type p53. Autophagy 7, 1348–1358.

Kanno, S., Kurauchi, K., Tomizawa, A., Yomogida, S., Ishikawa, M., 2011. Albumin modulates docosahexaenoic acid-induced cytotoxicity in human hepatocellular carcinoma cell lines. Toxicol. Lett. 200, 154–161.

Kawaratani, H., Tsujimoto, T., Douhara, A., Takaya, H., Moriya, K., Namisaki, T., Noguchi, R., Yoshiji, H., Fujimoto, M., Fukui, H., 2013. The effect of inflammatory cytokines in alcoholic liver disease. Mediators Inflamm. 2013, 495156.

Kensler, T.W., Chen, J.G., Egner, P.A., Fahey, J.W., Jacobson, L.P., Stephenson, K.K., Ye, L., Coady, J.L., Wang, J.B., Wu, Y., Sun, Y., Zhang, Q.N., Zhang, B.C., Zhu, Y.R., Qian, G.S., Carmella, S.G., Hecht, S.S., Benning, L., Gange, S.J., Groopman, J.D., Talalay, P., 2005. Effects of glucosinolate-rich broccoli sprouts on urinary levels of aflatoxin- DNA adducts and phenan-threne tetraols in a randomized clinical trial in He Zuo township, Qidong, People's Republic of China. Cancer Epidemiol. Biomarkers Prev. 14, 2605–2613.

Kensler, T.W., Egner, P.A., Agyeman, A.S., Visvanathan, K., Groopman, J.D., Chen, J.G., Chen, T.Y., Fahey, J.W., Talalay, P., 2013. Keap1-nrf2 signaling: a target for cancer prevention by sul-foraphane. Top Curr. Chem. 329, 163–177.

Kim, H., Vosseler, C.A., Weber, P.C., Erl, W., 2005. Docosahexaenoic acid induces apoptosis in proliferating human endothelial cells. J. Cell Physiol. 204, 881–888.

Kris-Etherton, P.M., Harris, W.S., Appel, L.J., 2002. Fish consumption, fish oil, omega-3 fatty acids and cardiovascular disease. Circulation 106, 2747–2757.

Krishnan, A.V., Moreno, J., Nonn, L., Malloy, P., Swami, S., Peng, L., Peehl, D.M., Feldman, D., 2007. Novel pathways that contribute to the anti-proliferative and chemopreventive activities of calcitriol in prostate cancer. J. Steroid Biochem. Mol. Biol. 103, 694–702.

Kromhout, D., Giltay, E.J., Geleijnse, J.M., 2010. n-3 fatty acids and cardiovascular events after myocardial infarction. New England J. Med. 363, 2015–2016.

Kwak, S.M., Myung, S.K., Lee, Y.J., Seo, H.G. Korean Metaanalysis Study Group. Efficacy of omega-3 fatty acid supplements (eicosapentaenoic acid and docosahexaenoic acid) in the secondary prevention of cardiovascular disease: a meta-analysis of randomized, double-blind, placebo-controlled trials. Arch Intern Med. 172, pp. 686–694.

La Vecchia, C., 2005. Coffee, liver enzymes, cirrhosis and liver cancer. J. Hepatol. 42, 444–446.

La Vecchia, C., 2007. Alcohol and liver cancer. Eur. J. Cancer Prev. 16, 495–497.

Lai, C.L., Yuen, M.F., 2013. Prevention of hepatitis B virus-related hepatocellular carcinoma with anti-viral therapy. Hepatology 57, 399–408.

Lambert, J.R., Kelly, J.A., Shim, M., Huffer, W.E., Nordeen, S.K., Baek, S.J., Eling, T.E., Lucia, M.S., 2006. Prostate derived factor in human prostate cancer cells: gene induction by vitamin D via a p53-dependent mechanism and inhibition of prostate cancer cell growth. J. Cell Physiol. 208, 566–574.

Lappe, J.M., Heaney, R.P., 2012. Why randomized controlled trials of calcium and vitamin D sometimes fail. Dermatoendocrinol. 4, 95–100.

Lee, J.Y., Plakidas, A., Lee, W.H., Heikkinen, A., Chanmugam, P., Bray, G., Hwang, D.H., 2003. Differential modulation of Toll-like receptors by fatty acids: preferential inhibition by n-3 polyunsaturated fatty acids. J. Lipid Res. 44, 479–486.

Lee, C.Y., Sit, W.H., Fan, S.T., Man, K., Jor, I.W., Wong, L.L., Wan, M.L., Tan-Un, K.C., Wan, J.M., 2010. The cell cycle effects of docosahexaenoic acid on human metastatic hepatocellular carcinoma proliferation. Int. J. Oncol. 36, 991–998.

Levy, J.R., Clore, J.N., Stevens, W., 2004. Dietary n-3 polyunsaturated fatty acids decrease hepatic triglycerides in Fischer 344 rats. Hepatology 39, 608–616.

Li, S., Qin, J., Tian, C., Cao, J., Fida, G., Wang, Z., Chen, H., Qian, Z., Chen, W.R., Gu, Y., 2014. The targeting mechanism of DHA ligand and its conjugate with Gemcitabine for the enhanced tumor therapy. Onco. target 15, 3622–3635.

Liaw, Y.F., Sung, J.J., Chow, W.C., Farrell, G., Lee, C.Z., Yuen, H., Tanwandee, T., Tao, Q.M., Shue, K., Keene, O.N., Dixon, J.S., Gray, D.F., Sabbat, J., 2004. Lamivudine for patients with chronic hepatitis B and advanced liver disease. New England J. Med. 7, 1521–1531.

Lim, K., Han, C., Dai, Y., Shen, M., Wu, T., 2009. Omega-3 polyunsaturated fatty acids inhibit hepatocellular carcinoma cell growth through blocking beta-catenin and cyclooxygenase-2. Mol. Cancer Ther. 8, 3046–3055.

Llovet, J.M., Burroughs, A., Bruix, J., 2003. Hepatocellular carcinoma. Lancet 6, 1907–1917.

Marcelli, M., Cunningham, G.R., Haidacher, S.J., Padayatty, S.J., Sturgis, L., Kagan, C., Denner, L., 1998. Caspase-7 is activated during lovastatin-induced apoptosis of the prostate cancer cell line LNCaP. Cancer Res. 58, 76–83.

Marchioli, R., Levantesi, G., 2013. N-3 PUFAs in cardiovascular disease. Int. J. Cardiol. 170, S33–S38.

Maruyama, R., Aoki, F., Toyota, M., Sasaki, Y., Akashi, H., Mita, H., Suzuki, H., Akino, K., Ohe-Toyota, M., Maruyama, Y., Tatsumi, H., Imai, K., Shinomura, Y., Tokino, T., 2006. Comparative genome analysis identifies the vitamin D receptor gene as a direct target of p53-mediated transcriptional activation. Cancer Res. 66, 4574–4583.

Masterton, G.S., Plevris, J.N., Hayes, P.C., 2010. Omega-3 fatty acids - a promising novel therapy for non-alcoholic fatty liver disease. Aliment Pharmacol. Ther. 31, 679–692.

McCarty, M.F., 1996. Fish oil may impede tumour angiogenesis and invasiveness by down-regulating protein kinase C and modulating eicosanoid production. Med. Hypotheses 46, 107–115.

Meckling, K.A., 2007. Nutrient and Phytochemical Modulation of Cancer Therapy. In: Meckling, K.A. (Ed.), Nutrient-Drug Interactions. Taylor and Francis, Boca Raton, pp. 108–113.

Michelotti, G.A., Machado, M.V., Diehl, A.M., 2013. NAFLD, NASH and liver cancer. Nat. Rev. Gastroenterol. Hepatol. 10, 656–665.

Montain, S., 2015. Experimental Biology.

Morgan, T.R., Ghany, M.G., Kim, H.Y., Snow, K.K., Shiffman, M.L., De Santo, J.L., Lee, W.M., Di Bisceglie, A.M., Bonkovsky, H.L., Dienstag, J.L., Morishima, C., Lindsay, K.L., Lok, A.S., 2010. Outcome of sustained virological responders with histologically advanced chronic hepatitis C. Hepatology 52, 833–844.

Morgan, R.L., Baack, B., Smith, B.D., Yartel, A., Pitasi, M., Falck-Ytter, Y., 2013. Eradication of hepatitis C virus infection and the development of hepatocellular carcinoma: a meta-analysis of observational studies. Ann. Intern. Med. 158, 329–337.

Nagpa, S., Na, S., Rathnachalan, R., 2005. Noncalcemic actions of vitamin D receptor ligands. Endocr. Rev. 26, 662–687.

Narayanan, B.A., Narayanan, N.K., Reddy, B.S., 2001. Docosahexaenoic acid regulated genes and transcription factors inducing apoptosis in human colon cancer cells. Int. J. Oncol. 19, 1255–1262.

Noguchi, M., Rose, D.P., Earashi, M., Miyazaki, I., 1995. The role of fatty acids and eicosanoid synthesis inhibitors in breast carcinoma. Oncology 52, 265–267.

Nonn, L., Peng, L., Feldman, D., Peehl, D.M., 2006. Inhibition of p38 by vitamin D reduces interleukin-6 production in normal prostate cells via mitogen-activated protein kinase phosphatase 5: implications for prostate cancer prevention by vitamin D. Cancer Res. 66, 4516–4524.

Norrish, A.E., Skeaff, C.M., Arribas, G.L., Sharpe, S.J., Jackson, R.T., 1999. Prostate cancer risk and consumption of fish oils: a dietary biomarker-based case-control study. Br. J. Cancer 81, 1238–1242.

Okumura, T., 2010. Mechanisms by which thiazolidinediones induce anti-cancer effects in cancers in digestive organs. J. Gastroenterol. 45, 1097–1102.

ORIGIN Trial investigators, Bosch, J., et al., 2012. N-3 Fatty acids and cardiovascular outcomes in patients with dysglycemia. New England J. Med. 367, 309–318.

Orman, E.S., Odena, G., Bataller, R., 2013. Alcoholic liver disease: pathogenesis, management, and novel targets for therapy. J. Gastroenterol. Hepatol. 28, 77–84.

Parker, H.M., Johnson, N.A., Burdon, C.A., Cohn, J.S., O'Connor, H.T., George, J., 2012. Omega-3 supplementation and non-alcoholic fatty liver disease: a systematic review and meta-analysis. J. Hepatol. 56, 944–951.

Paula, H., Asrani, S.K., Boetticher, N.C., Pedersen, R., Shah, V.H., Kim, W.R., 2010. Alcoholic liver disease-related mortality in the United States: 1980–2003. Am. J. Gastroenterol. 105, 1782–1787.

Poulsen, M.M., Vestergaard, P.F., Clasen, B.F., Radko, Y., Christensen, L.P., Stødkilde-Jørgensen, H., Møller, N., Jessen, N., Pedersen, S.B., Jørgensen, J.O., 2013. High-dose resvera-trol supplementation in obese men: an investigator- initiated, randomized, placebo-controlled clinical trial of substrate metabolism, insulin sensitivity, and body composition. Diabetes 62, 1186–1195.

Rao, S., Porter, D.C., Chen, X., Herliczek, T., Lowe, M., Keyomarsi, K., 1999. Lovastatin-mediated G1 arrest is through inhibition of the proteasome, independent of hydroxymethyl glutaryl-CoA reductase. Proc. Natl. Acad. Sci. 96, 7797–7802.

Rauch, B., Schiele, R., Schneider, S., Diller, F., Victor, N., 2010. OMEGA, a randomized, placebo-controlled trial to test the effect of highly purified omega-3 fatty acids on top of modern guideline-adjusted therapy after myocardial infarction. Circulation 122, 2152–2159.

Raza, A., Sood, G.K., 2014. Hepatocellular carcinoma review: current treatment, and evidence-based medicine. World J. Gastroenterol. 20, 4115–4127.

Reddy, B.S., 1994. Chemoprevention of colon cancer by dietary fatty acids. Cancer Metastasis Rev. 13, 285–302.

Rehermann, B., Nascimbeni, M., 2005. Immunology of hepatitis B virus and hepatitis C virus infection. Nature Rev. Immunol. 5, 215–229.

Rizos, E.C., Ntzani, E.E., Bika, E., Kostapanos, M.S., Elisaf, M.S., 2012. Association between omega-3 fatty acid supplementation and risk of major cardiovascular disease events: a systematic review and meta-analysis. JAMA 308, 1024–1033.

Roncaglioni, M.C., Tombesi, M., Silletta, M.G., 2013. n-3 fatty acids in patients with cardiac risk factors. New England J. Med. 369, 781–782.

Rovito, D., Giordano, C., Vizza, D., Plastina, P., Barone, I., Casaburi, I., Lanzino, M., De Amicis, F., Sisci, D., Mauro, L., Aquila, S., Catalano, S., Bonofiglio, D., Ando, S., 2013. Omega-3 PUFA ethanolamides DHEA and EPEA induce autophagy through PPARγ activation in MCF-7 breast cancer cells. J. Cell Physiol. 228, 1314–1322.

Rubio, N., Coupienne, I., Di Valentin, E., Heirman, I., Grooten, J., Piette, J., Agostinis, P., 2012. Spatiotemporal autophagic degradation of oxidatively damaged organelles after photody-namic stress is amplified by mitochondrial reactive oxygen species. Autophagy 8, 1312–1324.

Sahasrabuddhe, V.V., Gunja, M.Z., Graubard, B.I., Trabert, B., Schwartz, L.M., Park, Y., Hollenbeck, A.R., Freedman, N.D., McGlynn, K.A., 2012. Nonsteroidal anti- inflammatory drug use, chronic liver disease, and hepatocellular carcinoma. J. Natl. Cancer Inst. 104, 1808–1814.

Sarrazin, C., Hezode, C., Zeuzem, S., Pawlotsky, J.M., 2012. Antiviral strategies in hepatitis C virus infection. J. Hepatol. 56, S88–S100.

Sasazuki, S., Inoue, M., Iwasaki, M., Sawada, N., Shimazu, T., Yamaji, T., Takachi, R., Tsugane, S., 2011. Intake of n-3 and n-6 polyunsaturated fatty acids and development of colorectal cancer by subsite: Japan public health center-based prospective study. Int. J. Cancer 129, 1718–1729.

Sawada, N., Inoue, M., Iwasaki, M., Sasazuki, S., Shimazu, T., Yamaji, T., Takachi, R., Tanaka, Y., Mizokami, M., Tsugane, S., 2012. Consumption of n-3 fatty acids and fish reduces risk of hepatocellular carcinoma. Gastroenterology 142, 1468–1475.

Schmitt, C.A., Fridman, J.S., Yang, M., Baranov, E., Hoffman, R.M., Lowe, S.W., 2002. Dissecting p53 tumor sup-pressor functions in vivo. Cancer Cell 1, 289–298.

Simopoulos, A.P., 1986. Summary of the conference on the health effects of polyunsaturated fatty acids in seafoods. J. Nutr. 116, 2350–2354.

Singh, S., Singh, A.G., Singh, P.P., Murad, M.H., Iyer, P.G., 2013a. Statins are associated with reduced risk of esophageal cancer, particularly in patients with Barrett's esophagus: a systematic review and meta-analysis. Clin. Gastroenterol. Hepatol. 11, 620–629.

Singh, S., Singh, P.P., Singh, A.G., Murad, M.H., Sanchez, W., 2013b. Statins are associated with a reduced risk of hepatocellular cancer: a systematic review and meta-analysis. Gastroenterology 144, 323–332.

Sitia, G., Aiolfi, R., Di Lucia, P., Mainetti, M., Fiocchi, A., Mingozzi, F., Esposito, A., Ruggeri, Z.M., Chisari, F.V., Iannacone, M., Guidotti, L.G., 2012. Antiplatelet therapy prevents hepatocellular carcinoma and improves survival in a mouse model of chronic hepatitis B. Proc. Natl. Acad. Sci. 109, E2165–E2172.

Smith, W.L., 2005. Cyclooxygenases, peroxide tone and the allure of fish oil. Curr. Opin. Cell Biol. 7, 174–182.

Smith, L.C., Dauchy, E.M., Dauchy, R.T., Sauer, L.A., Blask, D.E., Davidson, L.K., Krause, J.A., Lynch, D.T., 2006. Dietary fish oil deactivates a growth-promoting signaling pathway in hepatoma 7288CTC in Buffalo rats. Nutr. Cancer 56, 204–213.

Soni, K.B., Lahiri, M., Chackradeo, P., Bhide, S.V., Kuttan, R., 1997. Protective effect of food additives on aflatoxin-induced mutagenicity and hepatocarcinogenicity. Cancer Lett. 115, 129–133.

Storlien, L.H., Kraegen, E.W., Chisholm, D.J., Ford, G.L., Bruce, D.G., Pascoe, W.S., 1987. Fish oil prevents insulin resistance induced by high-fat feeding in rats. Science 237, 885–888.

Stubbs, C.D., Smith, A.D., 1984. The modification of mammalian membrane polyunsaturated fatty acid composition in relation to membrane fluidity and function. Biochim. Biophys. Acta 27, 89–137.

Sun, S.N., Jia, W.D., Chen, H., Ma, J.L., Ge, Y.S., Yu, J.H., Li, J.S., 2013. Docosahexaenoic acid (DHA) induces apoptosis in human hepatocellular carcinoma cells. Int. J. Clin. Exp. Pathol. 6, 281–289.

Sung, J.J., Tsoi, K.K., Wong, V.W., Li, K.C., Chan, H.L., 2008. Meta-analysis: treatment of hepatitis B infection reduces risk of hepatocellular carcinoma. Aliment Pharmacol. Ther. 28, 1067–1077.

Tanaka, T., Nishikawa, A., Shima, H., Sugie, S., Shinoda, T., Yoshimi, N., 1990. Inhibitory effects of chlorogenic acid, reserpine, polyprenoic acid (E-5166), or coffee on hepatocarcinogenesis in rats and hamsters. Basic Life Sci. 52, 429–440.

Tanaka, N., Sano, K., Horiuchi, A., Tanaka, E., Kiyosawa, K., Aoyama, T., 2008. Highly purified eicosapentaenoic acid treatment improves nonalcoholic steatohepatitis. J. Clin. Gastroenterol. 42, 413–418.

Tao, K.S., Wang, W., Wang, L., Cao, D.Y., Li, Y.Q., Wu, S.X., Dou, K.F., 2008. The multifac-eted mechanisms for coffee's anti-tumorigenic effect on liver. Med. Hypotheses 71, 730–736.

Terano, T., Tanaka, T., Tamura, Y., Kitagawa, M., Higashi, H., Saito, Y., Hirai, A., 1999. Eicosapentaenoic acid and docosahexaenoic acid inhibit vascular smooth muscle cell proliferation by inhibiting phosphorylation of Cdk2-cyclinE complex. Biochem. Biophys. Res. Commun. 19, 502–506.

Thun, M.J., Jacobs, E.J., Patrono, C., 2012. The role of aspirin in cancer prevention. Nat. Rev. Clin. Oncol. 9, 259–267.

Tilg, H., Moschen, A.R., 2010. Evolution of inflammation in nonalcoholic fatty liver disease: the multiple parallel hits hypothesis. Hepatology 52, 1836–1846.

Torres, D.M., Harrison, S.A., 2013. Is it time to write a prescription for coffee? Coffee and liver disease. Gastroenterology 144, 670–672.

Tsan, Y.T., Lee, C.H., Wang, J.D., Chen, P.C., 2012. Statins and the risk of hepatocellular carcinoma in patients with hepatitis B virus infection. J. Clin. Oncol. 30, 623–630.

Tsan, Y.T., Lee, C.H., Ho, W.C., Lin, M.H., Wang, J.D., Chen, P.C., 2013. Statins and the risk of hepatocellular carcinoma in patients with hepatitis C virus infection. J. Clin. Oncol. 31, 1514–1521.

Vanden Heuvel, J.P., 2012. Nutrigenomics and nutrigenetics of ω3 polyunsaturated fatty acids. Prog. Mol. Biol. Transl. Sci. 108, 75–112.

Wendel, M., Heller, A.R., 2009. Anticancer actions of omega-3 fatty acids–current state and future perspectives. Anticancer Agents Med. Chem. 9, 457–470.

Weylandt, K.H., Krause, L.F., Gomolka, B., Chiu, C.Y., Bilal, S., Nadolny, A., Waechter, S.F., Fischer, A., Rothe, M., Kang, J.X., 2011. Suppressed liver tumorigenesis in fat-1 mice with elevated omega-3 fatty acids is associated with increased omega-3 derived lipid mediators and reduced TNF-α. Carcinogenesis 32, 897–903.

Wree, A., Broderick, L., Canbay, A., Hoffman, H.M., Feldstein, A.E., 2013. From NAFLD to NASH to cirrhosis-new insights into disease mechanisms. Nat. Rev. Gastroenterol. Hepatol. 10, 627–636.

Wu, J., Wong, W.W., Khosravi, F., Minden, M.D., Penn, L.Z., 2004. Blocking the Raf/MEK/ERK path-way sensitizes acute myelogenous leukemia cells to lovastatin-induced apoptosis. Cancer Res. 64, 6461–6468.

Wu, C.W., Farrell, G.C., Yu, J., 2012a. Functional role of peroxisome-proliferator-activated receptor γ in hepatocellular carcinoma. J. Gastroenterol. Hepatol. 27, 1665–1669.

Wu, Z., Qin, J., Pu, L., 2012b. Omega-3 fatty acid improves the clinical outcome of hepatectomized patients with hepatitis B virus (HBV)-associated hepatocellular carcinoma. J. Biomed. Res. 26, 395–399.

Yang, J.D., Roberts, L.R., 2010. Hepatocellular carcinoma: a global view. Nat. Rev. Gastroenterol. Hepatol. 7, 448–458.

Yao, Q.H., Zhang, X.C., Fu, T., Gu, J.Z., Wang, L., Wang, Y., Lai, Y.B., Wang, Y.Q., Guo, Y., 2014. Omega-3 polyunsaturated fatty acids inhibit the proliferation of the lung adenocarcinoma cell line A549 in vitro. Mol. Med. Rep. 9, 401–406.

Ylikomi, T., Laaksi, I., Lou, Y.R., Martikainen, P., Miettinen, S., Pennanen, P., Purmonen, S., Syvälä, H., Vienonen, A., Tuohimaa, P., 2002. Antiproliferative action of vitamin D. Vitamins Hormones 64, 357–406.

Zhang, C.H., Xu, G.L., Jia, W.D., Li, J.S., Ma, J.L., Ge, Y.S., 2011. Effects of interferon treatment on development and progression of hepatocellular carcinoma in patients with chronic virus infection: a meta-analysis of randomized con-trolled trials. Int. J. Cancer 129, 1254–1264.

Zhang, W., Shu, X.O., Li, H., Yang, G., Cai, H., Ji, B.T., Gao, J., Gao, Y.T., Zheng, W., Xiang, Y.B., 2012. Vitamin intake and liver cancer risk: a report from two cohort studies in China. J. Natl. Cancer Inst. 104, 1173–1181.

Zhang, Y., Han, L., Qi, W., Cheng, D., Ma, X., Hou, L., Cao, X., Wang, C., 2015. Eicosapentaenoic acid (EPA) induced apoptosis in HepG2 cells through ROS-Ca (2 +)-JNK mitochondrial pathways. Biochem. Biophys. Res. Commun. 24, 926–932.

Zhong, J.H., Mo, X.S., Xiang, B.D., Yuan, W.P., Jiang, J.F., Xie, G.S., Li, L.Q., 2013. Postop-erative use of the chemopreventive vitamin K2 analog in patients with hepatocellular carcinoma. PLoS ONE 8, e58082.

Zhou, G., Myers, R., Li, Y., Chen, Y., Shen, X., Fenyk-Melody, J., Wu, M., Ventre, J., Doebber, T., Fujii, N., Musi, N., Hirshman, M.F., Goodyear, L.J., Moller, D.E., 2001. Role of AMP-activated protein kinase in mechanism of metformin action. J. Clin. Invest. 108, 1167–1174.

CHAPTER

24

Brain, Fish Oil-Enriched Diet, and Sphingolipids

N.A. Babenko

Department of Physiology of Ontogenesis, Institute of Biology, Kharkov Karazin National University, Kharkov, Ukraine

INTRODUCTION

The n–3 polyunsaturated fatty acids (n–3 PUFAs) are critical contributors to cell structure and function in the nervous system and essential for development of the central nervous system (Kidd, 2007; Sinclair et al., 2007; Lukiw and Bazan, 2008; Kim, 2008.). The n–3 PUFAs are important components of fish and fish oil. Dietary n–3 PUFAs can be rapidly accumulated into cellular phospholipids and affect a variety of membrane and cell functions. Docosahexaenoic acid (DHA) prevents apoptotic death of neuronal cells induced by serum starvation (Kim et al., 2000). DHA, increasing the phosphatidylserine (PS) content in the neuronal cells, initiates the interaction of the serine threonine kinase Akt with the plasma membrane and facilitates its translocation and phosphorylation, thus promoting the cell survival (Akbar et al., 2005). DHA is also required for the survival of retinal photoreceptors. By enhancing Bcl-2 expression and reducing the proapoptotic lipid ceramide levels, DHA prevents oxidative stress-induced apoptosis of photoreceptor and amacrine neurons (Rotstein et al., 1996). Increased dietary intake of n–3 PUFA reduces oxygen induced retinopathy, due at least in part, to suppression of the retinal inflammatory cytokine, TNFα. Moreover, adding DHA to a culture media of human retinal endothelial cells downregulates the basal and TNFα- or IL-1β-induced acid sphingomyelinase (ASMase) and neutral sphingomyelinase (NSMase) expression and activity (Opreanu et al., 2010). It is worth noting that due to activation of ASMase/NSMase activity the local concentration of proinflammatory and proapoptotic sphingolipid, ceramide, is dramatically increasing (Grassme et al., 2007; Holopainen et al., 1998; Kolesnick et al., 2000; Nurminen et al., 2002). The generation of ceramide-enriched membrane microdomains may be a critical factor for receptor clustering and downstream signaling. Clustering is shown to be important for several receptors that mediate inflammatory TNFα- and IL-1β-dependent signaling pathways in diabetic retinopathy (Ko et al., 1999; Martin and Wesche, 2002). Thus, it becomes evident that DHA, decreasing the ceramide production, can distract cytokine signaling in retina cells.

DHA supplementation prevented hippocampal cell death induced by ischemia–reperfusion (Cao et al., 2004). Adding DHA to the culture media significantly reduced apoptotic cell death in n–3 fatty acid-deficient embryonic hippocampal cultures (Akbar et al., 2005). In the Neuro 2A cells and embryonic hippocampal cultures the anti-apoptotic effect of DHA has been found to depend on its ability to suppress the caspase-3 activation and to induce the PS-dependent acceleration of protein kinase Akt translocation to membranes (Akbar et al., 2006; Kim et al., 2000).

A deficit in dietary DHA, the major n–3 fatty acid found in brain, contributes to inflammation, apoptosis, neuronal dysfunction, and neurological disorders. Memory deficit (Gamoh et al., 1999), learning disability (Yoshida et al., 1997; Carrie et al., 1999) and loss of visual activity (Neuringer, 2000) are often associated with n–3 PUFA deficiency. Interrelationship between n–3 PUFA intake and risk of cognitive impairment was determined in humans (Cherubini et al., 2007). Generalized peroxisomal disorders and Alzheimer's disease are associated with low levels of DHA in brain (Martinez, 1990; Soderberg et al., 1991). In patients with Alzheimer's disease the low level of n–3 PUFA in blood serum and cells was found to be responsible for a higher risk of memory loss and cognitive dysfunction (Conquer et al., 2000), while dietary supply of DHA reduced neuronal injury in Alzheimer's disease

Fish and Fish Oil in Health and Disease Prevention. http://dx.doi.org/10.1016/B978-0-12-802844-5.00024-5

(Calon et al., 2004) and brain ischemia (Choi-Kwon et al., 2004; Okada et al., 1996), and improved some symptoms in patients with peroxisomal disorders (Martínez et al., 2000). Fish oil supplementation improved the reference memory or working memory in DHA-deficient state (Chung et al., 2008), normalized an age-related decrease of cognitive function and ceramide content and resulted in a production of new polyunsaturated PS species in the brain cortex and hippocampus (Babenko and Semenova, 2008, 2010). Moreover, feeding old rats with a fish oil-enriched diet prevented the development of spontaneous amyloidosis (Firląg et al., 2015). Fish oil supplementation avoided amyloid-β deposition on the cerebral vessel walls and in the brain cortex degenerating neuronal structures, as well as in microglia and astrocytes. Thus, it becomes evident that n–3 PUFA, and especially DHA, were shown to be extremely important in the neuronal cells survival under extreme conditions and brain functioning. The beneficial actions of n–3 PUFA on neuronal cells and brain structures which is often associated with reduction of elevated level of proapoptotic and proinflammatory sphingolipid and ceramide at pathological states, the effects of dietetic n–3 PUFA on sphingolipid turnover in the hippocampus and brain cortex, and cognitive dysfunction have all been analyzed in the present Chapter. Much attention was given to the improvement of the age-dependent and age-associated brain pathologies by dietetic fish oil. The mechanism triggering sphingolipid metabolism in the neuronal cells by fish oil n–3 fatty acids has been discussed.

SPHINGOLIPID TURNOVER AND BRAIN PATHOLOGY

Sphingolipids are structural components of biological membranes and involved in the regulation of cell growth and death. Defects in sphingolipid metabolism contribute to the development of many pathological states. Disruptions in sphingolipid turnover and ceramide accumulations have been recently reported in individuals with Alzheimer's disease, amyotrophic lateral sclerosis, and HIV-associated dementia (Cutler et al. 2002, 2004; Haughey et al. 2004). Sphingolipids, such as ceramides, represent a novel class of bioeffector molecules, participating in raft formation and accumulating in the cell in response to the stress stimuli (Hannun and Obeid, 2002, 2008; Gault et al., 2010; Sawai and Hannun, 1999). Ceramides can be produced via intercellular de novo synthesis and SMases activation.

Mice with a transgene for ASMase (tgASM) showed a depression/anxiety-like phenotype, high ASM activity and ceramide accumulation in the hippocampus, as well as a decline of such depression-related neuronal markers, as neurogenesis, neuronal maturation and neuronal survival (Gulbins et al., 2013). Moreover, the dysregulation of hippocampal neurogenesis was associated with a reduction in Akt phosphorylation at Ser473, while PC12 cells with AktS473 mutation were resistant to inhibitory action of C16-ceramide on cell proliferation. Thus, negative effects of ceramide on hippocampal neurons can coincide with Akt inhibition. Direct injections of C16-ceramide into hippocampus of wild type mice caused ceramide accumulation, reduced rates of neuronal proliferation, maturation and survival and also lead to the development of depression-like behavior (Gulbins et al., 2013). A significant increase of ceramide content in the hippocampus' of wild type mice was observed, as well as in ASMase-deficient animals under chronic stress. Stress-induced ceramide accumulation was followed by reduction of neurogenesis and neuronal maturation and can be normalized in wild type, but not in ASMase-deficient mice by known functional inhibitors of ASMase (Albouz et al., 1986; Kornhuber et al., 2010, 2011), amitriptyline and fluoxetine. Moreover, the antidepressant drugs improved depression-like behavior in corticosterone-stressed mice.

It is noteworthy that elevated ceramide levels have been found in the white matter of patients with bipolar disorder (Schwarz et al., 2008) and in patients with a diagnosis of major depression, regardless of dementia status (Gracia-Garcia et al., 2011). In patients with Parkinson (Mielke et al., 2013) or other diseases, (Demirkan et al., 2013) increased ceramide levels are positively associated with depressive symptoms. Sphingolipid storage diseases, such as Tay–Sachs (MacQueen et al., 1998), Fabry (Cole et al., 2007; Laney et al., 2010; Sadek et al., 2004) and Gaucher (Packman et al., 2006), usually coincide with a depressive state. Ceramide accumulation and increased ASM activity were found in the blood of patients with post-traumatic stress disorder (Hammad et al., 2012) which is frequently associated with depression. In addition, activated ASMase activity has been found in the peripheral blood mononuclear cells of patients with major depressive disorder (Kornhuber et al., 2005). The ASMase activity was higher in patients with severe symptoms compared to other depressive patients. All together, these results strongly suggest the important role of ASMase/ceramide pathway in the development of depression-like behavior and in the dysregulation of such important hippocampal function as neurogenesis.

Ceramide levels in mammalian cells can be elevated by ceramide synthases, as well as NSMase activation. Ceramide synthase 1 is mainly expressed in the brain and catalyzes the synthesis of C18-ceramide. A spontaneous deficiency in ceramide synthase 1 activity in fincher mice and toppler mice resulted in reduced ceramide synthase 1 activity and C18-ceramide synthesis and C18-ceramide levels in the brain (Zhao et al., 2011). At the same time, ceramide synthase 1 deficiency was associated with elevated C14- and C16-ceramide content in the cerebellum, progressive ataxia and loss of cerebellar Purkinje cells. In addition, loss of ceramide synthase 1 led to storage of lipofuscin, usually present in aging brains and in brains of patients with neurodegenerative disorders. Intracerebroventricular administration of an inhibitor of ceramide synthase, fumonisin B1, caused acute neurodegeneration (Osuchowski et al., 2005). Using ceramide synthase 1-deficient mice, it has been demonstrated that synthesis of gangliosides and expression of myelin-associated glycoprotein in the cerebellum and forebrain were both significantly decreased (Ginkel et al., 2012). In aged, ceramide synthase 1-deficient mice a significant decrease in levels of C18 and all other molecular species of sphingomyelin and hexosylceramides as well as a decrease in the level of substrates of ceramide synthases, sphinganine and sphingosine, were observed. These animals exhibited significant atrophy of cerebellar hemispheres and reduced size of the cerebellum as well as behavioral deficits such as: impaired exploration of novel objects, impaired locomotion, and impaired motor coordination. All together, these results suggest that not only an accumulation of ceramide, but also the lack of production of its separate molecular species and other more complex sphingolipids, can be harmful for brain and neuronal functions.

A progressive increase in ceramide and a decrease of sphingomyelin levels in the hippocampus and neocortex of rats during aging has been evaluated (Babenko and Semenova, 2010; Babenko and Shakhova, 2014). Age-dependent sphingolipid turnover dysregulation in the hippocampus and neocortex coincided with elevation of NSMase, but not ASMase activity in brain structures. NSMase-mediated ceramide accumulation in the hippocampus and brain cortex stimulated the rate of β-amyloid peptide production at old age (Costantini et al., 2005a). Ceramide regulates both the amyloid precursor protein processing and β-amyloid peptide synthesis by affecting the β-secretase (BACE1) stability (Puglielli et al., 2003). The chronic treatment of old animals with inhibitors of NSMase, manumycin (Costantini et al., 2005b) or N-acetylcysteine (Babenko and Shakhova, 2014), leads to NSMase inhibition and prevents ceramide accumulation in the brain cortex and hippocampus of the aged animals, while the inhibitor of ASMase, imipramine, was not successful. However, treatment of hippocampal neurons by β-amyloid peptide activates the NSMase as well as ASMase (He et al., 2010). In contrast, the fibrillar β-amyloid peptide-activated astroglia kill neurons via NSMase but not ASMase (Jana and Pahan, 2010). Inhibition of NSMase by a specific inhibitor, GW4869, or knockdown of neutral SMase by antisense oligonucleotides prevented the induction of proinflammatory molecules, activation of nuclear factor-*k*B in the activated astroglia and protected neurons from fibrillar β-amyloid peptide-induced death.

IMPROVEMENT OF BRAIN SPHINGOLIPID METABOLISM AND FUNCTIONS BY N–3 FATTY ACIDS OF THE FISH OIL

Important roles of dietary n–3 PUFAs have been well documented in brain development, processes of neuroplasticity, and learning and memory (Chalon et al., 1998; Moriguchi et al., 2000; Innis, 2007). Moreover, n–3 PUFAs play a strong neuroprotective role (Okada et al., 1996; Wu et al., 2004; Adibhatla and Hatcher, 2008). Neuroprotective effects of n–3 PUFAs under conditions of traumatic and ischemic damage to the brain as well as alcohol intoxication are both mediated by stimulation of the expression of antioxidant enzymes (catalases, glutathione peroxidases, and superoxide dismutases), induction of a neurotrophic factor (Wu et al., 2004), anti-inflammatory cytokines production, and inhibition of phospholipase A2 (PLA2) (Adibhatla and Hatcher, 2008). DHA and its metabolites such as docosatrienes, resolvins, and protectins help to prevent apoptosis of neurons in the brain and retina induced by oxidative stress (Sinclair et al., 2007; Kidd, 2007). DHA increases conversion of ceramide to glucosylceramide and thus results in a drop in content of endogenous ceramides in neurons of the retina photoreceptor system and prevents death of these cells (German et al., 2006). As it is known that ceramides themselves are prooxidant molecules, it cannot be excluded that DHA protects neurons from oxidative stress-induced apoptosis by reducing ceramide content in neurons. Feeding adult ethanol-treated rats with fish oil significantly reduced elevated ceramide and sphingosine levels and increased the level of the newly synthesized SM in the hippocampus up to that observed in control animals (Babenko, 2013). Supplementation of dietary fish oil normalized the ethanol-induced decrease of cognitive function and gave rise to a production of PS species, enriched by n–3 PUFAs, in the brain cortex and hippocampus (Babenko and Semenova, 2008). Ethanol increases levels of cytokines (TNF-α and IL-1β in the brain, liver, and blood serum (Qin et al., 2008). Ethanol also decreased the amount of inhibitor of NSMase, glutathione, in the cells (Addolorato et al., 1997). It becomes evident that ethanol-induced modifications of sphingolipid turnover in the hippocampus are mediated by the cytokines- and redox status-dependent NSMase activation. Taking into consideration that n–3 PUFAs of fish oil can reduce both cytokine production and NSMase activity, it is believed that the neuroprotective actions of fish oil depends to a large extent on the degree of stimulation of the antioxidant enzyme expression (Wu et al., 2004) and suppression of proinflammatory cytokine production (Adibhatla et al., 2008) and consequent NSMase inhibition.

DHA levels decrease in the diabetic retina (Futterman and Kupfer, 1968; Tikhonenko et al., 2010) and increased dietary intake of n–3 PUFAs prevents retinopathy in both type 1 and 2 diabetes (Opreanu et al., 2011; Tikhonenko et al., 2013) and a model of retinopathy (Connor et al., 2007). DHA plays a more active, preventive role among the different n–3 PUFAs due to its ability to modulate the retina capillary integrity, neovascularization and inflammation (San Giovanni and Chew, 2005). Treatment of diabetic animals with a DHA-enriched diet not only improved retinal health, but rat lifespan as well. Moreover, the beneficial effects of dietary n–3 PUFAs on diabetic human survival has also been defined (Hu et al., 2003). As vascular complications are the main cause of death in type 2 diabetes (Morrish et al., 2001) and are often associated with SMase overexpression and elevated ceramide production (Opreanu et al., 2011; Tikhonenko et al., 2013), it can be hypothesized that beneficial effects of dietary n–3 PUFAs are partly due to inhibition of sphingolipid turnover in cells. It is well documented that the anti-inflammatory effect of DHA in human retinal endothelial cells depends on n–3 PUFAs inhibitory action on both acid and neutral SMase (Opreanu et al., 2010, 2011). Retinal endothelial cells treatment by DHA decreased TNFα- and IL-1β-induced ASMase and NSMase expression and activity and cellular adhesion molecule expression (Opreanu et al., 2010). Anti-inflammatory effects of DHA can be imitated by siRNAs for ASMase and NSMase and by specific inhibitors of NSMase and ASMase activity, GW4869 and desipramine, respectively. In addition, DHA decreased ASMase activity can prevent both short- and long-term diabetes-induced changes in rat retina (Tikhonenko et al., 2013). Using the streptozotocin-induced type 1 diabetic rat model, it has been demonstrated that dietetic DHA prevented diabetes-induced up-regulation of inflammatory marker (vascular endothelial growth factor, intercellular adhesion molecule, and IL-1β) gene expression. Feeding 9-month old diabetic rats with DHA-enriched diet results in gene expression for ASMase and proinflammatory and proangiogenic mediators, IL-1β, and vascular endothelial growth factor, and protected the retina against vessel loss.

It is known that altered sphingolipid metabolism is a common feature of aged mammals and non-mammalian eukaryotes (Huang et al., 2014). Ceramide content dramatically increases in different tissues during aging (Babenko and Shakhova, 2006, 2014; Babenko and Semenova, 2010) and is related to the development of age-related diseases, including type 2 diabetes, cardiovascular and immune dysfunction and neurodegeneration (Cutler and Mattson, 2001; Nikolova-Karakashian et al., 2008; Jana et al., 2009; Guenther and Edinger, 2009; Ohno-Iwashita et al., 2010; Webb et al., 2010). There is a strong correlation between oxidative stress, inflammation, insulin resistance and ceramide accumulation, all of which are involved in the aging process and age-associated diseases (Mitsutake and Igarashi, 2013; Jiang et al., 2011; Vandanmagsar et al., 2011; Nikolova-Karakashian and Reid, 2011; Chavez and Summers, 2012; de la Monte, 2012; Bikman, 2012). Sustained increase of ceramide content in liver cells (Babenko and Kharchenko, 2012, 2015b), skeletal muscles (Babenko et al., 2015) and brain cortex (Babenko and Kharchenko, 2013, 2015a) at old age is associated with development of insulin resistance. The loss of target cell sensitivity to insulin action can be imitated by exogenous C2-ceramide or the ceramide precursor, palmitic acid, and ameliorated by the pretreatment of cells by specific inhibitors of ASMase (imipramine), NSMase (GW4869) and serine palmitoyltransferase (myriocin). Suggestions have been made, that accumulation of newly synthesized ceramide, as well as ceramide derived from sphingomyelin under SMases action, plays a specific role in the reduction of target cells sensitivity to insulin action at old age. Another recent study has shown that age-dependent dysfunction and type 2 diabetes dependent dysfunction of the insulin system in the CNS correlates with the development of neurodegenerative pathologies (de la Monte, 2009; Kapogiannis and Mattson, 2011). Among the signs for development of Alzheimer's disease are decreased intensity of glucose metabolism and insulin levels in the brain, increased expression of insulin receptors, and growing levels of insulin in the blood plasma (Kapogiannis and Mattson, 2011). We have also demonstrated that long-term treatment of rats with a fish oil-enriched diet suppressed ceramide and neutral lipids accumulation in the brain cortex (Fig. 24.1A) and classical insulin responsive tissues (liver and muscle) (Fig. 24.1b,c) of 24-month-old rats and increased cortex slices sensitivity to insulin action (unpublished data).

Taking into account that dietetic fish oil significantly decreased the ceramide/sphingomyelin ratio in the cortex and other tissues (Fig. 24.2), it cannot be ruled out that fish oil n–3 PUFAs, which inhibit the SMase activity, suppressed the age-dependent brain as well as liver and muscle insulin resistance.

The results, obtained on "old" brain cortex slices, pretreated with a specific inhibitor of NSMase, GW4869, supported this suggestion (unpublished data). Inhibition of NSMase activity by GW4869 was followed by a reduction of elevated ceramide content in the cortex and significantly increased sensitivity to insulin action. Inhibition of NSMase, but not the ASMase activity, by a specific inhibitor increased insulin-induced glucose uptake and glycogen synthesis in cortex slices of old rats. Other observations suggest the impact of NSMase in the age-dependent dysregulation of sphingolipid turnover in the brain cortex and hippocampus. Overexpression of NSMase, but not ASMase, was determined in the brain cortex and hippocampus of aged 24-month-old rats (Babenko and Shakhova, 2014). Treatment of old animals by inhibitor of NSMase, but not by inhibitor of ASMase, nullified the age-dependent changes

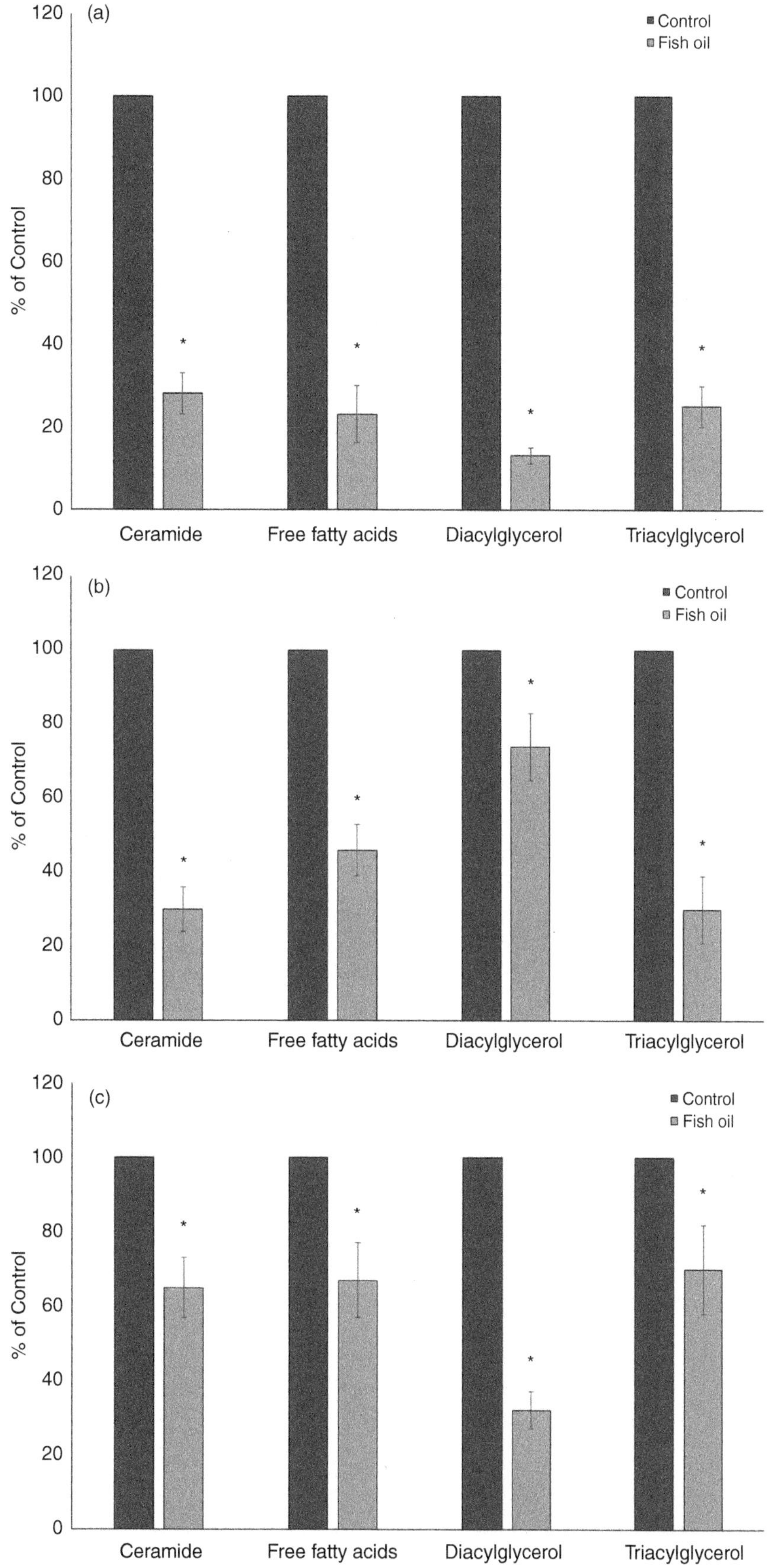

FIGURE 24.1 Long-term effect of a fish oil-enriched diet on ceramide, free fatty acids and neutral lipids contents in the brain cortex, liver and muscle tissues of 24-month-old rats. (a) Brain cortex. (b) Liver. (c) Diaphragm. Here and in the Fig. 24.2: the animals were fed by isocaloric diets enriched with fish oil (fish oil-fed) or sunflower oil/beef fat (control group) (Babenko and Semenova, 2010). Fish oil-fed and control groups of the rats were on the diets for 36 weeks. Results are mean ± SE of 6–8 individual experiments performed in duplicate. *$p < 0.05$, fish oil-fed versus control rats.

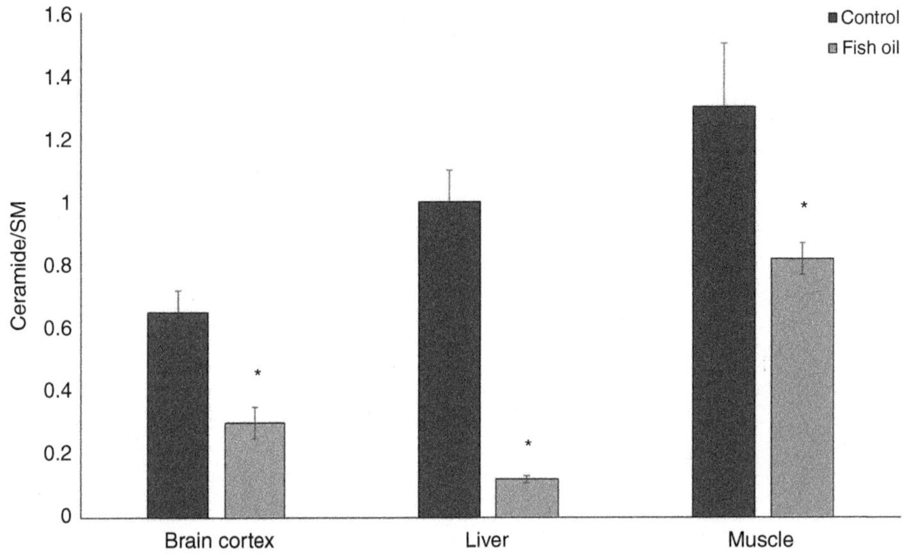

FIGURE 24.2 Long-term effect of a fish oil-enriched diet on ceramide/sphingomyelin ratio in the brain cortex, liver, and muscle tissues of 24-month-old rats. *SM*, sphingomyelin. *$p < 0.05$, fish oil-fed versus control rats.

of ceramide and sphingomyelin content in the brain structures. Treatment of animals with a diet enriched in fish oil reduced the elevated content of ceramide and the ceramide/sphingomyelin ratio in the hippocampus at old age (Babenko and Semenova, 2010). Dietetic eicosapentaenoic acid (EPA) and docosapentaenoic acid (DPA), which both can be primarily metabolized to DHA, significantly decreased the elevated NSMase activity in the brain cortex of 22-month-old rats to the level of 3-month-old animals and restored cognitive function and synaptic plasticity in aged rats. (Kelly et al. 2011). EPA or DPA supplementation reduced elevated content of C16- and C18-ceramide and increased sphingosine-1-phosphate content in the brain cortex of old, but not adult rats. Moreover, EPA as well as DPA levels significantly decreased, elevated by inflammatory stimulus activities of NSMase and caspase 3 in cortical neurons and thus shifted the balance towards an antiapoptotic state. The authors suggested that EPA and DPA improve age-related deficit in both long-term potentiation and spatial learning due to down-regulation of NSMase-dependent microglia activation and oxidative changes in DNA (Kelly et al. 2011).

Exogenous PS, as well as specific inhibitors of NSMase, imitated the effect of dietary fish oil on NSMase activity and the sphingolipid content in the hippocampus of old animals (Babenko and Semenova, 2010; Babenko and Shakhova, 2014). A fish oil enriched diet decreased the number of combinations of stimuli up to achievement of the conditioned active avoidance reflex criterion and latent period of avoidance, while the number of active avoidances in the shuttle box increased as compared with untreated rats (Babenko and Semenova, 2008). It is possible that dietetic n–3 PUFA, by reducing the NSMase activity by the PS-dependent pathway, can restore the sphingolipid turnover in the hippocampus and improve the cognitive capacities of aged rats. However, it is noteworthy that long-term treatment of rats with fish oil significantly reduced lipogenesis in the brain cortex, liver and muscle (Fig. 24.1a,b,c). A fish oil-enriched diet decreased synthesis of palmitic acid, the precursor of sphingolipid. Pretreatment of cortex slices, obtained from brain of aged rats, with myriocin, a specific inhibitor of serine palmitoyltransferase, decreased elevated ceramide content and increased insulin-stimulated glucose uptake and stimulation of glycogen synthesis by insulin (unpublished data). Based on these data, one may predict that fish oil, by decreasing both the NSMase activity and synthesis of ceramide de novo, can improve brain cortex sensitivity to insulin action at old age.

CONCLUSION

N-3 PUFAs are critical for cell membrane structure and function of the nervous system. Deficiency of n–3 PUFAs in the diet causes memory deficit, learning disability, and visual activity loss. Various neurological disease states, such as generalized peroxisomal disorders and Alzheimer's disease in human, are associated with a deficient n–3 PUFA status, while the dietary intake of n–3 PUFAs has been shown to reduce neuronal injury and to improve some symptoms in these patients. Dietary fish oil supplementation enhanced the reference or working memory in normal and n–3 PUFA-deficient animals. The n–3 PUFAs play an important role in control of such hippocampus-dependent neuronal functions as learning and memory. Dietary n–3 PUFAs of fish oil normalized an age-related decrease in cognitive function, ceramide content and polyunsaturated PS species in the brain cortex and hippocampus. Ceramide is a key molecule in sphingolipid metabolism. However, accumulation of ceramide in neurons and glial cells is associated with inflammation and neurodegeneration. The ceramide content progressively increasing in such brain structures as hippocampus and neocortex during aging is related to the development of age-associated pathologies, including type 2 diabetes, immune dysfunction and neurodegeneration. Experiments with a long-term treatment of animals by fish oil or culturing neuronal cells in the presence of n–3 PUFA demonstrated negative correlations between ceramide levels and cell survival under stress conditions. Neuroprotective actions of fish oil depend to a large extent on the down-regulation of NSMase which is activated by cytokines and oxidative stress. Age-dependent and type 2 diabetes-dependent dysfunction of insulin system in the CNS correlates with the development of neurodegenerative disorder and ceramide accumulation in the brain structures. Dietary fish oil can prevent age-dependent insulin resistance in brain cortex and restore the cognitive function and synaptic plasticity in aged rats via down regulation of ceramide production by NSMase and ceramide synthesis de novo. Thus, it is evident that alimentary n–3 PUFAs are powerful modulators of sphingolipid turnover. Among the targets of n–3 PUFAs in neuronal cells are key enzymes of sphingolipid metabolism, i.e. SMases and process of sphingolipid synthesis de novo. Increasing dietary n–3 PUFA makes it possible to diminish the accumulation of proinflammatory and proapoptotic ceramide accumulation in brain structures at old age and in stress conditions, thereby preventing cells from damage and pathophysiology.

References

Addolorato, G., Gasbarrini, A., Marcoccia, S., Simoncini, M., Baccarini, P., Vagni, G., Grieco, A., Sbriccoli, A., Granato, A., Stefanini, G.F., Gasbarrini, G., 1997. Prenatal exposure to ethanol in rats: effects on liver energy level and antioxidant status in mothers, fetuses, and newborns. Alcohol 14, 569–573.

Adibhatla, R.M., Hatcher, J.F., 2008. Altered lipid metabolism in brain injury and disorders. Subcell. Biochem. 49, 241–268.

Akbar, M., Baick, J., Calderon, F., Wen, Z., Kim, H.Y., 2006. Ethanol promotes neuronal apoptosis by inhibiting phosphatidylserine accumulation. J. Neurosci. Res. 83, 432–440.

Akbar, M., Calderon, F., Wen, Z., Kim, H.-Y., 2005. Docosahexaenoic acid: a positive modulator of Akt signaling in neuronal survival. Proc. Natl. Acad. Sci. USA. 102, 10858–10863.

Albouz, S., Le Saux, F., Wenger, D., Hauw, J.J., Baumann, N., 1986. Modifications of sphingomyelin and phosphatidylcholine metabolism by tricyclic antidepressants and phenothiazines. Life Sci. 38, 357–363.

Babenko, N., Shakhova, E., 2006. Effects of Chamomilla recutita flavonoids on age-related liver sphingolipid turnover in rats. Exp. Gerontol. 41, 32–39.

Babenko, N.A., Shakhova, E.G., 2014. Long-term food restriction prevents aging-associated sphingolipid turnover dysregulation in the brain. Arch. Gerontol. Geriatr. 58, 420–426.

Babenko, N.A., 2013. Fish oil n-3 fatty acids to prevent hippocampus and cognitive dysfunction in experimental alcoholism. In: Watson, R.R., Preedy, V.R., Zibadi, S. (Eds.), Alcohol, Nutrition, and Health Consequences. Humana Press, New York, pp. 227–240.

Babenko, N.A., Kharchenko, V.S., 2012. Ceramides inhibit phospholipase D-dependent insulin signaling in liver cells of old rats. Biochemistry (Moscow) 77, 180–186.

Babenko, N.A., Kharchenko, V.S., 2013. Age-related changes in the phospholipase D-dependent signal pathway of insulin in the rat neocortex. Neurophysiology 45, 120–127.

Babenko, N.A., Kharchenko, V.S., 2015a. Effects of aging and experimentally induced modifications of signal pathways on insulin-induced shifts of glucose metabolism in the rat neocortex. Neurophysiology 47, 16–22.

Babenko, N.A., Kharchenko, V.S., 2015b. Effects of inhibitors of key enzymes of sphingolipid metabolism on insulin-induced glucose uptake and glycogen synthesis in liver cells of old rats. Biochemistry (Moscow) 80, 104–112.

Babenko, N.A., Semenova, Y.A., 2008. Effect of the diet enriched in the polyunsaturatted fatty, acids of the fish oil on phospholipid turnover and cognitive function of the old rats. Rossiiskii fiziologicheskii zhurnal imeni I.M. Sechenova / Rossiiskaia akademiia nauk 94, 1400–1406.

Babenko, N.A., Semenova, Y.A., 2010. Effects of long-term fish oil-enriched diet on the sphingolipid metabolism in brain of old rats. Exp. Gerontol. 45, 375–380.

Babenko, N.A., Timofechuk, O.A., Beliy, A.N., 2015. Role of neutral sphingomyelinase in age-dependent muscle insulin resistance development and it improvement with N-acetylcysteine. Adv. Gerontol. 80, 104–112.

Bikman, B.T., 2012. A role for sphingolipids in the pathophysiology of obesity-induced inflammation. Cell. Mol. Life Sci. 69, 2135–2146.

Calon, F., Lim, G.P., Yang, F., Morihara, T., Teter, B., Ubeda, O., Rostaing, P., Triller, A., Salem, Jr., N., Ashe, K.H., Frautschy, S.A., Cole, G.M., 2004. Docosahexaenoic acid protects from dendritic pathology in an Alzheimer's disease mouse model. Neuron 43, 633–645.

Cao, D.H., Xu, J.F., Xue, R.H., Zheng, W.F., Liu, Z.L., 2004. Protective effect of chronic ethyl docosahexaenoate administration on brain injury in ischemic gerbils. Pharmacol. Biochem. Behav 79, 651–659.

Carrie, I., Clement, M., De Javel, D., Francès, H., Bourre, J.M., 1999. Learning de fi cits in fi rst generation OF1 mice de fi cient in (n-3) polyunsaturated fatty acids do not result from visual alteration. Neurosci. Lett. 266, 69–72.

Chalon, S., Delion-Vancassel, S., Belzung, C., 1998. Dietary fish oil affects monoaminergic transmission and behavior in rats. J. Nutrition 128, 2512–2519.

Chavez, J.A., Summers, S.A., 2012. A ceramide-centric view of insulin resistance. Cell. Metab. 15, 585–594.

Cherubini, A., Andres-Lacueva, C., Martin, A.J., Lauretani, F., Iorio, A.D., Bartali, B., Corsi, A., Bandinelli, S., Mattson, M.P., Ferrucci, L., 2007. Low plasma N-3 fatty acids and dementia in older persons: the InCHIANTI study. J. Gerontol. Ser. A 62, 1120–1126.

Choi-Kwon, S., Park, K.A., Lee, H.J., Park, M.S., Lee, J.H., Jeon, S.E., Choe, M.A., Park, K.C., 2004. Temporal changes in cerebral antioxidant enzyme activities after ischemia and reperfusion in a rat focal brain ischemia model: effect of dietary fish oil. Brain Res. Development. Brain Res. (Amsterdam) 152, 11–18.

Chung, W.L., Chen, J.J., Su, H.M., 2008. Fish oil supplementation of control and (n-3) fatty acid-de fi cient male rats enhances reference and working memory performance and increases brain regional docosahexaenoic acid levels. J. Nutr. 138, 1165–1171.

Cole, A.L., Lee, P.J., Hughes, D.A., Deegan, P.B., Waldek, S., Lachmann, R.H., 2007. Depression in adults with Fabry disease: a common and under-diagnosed problem. J. Inherited Metab. Dis. 30, 943–951.

Connor, K.M., Sangiovanni, J.P., Lofqvist, C., Aderman, C.M., Chen, J., Higuchi, A., Hong, S., Pravda, E.A., Majchrzak, S., Carper, D., Hellstrom, A., Kang, J.X., Chew, E.Y., Salem, Jr., N., Serhan, C.N., Smith, L.E., 2007. Increased dietary intake of omega-3-polyunsaturated fatty acids reduces pathological retinal angiogenesis. Nat. Med. 13, 868–873.

Conquer, J.A., Tierney, M.C., Zecevic, J., Bettger, W.J., Fisher, R.H., 2000. Fatty acid analysis of blood plasma of patients with Alzheimer's disease, other types of dementia, and cognitive impairment. Lipids 35, 1305–1312.

Costantini, C., Kolasani, R.M.K., Puglielli, L., 2005a. Ceramide and cholesterol: possible connections between normal aging of the brain and Alzheimer's disease. Just hypotheses or molecular pathways to be identified? Alzheimer's Dementia 1, 43–50.

Costantini, C., Weindruch, R., Della Valle, G., Puglielli, L., 2005b. A TrkA-to-p75 NTR molecular switch activates amyloidβ-peptide generation during aging. Biochem. J. 391, 59–67.

Cutler, R.G., Mattson, M.P., 2001. Sphingomyelin and ceramide as regulators of development and lifespan. Mech. Ageing Dev. 122, 895–908.

Cutler, R.G., Pedersen, W.A., Camandola, S., Rothstein, J.D., Mattson, M.P., 2002. Evidence that accumulation of ceramides and cholesterol esters mediates oxidative stress-induced death of motor neurons in amyotrophic lateral sclerosis. Annal. Neurol. (Boston, MA) 52, 448–457.

Cutler, R.G., Kelly, J., Storie, K., Pedersen, W.A., Tammara, A., Hatanpaa, K., Troncoso, J.C., Mattson, M.P., 2004. Involvement of oxidative stress-induced abnormalities in ceramide and cholesterol metabolism in brain aging and Alzheimer's disease. Proc. Natl. Acad. Sci. USA 101, 2070–2075.

de la Monte, S.M., 2009. Insulin resistance and Alzheimer's disease. BMB reports 42, 475–481.

de la Monte, S.M., 2012. Triangulated mal-signaling in Alzheimer's disease: roles of neurotoxic ceramides, ER stress, and insulin resistance reviewed. J. Alzheimer's Disease 30, S231–249.

Demirkan, A., Isaacs, A., Ugocsai, P., Liebisch, G., Struchalin, M., Rudan, I., Wilson, J.F., Pramstaller, P.P., Gyllensten, U., Campbell, H., Schmitz, G., Oostra, B.A., Van Duijn, C.M., 2013. Plasma phosphatidylcholine and sphingomyelin concentrations are associated with depression and anxiety symptoms in a Dutch family-based lipidomics study. J. Psychiatr. Res 47, 357–362.

Firląg, M., Kamaszewski, M., Adamek, D., Gajewska, M., Bałasińska B., 2015. Long-term consumption of fish oil partially protects brain tissue from age-related neurodegeneration. Postepy Higieny Medycyny Doswiadczalnej, Warszawa. Online, 69, pp. 188–196.

Futterman, S., Kupfer, C., 1968. The fatty acid composition of the retinal vasculature of normal and diabetic human eyes. Investig. Ophthalmol. 7, 105–108.

Gamoh, S., Hashimoto, M., Sugioka, K., Shahdat Hossain, M., Hata, N., Misawa, Y., Masumura, S., 1999. Chronic administration of docosahexaenoic acid improves reference memory-related learning ability in young rats. Neuroscience 93, 237–241.

Gault, C.R., Obeid, L.M., Hannun, Y.A., 2010. An overview of sphingolipid metabolism: from synthesis to breakdown. Adv. Exp. Med. Biol. 688, 1–23.

German, O.L., Miranda, G.E., Abrahan, C.E., Rotstein, N.P., 2006. Ceramide is a mediator of apoptosis in retina photoreceptors. Invest. Ophthalmol. Visual Sci. 47, 1658–1668.

Ginkel, Ch., Hartmann, D., vom Dorp, K., Zlomuzica, A., Farwanah, H., Eckhardt, M., Sandhoff, R., Degen, J., Rabionet, M., Dere, E., Dörmann, P., Sandhoff, K., Willecke, K., 2012. Ablation of neuronal ceramide synthase 1 in mice decreases ganglioside levels and expression of myelin-associated glycoprotein in oligodendrocytes. J. Biol. Chem. 287, 41888–41902.

Gracia-Garcia, P., Rao, V., Haughey, N.J., Banduru, V.V.R., Smith, G., Rosenberg, P.B., Lobo, A., Lyketsos, C.G., Mielke, M.M., 2011. Elevated plasma ceramides in depression. J. Neuropsychiatr. Clin. Neurosci. 23, 215–218.

Grassme, H., Riethmuller, J., Gulbins, E., 2007. Biological aspects of ceramide-enriched membrane domains. Prog. Lipid Res. 46, 161–170.

Guenther, G.G., Edinger, A.L., 2009. A new take on ceramide: starving cells by cutting off the nutrient supply. Cell Cycle 8, 1122–1126.

Gulbins, E., Palmada, M., Reichel, M., Lüth, A., Böhmer, C., Amato, D., Müller, C.P., Tschbirek, C.H., Groemer, T.W., Tabatabai, G., Becker, K., Tripal, P., Staedtler, S., Ackermann, T.F., van Brederode, J., Alzheimer, C., Weller, M., Lang, U.E., Kleuser, B., Grassmé, H., Kornhuber, J., 2013. Acid sphingomyelinase-ceramide system mediates effects of antidepressant drugs. Nat. Med. 19, 934–938.

Hammad, S.M., Truman, J.P., Al Gadban, M.M., Smith, K.J., Twal, W.O., Hamner, M.B., 2012. Altered blood sphingolipidomics and elevated plasma inflammatory cytokines in combat veterans with post-traumatic stress disorder. Neurobiol. Lipids 10, 2.

Hannun, Y.A., Obeid, L.M., 2002. The ceramide-centric universe of lipid-mediated cell regulation: stress encounters of the lipid kind. J. Biol. Chem. 277, 25847–25850.

Hannun, Y.A., Obeid, L.M., 2008. Principles of bioactive lipid signalling: lessons from sphingolipids. Nature Rev. Molecul. Cell. Biol. 9, 139–150.

Haughey, N.J., Cutler, R.G., Tamara, A., McArthur, J.C., Vargas, D.L., Pardo, C.A., Turchan, J., Nath, A., Mattson, M.P., 2004. Perturbation of sphingolipid metabolism and ceramide production in HIV-dementia. Ann. Neurol. 55, 257–267.

He, X., Huang, Y., Li, B., Gong, C.X., Schuchman, E.H., 2010. Deregulation of sphingolipid metabolism in Alzheimer's disease. Neurobiol. Aging 31, 398–408.

Holopainen, J.M., Subramanian, M., Kinnunen, P.K., 1998. Sphingomyelinase induces lipid microdomain formation in a fluid phosphatidylcholine/sphingomyelin membrane. Biochemistry 37, 17562–17570.

Hu, F.B., Cho, E., Rexrode, K.M., Albert, C.M., Manson, J.E., 2003. Fish and long-chain omega-3 fatty acid intake and risk of coronary heart disease and total mortality in diabetic women. Circulation 107, 1852–1857.

Huang, X., Withers, B.R., Dickson, R.C., 2014. Sphingolipids and lifespan regulation. Biochem. Biophys. Acta 1841, 657–664.

Innis, S.M., 2007. Dietary (n-3) fatty acids and brain development. J. Nutr. 137, 855–859.

Jana, A., Hogan, E.L., Pahan, K., 2009. Ceramide and neurodegeneration: susceptibility of neurons and oligodendrocytes to cell damage and death. J. Neurol. Sci. 278, 5–15.

Jana, A., Pahan, K., 2010. Fibrillar amyloid-β-activated human astroglia kill primary human neurons via neutral sphingomyelinase: Implications for Alzheimer's disease. J. Neurosci. 30, 12676–12689.

Jiang, X.C., Goldberg, I.J., Park, T.S., 2011. Sphingolipids and cardiovascular diseases: lipoprotein metabolism, atherosclerosis and cardiomyopathy. Adv. Exp. Med. Biol. 721, 19–39.

Kapogiannis, D., Mattson, M.P., 2011. Disrupted energy metabolism and neuronal circuit dysfunction in cognitive impairment and Alzheimer's disease. Lancet Neurol. 10, 187–198.

Kelly, L., Grehan, B., Chiesa, A.D., O'Mara, Sh.M., Downer, E., Sahyoun, G., Massey, K.A., Nicolaou, A., Lynch, M.A., 2011. The polyunsaturated fatty acids, EPA and DPA exert a protective effect in the hippocampus of the aged rat. Neurobiol. Aging 32, 2318e1–2318e15.

Kidd, P.M., 2007. Omega-3 DHA and EPA for cognition, behavior, and mood: clinical findings and structuralfunctional synergies with cell membrane phospholipids. Alternativ. Med. Rev. 12, 207–227.

Kim, H.Y., 2008. Biochemical and biological functions of docosahexaenoic acid in the nervous system: modulation by ethanol. Chem. Phys. Lipids 153, 34–46.

Kim, H.Y., Akbar, M., Lau, A., Edsall, L., 2000. Inhibition of neuronal apoptosis by docosahexaenoic acid (22:6n-3): role of phosphatidylserine in antiapoptotic effect. J. Biol. Chem. 275, 35215–35223.

Ko, Y.G., Lee, J.S., Kang, Y.S., Ahn, J.H., Seo, J.S., 1999. TNF-alpha-mediated apoptosis is initiated in caveolae-like domains. J. Immunol. 162, 7217–7223.

Kolesnick, R.N., Goni, F.M., Alonso, A., 2000. Compartmentalization of ceramide signaling: physical foundations and biological effects. J. Cell. Physiol. 184, 285–300.

Kornhuber, J., Medlin, A., Bleich, S., Jendrossek, V., Henkel, A.W., Wiltfang, J., Gulbins, E., 2005. High activity of acid sphingomyelinase in major depression. J. Neural Transm. 112, 1583–1590.

Kornhuber, J., Muehlbacher, M., Trapp, S., Pechmann, S., Friedl, A., Reichel, M., Mühle, C., Terfloth, L., Groemer, T.W., Spitzer, G.M., Liedl, K.R., Gulbins, E., Tripal, P., 2011. Identification of novel functional inhibitors of acid sphingomyelinase. PLoS One 6, e23852.

Kornhuber, J., Tripal, P., Reichel, M., Mühle, C., Rhein, C., Muehlbacher, M., Groemer, T.W., Gulbins, E., 2010. Functional inhibitors of acid sphingomyelinase (FIASMAs): a novel pharmacological group of drugs with broad clinical applications. Cell. Physiol. Biochem. 26, 9–20.

Laney, D.A., Gruskin, D.J., Fernhoff, P.M., Cubells, J.F., Ousley, O.Y., Hipp, H., Mehta, A.J., 2010. Social-adaptive and psychological functioning of patients affected by Fabry disease. J. Inherited Metab. Dis. 33, S73–S81.

Lukiw, W.J., Bazan, N.G., 2008. Docosahexaenoic acid and the aging brain. J. Nutr. 138, 2510–2514.

MacQueen, G.M., Rosebush, P.I., Mazurek, M.F., 1998. Neuropsychiatric aspects of the adult variant of Tay-Sachs disease. J. Neuropsychiatr. Clin. Neurosci. 10, 10–19.

Martin, M.U., Wesche, H., 2002. Summary and comparison of the signaling mechanisms of the Toll/interleukin-1 receptor family. Biochem. Biophys. Acta 1592, 265–280.

Martinez, M., 1990. Severe deficiency of docosahexaenoic acid in peroxisomal disorders: a defect of Æ4-desaturation? Neurology 40, 1292–1298.

Martínez, M., Vázquez, E., García-Silva, M.T., Manzanares, J., Bertran, J.M., Castelló, F., Mougan, I., 2000. Therapeutic effects of docosahexaenoic acid ethyl ester in patients with generalized peroxisomal disorders. Am. J. Clin. Nutr. 71, 376S–385S.

Mielke, M.M., Maetzler, W., Haughey, N.J., Banduru, V.V.R., Savica, R., Deuschle, C., Gasser, T., Hauser, A.K., Gräber-Sultan, S., Schleicher, E., Berg, D., Liepelt-Scarfone, I., 2013. Plasma ceramide and glucosylceramide metabolism is altered in sporadic Parkinson's disease and associated with cognitive impairment: a pilot study. PLoS One 8, e73094.

Mitsutake, S., Igarashi, Y., 2013. Sphingolipids in lipid microdomains and obesity. Vitam. Horm. 91, 271–284.

Moriguchi, T., Greiner, R.S., Salem, Jr., N., 2000. Behavioral deficits associated with dietary induction of decreased brain docosahexaenoic acid concentration. J. Neurochem. 75, 2563–2573.

Morrish, N.J., Wang, S.L., Stevens, L.K., Fuller, J.H., Keen, H., 2001. Mortality and causes of death in the WHO multinational study of vascular disease in diabetes. Diabetologia 44, S14–21.

Neuringer, M., 2000. Infant vision and retinal function in studies of dietary long-chain polyunsaturated fatty acids: methods, results, and implications. Am. J. Clin. Nutr. 71, 256S–267S.

Nikolova-Karakashian, M., Karakashian, A., Rutkute, K., 2008. Role of neutral sphingomyelinases in aging and inflammation. Subcell. Biochem. 49, 469–486.

Nikolova-Karakashian, M.N., Reid, M.B., 2011. Sphingolipid metabolism, oxidant signaling, and contractile function of skeletal muscle. Antioxid. Redox Signaling 15, 2501–2517.

Nurminen, T.A., Holopainen, J.M., Zhao, H., Kinnunen, P.K., 2002. Observation of topical catalysis by sphingomyelinase coupled to microspheres. J. Am. Chem. Soc. 124, 12129–12134.

Ohno-Iwashita, Y., Shimada, Y., Hayashi, M., Inomata, M., 2010. Plasma membrane microdomains in aging and disease. Geriatr. Gerontol. Int. 10, S41–S52.

Okada, M., Amamoto, T., Tomonaga, M., Kawachi, A., Yazawa, K., Mine, K., Fujiwara, M., 1996. The chronic administration of docosahexaenoic acid reduces the spatial cognitive deficit following transient forebrain ischemia in rats. Neuroscience 71, 17–25.

Opreanu, M., Lydic, T.A., Reid, G.E., McSorley, K.M., Esselman, W.J., Busik, J.V., 2010. Inhibition of cytokine signaling in human retinal endothelial cells through downregulation of sphingomyelinases by docosahexaenoic acid. Invest. Ophthalmol. Visual Sci. 51, 3253–3263.

Opreanu, M., Tikhonenko, M., Bozack, S., Lydic, T.A., Reid, G.E., McSorley, K.M., Sochacki, A., Perez, G.I., Esselman, W.J., Kern, T., Kolesnick, R., Grant, M.B., Busik, J.V., 2011. The unconventional role of acid sphingomyelinase in regulation of retinal microangiopathy in diabetic human and animal models. Diabetes 60, 2370–2378.

Osuchowski, M.F., Edwards, G.L., Sharma, R.P., 2005. Fumonisin B1-induced neurodegeneration in mice after intracerebroventricular infusion is concurrent with disruption of sphingolipid metabolism and activation of proinflammatory signaling. Neurotoxicology 26, 211–221.

Packman, W., Wilson Crosbie, T., Riesner, A., Fairley, C., Packman, S., 2006. Psychological complications of patients with Gaucher disease. J. Inherited Metab. Dis. 29, 99–105.

Puglielli, L., Ellis, B.C., Saunders, A.J., Kovacs, D.M., 2003. Ceramide stabilizes beta-site amyloid precursor protein-cleaving enzyme 1 and promotes amyloid beta-peptide biogenesis. J. Biol. Chem. 278, 19777–19783.

Qin, L., He, J., Hanes, R.N., Pluzarev, O., Hong, J.S., Crews, F.T., 2008. Increased systemic and brain cytokine production and neuroinflammation by endotoxin following ethanol treatment. J. Neuroinflammation 5, 10–26.

Rotstein, N.P., Aveldaño, M.I., Barrantes, F.J., Politi, L.E., 1996. Docosahexaenoic acid is required for the survival of rat retinal photoreceptors in vitro. J. Neurochem. 66, 1851–1859.

Sadek, J., Shellhaas, R., Camfield, C.S., Camfield, P.R., Burley, J., 2004. Psychiatric findings in four female carriers of Fabry disease. Psychiatr. Genet. 14, 199–201.

San Giovanni, J.P., Chew, E.Y., 2005. The role of omega-3 long-chain polyunsaturated fatty acids in health and disease of the retina. Prog. Retina. Eye Res. 24, 87–13.

Sawai, H., Hannun, Y.A., 1999. Ceramide and sphingomyelinases in the regulation of stress responses. Chem. Phys. Lipids 102, 141–147.

Schwarz, E., Prabakaran, S., Whitfield, P., Major, H., Leweke, F.M., Koethe, D., McKenna, P., Bahn, S., 2008. High throughput lipidomic profiling of schizophrenia and bipolar disorder brain tissue reveals alterations of free fatty acids, phosphatidylcholines, and ceramides. J. Proteome Res. 7, 4266–4277.

Sinclair, A.J., Begg, D., Mathai, M., Weisinger, R.S., 2007. Omega 3 fatty acids and the brain: review of studies in depression. Asia Pac. J. Clin. Nutr. 16, 391–397.

Soderberg, M., Edlund, C., Kristensson, K., Dallner, G., 1991. Fatty acid composition of brain phospholipids in aging and in Alzheimer's disease. Lipids 26, 421–425.

Tikhonenko, M., Lydic, T.A., Opreanu, M., Li Calzi, S., Bozack, S., McSorley, K.M., Sochacki, A.L., Faber, M.S., Hazra, S., Duclos, Sh., Guberski, D., Reid, G.E., Grant, M.B., Busik, J.V., 2013. N-3 polyunsaturated fatty acids prevent diabetic retinopathy by inhibition of retinal vascular damage and enhanced endothelial progenitor cell reparative function. PLoS One 8, e55177.

Tikhonenko, M., Lydic, T.A., Wang, Y., Chen, W., Opreanu, M., Sochacki, A., McSorley, K.M., Renis, R.L., Kern, T., Jump, D.B., Reid, G.E., Busik, J.V., 2010. Remodeling of retinal Fatty acids in an animal model of diabetes: a decrease in long-chain polyunsaturated fatty acids is associated with a decrease in fatty acid elongases Elovl2 and Elovl4. Diabetes 59, 219–227.

Vandanmagsar, B., Youm, Y.H., Ravussin, A., Galgani, J.E., Stadler, K., Mynatt, R.L., Ravussin, E., Stephens, J.M., Dixit, V.D., 2011. The NLRP3 inflammasome instigates obesity-induced inflammation and insulin resistance. Nat. Med. 17, 179–188.

Webb, L.M., Arnholt, A.T., Venable, M.E., 2010. Phospholipase D modulation by ceramide in senescence. Mol. Cell. Biochem. 337, 153–158.

Wu, A., Ying, Z., Gomez-Pinilla, F., 2004. Dietary omega-3 fatty acids normalize BDNF levels, reduce oxidative damage, and counteract learning disability after traumatic brain injury in rats. J. Neurotr. 21, 1457–1467.

Yoshida, S., Yasuda, A., Kawazato, H., Sakai, K., Shimada, T., Takeshita, M., Yuasa, S., Kobayashi, T., Watanabe, S., Okuyama, H., 1997. Synaptic vesicle ultrastructural changes in the rat hippocampus induced by a combination of alpha-linolenate deficiency and a learning task. J. Neurochem. 68, 1261–1268.

Zhao, L., Spassieva, S.D., Jucius, T.J., Shultz, L.D., Shick, H.E., Macklin, W.B., Hannun, Y.A., Obeid, L.M., Ackerman, S.L., 2011. A deficiency of ceramide biosynthesis causes cerebellar purkinje cell neurodegeneration and lipofuscin accumulation. PLoS Genetic. 7, e1002063.

CHAPTER

25

Liver Disease and Parenteral Fish Oil

G.L. Fell*, K.M. Gura**, M. Puder*

*Department of Surgery and Vascular Biology Program, Boston Children's Hospital, Boston, Massachusetts, United States; **Department of Pharmacy, Boston Children's Hospital, Boston, Massachusetts, United States

INTRODUCTION

Cholestasis and liver failure are potential complications of parenteral nutrition (PN) administration. Lipid emulsions provide the source of fat for PN-dependent patients. Each lipid emulsion available for parenteral use contains a unique profile of fatty acids and additives that can impact hepatic fat metabolism and modulate the risk of developing parenteral nutrition-associated liver disease (PNALD). This chapter discusses the role of fat emulsions in PN, describes PNALD, and focuses on the role of plant oil-based lipid emulsions in the pathophysiology of PNALD as well as the role of fish oil lipid emulsions in the treatment of PNALD.

PARENTERAL NUTRITION AND THE IMPORTANCE OF FAT EMULSIONS

Patients with intestinal failure (IF) have insufficient bowel length or function to enterally absorb the energy and nutrients required to fuel growth, development, and daily activities. These patients therefore require PN for survival. IF can be acquired in adulthood in settings such as intestinal trauma, abdominal tumors, Crohn's disease, or mesenteric ischemia requiring extensive bowel resection. However, many of the conditions that result in IF begin at or shortly after birth (Goulet and Ruemmele, 2006). Etiologies of IF in children include congenital intestinal atresias that result in short bowel length, congenital motility or enterocyte defects such as Hirschsprung's disease or microvillus inclusion disease, and acquired conditions that result in the need for extensive bowel resection such as necrotizing enterocolitis or midgut volvulus. PN is lifesaving for infants who develop IF given the importance of adequate nutrition during the rapid growth and development that characterize this phase of life. Infants with IF who initiate PN in the neonatal period often require PN over a long term, on the order of months to years. For most patients, intestinal adaptation and enteral autonomy eventually occur (Dowling and Booth, 1966; Fallon et al., 2014; Kurkchubasche et al., 1993). However, for patients who cannot meet caloric requirements to support growth and metabolic demands through an exclusively enteral diet, the need for PN may be lifelong.

PN is a means of supplying nutrition intravenously and bypassing the digestive system. It is composed of both macro- and micronutrients. Among the macronutrients, dextrose serves as the carbohydrate source, and protein is provided as crystalline amino acids. Parenteral fat is administered as a triglyceride-rich oil in water emulsion. Fat emulsions can be combined with the carbohydrates and amino acids for administration as a total nutrient admixture, or they can be administered separately from the carbohydrate/amino acid mixture. Typical micronutrients include electrolytes, minerals, vitamins, and trace elements.

Fat is an important component of PN. Parenteral fat provides a dense source of calories that decreases the amount of carbohydrate required to meet energy demands. Administration of fat free PN can induce hepatic de novo lipogenesis (Kalish et al., 2013b; Ling et al., 2011), in which carbohydrate calories in excess of what is immediately utilized to generate adenosine triphosphate (ATP) or stored as glycogen are converted to fat (Baker et al., 1978; Walli, 1978). PN devoid of an exogenous fat source results in the development of hepatosteatosis in animal models (Alwayn et al., 2005; Li et al., 1988; Yeh et al., 1995) and humans (Tulikoura and Huikuri, 1982).

Fish and Fish Oil in Health and Disease Prevention. http://dx.doi.org/10.1016/B978-0-12-802844-5.00025-7

Fats are also a necessary component of PN because they provide the essential long-chain polyunsaturated fatty acids (PUFAs) that humans cannot synthesize de novo. Due to a lack of enzymes to generate the n–3 fatty acid α-linolenic acid (ALA) and the n–6 fatty acid linoleic acid (LA) and their metabolites, these fatty acids must be supplied in the diet. Enteral and parenteral diets lacking these fatty acids result in the development of essential fatty acid deficiency (EFAD), characterized by growth and developmental impairments, fatigue, a characteristic dermatitis, infertility, and in some cases pulmonary insufficiency (Friedman and Rosenberg, 1979; Jeppesen et al., 1998; Kyriakides et al., 1976; Roqueta-Rivera et al., 2011). EFAD can be biochemically diagnosed given that the same enzymes act on ALA to generate eicosapentaenoic acid (EPA) and docosahexaenoic acid (DHA), LA to general arachidonic acid (ARA) and certain nonessential fatty acids, including the monounsaturated oleic acid (OA) to generate mead acid (MA). In a state of EFA sufficiency, these enzymes act on the ALA or LA and metabolites that are available as substrate, and the ratio of the products MA (a triene) to ARA (a tetraene) is low. In EFAD, when there are low levels of LA, ALA, or their metabolites for substrate, these enzymes act on MA precursors to produce MA and elevate the triene:tetraene ratio. Fatty acid levels can be monitored and the triene:tetraene ratio calculated. A biochemical diagnosis of EFAD is considered when the triene:tetraene is greater than 0.2 (Mascioli et al., 1996), but clinical symptoms do not appear until the triene:tetraene ratio reaches 0.4.

Fat emulsions used in PN must be derived from oil sources containing sufficient amounts of essential fatty acids (EFAs) to prevent the development of EFAD. Several types of plant oil as well as fish oil meet this criterion, however these oils differ with respect to EFA composition and additives. Additives include phytosterols and α-tocopherol. Phytosterols are plant-based sterols structurally similar to cholesterol but poorly metabolized in mammals. Alpha-tocopherol is an antioxidant that is a member of the vitamin E family. Each of these additives may contribute to the development of PNALD.

Soybean oil was used in the first commercial intravenous fat emulsion in 1961 (Schuberth and Wretlind, 1961), and today soybean oil lipid emulsions (SOLE) remain the most widely used plant-based fat emulsions. A majority of the EFA content in SOLE are n–6 fatty acids, with LA comprising 50% of the total fatty acids. SOLE is abundant in phytosterols and contains small amounts of α-tocopherol. Olive oil is another plant-based oil used in parenteral fat emulsions. It is abundant in phytosterols, low in α-tocopherol, and its fatty acid content is rich in the nonessential fatty acid OA with very few EFAs. In order to meet EFA requirements, it is available as a combination olive oil/soybean oil emulsion for use in PN. Fish oil is the only animal-based fat emulsion. The EFA composition of fish oil lipid emulsions (FOLE) is high in n–3 fatty acids and low in n–6 fatty acids. FOLE is abundant in α-tocopherol and contains minimal phytosterols.

PARENTERAL NUTRITION-ASSOCIATED LIVER DISEASE

Although PN is a critically important mode of nutrition for patients with IF, there are many associated risks. These include complications related to the indwelling central venous catheter (CVC) necessary for PN delivery, such as infection or thrombosis, and metabolic derangements from suboptimal PN formulations. PNALD is a complication of long-term PN-dependence that is characterized by the development of hepatic inflammation and cholestasis that can progress to fibrosis, cirrhosis, and end-stage liver disease. Untreated end-stage liver disease in the setting of PNALD can often result in liver transplant or death. Jaundice in a patient who has been receiving PN is frequently the first indication of the disease. The gold standard for diagnosing PNALD is the presence of cholestasis on liver biopsy, however PNALD can also be biochemically detected as a serum direct bilirubin of 2 mg/dL or greater (Christensen et al., 2007; Duro et al., 2011; Koseesirikul et al., 2012). Other laboratory markers that may be abnormal in the presence of PNALD include elevations in gamma glutamyl transferase (GGT), alanine aminotransferase (ALT), and aspartate aminotransferase (AST).

PNALD occurs in ~25%–50% of PN-dependent neonates (Javid et al., 2011; Koseesirikul et al., 2012; Lauriti et al., 2014). Historically, the most reliable way to stop progression of the disease was to stop PN and rely solely on enteral feeding. In patients who could not achieve enteral autonomy to stop progression of the disease, mortality or liver transplant rates approached 50% (Squires et al., 2012). PN-dependent infants who are at highest risk of developing PNALD are those born prematurely, of low birth weight, on PN over a longer term, lack enteral feeding, and undergo gastrointestinal surgical procedures (Christensen et al., 2007; Koseesirikul et al., 2012). The parenteral fat source can modulate the effect of PN on the liver. SOLE can increase the risk of developing PNALD while FOLE can reverse biochemical PNALD and stop progression of disease in patients who develop PNALD while receiving SOLE. The following sections of this chapter will discuss the role of SOLE in the development of PNALD and the role for FOLE in its management.

THE ROLE OF PARENTERAL SOYBEAN OIL EMULSIONS IN THE PATHOGENESIS OF PNALD

Over the last decade, clinical studies and research in animal models have shown that the use of SOLE as a parenteral fat source can increase the risk of developing PNALD. Initial studies in a rodent model of PN-induced hepatosteatosis showed that transitioning from an intravenous to an enteral route of SOLE administration could prevent the development of steatosis, suggesting that the route of fat administration matters in modulating the effect of PN on the liver (Javid et al., 2005). It was later shown in the same model that changing the intravenous lipid from SOLE to FOLE could also prevent the development of PN-induced steatosis (Alwayn et al., 2005; Meisel et al., 2011). More recently, studies have focused on understanding the properties of SOLE that promote the development of PNALD when administered intravenously as a fat source. There are several mechanisms that have been proposed, each of which may contribute to the role of SOLE in the pathogenesis of PNALD.

The EFA composition of SOLE is high in n–6 fatty acids, and it has been hypothesized that the high, approximately 5:1, n–6:n–3 fatty acid ratio may contribute to the inflammation associated with PNALD. Although n–3 and n–6 fatty acids are both essential in mammals, they differ with respect to the physiologic effects of their metabolites. The n–6 fatty acid LA metabolite ARA is a precursor for the synthesis of the proinflammatory mediators 2-series prostaglandins and 4-series leukotrienes. The n–3 fatty acid metabolites EPA and DHA, conversely, are precursors of the antiinflammatory 3-series prostaglandins and 5-series leukotrienes, as well as other antiinflammatory lipid mediators including resolvins, protectins, and maresins (Kalish et al., 2013a; Serhan et al., 2000). While some n–6 fatty acid metabolites, such as docosapentaenoic acid (DPA), do have antiinflammatory properties (Dangi et al., 2009), diets high in n–6:n–3 fatty acid ratio are overall more proinflammatory than diets containing a more balanced 1:1 ratio of n–6:n–3 fatty acids (Duan et al., 2013). High fat diets with fat sources low in n–6 fatty acids and high in n–3 fatty acids can mitigate hepatic injury and histologic evidence of steatosis in murine models of nonalcoholic fatty liver disease (Lazic et al., 2014). One study in a guinea pig model of PN dependence demonstrated that SOLE administration with PN increases hepatic markers of oxidative stress and inflammation (Miloudi et al., 2012). In other models of acute inflammation and in humans following a lipopolysaccharide challenge, infusion of SOLE increased inflammatory markers, leukocyte recruitment, and vascular extravasation compared to infusion of fat emulsions containing lower n–6:n–3 ratios (Buschmann et al., 2015; Hecker et al., 2015; Schaefer et al., 2007). One study of the effect of enteral soybean-based fat on recovery from protein malnutrition in utero and during lactation in rats demonstrated that initiation of enteral SOLE resulted in increased expression of the cytokine TNFα and the proinflammatory transcription factor NF-κB (Reis et al., 2015). These studies underscore the proinflammatory properties of n–6 fatty acids and highlight the inflammatory potential of n–6 fatty acid-rich SOLE that may contribute to the development of PNALD in PN-dependent patients.

Phytosterols are abundant in SOLE and may contribute to the development of PNALD. Parenteral administration of phytosterol-containing fat emulsions in animal models results in phytosterol accumulation in the blood, bile, and liver (Clayton et al., 1998; Iyer et al., 1998). The serum phytosterol:cholesterol ratio in PN-dependent children with IF is directly correlated with portal inflammation, cholestasis, and serum bile acid level (Mutanen et al., 2014). One recent study demonstrated that phytosterols may contribute to the development of hepatic inflammation and cholestasis through inhibition of the Farsenoid-X receptor, a key nuclear receptor transcription factor that upregulates expression of genes important for bile flow (Carter et al., 2007). Another group reported that infusion of stigmasterol, one of the principle phytosterols in SOLE, results in hepatic macrophage activation as measured by expression of the cytokine Interleukin-6 (El Kasmi et al., 2013).

FOLE is an alternative parenteral fat source that can reverse PN-induced liver damage in animal models and reverse PNALD in PN-dependent infants and children. Over the last decade several FOLE-based strategies have been developed with the aim of achieving a standard of care for the treatment or prevention of PNALD. These parenteral FOLE-based strategies are discussed below, but despite the promise of FOLE in the management of PNALD, SOLE continues to be the most widely used first-line parenteral fat source.

FISH OIL MONOTHERAPY IN PNALD

FOLE in the Treatment of PNALD

Use of parenteral FOLE as a sole fat source for PN-dependent patients was first reported in 2005 in a soy allergic patient (Gura et al., 2005) who could not receive intravenous SOLE and developed EFAD. Parenteral FOLE was well tolerated and effectively reversed both clinical and biochemical evidence of EFAD. Soon thereafter it was shown in a murine model that parenteral FOLE could protect from PN-induced hepatosteatosis (Alwayn et al., 2005). In 2006, it was first reported that parenteral FOLE could reverse PNALD in 2 PN-dependent infants (Gura et al., 2006). Since then, parenteral FOLE use has been permitted in the United States through compassionate use protocols for PN-dependent patients who develop cholestasis while receiving SOLE.

Over the last decade, there have been several reports of successful use of FOLE monotherapy to reverse cholestasis in PNALD. In an open-label trial of FOLE therapy at a dose of 1 g/kg per day in 42 infants with IF who developed PNALD, cholestasis reversed in 19 patients, 3 patients died, and 1 underwent liver transplant. This was compared to a historical cohort of 49 infants who developed biochemical PNALD but remained on SOLE, among whom cholestasis reversed in 2, 12 died, and 6 underwent liver transplant (Puder et al., 2009). No adverse effects were reported. More recently, other centers have adopted FOLE monotherapy for the treatment of PNALD, and have reported similar results. (Calkins et al., 2013; Lam et al., 2014; Park et al., 2014; Premkumar et al., 2014, 2013).

There is only one prospective, double-blind, randomized controlled trial testing the use of FOLE monotherapy in the treatment of PNALD (Lam et al., 2014). In this study, 16 infants who developed PNALD were randomized to receive 1.5 g/kg per day of FOLE or SOLE. Over a 4-month follow-up period there was no difference in the rates of reversal between the groups, with 3 of 9 infants in the FOLE-treated group reversing while on PN compared to 0 of 7 infants in the SOLE-treated group. None of the infants in the FOLE-treated group died, while 2 of 7 died in the SOLE-treated group. The rate of increase in direct bilirubin and ALT in the SOLE-treated group trended higher than in the FOLE-treated group. While the results of this study were suggestive of beneficial effects of FOLE monotherapy in the treatment of PNALD, the results failed to reach statistical significance in the setting of a small sample size.

FOLE in the Prevention of PNALD

The ability of FOLE to prevent PN-induced liver injury in animal models has been well established. FOLE has prevented PN-induced hepatosteatosis in mice (Alwayn et al., 2005; Meisel et al., 2011). In a mouse model of dextran sulfate sodium-induced bowel injury and PN-dependence, FOLE can prevent elevations in serum total bilirubin, AST, ALT, and bile acids (El Kasmi et al., 2013). In a preterm piglet model of PN-dependence, FOLE prevents elevations in serum total and direct bilirubin, AST, ALT, GGT, and bile acids; prevents development of hepatosteatosis; and reduces hepatic triglyceride levels (Vlaardingerbroek et al., 2014). Despite the data supporting the ability of FOLE to prevent PN-induced liver injury in animal models, minimal data reporting FOLE as a first-line parenteral fat source for the prevention of PNALD in PN-dependent infants exists. One study of 19 PN-dependent infants randomized to receive SOLE or FOLE for parenteral fat provision aimed to test whether FOLE, as an initial parenteral fat source, could prevent PNALD. Among enrolled infants, the rate of cholestasis development was lower than expected, and the study was not adequately powered to detect differences in development of PNALD. This study did demonstrate that infants provided intravenous FOLE as the parenteral fat source from the onset of PN-dependence had normal growth and neurodevelopmental outcomes at 6 and 24 months with no increased risk of hypertriglyceridemia, coagulopathy, infection, or EFAD compared to infants administered SOLE (Nehra et al., 2014).

Some have suggested that the reason PNALD resolves with the transition from SOLE to FOLE is that the 1 g/kg per day dose of FOLE administered is lower than the usual 2-3 g/kg per day dosing of SOLE. Other PNALD prevention studies have demonstrated that SOLE administered at a dose of 1 g/kg per day rather than 3 g/kg per day could not prevent the development of PNALD in PN-dependent neonates (Calkins et al., 2015; Levit et al., 2014). In the preterm piglet model of PN-dependence, addition of α-tocopherol, an antioxidant found in FOLE, to SOLE was able to prevent the development of PN-induced liver injury (Ng et al., 2015). While studies in animal models suggest that FOLE may be able to prevent PN-induced liver injury and that particular components of FOLE may play a role, more studies are needed to ascertain whether FOLE can protect infants with IF from PNALD.

Mechanisms of FOLE Therapy in PNALD

Several studies have focused on understanding the mechanisms by which FOLE mediates reversal of cholestasis in infants who develop PNALD. Several mechanisms of FOLE-mediated hepato-protection have been proposed, each of which may contribute to reversal of PN-induced cholestasis by FOLE.

FOLE is abundant in n–3 fatty acids, with a lower n–6:n–3 fatty acid ratio than SOLE. Depending on the fish oil source, FOLE fatty acid composition is 20%–40% n–3 fatty acids in the form of ALA, EPA, and DHA and only 1–3% n–6 fatty acids in the form of LA and ARA. High n–3 fatty acid content gives FOLE antiinflammatory potential. In both in vitro and in vivo studies, fish oil has demonstrated the ability to suppress responses to inflammatory stimuli

(De Nardi et al., 2008; Garib et al., 2013; Manzoni Jacintho et al., 2009). One in vitro study using cultured hepatic epithelial cells demonstrated the ability of fish oil to suppress TGFβ-induced epithelial-to-mesenchymal transition that characterizes hepatic fibrosis (Pastor-Clerigues et al., 2014). Infants transitioned from SOLE to FOLE after developing PNALD demonstrated systemic increases in antiinflammatory lipid mediators with FOLE therapy (Kalish et al., 2013a). These studies highlight the antiinflammatory properties of fish oil and the potential of FOLE to reduce the hepatic inflammation associated with PNALD.

In addition to differences in EFA content between SOLE and FOLE, there are also differences in additives that may contribute to FOLE-mediated hepatic protection. FOLE contains minimal phytosterols that have been implicated in the contribution of SOLE to the onset of cholestasis. In addition, FOLE contains an abundance of the anti-oxidant α-tocopherol, at a concentration of ~200 mg/L. It has been proposed that the α-tocopherol in FOLE contributes to FOLE-mediated reversal of PN-induced cholestasis. A-tocopherol and other members of the vitamin E family have antiinflammatory properties that can be beneficial in reducing systemic inflammation (Saboori et al., 2015) as well as inflammation associated with specific disease states, including atherosclerosis, allergies, vasculitis, and seizure disorders (Abdala-Valencia et al., 2014; Ambrogini et al., 2014; Hsieh et al., 2014; Shing et al., 2014). Ng and coworkers demonstrated in preterm piglets administered PN that addition of 251 mg/L α-tocopherol to SOLE could prevent hyperbilirubinemia, elevations in GGT, and increases in hepatic fat content associated with PN-induced hepatic injury, suggesting that the α-tocopherol contained in FOLE may play an important role in the reversal of PN-induced cholestasis (Ng et al., 2015).

Concerns about FOLE Monotherapy

Despite the efficacy of FOLE in the treatment of PNALD that has been demonstrated in both preclinical model systems and clinical studies, there remains debate over the safety of FOLE monotherapy in the management of PNALD. There are reports detailing potential complications of FOLE monotherapy, as well as research efforts to define the mechanisms by which FOLE monotherapy may mediate these complications.

One concern that has been raised is the EFAD potential of FOLE monotherapy. FOLE therapy in infants who develop PNALD is generally dosed at 1 g/kg per day, in contrast to the ~2–3 g/kg per day of fat recommended for this age group. Additionally, FOLE contains very little n–6 fatty acids, and it has been suggested that although sufficient amounts of n–3 fatty acids are supplied by FOLE, there may be a physiologic deficiency of n–6 fatty acids with FOLE monotherapy. One study in a murine model of EFAD demonstrated that supplementation of lipid containing a 20:1 ratio of the n–3 fatty acid DHA to the n–6 fatty acid ARA resulted in resolution of biochemical EFAD (Le et al., 2012). Prospectively followed PN-dependent infants receiving 1 g/kg per day FOLE monotherapy demonstrated no biochemical or clinical evidence of EFAD, and no adverse effects in growth parameters over a median 3.8-month follow-up time (de Meijer et al., 2010).

Others have expressed concerns about physiologically significant bleeding due to n–6 fatty acid paucity with FOLE monotherapy. The n–6 fatty acid ARA is a precursor of thromboxanes and prostacyclins that mediate platelet aggregation and promote clotting. Reports of Eskimo populations with diets high in n–3 fatty acids and low in n–6:n–3 fatty acid ratios showed increased bleeding times and decreased platelet aggregation, (Dyerberg and Bang, 1979), however other studies have demonstrated no significant bleeding with high n–3 fatty acid consumption (Simopoulos, 2002; Wachira et al., 2014). The American Heart Association has stated there is no clinical bleeding risk from high doses of fish oil, even when taken in combination with other medications known to impact a variety of coagulation parameters (Kris-Etherton et al., 2003). Dicken et al. reported significant bleeding in an infant receiving FOLE monotherapy over 26 days following removal of a femoral CVC and insertion of a new subclavian CVC. The authors attributed the bleeding event to FOLE monotherapy, and followed-up with thromboelastography studies in pigs receiving FOLE. There was a doubling of clot formation time and inhibition of platelet agonists in the FOLE-treated group compared to controls and no bleeding complications in the FOLE-treated pigs (Dicken et al., 2014). In studies of larger cohorts of infants receiving FOLE monotherapy for treatment of PNALD over longer periods of time, it has been reported that in the absence of cirrhosis, these children do not develop biochemical coagulopathies (Calkins et al., 2013; Puder et al., 2009). Large scale studies with the goals of assessing bleeding parameters and occurrence of clinically significant bleeding with FOLE monotherapy compared to alternative parenteral fat sources are required to settle this debate.

Additional concerns have been raised regarding hepatic disease progression despite biochemical resolution of cholestasis in PN-dependent infants receiving FOLE monotherapy. Soden and coworkers reported failure of portal fibrosis resolution in two infants despite normalization of serum direct bilirubin with FOLE monotherapy. The pre-FOLE liver biopsies in these infants were performed several months prior to the transition from SOLE to FOLE therapy and did not correlate with the timing of FOLE initiation. Fibrosis may have progressed in the months between the initial biopsy and FOLE initiation, thus conclusions regarding the effect of FOLE therapy on hepatic fibrosis cannot be definitively drawn from this report (Soden et al., 2010). In another report assessing serial liver biopsies in six PN-dependent infants receiving FOLE for PNALD, while all six infants had normalized direct bilirubin levels and had preserved hepatic synthetic function, histologic fibrosis progressed in three, remained unchanged in two, and regressed in one case (Mercer et al., 2013). Matsumoto and coworkers reported biopsy findings of seven explanted livers from infants who had received FOLE monotherapy for PNALD and then underwent combined liver-intestinal transplants. All infants had biochemical resolution of cholestasis on FOLE therapy, but upon explant pathologic examination, each had advanced fibrosis, similar to the fibrosis detected in matched controls that were maintained on SOLE therapy prior to transplant. No patients in this study had biopsy data prior to initiating FOLE therapy, thus no conclusions can be made regarding the effect of FOLE on fibrosis progression (Matsumoto et al., 2014). Several studies have demonstrated that portal fibrosis occurs early in PNALD and can progress rapidly (Moss et al., 1993; Mullick et al., 1994; Zambrano et al., 2004), and thus may be present prior to biochemical evidence of cholestasis and the initiation of FOLE therapy. In a recent prospective study of 51 infants diagnosed with cirrhosis due to PNALD prior to initiating FOLE monotherapy from 2004–12, 76% had biochemical resolution of cholestasis, none of the patients required liver transplant, none of the patients died of end-stage liver disease, and there was a normalization in Pediatric End-Stage Liver Disease score for the cohort that persisted over the study period (Nandivada et al., 2013). This suggests that although biochemical resolution of cholestasis may occur with FOLE monotherapy while histologic resolution of fibrosis may not, persistence of fibrosis on histology after reversal of cholestasis does not affect the clinical outcome in this population of patients.

ADDITION OF FOLE TO SOLE TO TREAT PNALD

An alternative strategy to FOLE monotherapy is to add FOLE to SOLE in PN-dependent infants who develop PNALD. This strategy is attractive because it provides the antioxidants and n–3 fatty acids of fish oil and offers a more balanced ratio of n–6:n–3 fatty acids. Diamond and coworkers reported their experience utilizing this strategy in 12 PN-dependent children who developed PNALD. Patients received 1 g/kg per day SOLE mixed with 1 g/kg per day FOLE to target an n–6:n–3 fatty acid ratio of 1:1 to 2:1. In all, four patients experienced resolution of their hyperbilirubinemia, five patients required transition to FOLE monotherapy in order to achieve resolution of cholestasis, and three patients failed and underwent liver transplantation (Diamond et al., 2009). In this small case series, it appears that while this strategy may be effective for some patients, others may require transition to FOLE monotherapy the achieve reversal of PNALD. The use of FOLE monotherapy rather than a 50:50 blend of SOLE and FOLE to treat PNALD is further supported in the recently published peer reviewed position paper on alternative lipid emulsions issued by the American Society of Parenteral and Enteral Nutrition (Vanek et al., 2012).

Another strategy that has been explored is utilization of FOLE combined with an 80%/20% soybean oil/olive oil fat emulsion. Olive oil is composed mostly of the nonessential monounsaturated fatty acid OA, which is less immunologically active compared to the essential fatty acids, but that is also a good source of calories. In a retrospective study, Angsten and coworkers evaluated 20 infants with PNALD that were treated with the FOLE/soybean oil/olive oil combination. Fourteen patients had biochemical reversal of cholestasis and survived, four patients died of causes unrelated to liver disease, and two patients died of liver failure. This was compared to a historical cohort of 18 infants who developed PNALD but remained on SOLE in which 6 patients died of liver failure and only 2 achieved normal serum direct bilirubin levels (Angsten et al., 2012). Another group reported reversal of cholestasis in five infants who developed PNALD with administration of a mixture to FOLE and soybean oil/olive oil (Lilja et al., 2011). Pawlik and coworkers compared development of cholestasis in 60 PN-dependent infants treated with a combination of FOLE and olive oil/soybean oil to 70 PN-dependent infants receiving soybean oil/olive oil alone. They reported development of cholestasis in 20 patients receiving the soybean oil/olive oil combination compared to only 3 patients in the FOLE/soybean oil/olive oil group that developed cholestasis (Pawlik et al., 2014). Overall, the strategies combining FOLE with plant oil-based lipid emulsions have been reported in only a few small studies with mixed results, and studies with larger cohorts are required to define the clinical circumstances in which these strategies may be clinically most useful.

COMBINATION EMULSIONS CONTAINING FISH OIL IN THE MANAGEMENT OF PNALD

In an effort to improve the balance of fatty acid content of lipid emulsions, several products have been introduced. The newest generation lipid emulsions include FOLE in combination with one or more of the oils used in previous generation lipid emulsions. FOLE is rich in n–3 fatty acids, which are highly bioactive compared to other oil sources including medium-chain triglycerides (MCT) and olive oil. SMOFLipid (Fresenius Kabi AG, Uppsala, Sweden) is a 20% oil emulsion comprised of 4 oil types including 30% soybean oil, 30% MCT, 25% olive oil, and 15% fish oil. It has been studied for use in both treating and preventing PNALD in PN-dependent infants and has a favorable safety profile compared to standard SOLE (Tomsits et al., 2010). SMOFLipid is not currently approved for use in the United States.

SMOFLipid in the Treatment of PNALD

Despite containing only a small amount of fish oil, there is some evidence to indicate that SMOFLipid may be effective for certain patients in the treatment of PNALD. In a retrospective study of 17 PN-dependent infants who developed PNALD of which 8 were transitioned to SMOFLipid and 9 continued to receive SOLE, biochemical cholestasis resolved in 5 of the 8 infants administered SMOFLipid and in only 2 of the 9 infants administered SOLE (Muhammed et al., 2012). This study suggests that in a portion of patients or in certain clinical circumstances, SMOFLipid can reverse PN-induced cholestasis. More studies are required to define the patients and clinical circumstances in which SMOFLipid may be beneficial.

SMOFLipid in the Prevention of PNALD

Several studies report the use of SMOFLipid as a first-line parenteral fat source in PN-dependent patients for the prevention of PNALD. In one study in which 60 infants requiring PN were randomized to receive either SMOFLipid or SOLE as a parenteral fat source, the SMOFLipid-treated group had a significantly lower GGT after 14 days of therapy compared to the SOLE-treated group (Tomsits et al., 2010). Another group reported development of cholestasis in two PN-dependent infants receiving SMOFLipid. These infants were transitioned to FOLE monotherapy and experienced resolution of their liver disease (Lee et al., 2015). In a study in which infants requiring PN were randomized to receive SOLE, SOLE/MCT, SOLE/MCT/FOLE, or SMOFLipid as a parenteral fat source over 21 days, cholestasis rarely developed in any of the groups, although the follow-up period was short (Savini et al., 2013). In animal models of PN dependence, the effects of intravenous lipid emulsions indicate that SMOFLipid does not prevent PN-induced liver injury as well as FOLE, however SMOFLipid appears to result in improved histologic outcomes compared to SOLE (Meisel et al., 2011). In a piglet model of PNALD, SMOFLipid can prevent the development of biochemical cholestasis and histologic steatosis, and results in less accumulation of hepatic and plasma bile acids compared to SOLE (Vlaardingerbroek et al., 2014).

Currently the existing studies testing the effect of SMOFLipid in the prevention and treatment of PNALD are in small cohorts of patients over short follow-up periods on the order of days to weeks. More long-term studies in larger cohorts of patients are required to determine the efficacy of SMOFLipid in both the prevention and treatment of PNALD.

CONCLUSION

Parenteral FOLE appears to have efficacy as monotherapy for the treatment of PNALD in infants dependent on PN for survival. Despite this, debate still exists whether FOLE monotherapy is safe. These concerns have fueled studies aimed at understanding the underlying etiology of PNALD as well as the development of alternative FOLE-based strategies for the management of PNALD. Future work will be aimed at defining the utility of novel combination emulsions and mixtures of existing parenteral fat emulsions in the management of PN-induced liver injury. It appears that the anti-inflammatory and anti-oxidant properties of fish oil, as well as minimization of phytosterols confer properties that may protect the liver from injury when administered intravenously, and it is likely that fish oil will remain important in PNALD management and a component of newly emerging therapies.

References

Abdala-Valencia, H., Berdnikovs, S., Soveg, F.W., Cook-Mills, J.M., 2014. α-Tocopherol supplementation of allergic female mice inhibits development of CD11c+CD11b+ dendritic cells in utero and allergic inflammation in neonates. Am. J. Physiol. Lung Cell. Mol. Physiol. 307, L482–L496.

Alwayn, I.P., Gura, K., Nose, V., Zausche, B., Javid, P., Garza, J., Verbesey, J., Voss, S., Ollero, M., Andersson, C., Bistrian, B., Folkman, J., Puder, M., 2005. Omega-3 fatty acid supplementation prevents hepatic steatosis in a murine model of nonalcoholic fatty liver disease. Pediatr. Res. 57, 445–452.

Ambrogini, P., Minelli, A., Galati, C., Betti, M., Lattanzi, D., Ciffolilli, S., Piroddi, M., Galli, F., Cuppini, R., 2014. Post-seizure α-tocopherol treatment decreases neuroinflammation and neuronal degeneration induced by status epilepticus in rat hippocampus. Mol. Neurobiol. 50, 246–256.

Angsten, G., Finkel, Y., Lucas, S., Kassa, A.-M., Paulsson, M., Lilja, H.E., 2012. Improved outcome in neonatal short bowel syndrome using parenteral fish oil in combination with ω-6/9 lipid emulsions. JPEN J. Parenter. Enteral Nutr. 36, 587–595.

Baker, N., Learn, D.B., Bruckdorfer, K.R., 1978. Re-evaluation of lipogenesis from dietary glucose carbon in liver and carcass of mice. J. Lipid Res. 19, 879–893.

Buschmann, K., Poeschl, J., Braach, N., Hudalla, H., Kuss, N., Frommhold, D., 2015. The olive oil-based lipid clinoleic blocks leukocyte recruitment and improves survival during systemic inflammation: a comparative in vivo study of different parenteral lipid emulsions. Mediators Inflamm. 2015, 757059.

Calkins, K.L., Dunn, J.C.Y., Shew, S.B., Reyen, L., Farmer, D.G., Devaskar, S.U., Venick, R.S., 2013. Pediatric intestinal failure-associated liver disease is reversed with 6 months of intravenous fish oil. JPEN J. Parenter. Enteral Nutr. 38, 682–692.

Calkins, K.L., Havranek, T., Kelley-Quon, L.I., Cerny, L., Flores, M., Grogan, T., Shew, S.B., 2015. Low-dose parenteral soybean oil for the prevention of parenteral nutrition-associated liver disease in neonates with gastrointestinal disorders: a multicenter randomized controlled pilot study. JPEN J. Parenter. Enteral Nutr., pii: 0148607115588334.

Carter, B.A., Taylor, O.A., Prendergast, D.R., Zimmerman, T.L., Von Furstenberg, R., Moore, D.D., Karpen, S.J., 2007. Stigmasterol, a soy lipid-derived phytosterol, is an antagonist of the bile acid nuclear receptor FXR. Pediatr. Res. 62, 301–306.

Christensen, R.D., Henry, E., Wiedmeier, S.E., Burnett, J., Lambert, D.K., 2007. Identifying patients, on the first day of life, at high-risk of developing parenteral nutrition-associated liver disease. J. Perinatol. 27, 284–290.

Clayton, P.T., Whitfield, P., Iyer, K., 1998. The role of phytosterols in the pathogenesis of liver complications of pediatric parenteral nutrition. Nutrition 14, 158–164.

Dangi, B., Obeng, M., Nauroth, J.M., Teymourlouei, M., Needham, M., Raman, K., Arterburn, L.M., 2009. Biogenic synthesis, purification, and chemical characterization of anti-inflammatory resolvins derived from docosapentaenoic acid (DPAn-6). J. Biol. Chem. 284, 14744–14759.

de Meijer, V.E., Le, H.D., Meisel, J.A., Gura, K.M., Puder, M., 2010. Parenteral fish oil as monotherapy prevents essential fatty acid deficiency in parenteral nutrition-dependent patients. J. Pediatr. Gastroenterol. Nutr. 50, 212–218.

De Nardi, L., Bellinati-Pires, R., Torrinhas, R.S., Bacchi, C.E., Arias, V., Waitzberg, D.L., 2008. Effect of fish oil containing parenteral lipid emulsions on neutrophil chemotaxis and resident-macrophages' phagocytosis in rats. Clin. Nutr. 27, 283–288.

Diamond, I.R., Sterescu, A., Pencharz, P.B., Kim, J.H., Wales, P.W., 2009. Changing the paradigm: omegaven for the treatment of liver failure in pediatric short bowel syndrome. J. Pediatr. Gastroenterol. Nutr. 48, 209–215.

Dicken, B.J., Bruce, A., Samuel, T.M., Wales, P.W., Nahirniak, S., Turner, J.M., 2014. Bedside to bench: The risk of bleeding with parenteral omega-3 lipid emulsion therapy. J. Pediatr. 164, 652–654.

Dowling, R.H., Booth, C.C., 1966. Functional compensation after small-bowel resection in man. Demonstration by direct measurement. Lancet 2, 146–147.

Duan, Y., Li, F., Li, L., Fan, J., Sun, X., Yin, Y., 2013. n-6:n-3 PUFA ratio is involved in regulating lipid metabolism and inflammation in pigs. Br. J. Nutr. 111, 445–451.

Duro, D., Mitchell, P.D., Kalish, L.A., Martin, C., McCarthy, M., Jaksic, T., Dunn, J., Brandt, M.L., Nobuhara, K.K., Sylvester, K.G., Moss, R.L., Duggan, C., 2011. Risk factors for parenteral nutrition–associated liver disease following surgical therapy for necrotizing enterocolitis: a Glaser Pediatric Research Network Study (corrected). J. Pediatr. Gastroenterol. Nutr. 52, 595–600.

Dyerberg, J., Bang, H.O., 1979. Haemostatic function and platelet polyunsaturated fatty acids in Eskimos. Lancet 2, 433–435.

El Kasmi, K.C., Anderson, A.L., Devereaux, M.W., Vue, P.M., Zhang, W., Setchell, K.D.R., Karpen, S.J., Sokol, R.J., 2013. Phytosterols promote liver injury and Kupffer cell activation in parenteral nutrition-associated liver disease. Sci. Transl. Med. 5, 206ra137.

Fallon, E.M., Mitchell, P.D., Nehra, D., Potemkin, A.K., O'Loughlin, A.A., Gura, K.M., Puder, M., 2014. Neonates with short bowel syndrome: an optimistic future for parenteral nutrition independence. JAMA Surg. 149, 663–670.

Friedman, Z., Rosenberg, A., 1979. Abnormal lung surfactant related to essential fatty acid deficiency in a neonate. Pediatrics 63, 855–859.

Garib, R., Garla, P., Torrinhas, R.S., Bertevello, P.L., Logullo, A.F., Waitzberg, D.L., 2013. Effects of parenteral fish oil lipid emulsions on colon morphology and cytokine expression after experimental colitis. Nutr. Hosp. 28, 849–856.

Goulet, O., Ruemmele, F., 2006. Causes and management of intestinal failure in children. Gastroenterology 130, S16–S28.

Gura, K.M., Duggan, C.P., Collier, S.B., Jennings, R.W., Folkman, J., Bistrian, B.R., Puder, M., 2006. Reversal of parenteral nutrition-associated liver disease in two infants with short bowel syndrome using parenteral fish oil: implications for future management. Pediatrics 118, e197–e201.

Gura, K.M., Parsons, S.K., Bechard, L.J., Henderson, T., Dorsey, M., Phipatanakul, W., Duggan, C., Puder, M., Lenders, C., 2005. Use of a fish oil-based lipid emulsion to treat essential fatty acid deficiency in a soy allergic patient receiving parenteral nutrition. Clin. Nutr. 24, 839–847.

Hecker, M., Linder, T., Ott, J., Walmrath, H.-D., Lohmeyer, J., Vadász, I., Marsh, L.M., Herold, S., Reichert, M., Buchbinder, A., Morty, R.E., Bausch, B., Fischer, T., Schulz, R., Grimminger, F., Witzenrath, M., Barnes, M., Seeger, W., Mayer, K., 2015. Immunomodulation by lipid emulsions in pulmonary inflammation: a randomized controlled trial. Crit. Care 19, 226.

Hsieh, C.-Y., Hsiao, G., Hsu, M.-J., Wang, Y.-H., Sheu, J.-R., 2014. PMC, a potent hydrophilic α-tocopherol derivative, inhibits NF-κB activation via PP2A but not IκBα-dependent signals in vascular smooth muscle cells. J. Cell. Mol. Med. 18, 1278–1289.

Iyer, K.R., Spitz, L., Clayton, P., 1998. BAPS prize lecture: new insight into mechanisms of parenteral nutrition-associated cholestasis: role of plant sterols. British Association of Paediatric Surgeons. J. Pediatr. Surg. 33, 1–6.

Javid, P.J., Greene, A.K., Garza, J., Gura, K., Alwayn, I.P.J., Voss, S., Nose, V., Satchi-Fainaro, R., Zausche, B., Mulkern, R.V., Jaksic, T., Bistrian, B., Folkman, J., Puder, M., 2005. The route of lipid administration affects parenteral nutrition-induced hepatic steatosis in a mouse model. J. Pediatr. Surg. 40, 1446–1453.

Javid, P.J., Malone, F.R., Dick, A.A.S., Hsu, E., Sunseri, M., Healey, P., Horslen, S.P., 2011. A contemporary analysis of parenteral nutrition-associated liver disease in surgical infants. J. Pediatr. Surg. 46, 1913–1917.

Jeppesen, P.B., Høy, C.E., Mortensen, P.B., 1998. Essential fatty acid deficiency in patients receiving home parenteral nutrition. Am. J. Clin. Nutr. 68, 126–133.

Kalish, B.T., Le, H.D., Fitzgerald, J.M., Wang, S., Seamon, K., Gura, K.M., Gronert, K., Puder, M., 2013a. Intravenous fish oil lipid emulsion promotes a shift toward anti-inflammatory proresolving lipid mediators. Am. J. Physiol. Gastrointest. Liver Physiol. 305, G818–G828.

Kalish, B.T., Le, H.D., Gura, K.M., Bistrian, B.R., Puder, M., 2013b. A metabolomic analysis of two intravenous lipid emulsions in a murine model. PLoS One 8, e59653.

Koseesirikul, P., Chotinaruemol, S., Ukarapol, N., 2012. Incidence and risk factors of parenteral nutrition-associated liver disease in newborn infants. Pediatr. Int. 54, 434–436.

Kris-Etherton, P.M., Harris, W.S., Appel, L.J., 2003. Fish consumption, fish oil, omega-3 fatty acids, and cardiovascular disease. Arterioscler. Thromb. Vasc. Biol. 23, e20–e30.

Kurkchubasche, A.G., Rowe, M.I., Smith, S.D., 1993. Adaptation in short-bowel syndrome: reassessing old limits. J. Pediatr. Surg. 28, 1069–1071.

Kyriakides, E.C., Beeler, D.A., Edmonds, R.H., Balint, J.A., 1976. Alterations in phosphatidylcholine species and their reversal in pulmonary surfactant during essential fatty-acid deficiency. Biochim. Biophys. Acta 431, 399–407.

Lam, H.S., Tam, Y.H., Poon, T.C.W., Cheung, H.M., Yu, X., Chan, B.P.L., Lee, K.H., Lee, B.S.C., Ng, P.C., 2014. A double-blind randomised controlled trial of fish oil-based versus soy-based lipid preparations in the treatment of infants with parenteral nutrition-associated cholestasis. Neonatology 105, 290–296.

Lauriti, G., Zani, A., Aufieri, R., Cananzi, M., Chiesa, P.L., Eaton, S., Pierro, A., 2014. Incidence, prevention, and treatment of parenteral nutrition-associated cholestasis and intestinal failure-associated liver disease in infants and children: a systematic review. JPEN J. Parenter. Enteral Nutr. 38, 70–85.

Lazic, M., Inzaugarat, M.E., Povero, D., Zhao, I.C., Chen, M., Nalbandian, M., Miller, Y.I., Cherñavsky, A.C., Feldstein, A.E., Sears, D.D., 2014. Reduced dietary omega-6 to omega-3 fatty acid ratio and 12/15-lipoxygenase deficiency are protective against chronic high fat diet-induced steatohepatitis. PLoS One 9, e107658.

Le, H.D., Meisel, J.A., de Meijer, V.E., Fallon, E.M., Gura, K.M., Nose, V., Bistrian, B.R., Puder, M., 2012. Docosahexaenoic acid and arachidonic acid prevent essential fatty acid deficiency and hepatic steatosis. JPEN J. Parenter. Enteral Nutr. 36, 431–441.

Lee, S., Park, H.J., Yoon, J., Hong, S.H., Oh, C.-Y., Lee, S.-K., Seo, J.-M., 2015. Reversal of intestinal failure-associated liver disease by switching from a combination lipid emulsion containing fish oil to fish oil monotherapy. J. Parenter. Enter. Nutr. 40 (3), 437–440.

Levit, O.L., Calkins, K.L., Gibson, L.C., Kelley-Quon, L., Robinson, D.T., Elashoff, D.A., Grogan, T.R., Li, N., Bizzarro, M.J., Ehrenkranz, R.A., 2014. Low-dose intravenous soybean oil emulsion for prevention of cholestasis in preterm neonates. JPEN J. Parenter. Enteral Nutr. 40 (3), 374–382.

Li, S.J., Nussbaum, M.S., McFadden, D.W., Gapen, C.L., Dayal, R., Fischer, J.E., 1988. Addition of glucagon to total parenteral nutrition (TPN) prevents hepatic steatosis in rats. Surgery 104, 350–357.

Lilja, H.E., Finkel, Y., Paulsson, M., Lucas, S., 2011. Prevention and reversal of intestinal failure-associated liver disease in premature infants with short bowel syndrome using intravenous fish oil in combination with omega-6/9 lipid emulsions. J. Pediatr. Surg. 46, 1361–1367.

Ling, P.-R., Andersson, C., Strijbosch, R., Lee, S., Silvestri, A., Gura, K.M., Puder, M., Bistrian, B.R., 2011. Effects of glucose or fat calories in total parenteral nutrition on fat metabolism and systemic inflammation in rats. Metabolism 60, 195–205.

Manzoni Jacintho, T., Gotho, H., Gidlund, M., García Marques, C., Torrinhas, R., Mirtes Sales, M., Linetzky Waitzberg, D., 2009. Anti-inflammatory effect of parenteral fish oil lipid emulsion on human activated mononuclear leukocytes. Nutr. Hosp. 24, 288–296.

Mascioli, E.A., Lopes, S.M., Champagne, C., Driscoll, D.F., 1996. Essential fatty acid deficiency and home total parenteral nutrition patients. Nutrition 12, 245–249.

Matsumoto, C.S., Kaufman, S.S., Island, E.R., Kallakury, B., Yazigi, N.A., Khan, K.M., Fishbein, T.M., 2014. Hepatic explant pathology of pediatric intestinal transplant recipients previously treated with omega-3 fatty acid lipid emulsion. J. Pediatr. 165, 59–64.

Meisel, J.A., Le, H.D., de Meijer, V.E., Nose, V., Gura, K.M., Mulkern, R.V., Akhavan Sharif, M.R., Puder, M., 2011. Comparison of 5 intravenous lipid emulsions and their effects on hepatic steatosis in a murine model. J. Pediatr. Surg. 46, 666–673.

Mercer, D.F., Hobson, B.D., Fischer, R.T., Talmon, G.A., Perry, D.A., Gerhardt, B.K., Grant, W.J., Botha, J.F., Langnas, A.N., Quiros-Tejeira, R.E., 2013. Hepatic fibrosis persists and progresses despite biochemical improvement in children treated with intravenous fish oil emulsion. J. Pediatr. Gastroenterol. Nutr. 56, 364–369.

Miloudi, K., Comte, B., Rouleau, T., Montoudis, A., Levy, E., Lavoie, J.-C., 2012. The mode of administration of total parenteral nutrition and nature of lipid content influence the generation of peroxides and aldehydes. Clin. Nutr. 31, 526–534.

Moss, R.L., Das, J.B., Raffensperger, J.G., 1993. Total parenteral nutrition-associated cholestasis: clinical and histopathologic correlation. J. Pediatr. Surg. 28, 1270–1274.

Muhammed, R., Bremner, R., Protheroe, S., Johnson, T., Holden, C., Murphy, M.S., 2012. Resolution of parenteral nutrition–associated jaundice on changing from a soybean oil emulsion to a complex mixed-lipid emulsion. J. Pediatr. Gastroenterol. Nutr. 54, 797–802.

Mullick, F.G., Moran, C.A., Ishak, K.G., 1994. Total parenteral nutrition: a histopathologic analysis of the liver changes in 20 children. Mod. Pathol. 7, 190–194.

Mutanen, A., Nissinen, M.J., Lohi, J., Heikkila, P., Gylling, H., Pakarinen, M.P., 2014. Serum plant sterols, cholestanol, and cholesterol precursors associate with histological liver injury in pediatric onset intestinal failure. Am. J. Clin. Nutr. 100, 1085–1094.

Nandivada, P., Chang, M.I., Potemkin, A.K., Carlson, S.J., Cowan, E., O'loughlin, A.A., Mitchell, P.D., Gura, K.M., Puder, M., 2013. The natural history of cirrhosis from parenteral nutrition-associated liver disease after resolution of cholestasis with parenteral fish oil therapy. Ann. Surg. 261 (1), 172–179.

Nehra, D., Fallon, E.M., Potemkin, A.K., Voss, S.D., Mitchell, P.D., Valim, C., Belfort, M.B., Bellinger, D.C., Duggan, C., Gura, K.M., Puder, M., 2014. A comparison of 2 intravenous lipid emulsions: interim analysis of a randomized controlled trial. JPEN J. Parenter. Enteral Nutr. 38, 693–701.

Ng, K., Stoll, B., Chacko, S., Saenz de Pipaon, M., Lauridsen, C., Gray, M., Squires, E.J., Marini, J., Zamora, I.J., Olutoye, O.O., Burrin, D.G., 2015. Vitamin E in new-generation lipid emulsions protects against parenteral nutrition-associated liver disease in parenteral nutrition-fed preterm pigs. JPEN J. Parenter. Enteral Nutr., pii: 0148607114567900.

Park, H.W., Lee, N.M., Kim, J.H., Kim, K.S., Kim, S.-N., 2014. Parenteral fish oil-containing lipid emulsions may reverse parenteral nutrition-associated cholestasis in neonates: a systematic review and meta-analysis. J. Nutr. 145, 277–283.

Pastor-Clerigues, A., Marti-Bonmati, E., Milara, J., Almudever, P., Cortijo, J., 2014. Anti-inflammatory and anti-fibrotic profile of fish oil emulsions used in parenteral nutrition-associated liver disease. PLoS One 9, e115404.

Pawlik, D., Lauterbach, R., Walczak, M., Hurkała, J., Sherman, M.P., 2014. Fish-oil fat emulsion supplementation reduces the risk of retinopathy in very low birth weight infants: a prospective, randomized study. JPEN J. Parenter. Enteral Nutr. 38, 711–716.

Premkumar, M.H., Carter, B.A., Hawthorne, K.M., King, K., Abrams, S.A., 2013. High rates of resolution of cholestasis in parenteral nutrition-associated liver disease with fish oil-based lipid emulsion monotherapy. J. Pediatr. 162, 793–798.

Premkumar, M.H., Carter, B.A., Hawthorne, K.M., King, K., Abrams, S.A., 2014. Fish oil-based lipid emulsions in the treatment of parenteral nutrition-associated liver disease: an ongoing positive experience. Adv. Nutr. 5, 65–70.

Puder, M., Valim, C., Meisel, J.A., Le, H.D., de Meijer, V.E., Robinson, E.M., Zhou, J., Duggan, C., Gura, K.M., 2009. Parenteral fish oil improves outcomes in patients with parenteral nutrition-associated liver injury. Ann. Surg. 250, 395–402.

Reis, S.R. de L., Feres, N.H., Ignacio-Souza, L.M., Veloso, R.V., Arantes, V.C., Kawashita, N.H., Colodel, E.M., Botosso, B.L., Reis, M.A. de B., Latorraca, M.Q., 2015. Nutritional recovery with a soybean diet after weaning reduces lipogenesis but induces inflammation in the liver in adult rats exposed to protein restriction during intrauterine life and lactation. Mediators Inflamm. 2015, 781703.

Roqueta-Rivera, M., Abbott, T.L., Sivaguru, M., Hess, R.A., Nakamura, M.T., 2011. Deficiency in the omega-3 fatty acid pathway results in failure of acrosome biogenesis in mice. Biol. Reprod. 85, 721–732.

Saboori, S., Shab-Bidar, S., Speakman, J.R., Yousefi Rad, E., Djafarian, K., 2015. Effect of vitamin E supplementation on serum C-reactive protein level: a meta-analysis of randomized controlled trials. Eur. J. Clin. Nutr. 69 (8), 867–873.

Savini, S., D'Ascenzo, R., Biagetti, C., Serpentini, G., Pompilio, A., Bartoli, A., Cogo, P.E., Carnielli, V.P., 2013. The effect of 5 intravenous lipid emulsions on plasma phytosterols in preterm infants receiving parenteral nutrition: a randomized clinical trial. Am. J. Clin. Nutr. 98, 312–318.

Schaefer, M.B., Ott, J., Mohr, A., Bi, M.H., Grosz, A., Weissmann, N., Ishii, S., Grimminger, F., Seeger, W., Mayer, K., 2007. Immunomodulation by n-3- versus n-6-rich lipid emulsions in murine acute lung injury—role of platelet-activating factor receptor. Crit. Care Med. 35, 544–554.

Schuberth, O., Wretlind, A., 1961. Intravenous infusion of fat emulsions, phosphatides and emulsifying agents. Acta Chir. Scand. Suppl. 278, 1–12.

Serhan, C.N., Clish, C.B., Brannon, J., Colgan, S.P., Chiang, N., Gronert, K., 2000. Novel functional sets of lipid-derived mediators with antiinflammatory actions generated from omega-3 fatty acids via cyclooxygenase 2-nonsteroidal antiinflammatory drugs and transcellular processing. J. Exp. Med. 192, 1197–1204.

Shing, C.M., Fassett, R.G., Peake, J.M., Coombes, J.S., 2014. Effect of tocopherol on atherosclerosis, vascular function, and inflammation in apolipoprotein E knockout mice with subtotal nephrectomy. Cardiovasc. Ther. 32, 270–275.

Simopoulos, A.P., 2002. Omega-3 fatty acids and cardiovascular disease: the epidemiological evidence. Environ. Health Prev. Med. 6, 203–209.

Soden, J.S., Lovell, M.A., Brown, K., Partrick, D.A., Sokol, R.J., 2010. Failure of resolution of portal fibrosis during omega-3 fatty acid lipid emulsion therapy in two patients with irreversible intestinal failure. J. Pediatr. 156, 327–331.

Squires, R.H., Duggan, C., Teitelbaum, D.H., Wales, P.W., Balint, J., Venick, R., Rhee, S., Sudan, D., Mercer, D., Martinez, J.A., Carter, B.A., Soden, J., Horslen, S., Rudolph, J.A., Kocoshis, S., Superina, R., Lawlor, S., Haller, T., Kurs-Lasky, M., Belle, S.H., 2012. Natural history of pediatric intestinal failure: initial report from the Pediatric Intestinal Failure Consortium. J. Pediatr. 161, e2723–e2728.

Tomsits, E., Pataki, M., Tölgyesi, A., Fekete, G., Rischak, K., Szollár, L., 2010. Safety and efficacy of a lipid emulsion containing a mixture of soybean oil, medium-chain triglycerides, olive oil, and fish oil: a randomised, double-blind clinical trial in premature infants requiring parenteral nutrition. J. Pediatr. Gastroenterol. Nutr. 51, 514–521.

Tulikoura, I., Huikuri, K., 1982. Morphological fatty changes and function of the liver, serum free fatty acids, and triglycerides during parenteral nutrition. Scand. J. Gastroenterol. 17, 177–185.

Vanek, V.W., Seidner, D.L., Allen, P., Bistrian, B., Collier, S., Gura, K., Miles, J.M., Valentine, C.J., Kochevar, M., 2012. A. S. P. E. N. Position Paper: Clinical Role for Alternative Intravenous Fat Emulsions. Nutr. Clin. Pract. 27, 150–192.

Vlaardingerbroek, H., Ng, K., Stoll, B., Benight, N., Chacko, S., Kluijtmans, L.A.J., Kulik, W., Squires, E.J., Olutoye, O., Schady, D., Finegold, M.L., van Goudoever, J.B., Burrin, D.G., 2014. New generation lipid emulsions prevent PNALD in chronic parenterally fed preterm pigs. J. Lipid Res. 55, 466–477.

Wachira, J.K., Larson, M.K., Harris, W.S., 2014. n-3 Fatty acids affect haemostasis but do not increase the risk of bleeding: clinical observations and mechanistic insights. Br. J. Nutr. 111, 1652–1662.

Walli, R.A., 1978. Interrelation of aerobic glycolysis and lipogenesis in isolated perfused liver of well-fed rats. Biochim. Biophys. Acta 539, 62–80.

Yeh, S.L., Chen, W.J., Huang, P.C., 1995. Effects of L-glutamine on induced hepatosteatosis in rats receiving total parenteral nutrition. J. Formos. Med. Assoc. 94, 593–599.

Zambrano, E., El-Hennawy, M., Ehrenkranz, R.A., Zelterman, D., Reyes-Múgica, M., 2004. Total parenteral nutrition induced liver pathology: an autopsy series of 24 newborn cases. Pediatr. Dev. Pathol. 7, 425–432.

CHAPTER

26

Fish Oil Supplementation and Cancer Cachexia

M. Seelaender

Department of Cell and Developmental Biology, Institute of Biomedical Sciences and Department of Surgery, Faculdade de Medicina, University of São Paulo, São Paulo, Brazil

Cachexia has been recently proposed to be a comorbidity of cancer (Muscaritoli et al., 2015), a disease that affects an ever increasing number of patients (in the EU, each year around 2.9 million people are diagnosed and 1.7 million deaths are associated with the disease (Boyle and Ferlay, 2005). In the United States (Kumar et al., 2010), around 5 million people suffered from cancer cachexia. Despite the high prevalence of cachexia (50%–80% of all cancer patients, as reviewed by Kumar et al. (2010) and devastating consequences) it is an independent predictor of treatment failure and decreased survival (Jatoi et al., 2004); this multifaceted syndrome is underestimated and underdiagnosed by health professionals in cancer management. Indeed, only around 2.2% of international oncological society's guidelines provide information on how to recognize and manage cachexia (Del Fabbro et al., 2015; Mauri et al., 2013). In a scenario in which cachexia appears as the direct cause of death in more than 20% of all cancer patients (Bennani-Baiti and Walsh, 2009), the relevance of providing treatment is unquestionable. Nevertheless, owing to its complex plethora of symptoms and partly undefined mechanisms, successful intervention remains a challenge.

The clinical aspects of this syndrome include marked involuntary weight loss (lean and fat mass wasting), decreased appetite, intestinal malabsorption, nausea, anemia, hypoalbuminemia, weakness, fatigue, disruption of carbohydrate, lipid, and protein metabolism, compromised immune cell function, endocrine alterations, systemic inflammation, depression, and decreased quality of life (Argilés et al., 2015; Klein et al., 2013; Muscaritoli et al., 2006). These symptoms may be also present in cachexia associated with other chronic diseases. For instance, chronic obstructive pulmonary disease, rheumatoid arthritis, and chronic heart failure patients are all at risk for developing cachexia, with similar consequences of poorer prognosis and shorter survival (von Haehling and Anker, 2014).

In cancer, the tumor type may be related to higher cachexia prevalence (Mantovani et al., 2006; Mantovani and Madeddu, 2006); patients with pancreatic and upper gastrointestinal tract tumors are the most affected (up to 83%), followed by colorectal, head and neck, prostate, and lung tumors (50–72%). Breast cancer patients show the lowest prevalence (10–35%). Nevertheless, cancer treatment may add to the onset and aggravation of cachexia-like symptoms.

Unfortunately, cachexia is only recognized by most health professionals when it is a fully established condition and major weight loss has occurred. In addition, the global obesity epidemic renders weight loss cutoff establishment a challenge. In an international effort to improve awareness on the importance of early diagnosis and intervention, Fearon et al. (2011) proposed the definition of cachexia as "a multifactorial syndrome characterized by ongoing loss of muscle mass, paralleled or not by fat mass loss, that cannot be fully reversed by conventional nutritional support and leads to progressive functional impairment." This consensus also supported the classification of cachexia into three stages: precachexia (weight loss < 5%; anorexia, metabolic alterations); cachexia [systemic inflammation, >5% weight loss or weight loss (>2%), accompanied by BMI < 20 kg/m^2 and sarcopenia]; and refractory cachexia (patients no longer responsive to anti-cancer treatment, catabolism and survival expectancy <3 months). Therefore, if intervention is carried out at the early stages, it is possible that the disease-related disturbances may be mitigated.

While weight loss may be commonly perceived as a result of anorexia and tumor growth energetic demand, it is rather clear that these are not the culprits. Cachexia may be found in the absence of marked reductions in appetite

Fish and Fish Oil in Health and Disease Prevention. http://dx.doi.org/10.1016/B978-0-12-802844-5.00026-9

and food intake, although these symptoms greatly contribute to aggravating the condition. On the other hand, conventional nutritional support has failed to control the progression of cachexia, as emphasized in the very definition proposed for the paraneoplastic syndrome. Caloric supplementation per se should not be discarded (Morley, 2009), as it is recognized to decrease hospital stay length, yet the employment of specific nutrients seems to yield better results. Indeed, it seems that nutrients that are capable of downregulating inflammation, such as the long chain omega-3 fatty acids (LCn–3), are related with the best outcomes in cachexia.

Systemic and central inflammation is a fundamental aspect of the syndrome (Klein et al., 2013; Mantovani and Madeddu, 2006; Meriggi, 2015; Molfino et al., 2015), and inflammatory factors such as cytokines, orchestrate the cachexia continuum. Nutrients that modulate immune function and inflammation are of great interest in the management of cancer-associated wasting, hence the relevance of LCn–3 supplementation. Moreover, these fatty acids have the capacity to modulate immune system function, central nervous system (CNS) biochemistry and function and even cachectic patient microbiota, what suggests an immense potential in adjuvant cancer therapy. In this chapter the effects of the fish oil derived LCn–3 fatty acids, eicosahexaenoic acid (EPA, 20:5n–3) and docosahexaenoic acid (DHA, 22:6n–3) in experimental cachexia models and in human cancer cachexia will be examined, and the underlying mechanisms, discussed.

CLINICAL STUDIES

LCn–3 Supplementation in Cancer Cachexia

The protective role of LCn–3 supplementation in cancer initiation and progression is not clear, due to the inherent difficulties in analyzing epidemiological studies, which present too many uncontrolled variables (Molfino et al., 2015). However, higher marine n–3 fatty acid consumption was shown to decrease pancreatic cancer incidence (by 30%) in a study with over eighty-thousand individuals in Japan (Hidaka et al., 2015). Similarly, Sawada et al. (2012) showed that fish oil intake in the 90,296 individuals studied, was associated with protection from hepatocellular cancer development in a dose-dependent manner. Pham et al. (2012), nevertheless, failed to detect a beneficial effect of LCn–3 for colorectal cancer patients. Therefore, it seems that high (4 g/day) fish oil consumption may present an anticarcinogenic effect upon some specific types of cancer. A comprehensive review on the antitumor properties of n–3 fatty acid is provided by Nabavi et al. (2015).

Once neoplastic disease has developed, the aims are to counteract its progression, to ensure optimal anticancer treatment outcome and to warrant quality of life. In order to fulfil these, cachexia must be at all costs be prevented or, when already established, attenuated. Omega-3 fatty acids could potentially interfere with many of the most relevant alterations reported for the syndrome, and in special cases, with those associated with cachexia-related chronic systemic inflammation. However, the compartment(s) initiating systemic inflammation is (are) still under debate.

In the last few decades, evidence for a teleological relationship between systemic and neuroinflammation and cachexia symptoms is emerging, as pointed out by Molfino et al. (2015). As proposed by the authors, the vagus nerve senses the inflammatory signals released by the tumor and by the host tissues response to neoplastic growth; this ultimately leads to activation of the hypothalamic melanocortin system, thereby inducing the expression of cytokines involved in food intake and body composition dysregulation (Molfino et al. 2015). Fish oil-derived EPA has been shown to modulate inflammation in cachexia, and an increasing number of studies address this property. Jatoi et al., 2004 demonstrated in a double-blind randomized trial (in which EPA supplementation was compared to megestrol acetate and with the combined treatment in 412 patients), that cachectic patients (63%) receiving 1.09 g EPA/day showed improved appetite, with some of the patients having a 10% increase in body weight. Similarly, Bauer et al. (2005) reported increased appetite and nutrition-related outcomes in unresectable pancreatic cancer patients, who consumed 2.2 g/day EPA as part of a protein and energy dense supplement. Indeed, supplementation with marine n–3 fatty acids seems to improve appetite even in healthy subjects (Damsbo-Svendsen et al., 2013). Perioperative total body and lean mass gain was also reported (Weed et al., 2011) after an EPA-enriched supplement (1.08 g) was given to patients with head and neck squamous cell cancer, 2 weeks prior to surgery. Bayram et al. (2009) described decreased weight loss and higher remission rates at 3 months when pediatric cancer patients received 1.09 g EPA/day.

It is apparent therefore, that fish oil supplementation may contribute to cessation of weight loss and an increase in appetite. In a scenario in which every gram of weight is precious, even small enhancements cannot be ignored. The fact that some studies point to enhancement of lean body mass, is even more encouraging. An interesting study (Kumar et al., 2010) showed that Lovaza® (90% n–3 fatty acid ethyl esters) supplementation of 4 g/day for 6 weeks was able to significantly improve serum albumin, transferrin, functional status and physical activity in cancer patients with initial signs of cachexia (the proposed precachectic stage). The supplement was found to inhibit proteasome activity in the serum of patients. The ubiquitin proteasome pathway is involved in the catabolism of proteins and its activity is enhanced in the skeletal muscle of patients with cachexia (Bowen et al., 2015).

Both well and malnourished colon cancer patients, who received 18 g/day of fish oil (5.1 g EPA and DHA) combined with vitamin E (200 mg/day) demonstrated prolonged survival, as compared with the patients consuming placebo (Gogos et al., 1998). Earlier studies (Wigmore et al., 1997; Wigmore et al., 1996) showed cachectic pancreatic cancer patients to benefit from fish oil supplementation (12 g/day), as a consequence of the antiinflammatory effect of the treatment upon IL-6 and acute phase proteins. The antiinflammatory and antioxidant action of fish-derived LCn–3 supplements was confirmed in a small double-blind randomized trial (33 patients with advanced lung cancer receiving chemotherapy): after 66 days, C-reactive protein and IL-6 levels were reduced in the treated patients (0.51 g and 0.34 g/day of EPA and DHA, respectively) versus control (placebo), while the presence of reactive oxygen species (ROS) was found to be higher in the latter. These changes resulted in an increase of body weight in the supplemented group. In opposition, a pilot study (Persson et al., 2005) with advanced gastrointestinal patients, did not provide evidence for alteration in plasma cytokine profile after 4 weeks of fish oil supplementation (4.9 g EPA, 3.2 g DHA/day). The Phase II study performed by Mantovani et al. (2006) exhibited significant results in regard to reduction of IL-6 and TNF-alpha in cachectic patients. However, supplementation was offered as a combination of many active ingredients in addition to 1.1 g EPA and 0.46 g DHA, what prevents the isolated analysis of LCn–3 action. In a more recent Phase III trial, the same group examined five treatment arms (Mantovani et al., 2010). The authors' conclusion was that combination of agents, including EPA (2.2 g/day) was the most effective strategy, ameliorating life questionnaires scores, and downregulating inflammation.

Another interesting aspect of offering n–3 fatty acids to cachectic patients is to modify n–3:n–6 fatty acid ratio, driving the body into a more antiinflammatory profile, as suggested by Yeh et al. (2013), who found that advanced cachexia-related weight loss in head and neck cancer patients was reduced by supplementation. Recent small trials have found that EPA supplementation is able to change functional status and life quality parameters in the presence of advanced disease. van der Meij et al. (2012) examined the effect of 2.02 g EPA and 0.92 g DHA/day administration to lung cancer (stage III) patients and reported relevant improvement in quality of life, performance status and physical activity. The same was found by Gómez-Candela et al. (2011), who supplemented 61 cancer patients for a month with 1.5 g EPA/day. The authors emphasize the efficiency and safety of the strategy, which induced a significant reduction in plasma interferon gamma, a potent proinflammatory cytokine, combined with enhanced quality of life. In a small trial of 16 patients, Barber et al. (2000) were able to detect improved metabolic response and normalized body energy expenditure after 3 weeks of EPA-enriched (2 g/day) food consumption. In another study, Barber et al. (2004) demonstrated that 2 g/day EPA, associated with an oral nutritional supplement for 3 weeks, contributed to whole body anabolism in pancreatic cancer patients studied at baseline and after the treatment.

LCn-3 Supplementation in Chemotherapy

Chemotherapy has extremely unwelcome side effects, adding to cachexia consequences. In this regard, LCn–3 fatty acids may also be helpful, as suggested by some studies. Bougnoux et al. (2009) explored one such potential, by treating breast cancer patients with 1.8 g DHA in association with anthracycline. The fatty acid functioned as a tumor cell sensitizer, improving therapy efficacy. In accordance, other studies also reported fish oil to improve chemotherapy outcome while at the same time enhancing lean mass (Murphy et al., 2011). Furthermore, high grade leukopenia after chemotherapy was not a common finding in esophageal cancer patients supplemented with n–3 fatty acids (Miyata et al., 2012).

The tolerated dose of 12 g/day of fish oil (~2 g EPA, 1.5 g DHA) was commonly associated with nausea, moderate abdominal discomfort, flatulence, and steatorrhea in cachectic patients (Harvie, 2014). Testing different forms of fish oil lipid administration is an important aspect that should be addressed in future trials. For instance, marine phospholipids seem to be well tolerated (Taylor et al., 2010), and when supplemented for 6 weeks (1.5 g/day) induced positive changes in the n–6:n–3 ratios, stabilization of body mass, concomitantly increasing appetite and quality of life.

Taken together, the results of the studies add to the concept that fish oil lipids supplementation, combined with adequate caloric support, may contribute to the management of human cancer cachexia (Bozzetti, 2013). The encouraging results with early (pre) cachectic patients (Kumar et al., 2010) further extend the potential of interrupting the cachexia continuum. The findings of Bruera et al. (2003) suggest that long term supplementation with at least 2–6 g fish oil should be performed, as lower dose and time (2 weeks) employed in the study could not elicit changes, as compared with the placebo. Indeed, Burns et al. (2004) recommended higher doses in the treatment of cachexia. Nevertheless, it is clear that fish oil fatty acids show broad therapeutic potential to treat this paraneoplastic syndrome, starting from the preparation of patients to surgery, and in the whole trajectory of cancer treatment (Murphy et al., 2012).

The mechanisms of fish oil derived lipids in cancer cachexia are nonetheless, still not well known. As proposed, they may interfere with cachexia-related inflammation, but many other possibilities deserve attention. In this regard, animal studies have shed some light into other possible effects, some of which are commented on in this chapter.

ANIMAL STUDIES

Animal models of cachexia are often criticized on the basis that they may not be comparable to human disease as the animals tend to have a faster and more dramatic onset and progression of the symptoms, leading rapidly to death. Yet, despite differences in intensity, the nature of the symptoms is, in many cases, very similar to that in humans. Therefore, rather than counting them as an unsuitable form of study, models may be envisaged as a possibility to examine whether treatments will be efficient even in fast-setting and aggravated cachexia. Rodent models are the most common form of approaching the syndrome, but the literature also provides results with other species. For instance, Ogilvie et al. (2000) reported that dogs with lymphomas showed decreased plasma lactic acid content, along prolonged survival and disease free interval, after receiving a fish oil-enriched diet. Long term research with animal models has demonstrated that in rodents, LCn–3 fatty acids supplementation increases survival and counteracts wasting. This outcome is mediated, at least partially, by enhanced balance of immune cell function, decreased pro-inflammatory cytokine expression, modulation of tumor-derived catabolic factors, improved insulin sensitivity and decreased muscle breakdown.

The MAC16 murine tumor model is broadly adopted in the study of cachexia. Studies with this model provide evidence for the capacity of EPA to reduce prostaglandin E2 expression in muscle cells and to suppress lipid mobilization in white adipocytes, through modulation of cAMP generating pathways (Nabavi et al., 2015). Babcock et al. (2000) suggested EPA as the principal contributor to fish oil effects in rodent cachexia. EPA was shown to inhibit tumor growth in a dose-dependent fashion (Tisdale, 1996). Decreased muscle protein breakdown in association with increased anabolism was also reported after EPA supplementation (Babcock et al., 2000). Similarly, tumor-bearing mice treated with chemotherapic agents, experienced mitigation of the cachexia/chemotherapy-related increase in IL-6, TNF- alpha, and myostatin, causing muscle wasting to cease, after administration of fish oil combined with selenium (Wang et al., 2015). Indeed, Smith et al. (2004) reported that both protein synthesis and protein catabolism were modulated by EPA and amino acid supplementation in cachectic mice. The same was observed by van Norren et al. (2009), who added that functional performance was also improved. Lipolysis was reduced in cachectic mice consuming EPA-enriched phospholipids in association with decreased IL-6 and TNF-alpha serum levels, resulting in milder cachexia (Du et al., 2015). In rat models of cachexia (Walker 256 carcinosarcoma) attenuation of tumor growth was described after lifelong consumption of fish oil (Pinto et al., 2004). Iagher et al. (2013) compared the effect of shark liver and fish oils in mice. Both treatments showed antitumoral effects (lower mass, higher apoptosis), in addition to normalizing the biochemical parameters affected by cachexia. Blood glucose was found to be increased after supplementation, while the hypertriglyceridemic effect of cachexia was decreased, along with the concentration of inflammatory markers (Schiessel et al., 2015). The same Brazilian group (Coelho et al., 2012; Fernandez et al., 2004) also addressed renal function in cachectic animals. Fish oil oral treatment was able to partially recover glomerular filtration and urine osmolarity, to recover fractional sodium excretion patterns, proximal sodium reabsorption, and decrease inflammatory cell presence in the kidney. Folador et al. (2009) evaluated immune function in cachectic rats after fish oil consumption for two generations and reported that the anticachectic effects might be correlated with modulation of lymphocyte function.

CONCLUSION

Clinical and animal studies clearly show the broad spectrum of the beneficial effects of fish oil on cancer cachexia. It seems clear that fish oil supplementation is safe for patients, contributing to improvements in all steps of cancer treatment and in mitigating cachexia symptoms. Nevertheless, the form, treatment time, and dose of the supplementation should be evaluated in further research in well-designed clinical trials. Animal models can contribute to the understanding of the molecular mechanisms of action in cancer cachexia. Future perspectives involve the interesting potential of these lipids to modulate microbial translocation/gut barrier dysfunction that occur in cachexia (Klein et al., 2013) and the influence on central inflammation and depression.

References

Argilés, J.M., Stemmler, B., López-Soriano, F.J., Busquets, S., 2015. Nonmuscle tissues contribution to cancer cachexia. Mediat. Inflamm. 2015, 182872.

Babcock, T., Helton, W.S., Espat, N.J., 2000. Eicosapentaenoic acid (EPA): an antiinflammatory omega-3 fat with potential clinical applications. Nutrition 16, 1116–1118.

Barber, M.D., McMillan, D.C., Preston, T., Ross, J.A., Fearon, K.C., 2000. Metabolic response to feeding in weight-losing pancreatic cancer patients and its modulation by a fish-oil-enriched nutritional supplement. Clin. Sci. (London) 98, 389–399.

Barber, M.D., Preston, T., McMillan, D.C., Slater, C., Ross, J.A., Fearon, K.C., 2004. Modulation of the liver export protein synthetic response to feeding by an n-3 fatty-acid-enriched nutritional supplement is associated with anabolism in cachectic cancer patients. Clin. Sci. (London) 106, 359–364.

Bauer, J., Capra, S., Battistutta, D., Davidson, W., Ash, S., Group, C.C.S., 2005. Compliance with nutrition prescription improves outcomes in patients with unresectable pancreatic cancer. Clin. Nutr. 24, 998–1004.

Bayram, I., Erbey, F., Celik, N., Nelson, J.L., Tanyeli, A., 2009. The use of a protein and energy dense eicosapentaenoic acid containing supplement for malignancy-related weight loss in children. Pediatr. Blood Cancer 52, 571–574.

Bennani-Baiti, N., Walsh, D., 2009. What is cancer anorexia-cachexia syndrome? A historical perspective. J. R. Coll. Phys. Edinburg 39, 257–262.

Bougnoux, P., Hajjaji nN, Ferrasson, M.N., Giraudeau, B., Couet, C., LeFloch, O., 2009. Improving outcome of chemotherapy of metastatic breast cancer by docosahexaenoic acid: a phase II trial. Br. J. Cancer 101, 1978–1985.

Bowen, T.S., Schuler, G., Adams, V., 2015. Skeletal muscle wasting in cachexia and sarcopenia: molecular pathophysiology and impact of exercise training. J. Cachexia Sarcopenia Muscle 6, 197–207.

Boyle, P., Ferlay, J., 2005. Cancer incidence and mortality in Europe. Ann. Oncol. 16, 481–488.

Bozzetti, F., 2013. Nutritional support of the oncology patient. Crit. Rev. Oncol. Hematol. 87, 172–200.

Bruera, E., Strasser, F., Palmer, J.L., Willey, J., Calder, K., Amyotte, G., Baracos, V., 2003. Effect of fish oil on appetite and other symptoms in patients with advanced cancer and anorexia/cachexia: a double-blind, placebo-controlled study. J. Clin. Oncol. 21, 129–134.

Burns, C.P., Halabi, S., Clamon, G., Kaplan, E., Hohl, R.J., Atkins, J.N., Schwartz, M.A., Wagner, B.A., Paskett, E., 2004. Phase II study of high-dose fish oil capsules for patients with cancer- related cachexia. Cancer 101, 370–378.

Coelho, I., Casare, F., Pequito, D.C., Borghetti, G., Yamazaki, R.K., Brito, G.A., Kryczyk, M., Fernandes, L.C., Coimbra, T.M., Fernandez, R., 2012. Fish oil supplementation reduces cachexia and tumor growth while improving renal function in tumor-bearing rats. Lipids 47, 1031–1041.

Damsbo-Svendsen, S., Rønsholdt, M.D., Lauritzen, L., 2013. Fish oil-supplementation increases appetite in healthy adults. A randomized controlled cross-over trial. Appetite 66, 62–66.

Del Fabbro, E., Jatoi, A., Davis, M., Fearon, K., di Tomasso, J., Vigano, A., 2015. Health professionals' attitudes toward the detection and management of cancer-related anorexia-cachexia syndrome, and a proposal for standardized assessment. J. Commun. Support Oncol. 13, 181–187.

Du, L., Yang, Y.H., Wang, Y.M., Xue, C.H., Kurihara, H., Takahashi, K., 2015. EPA-enriched phospholipids ameliorate cancer-associated cachexia mainly via inhibiting lipolysis. Food Funct. 6 (12), 3652–3662.

Fearon, K., Strasser, F., Anker, S.D., Bosaeus, I., Bruera, E., Fainsinger, R.L., Jatoi, A., Loprinzi, C., MacDonald, N., Mantovani, G., Davis, M., Muscaritoli, M., Ottery, F., Radbruch, L., Ravasco, P., Walsh, D., Wilcock, A., Kaasa, S., Baracos, V.E., 2011. Definition and classification of cancer cachexia: an international consensus. Lancet Oncol. 12, 489–495.

Fernandez, R., Piechnik, J., Fabris, R., Malnic, G., Fernandes, L.C., 2004. Effect of chronic fish oil supplementation on renal function of normal and cachectic rats. Braz. J. Med. Biol. Res. 37, 1481–1489.

Folador, A., de Lima-Salgado, T.M., Hirabara, S.M., Aikawa, J., Yamazaki, R.K., Martins, E.F., de Oliveira, H.H., Pizatto, N., Kanunfre, C.C., Peres, C.M., Fernandes, L.C., Curi, R., 2009. Effect of fish oil supplementation for two generations on changes of lymphocyte function induced by Walker 256 cancer cachexia in rats. Nutr. Cancer 61, 670–679.

Gogos, C.A., Ginopoulos, P., Salsa, B., Apostolidou, E., Zoumbos, N.C., Kalfarentzos, F., 1998. Dietary omega-3 polyunsaturated fatty acids plus vitamin E restore immunodeficiency and prolong survival for severely ill patients with generalized malignancy: a randomized control trial. Cancer 82, 395–402.

Gómez-Candela, C., Villarino Sanz, M., Horrisberger, A., Loria Kohen, V., Bermejo, L.M., Zamora Auñón, P., 2011. Efficacy evaluation of an oral powder supplement enriched with eicosapentaenoic acid in cancer patients. Nutr. Hosp. 26, 1385–1393.

Harvie, M., 2014. Nutritional supplements and cancer: potential benefits and proven harms. Am. Soc. Clin. Oncol. Educ. Book 2014, e478–e486.

Hidaka, A., Shimazu, T., Sawada, N., Yamaji, T., Iwasaki, M., Sasazuki, S., Inoue, M., Tsugane, S., Japan Public Health Center–based Prospective Study Group, 2015. Fish, n-3 PUFA consumption, and pancreatic cancer risk in Japanese: a large, population-based, prospective cohort study. Am. J. Clin. Nutr. 102 (6), 1490–1497.

Iagher, F., de Brito Belo, S.R., Souza, W.M., Nunes, J.R., Naliwaiko, K., Sassaki, G.L., Bonatto, S.J., de Oliveira, H.H., Brito, G.A., de Lima, C., Kryczyk, M., de Souza, C.F., Steffani, J.A., Nunes, E.A., Fernandes, L.C., 2013. Antitumor and anti-cachectic effects of shark liver oil and fish oil: comparison between independent or associative chronic supplementation in Walker 256 tumor-bearing rats. Lipids Health Dis. 12, 146, 2013.

Jatoi, A., Rowland, K., Loprinzi, C.L., Sloan, J.A., Dakhil, S.R., MacDonald, N., Gagnon, B., Novotny, P.J., Mailliard, J.A., Bushey, T.I., Nair, S., Christensen, B., 2004. An eicosapentaenoic acid supplement versus megestrol acetate versus both for patients with cancer-associated wasting: a North Central Cancer Treatment Group and National Cancer Institute of Canada collaborative effort. J. Clin. Oncol. 22, 2469–2476.

Klein, G.L., Petschow, B.W., Shaw, A.L., Weaver, E., 2013. Gut barrier dysfunction and microbial translocation in cancer cachexia: a new therapeutic target. Curr. Opin. Support Palliat. Care 7, 361–367.

Kumar, N.B., Kazi, A., Smith, T., Crocker, T., Yu, D., Reich, R.R., Reddy, K., Hastings, S., Exterman, M., Balducci, L., Dalton, K., Bepler, G., 2010. Cancer cachexia: traditional therapies and novel molecular mechanism-based approaches to treatment. Curr. Treat Options Oncol. 11, 107–117.

Mantovani, G., Macciò, A., Madeddu, C., Gramignano, G., Lusso, M.R., Serpe, R., Massa, E., Astara, G., Deiana, L., 2006. A phase II study with antioxidants, both in the diet and supplemented, pharmaconutritional support, progestagen, and anti-cyclooxygenase-2 showing efficacy and safety in patients with cancer-related anorexia/cachexia and oxidative stress. Cancer Epidemiol. Biomarkers Prev. 15, 1030–1034.

Mantovani, G., Macciò, A., Madeddu, C., Serpe, R., Massa, E., Dessì, M., Panzone, F., Contu, P., 2010. Randomized phase III clinical trial of five different arms of treatment in 332 patients with cancer cachexia. Oncologist 15, 200–211.

Mantovani, G., Madeddu, C., 2006. In: Mantovani, G. (Ed.), Epidemiology of Cachexia. Cachexia and Wasting: A Modern Approach Springer, Cagliari, Italy, pp. 39–43.

Mauri, D., Tsiara, A., Valachis, A., Kalopita, K., Tsali, L., Tolis, P., Polyzos, N.P., 2013. Cancer cachexia: global awareness and guideline implementation on the web. BMJ Support Palliat. Care 3, 155–160.

Meriggi, F., 2015. Cancer cachexia: one step ahead. Rev. Recent Clin. Trials 10, 246–250.

Miyata, H., Yano, M., Yasuda, T., Hamano, R., Yamasaki, M., Hou, E., Motoori, M., Shiraishi, O., Tanaka, K., Mori, M., Doki, Y., 2012. Randomized study of clinical effect of enteral nutrition support during neoadjuvant chemotherapy on chemotherapy-related toxicity in patients with esophageal cancer. Clin Nutr. 31, 330–336.

Molfino, A., Gioia, G., Rossi Fanelli, F., Laviano, A., 2015. Contribution of neuroinflammation to the pathogenesis of cancer cachexia. Mediat. Inflamm. 2015, 801685.

Morley, J.E., 2009. Calories and cachexia. Curr. Opin. Clin. Nutr. Metab. Care 12, 607–610.

Murphy, R.A., Mourtzakis, M., Mazurak, V.C., 2012. n-3 polyunsaturated fatty acids: the potential role for supplementation in cancer. Curr. Opin. Clin. Nutr. Metab Care 15, 246–251.

Murphy, R.A., Yeung, E., Mazurak, V.C., Mourtzakis, M., 2011. Influence of eicosapentaenoic acid supplementation on lean body mass in cancer cachexia. Br. J. Cancer 105, 1469–1473.

Muscaritoli, M., Bossola, M., Aversa, Z., Bellantone, R., Rossi Fanelli, F., 2006. Prevention and treatment of cancer cachexia: new insights into an old problem. Eur. J. Cancer 42, 31–41.

Muscaritoli, M., Molfino, A., Lucia, S., Rossi Fanelli, F., 2015. Cachexia: a preventable comorbidity of cancer. A T.A.R.G.E.T. approach. Crit. Rev. Oncol. Hematol. 94, 251–259.

Nabavi, S.F., Bilotto, S., Russo, G.L., Orhan, I.E., Habtemariam, S., Daglia, M., Devi, K.P., Loizzo, M.R., Tundis, R., Nabavi, S.M., 2015. Omega-3 polyunsaturated fatty acids and cancer: lessons learned from clinical trials. Cancer Metastasis Rev. 34, 359–380.

Ogilvie, G.K., Fettman, M.J., Mallinckrodt, C.H., Walton, J.A., Hansen, R.A., Davenport, D.J., Gross, K.L., Richardson, K.L., Rogers, Q., Hand, M.S., 2000. Effect of fish oil, arginine, and doxorubicin chemotherapy on remission and survival time for dogs with lymphoma: a double-blind, randomized placebo-controlled study. Cancer 88, 1916–1928.

Persson, C., Glimelius, B., Rönnelid, J., Nygren, P., 2005. Impact of fish oil and melatonin on cachexia in patients with advanced gastrointestinal cancer: a randomized pilot study. Nutrition 21, 170–178.

Pham, N.M., Mizoue, T., Tanaka, K., Tsuji, I., Tamakoshi, A., Matsuo, K., Ito, H., Wakai, K., Nagata, C., Sasazuki, S., Inoue, M., Tsugane, S., Japan, R.G.f.t.D.a.E.o.C.P.S.i., 2012. Physical activity and colorectal cancer risk: an evaluation based on a systematic review of epidemiologic evidence among the Japanese population. Jpn. J. Clin. Oncol. 42, 2–13.

Pinto, J.A., Folador, A., Bonato, S.J., Aikawa, J., Yamazaki, R.K., Pizato, N., Facin, M., Grohs, H., de Oliveira, H.H., Naliwaiko, K., Ferraz, A.C., Nishiyama, A., Fernandez, R., Curi, R., Fernandes, L.C., 2004. Fish oil supplementation in F1 generation associated with naproxen, clenbuterol, and insulin administration reduce tumor growth and cachexia in Walker 256 tumor-bearing rats. J. Nutr. Biochem. 15, 358–365.

Sawada, N., Inoue, M., Iwasaki, M., Sasazuki, S., Shimazu, T., Yamaji, T., Takachi, R., Tanaka, Y., Mizokami, M., Tsugane, S., Group, J.P.H.C.-B.P.S., 2012. Consumption of n-3 fatty acids and fish reduces risk of hepatocellular carcinoma. Gastroenterology 142, 1468–1475.

Schiessel, D.L., Yamazaki, R.K., Kryczyk, M., Coelho, I., Yamaguchi, A.A., Pequito, D.C., Brito, G.A., Borghetti, G., Fernandes, L.C., 2015. α-Linolenic Fatty Acid Supplementation Decreases Tumor Growth and Cachexia Parameters in Walker 256 Tumor-Bearing Rats. Nutr. Cancer 67, 839–846.

Smith, H.J., Greenberg, N.A., Tisdale, M.J., 2004. Effect of eicosapentaenoic acid, protein and amino acids on protein synthesis and degradation in skeletal muscle of cachectic mice. Br. J. Cancer 91, 408–412.

Taylor, L.A., Pletschen, L., Arends, J., Unger, C., Massing, U., 2010. Marine phospholipids--a promising new dietary approach to tumor-associated weight loss. Support Care Cancer 18, 159–170.

Tisdale, M.J., 1996. Inhibition of lipolysis and muscle protein degradation by EPA in cancer cachexia. Nutrition 12, S31–S33.

van der Meij, B.S., Langius, J.A., Spreeuwenberg, M.D., Slootmaker, S.M., Paul, M.A., Smit, E.F., van Leeuwen, P.A., 2012. Oral nutritional supplements containing n-3 polyunsaturated fatty acids affect quality of life and functional status in lung cancer patients during multimodality treatment: an RCT. Eur. J. Clin. Nutr. 66, 399–404.

van Norren, K., Kegler, D., Argilés, J.M., Luiking, Y., Gorselink, M., Laviano, A., Arts, K., Faber, J., Jansen, H., van der Beek, E.M., van Helvoort, A., 2009. Dietary supplementation with a specific combination of high protein, leucine, and fish oil improves muscle function and daily activity in tumour-bearing cachectic mice. Br. J. Cancer 100, 713–722.

von Haehling, S., Anker, S.D., 2014. Prevalence, incidence and clinical impact of cachexia: facts and numbers-update 2014. J. Cachexia Sarcopenia Muscle 5, 261–263.

Wang, H., Li, T.L., Hsia, S., Su, I.L., Chan, Y.L., Wu, C.J., 2015. Skeletal muscle atrophy is attenuated in tumor-bearing mice under chemotherapy by treatment with fish oil and selenium. Oncotarget 6, 7758–7773.

Weed, H.G., Ferguson, M.L., Gaff, R.L., Hustead, D.S., Nelson, J.L., Voss, A.C., 2011. Lean body mass gain in patients with head and neck squamous cell cancer treated perioperatively with a protein- and energy-dense nutritional supplement containing eicosapentaenoic acid. Head Neck 33, 1027–1033.

Wigmore, S.J., Fearon, K.C., Maingay, J.P., Ross, J.A., 1997. Down-regulation of the acute-phase response in patients with pancreatic cancer cachexia receiving oral eicosapentaenoic acid is mediated via suppression of interleukin-6. Clin. Sci. (London) 92, 215–221.

Wigmore, S.J., Ross, J.A., Falconer, J.S., Plester, C.E., Tisdale, M.J., Carter, D.C., Fearon, K.C., 1996. The effect of polyunsaturated fatty acids on the progress of cachexia in patients with pancreatic cancer. Nutrition 12, S27–S30.

Yeh, K.Y., Wang, H.M., Chang, J.W., Huang, J.S., Lai, C.H., Lan, Y.J., Wu, T.H., Chang, P.H., Wang, H., Wu, C.J., Hsia, S., Wang, C.H., 2013. Omega-3 fatty acid-, micronutrient-, and probiotic-enriched nutrition helps body weight stabilization in head and neck cancer cachexia. Oral Surg. Oral Med. Oral Pathol. Oral Radiol. 116, 41–48.

CHAPTER

27

Utilization of Fish Oil for the Prevention and Treatment of Traumatic Brain Injury

M.D. Lewis

Brain Health Education and Research Institute, Potomac, Maryland, United States

INTRODUCTION

Omega-3 polyunsaturated fatty acids (n–3FA), particularly docosahexaenoic acid (DHA), are structural components of cell membranes, most concentrated in the brain and retina. Emerging science on the ability of n–3FA to be beneficial to the nervous system during and after acute traumatic brain injury (TBI) is acknowledged, mainly in preclinical studies, but now in clinical experience and case reports. TBI has long been recognized as a leading cause of traumatic death and disability (Selassie et al., 2008). TBI is caused by a bump, blow or jolt to the head or a penetrating head injury that disrupts the normal function of the brain. Over 3.5 million TBI's occur annually, approximately 52,000 deaths, and more than 300,000 hospitalizations in the United States alone (Coronado et al., 2012). TBI, most often from falls, vehicle accidents, and violence, accounts for almost one third of all injury-related deaths and males sustain TBI more frequently than do females (Faul et al., 2010). There is an increasing awareness of mild TBI, or concussions, and the longer term effects over the past decade due to the number of military service members returning from the wars in Iraq and Afghanistan, as well as a number of high profile deaths of professional American football players (Turner et al., 2012). TBI is a major healthcare concern, constituting a major cause of death, and disability not just in the United States, but throughout the world. Motor bikes are major causes, increasing in significance in developing countries as other causes reduce (Reilly, 2007). Some consider TBI a global public health epidemic (Rodríguez-Rodríguez et al., 2014).

TBI can cause a wide range of functional short- or long-term changes affecting thinking, sensation, language, or emotions (NINDS, 2002; Table 27.1). It is believed that 80% or more of persons suffering a TBI would be classified as mild and do not seek medical attention (Coronado et al., 2012). Most of those improve over the first few hours to days, but 5–20% may continue to have postconcussion symptoms (PCS) for an extended period following the initial injury (Jotwani and Harmon, 2010). Patients with PCS often present with ongoing and persistent headaches, fatigue, sleep disturbance, vertigo, irritability, anxiety, depression, apathy, and difficulty with concentration and exercise (Willer and Leddy, 2006). Although much has been learned about the molecular and cellular mechanisms of TBI in the past two decades, these advances have failed to translate into a successful clinical trial and no significant improvement in treatment beyond the acute setting (Ling and Marshall, 2008).

Classification of TBI

Most commonly, TBI is classified using mild, moderate, and severe categories. The Glasgow Coma Scale (GCS), the most commonly used system, grades a person's level of consciousness on a scale of 3–15 based on verbal, motor, and eye-opening reactions to stimuli. A GCS of 13 or above is considered mild, 9–12 moderate, and below 9 severe. Severe TBI is typically associated with significant neurological injury, often with abnormal neuroimaging (eg, head CT scan revealing skull fracture, intracranial hemorrhage, and early diffuse cerebral edema) and these patients require advanced medical care (Ling et al., 2009). Due to numerous problems, including timing of when the GCS is determined, the GCS grading system has limited ability to predict outcomes. Because of this, other classification systems are also used, but currently, there is no consensus.

Fish and Fish Oil in Health and Disease Prevention. http://dx.doi.org/10.1016/B978-0-12-802844-5.00027-0

TABLE 27.1 Signs and Symptoms of a Head Injury May Include the Following

Physical	Cognitive	Emotional	Sleep
• Headache • Nausea • Vomiting • Balance problems • Dizziness • Visual problems • Fatigue • Sensitivity to light • Sensitivity to noise • Numbness/tingling • Dazed or stunned	• Feeling mentally "foggy" • Feeling slowed down • Difficulty concentrating • Difficulty remembering • Forgetful of recent information or conversations • Confused about recent events • Answers questions slowly • Repeats questions	• Irritability • Sadness • More emotional • Nervousness	• Drowsiness • Sleeping less than usual • Sleeping more than usual • Trouble falling asleep

CDC (2015).

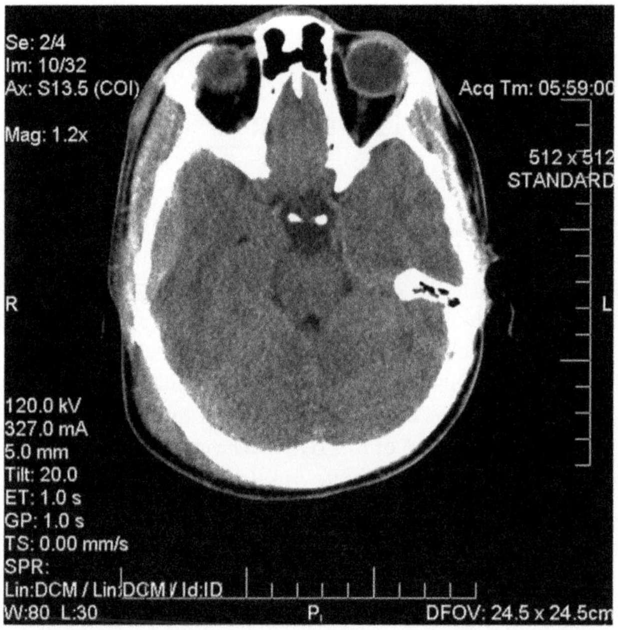

FIGURE 27.1 **CT scan of the patient approximately two hours after the motor vehicle accident and before neurosurgery.** Note the moderate-sized panhemispheric right subdural hematoma, a small right temporal epidural hematoma, subarachnoid hemorrhage, and 3-mm right to left shift of the midline. Source: *Lewis et al. (2013).*

Classically, TBI is described as occurring in two phases, or on the basis of the pathophysiologic mechanism. The primary or initial injury occurs as a direct result of the traumatic event itself. A secondary injury, or phase, occurs from multiple neuropathological processes that can continue for days to weeks following the initial insult.

Primary Injury

The primary injury is immediate and not amenable to treatment, only prevention. If severe enough, death can occur almost instantaneously. The damage that occurs from the primary injury is complete by the time medical care can be instituted. High-speed collisions with very rapid deceleration are particularly injurious, but sports-related injuries also can be devastating. Because the neuronal structures reside in a fluid-filled compartment, they often lag behind the bony structure as it moves during the sudden stopping of the body in motion. The brain often strikes both in the direct and opposite plane of motion against the inner bony table. This is the coup–contre–coup pattern, where contusions to the brain are seen at the site of skull impact and 180 degrees opposite the site of impact (Ling and Marshall, 2008).

By far, the most devastating complication of the primary injury in an acute TBI is the development of an intracranial hematoma. (Fig. 27.1) Early diagnosis and aggressive, often surgical management, may decrease or prevent some of the secondary problems from occurring. Computerized tomography (CT) scans are routinely used to identify

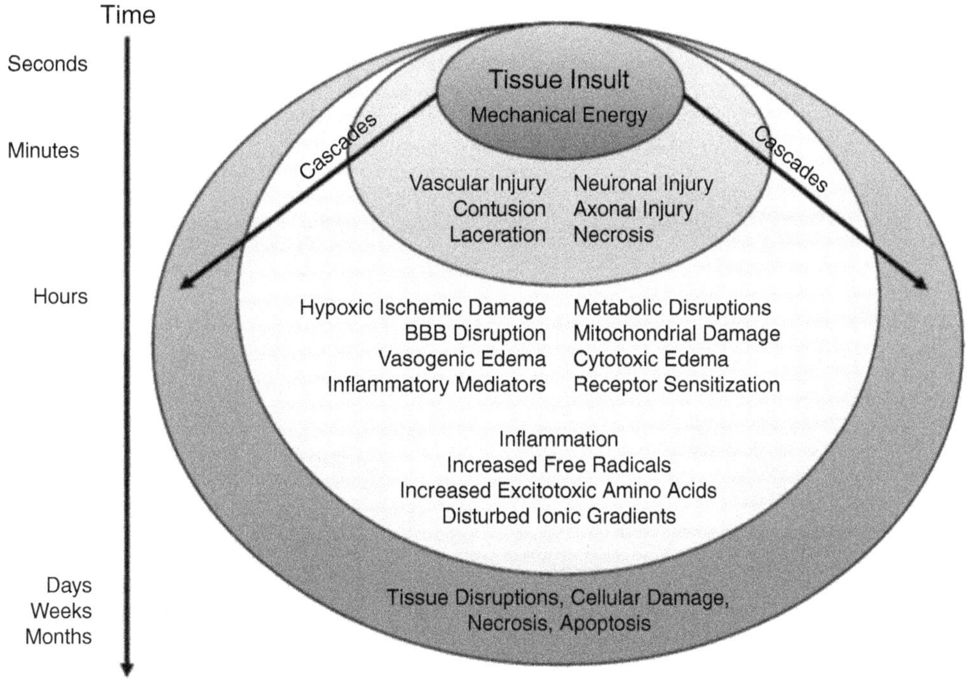

FIGURE 27.2 **The primary injury of TBI is caused by a transfer of mechanical injury to the brain tissue.** This is followed by the secondary injury that occurs over minutes to hours to days and even weeks and months. It is characterized by numerous metabolic and biochemical cascades that may cause more damage than the initial tissue insult itself.

intracranial hemorrhage and is essential to surgical planning. (Lee and Newberg, 2005) While magnetic resonance imaging (MRI) may be more sensitive, conventional CT scans are far more available and cost effective for detecting acute subarachnoid or acute parenchymal hemorrhage (Yealy and Hogan, 1991).

Secondary Injury

The secondary injury of TBI is a prolonged pathogenic process leading to cell death and worsening damage to the brain far beyond the primary injury (Michael-Titus, 2007). Secondary injury may include damage to the blood–brain barrier, ischemia, hypoxia, intracranial hypertension, hypercarbia, hyponatremia, seizures, neuroinflammation, free radical overload, and excitotoxicity (Saatman et al., 2008; Fig. 27.2).

Four categories of mechanisms can be defined in the secondary injury phase of TBI: (1) ischemia, excitotoxicity, and intracellular biochemical cascades; (2) axonal injury; (3) cerebral edema; and (4) inflammation and regeneration. Within each category, a constellation of mediators of secondary damage, neuroprotection, repair, and regeneration exist (Kochanek et al., 2007).

Ischemia

Besides the obvious causes of ischemia, underlying biochemical mechanisms leading to ischemia may also exist such as a reduction in vasodilatory response to nitric oxide and prostaglandins (Armstead, 1998, 1999). Of concern to the military population, blast TBI caused cerebral vasospasm are not uncommon even weeks after the injury (Armonda et al., 2006). The result of cerebral blood flow compromise results in metabolic responses such as increased anaerobic metabolism, and biochemical responses such as intracellular accumulation of calcium, activation of nitric oxide synthesis, and production of free radicals. These mechanisms begin to occur within minutes of the injury and progress hours and days following the insult, culminating in cell injury and tissue death (Williams et al., 2013). Glutamate overflow from damaged cells leads to excitotoxicity, affecting neurons and glia. The influx of calcium through glutamate receptors and voltage-gated calcium channels activates calcium-dependent proteases such as phospholipase A2 (PLA_2) which degrade membrane phospholipids, leading to the release of fatty acids, principally arachidonic acid (AA), an omega-6 fatty acid (n–6FA), and DHA, an n–3FA. Posttraumatic fatty acid alterations involve the release of both auto-destructive and neuroprotective cascades (Michael-Titus, 2007).

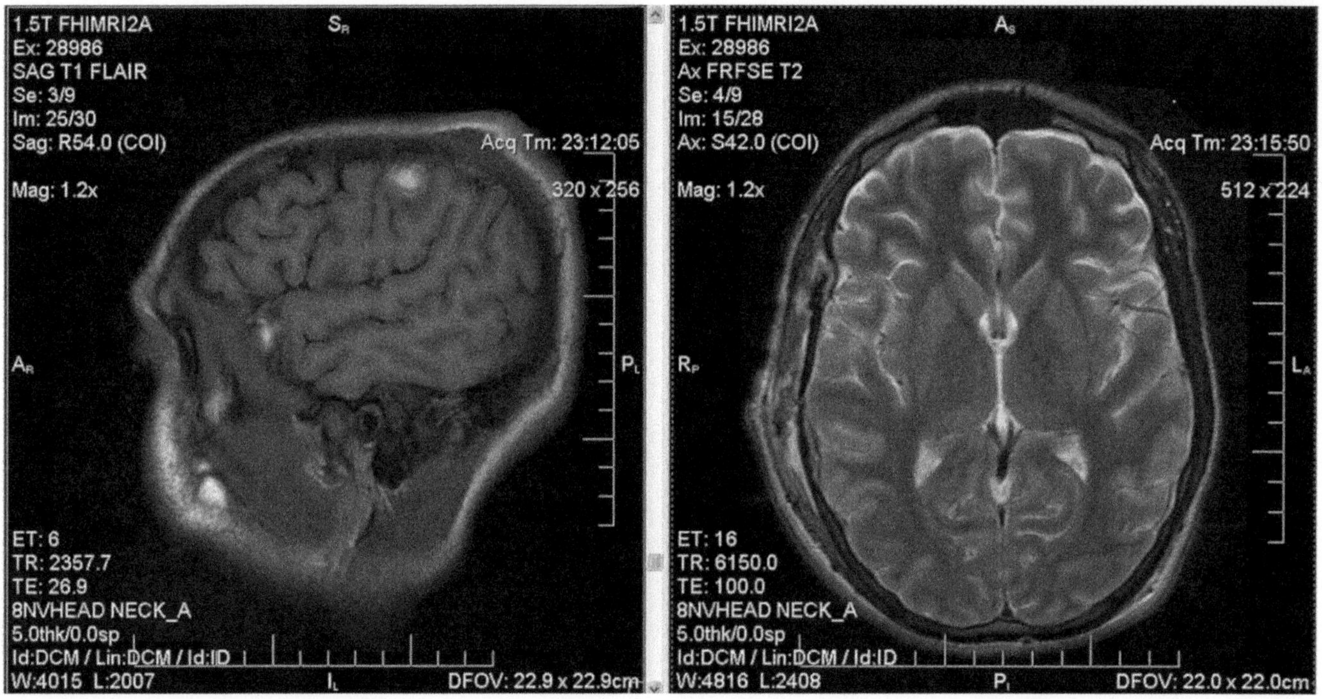

FIGURE 27.3 **T2-weighted magnetic resonance imaging (MRI) on hospital day 10.** Note the right cerebral convexity subdural hemorrhage, right postcentral gyrus and left temporal lobe parenchymal petechial hemorrhage, and small superior vermian subarachnoid hemorrhage in the image on the right. In addition, multiple zones of abnormal fluid-attenuated inversion recovery signals consistent with diffuse axonal injury (DAI) are present on both images. *Source: Lewis et al. (2013).*

Diffuse Axonal Injury

Diffuse axonal injury (DAI) is a frequent result of traumatic acceleration/deceleration or rotational injuries resulting in extensive lesions in white matter tracts. Rapid deceleration, most commonly a result of high-speed motor vehicle accidents, causes shearing, inflicted as tissues of differing densities within the brain slide over other tissues, stretching axons, especially at junctions between white and gray matter (Meythaler et al., 2001). Classically considered a result of the physical shearing during the primary injury, it is now understood that much of DAI occurs through secondary biochemical cascades in response to the primary injury, hours to days after the initial injury. Axons are normally elastic, but when rapidly stretched they become brittle, and the axonal cytoskeleton can be broken (Hemphill et al., 2011). Ultimately, death of the axon is brought on by the neurochemical pathology as described in the previous paragraph. The axon degrades causing it to draw back toward the cell body and form a bulb. This bulb is called a retraction ball, the hallmark of diffuse axonal injury (Smith and Meaney, 2000). Because DAI progresses over hours to days, often it is not found on CT scans done in the emergency setting (Fig. 27.1). Among patients with DAI, 50–80% demonstrate a normal CT scan in the acute setting (Wasserman et al., 2012). DAI is most likely to be diagnosed with MRI days to weeks following the TBI. Abnormal MRI signals, bright on T2-weighted images in characteristic multifocal locations, leaves little doubt about the diagnosis of DAI (Fig. 27.3) 3-Tesla diffusion tensor imaging (DTI) for white matter injury has been shown to be a more accurate imaging modality that even has utility for outcome prediction in the mild TBI (Yuh et al., 2014).

Cerebral Edema

Cerebral edema is a hallmark finding in severe TBI often resulting in intracranial hypertension unless aggressively managed, commonly through surgical and intensive care means. Intracranial hypertension as a result of edema can compromise cerebral blood flow and result in secondary ischemia or devastating herniation syndromes. In most TBI, cytotoxic (cellular) and vasogenic cerebral edema occur together. Vasogenic edema forms in the extracellular space due to a breakdown of the blood brain barrier. Osmotic swelling also may contribute to extracellular cerebral edema (Kochanek et al., 2007). It may be rapid and extensive. Cellular edema, however, may be of greatest importance. Swelling of neurons and astrocytes can occur following the breakdown of sodium and calcium pumps on cell membranes. Excess glutamate uptake coupled to glucose utilization causes sodium, calcium, and water to accumulate exacerbating intracellular edema (Rosenberg, 1999). Cerebral edema and intracranial hypertension are the main targets of concern and intervention in the acute intensive care setting.

Neuroinflammation

Neuroinflammation is complicated, beyond the scope of this chapter, and covered in detail in other chapters. Inflammation is essential following any injury yet may be detrimental if not properly modulated or appropriately sized in response to the injury. A critical balance exists between repair and proinflammatory factors that determine the outcome of neurodegenerative processes. Acute inflammation in the brain is characterized by rapid activation of the innate immune cells of the central nervous system, microglia and astrocytes (Streit et al., 2004). Not limited to just severe TBI, once activated, astrocytes, the most abundant cells in the brain, release various growth factors, cytokines, and chemokines that function as neuromodulators to regulate inflammation. Common cytokines produced in response to brain injury include: interleukin-6 (IL-6), which is produced during astrogliosis, and interleukin-1 beta (IL-1β) and tumor necrosis factor alpha (TNF-α), which can induce neuronal cytotoxicity. Although the pro-inflammatory cytokines may cause cell death and secondary tissue damage, they are necessary to repair the damaged tissue. For example, TNF-α contributes to tissue growth at later stages of inflammation (Ramesh et al., 2013).

Chronic Traumatic Encephalopathy

The concept that TBI can lead to neurodegenerative changes was first introduced almost a century ago in 1926 by neurologists Osnato and Giliberti. In 1928, a New Jersey pathologist, Harrison Martland, described "punch drunk syndrome" in retired boxers who developed chronic motor and neuropsychiatric symptoms. Millspaugh introduced the term "dementia pugilistica" in 1937 describing the neuropathological findings in the aftermath of repetitive TBI in boxing. The prevailing term used in modern day literature, chronic traumatic encephalopathy (CTE), was coined by British neurologist, Macdonald Critchley, in 1949 (Ling et al., 2015). Affected individuals often exhibit disordered memory and executive functioning, behavioral, and personality disturbances (eg, apathy, depression, irritability, impulsiveness, and suicidality), Parkinsonism, and, occasionally, motor neuron disease. Upon autopsy, the presence of hyperphosphorylated tau protein deposition, whether it be in the form of neurofibrillary tangles (NFTs), neuropil threads (NTs), or glial tangles (GTs), is a defining feature of CTE while neuritic β-amyloid plaques, common in Alzheimer's Disease, are found only in a minority of cases (Gavett et al., 2011). CTE in a retired professional American football player was first recognized in 2002 by Bennet Omalu when autopsying the brain of a deceased player (Omalu et al., 2005).

It has been widely believed that the blood–brain barrier completely separated the neuroimmune system from the rest of the body's immune system, thus the accumulation of toxins and pathological proteins were believed to be an issue of overproduction rather than poor clearance from the brain. Recently, a brain-wide network of paravascular channels, termed the "glymphatic" pathway, was defined that moves cerebralspinal fluid (CSF) into and through the brain parenchyma, facilitating the clearance of toxins and proteins including β-amyloid and tau from the brain. After TBI however, glymphatic pathway function was reduced by ~60%, with this impairment persisting for at least 1 month post injury. Such chronic impairment of glymphatic pathway function after TBI may be a key factor that renders the posttraumatic brain vulnerable to tau aggregation and the onset of neurodegeneration (Iliff et al., 2014). Subsequently, the recent discovery of microscopic lymphatic vessels connecting the brain to the immune system may have profound implications in many disease processes involving neuroinflammation, including TBI, where the clearance of toxins and protein complexes such as phosphylated tau and β-amyloid are paramount (Louveau et al., 2015).

Though nearly lost in the discussions of CTE and neurodegeneration after TBI has been the role of sustained neuroinflammation, even though this association has been well established pathologically since the 1950s and is strongly supported by preclinical and clinical studies. Manifested by extensive microglial and astroglial activation, neuroinflammation may be the most important cause of posttraumatic neurodegeneration. Preclinical studies indicate that persistent neuroinflammation and associated neurodegeneration may be treatable long after the initiating insults (Faden and Loane, 2015).

The importance of the secondary injury has gained widespread recognition as a potential target of such therapeutic intervention. Although much has been learned about the molecular and cellular mechanisms of TBI in the past two decades, these advances have failed to translate into a successful clinical trial and no significant improvement in treatment beyond the acute setting (Ling and Marshall, 2008).

Failure to Find Therapeutic Interventions for TBI

Tremendous advances in surgical and intensive care unit (ICU) management of TBI, including maintaining adequate oxygenation, controlling intracranial pressure (ICP), and ensuring proper cerebral perfusion, have resulted in reduced mortality (Ling et al., 2009). The increasing role of specialized intensive care units with neurologically trained medical and nursing providers using evidence-based clinical management has had a favorable impact on both the consistency and level of care. Advances in neuromonitoring, neuroimaging, and early aggressive neurosurgical interventions are important contributors to improved TBI outcome (Ling and Marshall, 2008).

The most definitive strategy to avoid short- or long-term detrimental effects of TBI is through primary prevention or avoidance of the injury in the first place. However, once a TBI occurs, the secondary injury represents a window of opportunity for therapeutic intervention with the potential to prevent and/or reduce brain damage and improve long-term patient outcome. Recently, treatments with broader, pleiotropic effects have been explored. Progesterone, unlike corticosteroids, is thought to not only reduce cerebral edema but to also have neuroprotective effects and was positively correlated with improved functional outcomes at up to 6 months follow-up in two randomized, double-blind, placebo-controlled phase II trials. Unfortunately, two multicenter, phase III clinical trials were recently halted due to futility. To date, no promising preclinical results have been translated into successful clinical trials (Stein, 2015). This may be due, in part, to the fact that most interventions target a single biochemical cascade rather than multiple mechanisms of injury.

Approaches that target multiple aspects of TBI are needed. The Western medical system evolved around the epidemiological triad of acute infectious diseases: one host–agent environment and subsequently one drug to cure. Pharmaceuticals by nature are aimed at disrupting single enzymatic processes. TBI is too complicated for such a narrow minded approach. What is needed is a broad spectrum, more holistic approach. Progesterone represented a good step in that direction. Progesterone was thought to exert its neuroprotective effects by protecting or rebuilding the blood-brain barrier, decreasing development of cerebral edema, down-regulating the inflammatory cascade, and limiting cellular necrosis and apoptosis (Stein et al., 2008). However, progesterone must be administered by continuous intravenous infusion over the first three days following injury. It cannot be given beyond that period, or orally, and does not have any neurorestorative properties that may improve neurological function after the patient survives the initial acute phase of TBI. Tragically, persistently negative clinical trial outcomes have led to disinvestment in new drug research by companies and policy-makers and disappointment for patients and their families (Stein, 2015).

Interventions targeting all aspects of the four mechanisms of secondary injury, plus repair, regeneration, and protection of the brain are desperately needed. Mechanisms that are potential drug targets include angiogenesis, axon remodeling, remyelination, neurogenesis, and synaptogenesis. Therapies may also target regeneration by enhancing the ability of pluripotent cells to differentiate into neurons, glia, and vascular endothelium. Effective interventions should also treat the persistent symptoms associated with the long-term effects of TBI (eg, memory disturbances, depression, headache; Diaz-Arrastia et al., 2014).

Omega-3 PUFAs and TBI

If one were to take a blank sheet of paper and design an intervention for TBI, it is possible it would look similar to omega-3 fatty acids (Table 27.2) EPA and DHA have the ability to impact all four main mechanisms of the secondary injury phase of TBI; have neuroregenerative properties; are well known to benefit cardiovascular and mental health; is well studied as a substance in the scientific literature; a safety profile beyond compare such that DHA is added to 100% of all infant formulations in the United States; is available in oral, enteral, and intravenous (in Europe) forms; can be given to a patient during the acute phase of injury and continued throughout the patient's entire

TABLE 27.2 Design of a "Perfect" TBI Drug

- Impacts all four main mechanisms of the secondary injury phase
- Has neuroregenerative properties
- Beneficial impact on cardiovascular and mental health
- Effective in treating long-term effects of TBI (postconcussive symptoms)
- Well studied as a substance in the scientific literature
- Strong safety profile
- Readily available in oral, enteral, and intravenous forms
- Can be given to a patient prehospital, acute phase of injury and can be continued throughout patient's chronic phase and rehabilitation
- Can be used prophylactically prior to injury in populations at risk of TBI

rehabilitation; and can be used prophylactically prior to injury in populations at risk of TBI. It is a ubiquitous substance that has been around longer than mankind and consumed by people worldwide. Some argue evolution of the human brain could not have occurred without the access to EPA and DHA from fish (Bradbury, 2011). The FDA recognizes n–3FA as generally recognizable as safe (GRAS) up to 3000 mg/day while the European Food Safety Authority recognizes up to 5000 mg (EFSA, 2012). In 2011, the FDA approved investigational new drug (IND) status for up to 9000 mg of EPA/DHA (Katz, 2011).

Preclinical Studies

Omega-3 for neurotrauma use in preclinical studies generally separates into several categories of interest to include TBI, stroke, and spinal cord injury, as well as postinjury treatment and preinjury administration.

Postinjury Administration

Gomez-Pinilla (2008) and coworkers have shown in several TBI treatment studies that dietary DHA following experimental TBI in rats counteracts broad and fundamental aspects of TBI pathology. In fluid percussion injury studies of rats, they demonstrated that DHA normalized levels of BDNF, synapsin I (Syn-1), cAMP-responsive element-binding protein (CREB), and calcium/calmodulin-dependent kinase II (CaMKII), and improved learning ability. The DHA diet counteracted the reduction of superoxide dismutase (SOD) and SIR-2 that follows TBI. Furthermore, DHA normalized levels of PLA2 and syntaxin-3, which may help preserve membrane homeostasis and function after injury (Gomez-Pinilla, 2008). Additionally, the same group found effects of TBI were optimally counteracted by the combination of DHA and exercise (Wu et al., 2007, 2011, 2013). Shin and Dixon also investigated the supplementation of n–3FA and found they restored dopamine transmission deficits after TBI (Shin and Dixon, 2011).

In two separate experiments using an impact acceleration injury model in rats, Bailes and Mills (2010) used four groups of animals: two groups that were injured then gavaged with 10 or 40 mg/kg per day of n–3FA consisting of EPA and DHA for thirty days; an unsupplemented control group that received an injury; and an unsupplemented sham group that was not injured (Mills et al., 2011a). A second study was done using DHA only (Bailes and Mills, 2010). In both studies, supplementation significantly reduced the number of β-amyloid precursor protein (APP)-positive axons at 30 days postinjury, in a dose-dependent manner, to levels similar to those in uninjured sham animals.

More recently, compelling experiments in TBI treatment using functional outcome measures were done by Schobe et al. (2015). They demonstrated that dietary DHA decreased cognitive impairment, oxidative stress, and white matter injury and improved cognitive, imaging and histologic outcomes in adult rats after TBI. DHA acutely decreased markers of oxidative stress and increased antiinflammatory interleukin-10 in the brains following controlled cortical impact. DHA improved Morris Water Maze performance and lesion volume late after injury while decreasing T2-imaging measures of cerebral edema and decreased radial diffusivity, an index of white matter injury (Schobe et al., 2015)

Eady et al. (2013) have a variety of preclinical studies which administered DHA following experimentally induced ischemia in a rodent stroke model. Animals were subjected to middle cerebral artery occlusion for two hours. Most recently, they demonstrated that DHA complexed to albumin (DHA-Alb) given three hours after onset of stroke is highly neuroprotective following focal cerebral ischemia in aged rats (Eady et al., 2014). Infarct volumes were significantly decreased and neurological scores improved. DHA also reduced microglia infiltration and increased the number of astrocytes and neurons. The same group had previously tested young rats with similar results (Belayev et al., 2005). Additionally, this group determined that DHA-Alb therapy is highly neuroprotective in permanent stroke (rather than transient) in rats (Eady et al., 2013). When they used DHA not complexed to albumin, in addition to the previously described findings, they found that DHA also modulates the neuroinflammatory response and triggers long term restoration of synaptic circuits, even when administered up to five hours after injury. When investigating the therapeutic window for using DHA-Alb, DHA-Alb led to improved neurological score and significant reductions of infarct volumes (especially in the cortical or penumbral region), even when treatment was initiated as late as seven hours after onset of temporary middle cerebral artery occlusion (Eady et al., 2012) and confers enduring neuroprotection for at least three weeks poststroke (Hong et al., 2013). Most recently, the same research group reported DHA improves neurologic deficits and attenuates blood-brain barrier injury induced by focal ischemia in rats (Hong et al., 2015).

When Williams et al. (2013) evaluated an n–3FA triglyceride emulsion administered before and after a hypoxic-ischemic (H/I) injury, they found a significantly (43%) reduced total infarct when administered 90 min prior to H/I and 47% when administered immediately after H/I. In post-H/I experiments, the triglyceride formulation containing only DHA, but not one with only EPA, exhibited neuroprotective effects. The DHA emulsion significantly decreased total infarct volume by 51% when administered at 0 h postinjury, 46% at 1 h, 51% at 2 h, and no protective effect at 4 h (Williams et al., 2013). Similarly, Berman et al. (2010) found significant improvement in functional outcome with DHA-Alb treatment following H/I in very young rats and when combined with hypothermia, even further functional improvement and reduced brain damage (Berman et al., 2013). In more recent studies, de Souza et al. (2015) concluded that n–3FA, especially in the triacylglycerol form (as opposed to thyl ester form), could be a promising therapy to prevent microvascular damage induced by ischemia/reperfusion and its consequent clinical sequelae (de Souza et al., 2015).

DHA lessens neurological damage following spinal cord injury (SCI) as well. Michael-Titus (2007) conducted a series of SCI experiments. First, they administered DHA 30 min after SCI induced by surgical hemisection in adult rats. One week after injury, they found reduced neuronal cell loss, oligodendrocyte loss, decreased apoptosis, as well as improved functional outcome. In contrast, when the n–6FA AA was administered after injury, it exacerbated injury, increased the size of the spinal cord lesion, decreased neuronal and glial cell survival and worsened functional outcome. Next, the same group used a more severe model of SCI, induced by compression, but also added DHA to the diet for six weeks following injury and injection at 30 min. Similar to the previous study, neuroprotection and maintenance of locomotion was greatly enhanced. Additional neuroprotective effects of the DHA-enriched diet, while not apparent the first week, were improved functional and histological outcomes even more than bolus alone at six weeks. Of note, when DHA was given within an hour of SCI, neuromotor function was maintained but the effect was lost when treatment was delayed four hours. These findings also support the idea that treatment with n–3FA represent a promising therapeutic approach for neurotrauma which would be easy to translate to the emergency patient-care arena considering the well documented safety and tolerability of these compounds (Michael-Titus, 2007; Paterniti et al., 2014).

Preinjury Administration

Preclinical studies also have demonstrated that n–3FA can be protective when administered prior to injury. When fish oil was administered 30 min prior to experimental TBI, it improved functional outcome after TBI and decreased disruption of the blood-brain barrier. When rats were fed fish oil for a longer period of time (4 weeks) a different research group found that in the fish oil group, as compared to placebo, spatial learning and cognitive function were significantly better using the Morris Water Maze and had a higher density of hippocampal neurons on autopsy (Wang et al., 2013b; Bailes and Mills, 2010), following their successful treatment experiments, repeated their acceleration injury model in rats using a 30-day preinjury gavage of DHA with no postinjury supplementation. Again, they found decreased numbers of APP positive axons, most significant at 40mg/kg/day, in addition to improved Morris Water Maze testing. (Mills et al., 2011b) If animals were deprived of DHA prior to TBI, decreased brain levels of DHA were associated with poorer sensorimotor outcomes (Russell et al., 2014). The effects of DHA depletion prior to TBI was confirmed by HY Kim and colleagues when they observed DHA depleted mice exhibited significantly slower recovery from motor deficits evaluated by the rotarod and the beam walk tests. Furthermore, the DHA deficient mice showed greater anxiety-like behavior tested in the open field test as well as cognitive deficits evaluated by an object recognition test (Desai et al., 2014).

With three days of prestroke treatment, DHA exhibited a neuroprotective effect against ischemic deficits by reduction of behavioral disturbance, brain infarction, edema and blood–brain barrier disruption (Chang et al., 2013). Berman's work includes pretreatment 90 min prior to H/I injury. They report DHA-Alb pretreatment improves functional outcome and reduces volume loss after H/I in neonatal rats (Berman et al., 2009). In another rat H/I study, DHA pretreatment was done one hour; three days; or daily for six weeks prior to injury. All three groups resulted in a reduction of blood–brain barrier disruption, brain edema, inflammatory cell infiltration, interleukin-6 (IL-6) expression and caspase-3 activity and an increase in antioxidative capacity (Pan et al., 2009).

Figueroa et al. (2013) performed several SCI prophylactic studies. When rats were fed a n–3FA enriched diet for eight weeks prior to sham or a contusion SCI operation, the n–3FA group exhibited significantly better functional outcomes including lower sensory deficits, autonomic bladder recovery, and early improvements in locomotion. They also found SCI triggers a marked DHA deficiency that was associated with dysfunction and corrected with the enriched diet. They conclude that n–3FA prophylaxis confers resiliency to SCI mediated, at least in part, by generating a neuroprotective and restorative neurolipidome (Figueroa et al., 2013).

Omega-3 Use in Human TBI

Unfortunately, there is a significant deficit of data demonstrating the use of n–3FA in human TBI. However, several case studies are recorded that can provide clinical guidance. In Jan. 2006, an explosion in the Sago Mine in central West Virginia resulted in 14 trapped miners. Two days later, one lone survivor was found and brought to medical care. He had suffered hypoxia and exposure to toxic gases, dehydration, and rhabdomyolysis. The patient demonstrated many classic features of carbon monoxide toxicity, including neurologic, cardiac, and renal dysfunction as well as respiratory failure. In addition to rapid resuscitation, dialysis, and hyperbaric oxygen therapy, starting on hospital day 8, the patient was treated with 21.2 g per day of n–3FA that contributed to his neurological recovery following an initial presentation in deep coma. On day 21, he was transferred to a rehabilitation facility and discharged to home 2 months later (Roberts et al., 2008).

The only case report in the scientific literature on the specific use of substantial amounts of n–3FA for TBI occurred four years later and was guided by the Sago Mine experience. In Mar. 2010, a teenager sustained a severe TBI in a motor vehicle accident. After prolonged extrication, he was resuscitated at the scene and flown to a Level I Trauma Center. His GCS score was three. CT scan revealed panhemispheric right subdural and small temporal epidural hematomas and a three millimeter midline shift (Fig. 27.1). The patient underwent emergency craniotomy and ICP monitor placement. The patient was rated at Rancho Los Amigos Cognitive Scale Level I and the attending neurosurgeon's impression was that the injury was likely lethal. On hospital day 10, T2 weighted magnetic resonance imaging (MRI) revealed right cerebral convexity subdural hemorrhage and abnormal FLAIR signals consistent with diffuse axonal injury (Fig. 27.3). Believed to be in a permanent vegetative state, a tracheotomy and percutaneous endoscopic gastrostomy (PEG) tube were placed for custodial care and enteral feedings were started. The following day, n–3FAs were added to enteral feedings. With the cooperation of the attending neurosurgeon and hospital pharmacy, the patient began receiving 19,212 mg total n–3FA daily via his PEG. On day 21, he was weaned off the ventilator and transported to a specialized rehabilitation institute. Notably, the patient attended his high school graduation 3 months after the injury. He was discharged to home 4 months after the injury (Lewis et al., 2013). The patient remained on this level of n–3FA for more than one year, experienced no adverse effects, and remains on 15-grams of fish oil orally per day. The patient is currently a full time college student and working two part-time jobs.

Subsequent to that case, and as a result of the media coverage of the previous two cases, when an 8-year-old girl sustained severe anoxic brain injury caused by prolonged cardiac and respiratory arrest secondary to a near drowning accident in Aug. 2012, high doses of n–3FA supplements were started postaccident day 82. The patient quickly moved from an unresponsive state to participating in in-patient rehabilitation and eventually home-care training with her parents. That case was reviewed by Sears, Bailes, and Asselin (Sears et al., 2013). Media coverage of the first two cases also resulted in additional case being reported in the media, this time a 16-year old male pedestrian hit-and-run victim who suffered a torn aorta, skull fractures, subarachnoid hemorrhage, compound bone fractures, and spinal fractures. When transferred to a rehabilitation hospital nine weeks postaccident, the patient, who had been on small doses of fish oil for several weeks, was put on 20-g per day of omega-3 concentrate. Two days following the increased dosage, the patient was capable of holding a complete, intelligent conversation with his mother (Smith, 2014).

GUIDELINES AND PROTOCOLS

Severe TBI Protocol

Without definitive clinical trial evidence, there is no way to know if n–3FA actually helps in any particular case of TBI. The clinical experience of the author and others is that the brain needs to be saturated with high doses of n–3FA in order for the brain to have the opportunity to heal. Without an optimal supply of n–3 fatty acids, healing is less likely to happen. The n–3FAs are not a drug and not a cure. Every situation is different and some patients may respond better than others. However, there is no downside to providing optimal levels of nutrition in order to give a patient the best opportunity to regain as much function as possible following a TBI.

The dose that was used in the case that was reported on CNN's Sanjay Gupta MD show ≪ http://www.cnn.com/2012/10/19/health/fish-oil-brain-injuries/ ≫ and also published in the American Journal of Emergency Medicine (Lewis et al., 2013) was: one tablespoon (15ml) concentrated fish oil twice a day for a total of 30ml per day in the feeding tube followed by a saline flush providing 9,756 mg EPA, 6,756 mg DHA, and19,212 mg total n–3FA daily. This dose has been used in adults. In pediatric patients, lower doses should be considered. A rudimentary, untested, and arbitrary rule used by Lewis is to divide the patient's weight in pounds by 10 to give the total number of milliliters to be given twice per day. For example, in a 100-lb child, 10ml twice a day for a total of 20ml should be considered. This dose has been frequently recommended by the author over the past five years without a single clinical report of side effects. Monitoring of applicable blood parameters should be implemented and include fatty acid profile analysis, liver functions, and bleeding time, prothrombin time (PT)/partial thromboplastin time (PTT), or as per local protocols.

Implications for critical or intensive care

Early nutritional intervention in TBI is underappreciated. Patients not fed within 5 and 7 days after TBI have a two- and four fold increased likelihood of death, respectively; and decreasing amount of nutrition in the first 5 days is related to increased mortality rates (Härtl et al., 2008). Early enteral nutrition after brain injury can be accomplished by PEG or nasogastric tube, even in the emergency department. Of the 49 total recommendations published by the America Society for Parenteral and Enteral Nutrition and the Society of Critical Care Medicine, only two warrant Grade A recommendations, both of which state that immune-enhancing enteral formulations with n–3FA should be used in critically ill surgical patients (including trauma; McClave et al., 2009). Similar recommendation exist in Europe (Weimann et al., 2006).

One recent metaanalysis concludes early initiation of nutritional support for TBI patients can decrease mortality, reduce complications and facilitate recovery. Wan et al. (2013) also concluded that parenteral nutrition appears to be superior to enteral and immune-modulating formulas seem to be superior to standard formulas in reducing infectious complications (Wang et al., 2013a). One reason why enteral nutrition is favored over parenteral nutrition in current clinical practice may be because of the formulations themselves. Unfortunately, the only available FDA-approved parenteral lipid emulsion in the United States is composed of soybean oil (Intralipid, Fresenius Kabi) whereas in Europe, several formulations currently contain fish oil (Nandivada et al., 2013). As noted previously, soybean oil is a major source of AA and the proinflammatory properties of AA likely are more harmful than good.

In 2006, Heller and his German colleagues report one study evaluating the use of a fish oil parenteral formulation in a total of 661 patients from 82 German hospitals. The retrospective study included 276 patients with abdominal sepsis, 59 after multiple trauma, and 18 with severe head injury. Administration of omega-3 fatty acid may reduce mortality, antibiotic use, and length of hospitalization (Heller et al., 2006). Mayer and Seeger reviewed the literature in 2008 and concluded that enteral nutrition with n–3FA improved ventilation time in patients with acute lung injury and reduced mortality in septic patients. They noted that using a high dose, short-term infusion of fish oil-based lipid emulsion improved immunologic parameters and decreased length of stay in surgical patients by balancing the negative effects of n–6FA (Mayer and Seeger, 2008). More recently, two reviews involving Heller and Mayer provide further evidence that parenteral nutrition with fish oil based emulsions are not only safe and effective in reducing the infection rate and hospital/ICU stay in surgical and ICU patients, but cost effective in Italian, French, German, and UK hospitals (Pradelli et al., 2012).

Since 2004, European fish oil based lipid parenteral emulsions have been used at Boston Children's Hospital under investigational new drug status for the treatment of parenteral nutrition-associated liver disease (PNALD) in neonates. The use of parenteral soybean oil is strongly associated with the development of PNALD, cholestasis, and cirrhosis. Without transplant, mortality in this population approaches 100%. Switching infants to a fish oil based emulsion results in resolution of cholestasis, stabilization or improvement of PNALD, and a noticeable impact on decreasing the incidence of morbidity and mortality (Chang et al., 2012; Nandivada et al., 2015).

The Omega Protocol for Brain Health

As noted previously, >80% of TBI are mild not requiring hospitalization and may not even seek medical treatment. These patients are typically capable of swallowing capsules, liquid, or gels on their own. Through several years of clinical experience, the Omega Protocol for Brain Health has been used, recommended, or experienced by thousands of people across the globe including a large number of American university athletic programs following a concussion as well as other brain health issues.

The protocol begins with fifteen (15) capsules a day divided into three doses of five (5) capsules (or one teaspoon of liquid concentrate) starting as soon as possible following an injury. This provides approximately 3000 mg of combined EPA and DHA per dose or a total of 9000 mg daily. It is suggested that patients stay on this dose for one week or until they no longer experience concussion or brain injury symptoms (Table 27.1). In some cases, this is less than a week, in others, greater than a week. A taper is suggested to decrease to two doses a day for a week before going to a single dose per week (Table 27.3). Clinically, many patients see a marked improvement in symptoms within 1–2 days. Every individual is different. This protocol has been developed as a guideline and patients and their healthcare provider may consider adjusting the dosage. For example, if the injury is more severe or happened months or years prior, the patient may find they need to be on the higher doses for a longer period of time.

While clinical experience is obviously important, scientific research needs to catch up to the anecdotal reports. There are several human clinical trials underway to evaluate n–3FA following a concussion or for PCS, but one of the first such studies published was done by Lewis and coworkers, looking at the use of five weeks of high dose n–3FA

TABLE 27.3 The Omega Protocol for Brain Health

Week 1: Take 3000 mg of combined EPA + DHA three times a day for seven days[a]
Week 2: Take 3000 mg of combined EPA + DHA two times a day for seven days[a]
Week 3 and beyond: Take 3000 mg of combined EPA + DHA one time a day[a]

[a] *The Omega-3 Protocol for Brain Health has not been approved by the US Food and Drug Administration. The FDA has classified Omega-3 fatty acids as "generally recognized as safe" (GRAS). The FDA has ruled that up to 3000 mg of EPA+DHA is safe to be included in the food supply of Americans without fear of adverse events. When using higher amounts of EPA and DHA, it is important for persons considering following this protocol to do so under the supervision of a healthcare provider.*

(9000 mg of combined EPA and DHA) in seven military veterans having sustained improvised explosive device (IED) blast injury and having a positive symptom history consistent with PCS for greater than 6 months. The veterans were evaluated pre- and post-therapy with a clinical interview and baseline 19 channel EEG and three lead electrocardiogram. The assessment results incorporated neurocognitive screening, quantitative electroencephalogram (qEEG), event related potentials (ERP), and heart rate variability (HRV) measures. Based on the significant results of n–3FA on HRV total power and auditory processing ERP, it appears that n–3FA have a positive impact on both central and autonomic nervous system functions in patients with PCS. Although other measures of HRV, sensory and cognitive ERP, and qEEG amplitude were not found to have a significant change from the intervention, the pilot study only assessed a small number of subjects but all measures were trending towards statistical improvement (Lewis et al., 2015).

Potential Harmful Effects

Potential harmful effects of n–3FA have been described in the literature (Hasadsri et al., 2013). By virtue of having several double bonds, n–3FA has high susceptibility to lipid peroxidation. However, this has never been shown to be an issue clinically. Development of a fatty liver is often cited as a potential issue as well, however, the experience at Boston Children's Hospital over the past decade demonstrates that n–3FA have a beneficial effect on liver health (Chang et al., 2012; Nandivada et al., 2015).

Due to the established antithrombotic action of these compounds, it is commonly believed they may increase the risk of excessive bleeding or even hemorrhagic stroke. Theoretically, the biochemistry of n–3FAs tells us this should be true. However, that has never been shown to be of clinical concern in any clinical trial reported in the literature. Several surgical studies covered previously using n–3FAs demonstrate their benefit without any adverse events (Heller et al., 2006; Mayer and Seeger, 2008; Pradelli et al., 2012).

The antithrombotic nature is one of the properties that makes n–3FAs effective in decreasing mortality, particularly cardiovascular mortality where the effect can be more beneficial than statins (Studer et al., 2005). Multiple clinical trials have shown that high dose fish oil consumption is safe, even in patients receiving other agents that may increase the risk of bleeding, such as Aspirin and Warfarin (Hasadsri et al., 2013). Clinical data suggests that DHA at doses at least up to 6 g/day does not have deleterious effects on platelet aggregation or other clotting parameters, and fish oil does not augment aspirin-induced inhibition of blood clotting.

This point is worth examining further. It is standard of care that most critically ill and injured patients are put on subcutaneous heparin, or similar, to prevent deep vein thrombosis while immobile. Recently, Farooqui and coworkers examined the use of blood thinning pharmaceuticals and concluded they are safe, do not increase the risk of intracranial hemorrhage, and decreases the rate of deep vein thrombosis and pulmonary embolism (Farooqui et al., 2013). Potent blood thinners used in this protocol (heparin and Lovenox) completely block the enzymes responsible for allowing the platelets to clot. The n–3FAs potentiate the body's natural anticlotting abilities rather than blocking enzymatic processes and add the ability to modulate neuroinflammation, decrease apoptosis, and start synaptogenesis. Ironically, most doctors will not use n–3FA citing that high doses of n–3FA decrease the ability of blood to clot and increase a patient's risk of bleeding, yet immediately put their ICU patients on potent pharmaceutical blood thinners that increase the risk far greater than that of n–3FA.

Conclusions and Future Directions

TBI, with its diverse heterogeneity and prolonged secondary pathogenesis, remains a clinical challenge to clinicians, patients, and their families. Current medical management of TBI patients appropriately focuses on specialized prehospital care, intensive acute clinical care, and long-term rehabilitation, but lacks clinically proven effective management with neuroprotective and neuroregenerative agents (Xiong et al., 2009). Clinical studies thus far have failed to identify an effective treatment strategy as they typically have targeted single enzymatic factors in an attempt to identify a pharmacologic target rather than considering multiple mechanisms of injury with a more holistic approach. The concept of a "magic bullet" focused on a single target is not helpful, and instead a combination of targets controlling aspects of neuroprotection, neuroinflammation, and regeneration is needed. The n–3FAs offer the advantage of this poly-target approach (Michael-Titus and Priestley, 2014).

Although further clinical trial research is needed to establish the true advantage of using n–3FA in severe TBI, mild TBI/concussions, and postconcussion syndrome, there is a growing body of strong preclinical evidence and clinical experience suggests that benefits may be possible from aggressively adding substantial amounts of n–3FA to optimize the nutritional foundation of severe TBI patients. Recovery from TBI may be hindered by our modern, pro-inflammatory diet. An optimal nutritional regimen to overcome the n–6FA dominance must be in place if the brain is to be given the best opportunity to repair itself.

Administration of substantial and optimal doses of n–3FA earlier in the course of TBI, even in preinjury phase of susceptible people such as soldiers and athletes, as well as the prehospital or emergency department setting, has the potential to improve outcomes from this potentially devastating public health problem. As the father of one severe TBI survivor says, "Conventional medicine only takes survivors of severe TBI so far, often ending at the nursing home door, or heavily medicated at home, facing long empty hours, and overwhelming family resources. Unconventional therapies are not merely a reasonable option, they are a necessity." (Goldstein, 2012). With evidence of unsurpassed safety and tolerability, n–3FA should be considered mainstream, conventional medicine, if conventional medicine can overcome its inherent bias against nutritional, nonpharmacologic therapies.

References

Armonda, R.A., Bell, R.S., Vo, A.H., Ling, G., DeGraba, T.J., Crandall, B., Campbell, W.W., 2006. Wartime traumatic cerebral vasospasm: recent review of combat casualties. Neurosurgery 59 (6), 1215–1225.

Armstead, W., 1998. Brain injury impairs prostaglandin cerebrovasodilation. J. Neurotrauma 15, 721–729.

Armstead, W., 1999. Superoxide generation links protein kinase C activation to impaired ATP-sensitive K+ channle function after brain injury. Stroke J. Cerebr. Circul. 30, 153–159.

Bailes, J.E., Mills, J.D., 2010. Docosahexaenoic acid reduces traumatic axonal injury in a rodent head injury model. J. Neurotrauma 27 (9), 1617–1624.

Belayev, L., Marcheselli, V.L., Khoutorova, L., Rodriguez De Turco, E.B., Busto, R., Ginsberg, M.D., Bazan, N.G., 2005. Docosahexaenoic acid complexed to albumin elicits high-grade ischemic neuroprotection. Stroke J. Cerebr. Circul. 36 (1), 118–123.

Berman, D., Liu, Y., Barks, J., Mozurkewich, E., 2010. Treatment with docosahexaenoic acid after hypoxia-ischemia improves forepaw placing in a rat model of perinatal hypoxia-ischemia. Am. J. Obstetrics Gynecol. 203 (4), 385, e1-5.

Berman, D., Mozurkewich, E., Liu, Y., Shangguan, Y., Barks, J., Silverstein, F., 2013. Docosahexaenoic acid augments hypothermic neuroprotection in a neonatal rat asphyxia model. Neonatology 104 (1), 71–78.

Berman, D.R., Mozurkewich, E., Liu, Y., Barks, J., 2009. Docosahexaenoic acid pretreatment confers neuroprotection in a rat model of perinatal cerebral hypoxia-ischemia. Am. J. Obstetrics Gynecol. 200 (3), 305, e1-e6.

Bradbury, J., 2011. Docosahexaenoic acid (DHA): an ancient nutrient for the modern human brain. Nutrients 3, 529–554.

Chang, C.Y., Kuan, Y., Li, J., Chen, W., Ou, Y., Pan, H., Chen, C., 2013. Docosahexaenoic acid reduces cellular inflammatory response following permanent focal cerebral ischemia in rats. J. Nutr. Biochem. 24 (12), 2127–2137.

Chang, M., Puder, M., Gura, K., 2012. The use of fish oil lipid emulsion in the treatment of intestinal failure associated liver disease. IFALD Nutrients 4 (12), 1828–1850.

Coronado, V.G., McGuire, L., Sarmiento, K., Bell, J., Lionbarger, M., Jones, C., Xu, L., 2012. Trends in traumatic brain injury in the U.S. and the public health response: 1995-2009. J. Safety Res. 43 (4), 299–307.

de Souza, M., Conde, C., Laflôr, C., Sicuro, F., Bouskela, E., 2015. n-3 PUFA induce microvascular protective changes during ischemia/reperfusion. Lipids 50 (1), 23–37.

Desai, A., Kevala, K., Kim, H., 2014. Depletion of brain docosahexaenoic acid impairs recovery from traumatic brain injury. PLoS One 27 (9), e86472.

Diaz-Arrastia, R., Kochanek, P., Bergold, P., Kenney, K., Marx, C., Grimes, J., Salzer, W., 2014. Pharmacotherapy of traumatic brain injury: state of the science and the road forward report of the department of defense neurotrauma pharmacology workgroup. J. Neurotrauma 31 (2), 135–158.

Eady, T., Khoutorova, L., Anzola, D., Hong, S., Obenaus, A., Mohd-Yusof, A., Belayev, L., 2013. Acute treatment with docosahexaenoic acid complexed to albumin reduces injury after a permanent focal cerebral ischemia in rats. PLoS One 8 (10), e77237.

Eady, T., Khoutorova, L., Atkins, K., Bazan, N., Belayev, L., 2012. Docosahexaenoic acid complexed to human albumin in experimental stroke: neuroprotective efficacy with a wide therapeutic window. Exp. Translational Stroke Med. 4 (1), 19.

Eady, T., Khoutorova, L., Obenaus, A., Mohd-Yusof, A., Bazan, N., Belayev, L., 2014. Docosahexaenoic acid complexed to albumin provides neuroprotection after experimental stroke in aged rats. Neurobiol. Dis. 62, 1–7.

EFSA, 2012. Scientific opinion on the tolerable upper intake level of eicosapentaenoic acid (EPA), docosahexaenoic acid (DHA) and docosapentaenoic acid (DPA). EFSA J., 10 (7), pp. 2815. http://www.efsa.europa.eu/en/efsajournal/pub/2815.htm

Faden, A., Loane, D., 2015. Chronic neurodegeneration after traumatic brain injury: alzheimer disease, chronic traumatic encephalopathy, or persistent neuroinflammation? Neurotherapeutics 12 (1), 143–150.

Farooqui, A., Hiser, B., Barnes, S., Litofsky, N., 2013. Safety and efficacy of early thromboembolism chemoprophylaxis after intracranial hemorrhage from traumatic brain injury. J. Neurosurg. 119 (6), 1576–1582.

Faul, M., Xu, L., Wald, M., and Coronado, V., 2010. Traumatic brain injury in the United States: emergency department visits, hospitalizations, and deaths 2002-2006. Centers for Disease Control and Prevention. http://www.cdc.gov/traumaticbraininjury/pdf/blue_book.pdf

Figueroa, J.D., Cordero, K., Llán, M.S., De Leon, M., 2013. Dietary omega-3 polyunsaturated fatty acids improve the neurolipidome and restore the dha status while promoting functional recovery after experimental spinal cord injury. J. Neurotrauma 16, 1–16.

Gavett, B., Stern, R., McKee, A., 2011. Chronic traumatic encephalopathy: a potential late effect of sport-related concussive and subconcussive head trauma. Clin. Sports Med. 30 (1), 179xi.

Goldstein, J., 2012. No Stone Unturned: A Father's Memoir of His Son's Encounter with Traumatic Brain Injury. Dulles. Potomac Books, Virginia, USA.

Gomez-Pinilla, F., 2008. The influences of diet and exercise on mental health through hormesis. Ageing Res. Rev. 7 (1), 49–62.

Härtl, R., Gerber, L.M., Ni, Q., Ghajar, J., 2008. Effect of early nutrition on deaths due to severe traumatic brain injury. J. Neurosurgery 109 (1), 50–56.

Hasadsri, L., Wang, B., Lee, J., Erdman, J., Llano, D., Barbey, A., Wang, H., 2013. Omega-3 fatty acids as a putative treatment for traumatic brain injury. J. Neurotrauma 1, 897–906, (30(11)).

Heller, A.R., Rössler, S., Litz, R.J., Stehr, S.N., Heller, S.C., Koch, R., Koch, T., 2006. Omega-3 fatty acids improve the diagnosis-related clinical outcome. Critical Care Med. 34 (4), 972–979.

Hemphill, M., Dabiri, B., Gabriele, S., Kerscher, L., Franck, C., Goss, J., Wanunu, M., 2011. A possible role for integrin signaling in diffuse axonal injury. PLoS ONE 6 (7), e2289.

Hong, S., Belayev, L., Khoutorova, L., Obenaus, A., Bazan, N., 2013. Docosahexaenoic acid confers enduring neuroprotection in experimental stroke. J. Neurol. Sci. 15, 135–141.

Hong, S., Khoutorova, L., Bazan, N., Belayev, L., 2015. Docosahexaenoic acid improves behavior and attenuates blood-brain barrier injury induced by focal cerebral ischemia in rats. Experiment. Translation. Stroke Med. 7 (1), 3–13.

Iliff, J., Chen, M., Plog, B., Zeppenfeld, D., Soltero, M., Yang, L., Nedergaard, M., 2014. Impairment of glymphatic pathway function promotes tau pathology after traumatic brain injury. J. Neurosci. 34 (49), 16180–16193.

Jotwani, V., Harmon, H., 2010. Postconcussion syndrome in athletes. Curr. Sports Med. Report 9 (1), 21–26.

Katz, R., 2011. Investigational New Drug submission. Silver Spring, MD.

Kochanek, P., Clark, R., Jenkins, L., 2007. TBI: Pathology. In: Zasler, N., Katz, D., Zafonte, R. (Eds.), Brain Injury Medicine: Principles and Practice. Demos Medical Publishing, LLC, New York, pp. 81–92.

Lee, B., Newberg, A., 2005. Neuroimaging in traumatic brain imaging. J. Am. Soc. Experiment. Neurotherapeutics 2, 372–383.

Lewis, M., Ghassemi, P., Hibbeln, J., 2013. Therapeutic use of omega-3 fatty acids in severe head trauma. Am. J. Emerg. Med. 31 (1), 5–8.

Lewis, M., Hagedorn, M., Hagedorn, C., Hagedorn, N., and Hagedorn, D., 2015. Electrophysiology improvements in veterans with post-concussive symptoms using omega-3 nutritional therapy: a pilot study. Military Medicine.

Ling, G., Bandak, F., Armonda, R., Grant, G., Ecklund, J., 2009. Explosive blast neurotrauma. J. Neurotrauma 26 (6), 815–825.

Ling, G., Marshall, S., 2008. Management of traumatic brain injury in the intensive care unit. Neurologic Clin. 26 (2), viii.

Ling, H., Hardy, J., Zetterberg, H., 2015. Neurological consequences of traumatic brain injuries in sports. Mol. Cell. Neurosci. 66 (Pt B), 114–122.

Louveau, A., Smirnov, I., Keyes, T., Eccles, J., Rouhani, S., Peske, J., Kipnis, J., 2015. Structural and functional features of central nervous system lymphatic vessels. Nature 523 (7560), 337–341.

Mayer, K., Seeger, W., 2008. Fish oil in critical illness. Curr. Op. Clin. Nutr. Metabolic Care 11 (2), 121–127.

McClave, S.A., Martindale, R.G., Vanek, V.W., McCarthy, M., Roberts, P., Taylor, B., Cresci, G., 2009. Guidelines for the Provision and Assessment of Nutrition Support Therapy in the Adult Critically Ill Patient: Society of Critical Care Medicine (SCCM) and American Society for Parenteral and Enteral Nutrition (A.S.P.E.N.). J. Parenteral Enteral Nutr. 33 (3), 277–316.

Meythaler, J., Peduzzi, J., Eleftheriou, E., Novack, T., 2001. Current concepts: diffuse axonal injury-associated traumatic brain injury. Arch. Phys. Med. Rehab. 82 (10), 1461–1471.

Michael-Titus, A., Priestley, J., 2014. Omega-3 fatty acids and traumatic neurological injury: from neuroprotection to neuroplasticity? Trends Neurosci. 37 (1), 30–38.

Michael-Titus, A.T., 2007. Omega-3 fatty acids and neurological injury. Prostagland. Leukotr. Essent. Fatty Acid. 77 (5–6), 295–300.

Mills, J.D., Bailes, J.E., Sedney, C.L., Hutchins, H., Sears, B., 2011a. Omega-3 fatty acid supplementation and reduction of traumatic axonal injury in a rodent head injury model. J. Neurosurg. 114 (1), 77–84.

Mills, J.D., Hadley, K., Bailes, J.E., 2011b. Dietary supplementation with the omega-3 fatty acid docosahexaenoic acid in traumatic brain injury. Neurosurgery 68 (2), 474–481.

Nandivada, P., Carlson, S., Chang, M., Cowan, E., Gura, K., Puder, M., 2013. Treatment of parenteral nutrition-associated liver disease: the role of lipid emulsions. Adv. Nutrition 4 (6), 711–717.

Nandivada, P., Chang, M., Potemkin, A., Carlson, S., Cowan, E., O'loughlin, A., Puder, M., 2015. The natural history of cirrhosis from parenteral nutrition-associated liver disease after resolution of cholestasis with parenteral fish oil therapy. Ann. Surg. 26 (1), 172–179.

Omalu, B., DeKosky, S., Minster, R., Kamboh, M., Hamilton, R., Wecht, C., 2005. Chronic traumatic encephalopathy in a National Football League playe. Neurosurgery 57 (1), 128–134.

Pan, H.-C., Kao, T.-K., Ou, Y.-C., Yang, D.-Y., Yen, Y.-J., Wang, C.-C., Chen, C.-J., 2009. Protective effect of docosahexaenoic acid against brain injury in ischemic rats. J. Nutr. Biochem. 20 (9), 715–725.

Paterniti, I., Impellizzeri, D., Di Paola, R., Esposito, E., Gladman, S., Yip, P., Cuzzocrea, S., 2014. Docosahexaenoic acid attenuates the early inflammatory response following spinal cord injury in mice: in-vivo and in-vitro studies. J. Neuroinflam. 11 (6), 1–18.

Pradelli, L., Eandi, M., Povero, M., Mayer, K., Muscaritoli, M., Heller, A., Fries-Schaffner, E., 2014. Cost-effectiveness of omega-3 fatty acid supplements in parenteral nutrition therapy in hospitals: A discrete event simulation mode. Clinical Nutr. 33 (5), 785–792.

Pradelli, L., Mayer, K., Muscaritoli, M., Heller, A., 2012. n-3 fatty acid-enriched parenteral nutrition regimens in elective surgical and ICU patients: a meta-analysis. Critical Care 16 (5), R184.

Ramesh, G., MacLean, A., Philipp, M., 2013. Cytokines and chemokines at the crossroads of neuroinflammation, neurodegeneration, and neuropathic pain. Mediators Inflamm. 2013, Article ID 480739, 20 pages.

Reilly, P., 2007. In: Weber, J. (Ed.), Neurotrauma: New Insights Into Pathology and Treatment. Academic Press, Amsterdam, pp. 5–7.

Roberts, L., Bailes, J., Dedhia, H., Zikos, A., Singh, A., McDowell, D., Carpenter, J., 2008. Surviving a mine explosion. J. Am. Coll. Surg. 207 (2), 276–283.

Rodríguez-Rodríguez, A., Egea-Guerrero, J., Murillo-Cabezas, F., Carrillo-Vico, A., 2014. Oxidative stress in traumatic brain injury. Curr. Med. Chem. 21 (10), 1201–1211.

Rosenberg, G., 1999. Ischemic brain edem. Prog. Cardiovascul. Dis. 42 (3), 209–216.

Russell, K., Berman, N., Gregg, P., Levant, B., 2014. Fish oil improves motor function, limits blood-brain barrier disruption, and reduces Mmp9 gene expression in a rat model of juvenile traumatic brain injury. Prostagland. Leukotr. Essent. Fatty Acid. 90 (1), 5–11.

Saatman, K., Duhaime, A., Bullock, R., Maas, A., Valadka, A., Manley, G., Members, W.S.T., A.P, 2008. Classification of traumatic brain injury for targeted therapies. J. Neurotrauma 25 (7), 719–738.

Schobe, M., Requena, D., Abdullah, O., Casper, T., Beachy, J., Malleske, D., Pauly, J., 2015. Dietary docosahexaenoic acid improves cognitive function, tissue sparing, and magnetic resonance imaging indices of edema and white matter injury in the immature rat after traumatic brain injury. J. Neurotrauma 32 (18), .

Sears, B., Bailes, J., Asselin, B., 2013. Therapeutic uses of high-dose omega-3 fatty acids to treat comatose patients with severe brain injury. PharmaNutrition 1, 86–89.

Selassie, A., Zaloshnja, E., Langlois, J., Miller, T., Jones, P., Steiner, C., 2008. Incidence of long-term disability following traumatic brain injury hospitalization, United States, 2003. J Head Trauma Rehab. 23 (2), 123–131.

Shin, S., Dixon, C., 2011. Oral fish oil restores striatal dopamine release after traumatic brain injury. Neurosci. Letters 496 (3), 168–171.

Smith, D., Meaney, D., 2000. Axonal damage in traumatic brain injury. Neuroscientist 6 (6), 483–495.

Smith, S., 2014. "He"s going to be better than he was before'. http://www.cnn.com/2014/01/18/health/fish-oil-recovery/

Stein, D., 2015. Embracing failure: what the phase III progesterone studies can teach about TBI clinical trials. Brain Injury 14 (8), 1–14.

Stein, D., Wright, D., Kellermann, A., 2008. Does progesterone have neuroprotective properties? Annals Emergency Med. 51 (2), 164–172.

Streit, W., Mrak, R., Griffin, W., 2004. Microglia and neuroinflammation: a pathological perspective. J. Neuroinflammation 1 (1), 14.

Studer, M., Briel, M., Leimenstoll, B., Glass, T., Bucher, H., Zuo, C., 2005. Effect of different antilipidemic agents and diets on mortality: a systematic review. Arch. Internal Med. 165 (7), 725–730.

NINDS, 2002. National institute of neurological disorders and stroke; traumatic brain injury: hope through research. National Institutes of Health, NIH Publication No.: 02-158.

Turner, R., Lucke-Wold, B., Robson, M., Omalu, B., Petraglia, A., Bailes, J., 2012. Repetitive traumatic brain injury and development of chronic traumatic encephalopathy: a potential role for biomarkers in diagnosis, prognosis, and treatment? Frontiers Neurol. 3 (186), 1–11.

CDC, United States Centers for Disease Control and Prevention, 2015. Facts for Physicians About Mild Traumatic Brain Inury (MTBI). http://www.cdc.gov/headsup/pdfs/providers/facts_for_physicians_booklet-a.pdf

Wang, X., Dong, Y., Han, X., Qi, X., Huang, C., Hou, L., 2013a. Nutritional support for patients sustaining traumatic brain injury: a systematic review and meta-analysis of prospective studies. PLoS One 8 (3), e58838.

Wang, T., Van, K., Gavitt, B., Grayson, J., Lu, Y., Lyeth, B., Pichakron, K., 2013b. Effect of fish oil supplementation in a rat model of multiple mild traumatic brain injuries. Restorative Neurol. Neurosci. 31 (5), 647–659.

Wasserman, J., Feldman, J., and Koenigsberg, R., 2012. Diffuse Axonal Injury Imaging. http://emedicine.medscape.com/article/339912

Weimann, a., Braga, M., Harsanyi, L., Laviano, a., Ljungqvist, O., Soeters, P., Vestweber, K.H., 2006. ESPEN guidelines on enteral nutrition: surgery including organ transplantation. Clinical Nutr. 25 (2), 224–244.

Willer, B., Leddy, J., 2006. Management of concussion and post-concussion syndrome. Curr. Treatment Options Neurol. 8 (5), 415–426.

Williams, J.J., Mayurasakorn, K., Vannucci, S.J., Mastropietro, C., Bazan, N.G., Ten, V.S., Deckelbaum, R.J., 2013. N-3 Fatty Acid rich triglyceride emulsions are neuroprotective after cerebral hypoxic-ischemic injury in neonatal mice. PloS One 8 (2), e56233.

Wu, A., Ying, Z., Gomez-Pinilla, F., 2007. Omega-3 fatty acids supplementation restores mechanisms that maintain brain homeostasis in traumatic brain injury. J. Neurotrauma 24 (10), 1587–1595.

Wu, A., Ying, Z., Gomez-Pinilla, F., 2011. The salutary effects of DHA dietary supplementation on cognition, neuroplasticity, and membrane homeostasis after brain trauma. J. Neurotrauma 28 (10), 2113–2122.

Wu, A., Ying, Z., Gomez-Pinilla, F., 2013. Exercise facilitates the action of dietary DHA on functional recovery after brain trauma. Neuroscience 248, 655–663.

Xiong, Y., Mahmood, A., Chopp, M., 2009. Emerging treatments for traumatic brain injury. Expert Op. Emergency Drugs 14 (1), 67–84.

Yealy, D., Hogan, D., 1991. Imaging after head trauma. Who needs what? Emergency Medical Clinics North Am. 9, 707–717.

Yuh, E., Cooper, S., Mukherjee, P., Yue, J., Lingsma, H., Gordon, W., INVESTIGATORS, T.-T., 2014. Diffusion tensor imaging for outcome prediction in mild traumatic brain injury: a TRACK-TBI study. J. Neurotrauma 31 (17), 1457–1477.

CHAPTER

28

Dietary Fish Oil Protects Against Gentamicin, Cisplatin, Uranyl Nitrate, and Nitric Oxide Donor/Metabolite-Induced Nephrotoxicity and Oxidative Damage in Rat Kidney

A.N.K. Yusufi, M.W. Khan**, S.A. Khan†, S. Priyamvada‡, F.N. Khan Yusufi§*

*Department of Biochemistry, Faculty of Life Sciences, Aligarh Muslim University, Aligarh, UP, India; ** DST-INSPIRE Faculty, Cell Biology & Physiology Division, CSIR-Indian Institute of Chemical Biology, Kolkata, India; †SVKMs Mithibai College, Bhakti Vedanta Swami Marg, Mumbai, India; ‡Division of Gastroenterology and Hepatology, Department of Medicine, University of Illinois at Chicago, Chicago, Illinois, United States; §Department of Statistics and Operations Research, Faculty of Science, Aligarh Muslim University, Aligarh, UP, India

INTRODUCTION

"Let food be thy medicine and medicine be thy food." This philosophy of Hippocrates (460 BC) is the underlying concept for the development of functional foods. From ancient times the physicians and scholars in Asia have understood that food has both preventive and therapeutic value and is an integral part of health. The concept of disease prevention using naturally occurring substances that can be included in the diet consumed by the human population is gaining much interest. Fish/fish oil (FO) rich in long chain n–3 (LCn3) polyunsaturated fatty acids (PUFA) provides one such dietary source of biologically active components that have been shown to be copreventive and cotherapeutic in a wide variety of ailments (Doughman et al., 2007). Early clues to the possible importance of unsaturated fatty acids, especially PUFA, came from studies showing that young humans and experimental animals experienced impaired growth when all fatty acids were removed from the diet. Small amounts of n–3 (α-linolenic acid; 18:3n–3) or n–6 (linoleic acid; 18:2n–6) fatty acids prevented impaired growth and thus were termed "essential fatty acids" (Burr and Burr, 1930).

We are exposed daily to numerous toxins that pose problems in the form of serious health risks. A number of environmental contaminants, chemicals, and drugs including heavy metals, organic solvents, antibiotics, antihypertensive, anticancer drugs, and nitric oxide donors and metabolites have been found to dramatically alter the structure and function of the kidney and other major organs and produce multiple adverse effects. (Banday et al., 2008a,b; Fatima et al., 2004, 2005; Khan et al., 2009a,b,c; Khan et al., 2012a,b, 2013; Priyamvada et al., 2008, 2010; Naqshbandi et al., 2012; Shahid et al., 2014; Khan et al., 2015). Histopathological and biochemical studies have revealed that exposure to certain drugs and/or chemicals including heavy metals; mercury, chromium, platinum, lead and uranium, trichloroethylene, aminoglycoside, nitric oxide donors/metabolites, etc., cause severe damage to the kidneys and alters the structure and functions of renal proximal tubule leading to acute renal failure (ARF; Sanchez et al., 2001;

Fish and Fish Oil in Health and Disease Prevention. http://dx.doi.org/10.1016/B978-0-12-802844-5.00028-2

Fatima et al., 2004, 2005; Barbier et al., 2005; Banday et al., 2008a,b; Khan et al., 2009a,b,c; Priyamvada et al., 2008, 2010; Khan et al., 2012a,b, 2013).

Several approaches and strategies using many different agents and different mechanisms have been attempted to prevent drug-/chemical-induced nephrotoxicity and oxidative damage, however, a clinically viable approach has not yet been established (Ali, 2003; Nagai and Takano, 2004; Ali and Al-Moundhri, 2006). In the past few years, much interest has been centered on the role of naturally occurring dietary substances for their ability to confer health and physiological benefits. It has been established that diets supplemented with FO containing LCn3 PUFA have profound beneficial health effects against various pathologies, including cancers, cardiovascular diseases, diabetes, depression, arthritis, asthma, and inflammatory and immune disorders of kidney and intestine (De Caterina et al., 1994; Barbosa et al., 2003; Bhattacharya et al., 2006). Recently, we have demonstrated that dietary FO protects against gentamicin (GM), cisplatin (CP), uranyl nitrate (UN), sodium nitroprusside (SNP), sodium nitrite (SNT), and arginine (ARG)-induced nephropathy in animal models (Priyamvada et al., 2008, 2010; Khan et al., 2012a,b, 2013; Naqshbandi et al., 2012). In this review article, we summarize the protective effects of dietary FO against drug- and chemical-induced nephrotoxicity and oxidative damage carried out in our laboratory in the past decade.

Beneficial Health Effects of FO Enriched in ω–3 PUFA From Marine Sources

The nature of the relationship between diet and disease is the subject of great controversy. Although, dietary and body fats are essential for life, they also affect our health in many different ways. The intake of saturated fat, trans-fat and refined oils are related to diseases such as cancer, diabetes, depression, hypertension, and heart disease (Anti et al., 1994; Yusufi and Siddiqi, 1974). However, the consumption of unsaturated fats, especially PUFA, was shown to have numerous health benefits (Simopoulos, 1991; Zamaria, 2004; Deckelbaum et al., 2006; Doughman et al., 2007). This stems from the observation of the lower prevalence of coronary heart disease and other chronic diseases (including psoriasis, bronchial asthma, diabetes mellitus, and thyrotoxicosis) in the Greenland Inuit (Eskimo) population relative to Western populations (Kromann and Green, 1980). Omega-3 PUFA from marine fish and mammals were indicated as the main dietary factor responsible for such differences (Dyerberg et al., 1975; Bang et al., 1976). Certain fish and/or FO contain a high proportion of n–3 PUFA, for example, eicosapentaenoic acid (EPA) and docosahexaenoic acid (DHA), which are responsible for the health benefits of fish/FO.

The role of fish oil/n–3 PUFA has been extensively investigated and received a great deal of attention in recent times as a therapeutic option in a number of clinical situations. A number of investigations have demonstrated that n–3 fatty acids present in fish/fish oil have beneficial effects against various pathologies including cancers (Larsson et al., 2004), cardiovascular (Leaf, 2008) and respiratory diseases, diabetes, depression (Hibbeln, 1998), arthritis, asthma, and inflammatory and immune disorders of kidney and intestine (De Caterina 1993; De Caterina et al., 1994; Donadio, 2001; Barbosa et al., 2003; Bhattacharya et al., 2006; Kakar et al., 2008). FO/n–3 fatty acids targeted cell cycle regulation/cell signaling may also underlie its protective effects (Yusufi et al., 2003; Siddiqui et al., 2003). Recently, it has been shown that FO may have a therapeutic potential as an adjunct therapy for human AIDS (Xi and Chen, 2000). DHA has been found to be essential in normal functional development of retina and brain (Simopoulos, 2000; Neuringer, 2000). The intake of n–3 PUFA/FO or consumption of fish was shown to have inverse association with growth and development and rate of depression (Small, 2002) and other mental deficiencies (Simopoulos, 1991; Carrie et al., 1999; Gamoh et al., 1999; Bourre, 2005). Some of the specific effects on renal disorders are given below.

Renal Health Effects of FO Enriched in n–3 PUFA from Marine Sources

Omega-3 fatty acids and renal disorders: Recent studies have demonstrated that dietary supplementation with n–3 PUFA retards renal disease progression in human and experimental animals (Donadio, 2001). In IgA nephropathy, the most common glomerulonephritis worldwide, the rate of renal disease progression was significantly reduced in patients given fish oil supplements (Donadio et al., 2001). Dietary n–3 competes for arachidonic acid oxygenation pathway resulting in formation of biologically inactive end products, thus exhibiting a favorable effect on glomerular injury, various forms of acute and chronic renal failure, allograft rejection, structural and functional renal damage in cyclosporine nephrotoxicity, hepatorenal syndrome, diabetic nephropathy, renal hypertension, vascular access thrombosis of end stage renal disease, idiopathic calcium urolithiasis, idiopathic immunoglobulin A nephropathy, and lupus nephritis (De Caterina and Craven, 1993; De Caterina et al., 1994; Donadio, 2001; Baggio et al., 2002). Fish oil was also linked to the management of type 2 diabetes (Montori et al., 2000; Mostad et al., 2006).

PROTECTIVE EFFECT OF DIETARY FISH OIL (FO) ON GENTAMICIN (GM), CISPLATIN (CP) AND URANYL NITRATE (UN) INDUCED NEPHROTOXICITY

Pathophysiology of GM, CP, and UN

Gentamicin Pathophysiology

Aminoglycoside such as GM are the most commonly used antibiotics worldwide in the treatment of gram-negative bacterial infections (Nagai and Takano, 2004). The high incidence of associated nephrotoxicity and ototoxicity (Lang and Liu, 1997) represents an important concern in the use of aminoglycoside antibiotics which have been implicated as one of the primary causes of drug induced ARF (Ali, 1995). The specificity of GM renal toxicity is apparently related to its accumulation in the renal proximal convoluted tubule causing a number of morphological and biochemical alterations in humans and experimental animals (Kacew and Bergeron, 1990; Ali, 1995; Mingeot-Leclercq and Tulkens, 1999a). GM has been shown to cause marked histological damage in particular to renal proximal convoluted tubules (S_1 and S_2 subsegments; Abdel-Gayoum et al., 1994) resulting in swelling, vacuolization and necrosis of epithelial cells and accumulation of myelin-like bodies (Ali and Bashir, 1994; Pedraza-Chaverri et al., 2000). The adverse interaction of the drug with critical intracellular processes leads to renal cortical phospholipidosis disrupting functions of membranes and organelles including BBM, BLM, mitochondria, lysosomes, and microsomes (Laurent et al., 1990; Sundin et al., 2001).

GM nephrotoxicity is often characterized by an increase in serum creatinine and blood urea nitrogen (BUN) associated with massive proteinuria, enzymuria, glucosuria, and phosphaturia (Banday et al., 2008a). Gentamicin has been reported to inhibit the oxidative phosphorylation in the isolated renal cortex and to decrease the total ATP content of rat kidney (Simmons et al., 1980). Recently, GM has been shown to affect various enzymes of carbohydrate metabolism including glycolysis, TCA cycle, HMP shunt pathway, and gluconeogenesis (Banday et al., 2008a). The damage caused by GM to lysosomes, BBM and BLM was demonstrated by decreases in the activities of their biomarker enzymes in renal cortex associated with their increase in the urine (Banday et al., 2008a). GM has been shown to generate ROS and produce oxidative stress leading to cellular injury (Walker et al., 1999; Cuzzocrea et al., 2002; Ali, 2003; Banday et al., 2008a). Decreased expression of multiple genes by GM treatment has been elucidated by toxicogenomic studies (Amin et al., 2004; Kramer et al., 2004).

Cisplatin Pathophysiology

Cisplatin (cis-diamminedichloroplatinum II, CP) is a potent antitumor agent and is highly effective agent against a diverse spectrum of malignancies (Cohen and Lippard, 2001). However, the use of this agent in combating cancer is limited by the development of nephrotoxicity and ototoxicity (Ward and Fauvie, 1976; Ali and Al-Moundhri, 2006), along with various untoward side effects including nausea, vomiting, diarrhea, and myelosuppression (McKeage, 1995; Markman, 2003).

Cisplatin-induced nephrotoxicity is associated with necrosis of the terminal portion of the proximal tubule and apoptosis, predominantly in cells in the distal nephron (Arany and Safirstein, 2003; Taguchi et al., 2005). Light and electron microscopy have shown that the CP-induced injury and necrosis in the rat kidney are predominantly localized in the S3 segment of proximal tubule in the cortical-medullary region with or without accompanying distal changes (Townsend et al., 2003). A spectrum of changes was seen including focal loss of brush border, cellular swelling, and condensation of nuclear chromatin and focal areas of necrosis (Dobyan et al., 1980). The mitochondria, lysosomes, and microsomes appeared to be critical targets of CP (Zhang and Lindup, 1993; Leibbrandt et al., 1995). Different studies have shown that CP-induced cytotoxicity is probably due to a combination of insults including peroxidation of cell membrane, inhibition of protein synthesis, and DNA damage in the kidney (Santos et al., 2007). It has been shown that CP induces renal damage by free radical generation, such as hydroxyl radical and superoxide anion, by altering arginine metabolism and by apoptosis (Fatima et al., 2004; Santos et al., 2007; Khan et al., 2009b). However, CP-induced oxidative stress was shown to be strongly involved in acute renal damage (Gonzales et al., 2005).

Uranyl Nitrate Pathophysiology

Uranium, the heaviest of the naturally occurring elements, is widely present in the environment as a result of leaching from natural deposits, industrial emissions, and weapons that contain uranium (Martinez et al., 2003; Bem and Bou-Rabee, 2004; Periyakaruppan et al., 2007). They are major environmental and occupational hazards (Barbier et al., 2005). Uranium is found in various chemical forms in all soils, rocks, sea, and bedrocks (Bosshard et al., 1992; Kurttio et al., 2002). It is also found in both food and drinking water and poses significant environmental and occupational hazards (Barbier et al., 2005; McDonald-Taylor et al., 1997). The major health effect of uranium is chemical kidney toxicity rather than a radiation hazard (Bem and Bou-Rabee, 2004; Taulan et al., 2004). Although, the kidney is major target organ, toxic effects were also observed in the liver, intestine, cardiovascular, respiratory and nervous systems, muscle, and skeleton (Gilman et al., 1998; Taulan et al., 2004; Guéguen et al., 2006; Periyakaruppan et al., 2007; Dublineau et al., 2007).

Uranium nephrotoxicity has been extensively studied in experimental animals using uranyl nitrate (UN) or uranyl acetate (Haley et al., 1982; Goldman et al., 2006). Histopathological studies have shown that UN-caused specific damage to renal proximal tubules (Haley et al., 1982) accompanied by tubular vacuolization and epithelial cell degeneration with focal loss of BBM, thickening and splitting of basolateral membrane (BLM) with significant increase in lysosomal and mitochondrial mass and occasionally cell necrosis (Blantz, 1975; McDonald-Taylor et al., 1997; Hamid, 2012). The pars recta (S_2 and S_3 subsegments) of proximal tubule in juxtamedullary region were predominantly damaged (Haley, 1982; Haley et al., 1982). Uranyl ions interact with enzyme protein sulfhydryl groups in the acidic luminal plasma membrane of pars recta or deplete intracellular glutathione causing phospholipids derangement and alterations in membrane structure and functions (Weiner and Jacobs, 1983). Thus, the pattern of injury caused by uranium more closely resembles that of cisplatin rather than mercury or GM (Mahmood and Waters, 1994). Banday et al. (2008b) demonstrated that UN administration caused specific alterations in biochemical parameters involving cellular metabolism, structural integrity, and functional capacity of BBM, BLM, lysosomes and mitochondria, and most importantly perturbation in antioxidant defense system. Recently, renal toxicogenomic studies revealed that UN causes alteration of many genes involved in cellular metabolism, oxidative stress, inflammatory response, protein and lipid metabolism, signal transduction, and in solute transporters (Taulan et al., 2004).

Protection Against Gentamicin, Cisplatin, and Uranyl Nitrate-Induced Nephrotoxicity and Oxidative Damage

Several approaches, utilizing different mechanisms, have been attempted to reduce nephrotoxicity of GM and related aminoglycoside antibiotics. These mechanisms include decreasing or preventing drug accumulation by the kidneys or decreasing binding to BBM (Mingeot-Leclercq and Tulkens 1999b). Many different agents and strategies have been reported to ameliorate GM nephrotoxicity in experimental animals (Ali, 2003; Nagai and Takano, 2004). Among them, protection against GM nephrotoxicity was mainly focused on the use of various antioxidant agents including the extracts from medicinal plants with antioxidant properties (Ali, 2003). Such medicinal plants include garlic (Pedraza-Chaverri et al., 2000), as well as diallyl sulfide, a compound isolated from garlic (Pedraza-Chaverrí et al., 2003) and *Nigella sativa* oil (Ali, 2004).

Several agents have been tested to ameliorate cisplatin-induced nephropathy and other adverse effects (Ali and Al-Moundhri, 2006). These include antioxidants, modulators of nitric oxide, agents interfering with metabolic pathways of CP, diuretics, cytoprotective and apoptotic agents (Ali and Al-Moundhri, 2006).

A variety of protective measures against UN-induced nephropathy and oxidative damage have been explored. These include certain complexing and chelating agents which form nonionized ring compounds with inorganic ions that are subsequently eliminated by the kidney (Durakoviae, 1999; Domingo et al., 1997). Recently, Banday et al. (2008b) has shown that UN-induced nephrotoxicity was mediated in part by oxidative stress mechanism as reported for GM- and cisplatin-induced nephrotoxicity (Chang et al., 2002; Banday et al., 2008a). In view of this, certain compounds having antioxidant properties were used to reduce UN nephrotoxicity. Kato et al. (1994) reported that hydroxyl radical scavengers: dimethyl thiourea (DMTU) and dimethyl sulfoxide (DMSO) significantly attenuate uranyl acetate (UA)-induced rise in serum creatinine and decreased renal tubular damage. Similarly, melatonin was shown to reduce UA induced damage in the kidney by increasing the antioxidant defense mechanism (Belles et al., 2007).

However, none of the above strategies and mechanisms were found to be safe for clinical practice in protecting GM/CP/UN-induced nephrotoxicity. An increasing number of studies have demonstrated that naturally occurring chemical moieties (neutraceuticals) hold great promise in combating several disorders. Green tea (GT) and LCn3 PUFA/fish oil are two examples of such biologically active dietary sources that have been shown to have extensive health benefits against several human pathologies (Simopoulos, 1991; Khan and Mukhtar, 2007). Preliminary reports showed that dietary fish oil prevents GM- and cyclosporine-induced nephrotoxicity (Abdel-Gayoum et al., 1995; Ali and Bashir, 1994; Thakkar et al., 2000). Recently, Khan et al. (2009a,b) have shown that GT consumption prevents GM- and CP-induced nephrotoxicity and oxidative damage whereas Priyamvada et al. (2008, 2010) have demonstrated protection against GM- and UN-induced nephropathies and Naqshbandi et al. (2012) against CP-induced nephropathies by dietary fish oil. In this report, we reviewed and discussed the protective effects of dietary fish oil (FO) against GM/CP/UN-induced nephrotoxicity and oxidative damage as summarized in the following pages.

TABLE 28.1 Effect of Dietary Fish Oil on Serum Parameters with; (1) Gentamicin (GM), (2) Cisplatin (CP), (3) Uranyl Nitrate (UN), (4) Sodium Nitrite (SNT), (5) Sodium Nitroprusside (SNP), (6) L-Arginine (ARG) Treatments

Groups	Creatinine (mg/dL)	BUN (mg/dL)	Cholesterol (mg/dL)	Phospholipids (mg/dL)	Phosphate (μmol/mL)	Glucose (mg/dL)
(1) GM	+79%	+93%	+35%	+83%	−27%	−38%
FOGM	−66%	−23%	−5%	+14%	+37%	+4%
(2) CP	+60%	+96%	+37%	+50%	−26%	−10%
FOCP	+21%	+49%	+14%	+12%	+14%	+22%
(3) UN	+97%	+103%	+33%	+93%	−39%	+113%
FOUN	−56%	−31%	−13%	+8%	+55%	+62%
(4) SNT	+54%	+85%	+18%	+46%	−32%	+25%
FOSNT	+12%	+16%	+1%	+10%	+7%	−7%
(5) SNP	+23%	+67%	−23%	−24%	−32%	−16%
FOSNP	+2%	−6%	−3%	−9%	+11%	+6%
(6) ARG	+28%	+29%	−8%	+21%	−27%	−29%
FOARG	−29%	−11%	+2%	−10%	+46%	−7%

Results are Mean ± SEM for five different preparations.
Values represent percent change from respective controls.

Effect of Dietary Fish oil (FO) on GM/CP/UN-Elicited Nephrotoxicity Parameters in Serum

As reported earlier (Banday et al., 2008a,b; Priyamvada et al., 2008, 2010; Naqshbandi et al., 2012), the administration of GM/CP/UN-caused nephrotoxicity in a similar manner as characterized by increased serum creatinine, blood urea nitrogen (BUN), cholesterol, and phospholipids accompanied by a decrease in inorganic phosphate (Pi). GM/CP also caused a decrease in serum glucose but was increased by UN administration (Table 28.1). FO diet alone significantly increased serum glucose, Pi, and phospholipids but decreased BUN (Priyamvada et al., 2008). Feeding of FO diet to GM/CP/UN rats, however, significantly lowered the increased concentration of creatinine, BUN and cholesterol indicating reduction in drug/chemical-induced nephropathy (Table 28.1). Serum glucose and Pi significantly increased by FO given to experimental rats (Table 28.1).

Effect of Dietary Fish oil (FO) on Brush Border Membrane (BBM) Enzymes in Cortical Homogenates and Isolated BBM Vesicles (BBMV)

The kidneys play an essential role in the maintenance of total body fluid volume, its composition, pH, and acid base balance by selective reabsorption of nutrients which is dependent on the integrity of BBM and available energy in the form of ATP supplied by various metabolic pathways. GM/CP/UN administration significantly, but differentially, decreased BBM enzymes alkaline phosphatase (ALP), γ-glutamyl transferase (GGTase), and leucine aminopeptidase (LAP), both in the homogenate and BBMV (Table 28.2). The extent of the effect, however, was much greater in BBMV. Since these enzymes are structural/function components embedded in the BBM (Yusufi et al., 1994), the decrease in these enzyme activities showed disruption of membrane structure as they were later excreted in the urine as part of the BBM which is known to be effaced by toxic insult, as reported earlier (Banday et al., 2008a,b). FO diet consumption alone markedly increased ALP and GGTase, but LAP was decreased by FO. FO in combination with GM/CP/UN caused marked reversal of toxic insult and increased levels of these enzymes suggesting overall improvement of BBM integrity (Priyamvada et al., 2008, 2010; Naqshbandi et al., 2012). Dietary LCn3 PUFAs are known to incorporate in cellular membranes and cause alterations in membrane organization, fluidity, and permeability that stabilize membrane bound components including enzymes and transport proteins and reduce lipid peroxidation (Kaur et al., 1996; Thakkar et al., 2000; Carrillo-Tripp and Feller, 2005). A similar effect of dietary n-3 PUFA present in FO has been shown to incorporate in the membranes that alter membrane organization and their properties (Katakura et al., 2014).

TABLE 28.2 Effect of Dietary Fish Oil on Biomarker Enzymes with; (1) Cisplatin (CP), (2) Uranyl Nitrate (UN), (3) Gentamicin (GM), (4) Sodium Nitrite (SNT), (5) Sodium Nitroprusside (SNP), (6) L-Arginine (ARG) Treatments in (a) Cortical BBMV and (b) Cortex Homogenate

Groups	ALP (μmol/mg protein per hour)	GGTase (μmol/mg protein per hour)	LAP (μmol/mg protein per hour)
(A) BBMV			
(1) GM	−67%	−62%	−58%
FOGM	+37%	+6%	−42%
(2) CP	−57%	−34%	−42%
FOCP	−22%	−17%	−12%
(3) UN	−53%	−64%	−52%
FOUN	+18%	+30%	−28%
(4) SNT	−67%	−53%	−61%
FOSNT	+19%	+7%	−15%
(5) SNP	−25%	−13%	−43%
FOSNP	−9%	+19%	+10%
(6) ARG	−47%	−45%	−40%
FOARG	+6%	−7%	+9%
(B) HOMOGENATE			
(1) GM	−45%	−27%	−37%
FOGM	+34%	+7%	−23%
(2) CP	−37%	−30%	−56%
FOCP	−27%	−8%	−12%
(3) UN	−39%	−51%	−42%
FOUN	+10%	+16%	−15%
(4) SNT	−35%	−57%	−56%
FOSNT	−7%	−26%	+13%
(5) SNP	+50%	−24%	−56%
FOSNP	−4%	−4%	+20%
(6) ARG	−28%	−27%	−29%
FOARG	+14%	+51%	+6%

Results are Mean ± SEM for five different preparations.
Values represent percent change from respective controls.

Effect of Dietary Fish Oil (FO) on GM/CP/UN-Induced Alterations in Carbohydrate Metabolism Enzymes in Renal Cortex and Medulla

The proximal tubule of the kidney along with lysosomes, microsomes, and mitochondria are the major target of toxic insult. Any alterations in cellular membranes would affect the transport capacity of various nutrients including Na^+ and Pi (Coux et al., 2001) and available energy in the form of ATP generated by various metabolic pathways (Khundmiri et al., 2004, 2005; Banday et al., 2008a,b). The various marker enzymes of carbohydrate metabolism involved in glycolysis, TCA cycle, gluconeogenesis, and HMP shunt pathway were selectively altered by GM/CP/UN administration in the cortex and medulla (Table 28.3). GM/CP/UN caused a significant increase in LDH, but decrease in MDH, G6Pase, and FBPase activities in renal cortex (Table 28.3). Although actual rates of the pathways were not determined, at least it appears from these observations that glycolysis, oxidative metabolism, and gluconeogenesis were affected. A marked decrease in MDH activity appears to be due to drug/chemical-induced mitochondrial dysfunction as shown earlier (Kuhlmann et al., 1997; Banday et al., 2008a,b). At the same time, the increase

TABLE 28.3 Effect of Dietary Fish Oil on Carbohydrate Metabolism Enzymes with; (1) Cisplatin (CP), (2) Uranyl Nitrate (UN), (3) Gentamicin (GM), (4) Sodium Nitrite (SNT), (5) Sodium Nitroprusside (SNP), (6) L-Arginine (ARG) Treatments in Cortex

Groups	LDH (μmol/mg protein/h)	MDH (μmol/mg protein/h)	G6Pase (μmol/ mg protein/h)	FBPase (μmol/ mg protein/h)	G6PDH (μmol/ mg protein/h)	ME (μmol/mg protein/h)
(i) GM	+28%	−31%	−23%	−17%	+24%	−64%
FOGM	+23%	+19%	−8%	+15%	−12%	−37%
(ii) CP	+70%	−46%	−23%	−19%	−43%	+35%
FOCP	+13%	−8%	+5%	+1%	0%	−14%
(iii) UN	+60%	−28%	−54%	−57%	−46%	+40%
FOUN	+31%	+22%	+13%	+5%	−35%	+9%
(iv) SNT	+29%	−35%	−41%	−18%	+42%	−19%
FOSNT	+4%	+3%	+6%	−5%	−11%	+9%
(v) SNP	+23%	−30%	−18%	−22%	+33%	−24%
FOSNP	+17%	+11%	+13%	+41%	+5%	+2%
(vi) ARG	+19%	−24%	−14%	−19%	−22%	−28%
FOARG	+9%	+18%	+3%	+9%	−6%	−9%

Results are Mean ± SEM for five different preparations.
Values represent percent change from respective controls.

in LDH appears to be a cellular adaptive response, changing energy dependence from aerobic to anaerobic metabolism also due to mitochondrial damage (Priyamvada et al., 2008, 2010; Khan et al., 2009a,b). The decrease of G6Pase and FBPase enzymes of gluconeogenesis may be the result of decreased MDH activity. The oxidative conversion of glucose by G6PDH (HMP shunt pathway) markedly decreased by CP/UN but increased by GM, however they have the opposite effect on NADP–malic enzyme (ME). Both these enzymes control cellular NADPH that is required, in part, for biosynthesis of cholesterol/phospholipids and plays a major role in oxidant/antioxidant balance (Banday et al., 2008a,b; Priyamvada et al., 2008, 2010; Khan et al., 2009a,b,c), Taken together the decrease in oxidative metabolism, serum Pi, and Na-dependent transport of Pi (data not shown; Fatima et al., 2004; Banday et al., 2008a,b) by the kidney indicates overall lower production of ATP and hence a decrease in kidney functions.

In contrast, FO consumption alone was shown to enhance the enzyme activities involved in glycolysis, TCA-cycle, gluconeogenesis, and HMP shunt pathway (Priyamvada et al., 2008, 2010). Feeding of FO-diet along with GM/CP/UN treatment caused marked reversal and prevented the effects of GM/CP/UN on the enzymes of carbohydrate metabolism and appears to improve energy metabolism and hence overall kidney functions (Table 28.3). This is also supported by the fact that a decrease in serum Pi and Na-dependent transport of Pi across BBM caused by toxic insult was profoundly increased by FO diet given to drug/chemical-treated animals (Priyamvada et al., 2008, 2010; Khan et al., 2012a,b, 2013). Similar results were obtained in the medulla (data not shown; Priyamvada et al., 2008, 2010; Naqshbandi et al., 2012).

Effect of Dietary Fish oil (FO) on GM/CP/UN-Induced Alterations in Antioxidant Defense Parameters in Renal Cortex and Medulla

It is well established that certain drugs and chemical toxicants, including GM/CP/UN exert their toxic effects by inducing generation of free radicals (ROS/RNOS) and by causing imbalances in oxidants and antioxidants levels resulting in oxidative damage to renal tissues. (Walker et al., 1999; Devipriya and Shyamaladevi, 1999; Banday et al., 2008a,b; Khan et al., 2009a,b,c). However, oxidative stress can occur by either increased lipid peroxidation and/or decreased activity of antioxidant enzymes, superoxide dismutase (SOD), catalase and glutathione peroxidase (GSH-Px). GM/CP/UN administration resulted in severe oxidative damage to the kidney as reflected by enhanced oxidative stress parameters and suppressed antioxidative parameters both in renal cortex and medulla (Table 28.4). GM/CP/UN markedly increased lipid peroxidation (LPO, measured in terms of malondialdehyde) and significantly decreased Total-SH levels indicating oxidative damage to the kidney tissues.

TABLE 28.4 Effect of Dietary Fish Oil on Antioxidant Enzymes with; (1) Cisplatin (CP), (2) Uranyl Nitrate (UN), (3) Gentamicin (GM), (4) Sodium Nitrite (SNT), (5) Sodium Nitroprusside (SNP), and (6) L-Arginine (ARG) Treatments in Cortex

Groups	LPO (nmol/g tissue)	Total SH (μmol/g tissue)	SOD (units/mg protein)	Catalase (μmol/mg protein/min)	GSH-Px (μmol/mg protein/min)
(1) GM	+47%	−33%	−67%	−44%	−40%
FOGM	−4%	+15%	+34%	−17%	+8%
(2) CP	+215%	−30%	−36%	−25%	−33%
FOCP	+55%	−17%	−12%	−9%	−29%
(3) UN	+67%	−32%	+72%	−37%	+49%
FOUN	+21%	+7%	+49%	+3%	+10%
(4) SNT	+46%	−29%	+58%	−16%	+31%
FOSNT	+10%	−7%	+42%	+30%	+6%
(5) SNP	+42%	−22%	+40%	−18%	−29%
FOSNP	+4%	+23%	+15%	−10%	−6%
(6) ARG	+43%	−16%	+68%	−9%	+37%
FOARG	+2%	+5%	+7%	+5%	+4%

Results are Mean ± SEM for five different preparations.
Values represent percent change from respective controls.

In agreement with previous reports (Banday et al., 2008a,b; Khan et al., 2009b), GM/CP decreased SOD, catalase and GSH-Px in the same manner whereas UN significantly increased SOD and GSH-Px but decreased catalase activity as shown by Priyamvada et al. (2010). These antioxidant enzymes protect the cell against cytotoxic ROS. In contrast, FO-diet alone significantly increased the activities of SOD, catalase, and GSH-Px in renal tissues (Priyamvada et al., 2008; Naqshbandi et al., 2012). FO diet along with GM/CP/UN administration enhanced antioxidant defense mechanism as evident by simultaneous increase of SOD, catalse, and GSH-Px along with associated lowering of LPO (Table 28.4). Thus, it appears that FO-diet offers a significant protection from GM/CP/UN-induced oxidative damage to the kidney and can be used as a safe option in clinical practice to prolong GM treatment against severe bacterial infection, CP treatment for certain cancers and against critical exposure to any toxic insult (Data not shown for medulla).

Protective Effect of Dietary Fish Oil (FO) on Nitric Oxide Donor/Metabolites, Sodium Nitroprusside (SNP), Sodium Nitrite (SNT), and Arginine (ARG)-Induced Nephrotoxicity

Nitric Oxide Donors and Metabolites

Overview: Besides oxygen, carbon, and hydrogen, nitrogen is an essential element that constitutes life. It is generally consumed as nitrate (NO^{3-}) or nitrite (NO^{2-}). Changes in patterns of agricultural practice, food processing, and industrialization have impacted accumulation of nitrates/nitrites in the environment. Nitrate is abundantly present in the environment (Hill, 1991) as fertilizer, sewage treatment, and nitrogenous bacteria product (Tannenbaum et al., 1978) besides being used as food preservatives and vasodilators. Nitric oxide (NO), which is synthesized in vivo from L-arginine (ARG), can be oxidized to nitrite or nitrate. Thus, man and animals are subjected to significant nitrate and nitrite levels in foods, feed, soil, and water as well as those formed in vivo.

Toxicity: Any toxicity linked with nitrate was found to be due to its bioconversion to nitrite by the bacteria in the soil, mouth, or stomach (Duncan et al., 1995; Lundberg and Govoni, 2004). The major health concerns with nitrite are the risk of methemoglobinaemia and its potential carcinogenic, mutagenic, and cytotoxic effects (Ger et al., 1996; Magee and Barnes, 1956; Spencer et al., 2000; Sun et al., 2006). It has now been documented that reactions of H_2O_2 with nitrite and of superoxide with NO have a common intermediate—peroxynitrite ($ONOO^-$) (Carmichael et al., 1993), which is responsible for nitration of proteins, DNA strand breaks and mutations, and with interference of protein functions (Sampson et al., 1998). Sodium nitroprusside (SNP), used as an antihypertensive agent has been documented to induce genotoxicity (Andreassi et al., 2001), mutagenicity (Asaka et al., 1997; Lin et al., 1998), apoptosis (Feldmann, 1997), and altered metabolism (Brown and Borutaite, 2002; Maletic et al., 2000). L-Arginine (ARG) is the substrate for the different nitric oxide synthase (NOS) isoforms which are responsible for the production of NO in vivo. ARG itself has very moderate toxicity, whatever harmful effects it manifests is mainly due to the overproduction of NO.

Nitric oxide is a double-edged sword, it serves as a key signaling molecule in physiological processes and on the other hand, excessive and unregulated NO synthesis has been implicated as causal or contributing to pathophysiological conditions including many lethal and debilitating human disorders: arthritis, atherosclerosis, cancer, diabetes, numerous degenerative neuronal diseases, stroke, and myocardial infarction to name a few (Culotta and Koshland, 1992; Gross and Wolin, 1995). Recently, both nitrates and nitrites have been recognized as key oxidation products of NO, which can be generated in the tissues by a number of enzymatic and nonenzymatic reactions (Lundberg et al., 2008). Therefore, they should now be viewed as storage pools for NO-like bioactivity, thereby complementing the NO synthase (NOS)-dependent pathway. The recognition of this mammalian nitrogen cycle (nitrate–nitrite–NO) has led researchers to explore the role of nitrate and nitrite in physiological and pathophysiological processes where NO is known to play a key role.

Protective effect of LCn3 PUFA on NO donor/metabolites induced nephrotoxicity: Fish oils high in n–3 PUFA (EPA and DHA) provide one such dietary source of biologically active components that has been shown to be copreventative and cotherapeutic in a wide variety of ailments (Doughman et al., 2007). Although n–3 PUFA have been shown to provide beneficial effects in many pathophysiological conditions, studies on their possible beneficial effects against drug/chemical-induced nephrotoxicity is very limited (Watkins et al., 2007; Priyamvada et al., 2008, 2010). Recently Khan et al., (2012a,b, 2013) showed that fish oil can ameliorate the toxic effects of NO donors/metabolites in rat kidney, possibly due to their intrinsic biochemical and antioxidant properties. In their study Khan and coworkers, have taken SNP/ARG as the NO donor and SNT as the metabolite. The increase in the tissue levels of nitrite in the kidney homogenates was a reflection of the possible toxic effects of NO donors/metabolites. All three chemical agents used in the study significantly increased the levels of nitrite in the kidney. NO donor/metabolite treatment to rats resulted in significant nephrotoxicity as evident by the increase in serum creatinine and blood urea nitrogen (Table 28.1) and profound phosphaturia, proteinuria, and glucosuria, accompanied by decrease in creatinine clearance. NO donors and metabolite treatment to rats resulted in perturbation of the glucose metabolism as evident by the activities of key metabolic enzymes of the glycolytic and mitochondrial tricarboxylic acid pathway (TCA). Khan et al. (2012a,b, 2013) observed a shift from aerobic to anaerobic glucose metabolism as evident by increased activity of LDH concomitant with decrease in TCA cycle enzyme activities (Table 28.3). The primary toxic effect of NO donors/metabolites is due to the production of free radicals such as NO and $ONOO^-$, that was evident by the damage to the membrane integrity. Key membrane enzymes such as alkaline phosphatase, γ-glutamyl transpeptidase, leucine aminopeptidase, and acid phosphatase activities were found to be significantly reduced in the cortex and enriched BBM preparation (Table 28.2). The fact that NO donors/metabolites extensively damage the cellular membranes was further corroborated by the decreased activity of the sodium-dependent phosphate transporter which pumps phosphate across the membrane using a sodium gradient. The oxidizing capability of NO donors/metabolites was further proved using the lipid peroxidation assay which shows a significant increase along with a concomitant decrease of the cellular reducing power measured by the levels of free thiol groups. The antioxidant enzyme systems were differentially affected by NO donors/metabolites. Superoxide dismutase (SOD) activity was found to be increased in cortical homogenates whereas the activities of catalase and GSH-Px were decreased by NO donors/metabolites (Table 28.4). In the medullary homogenates, the effect was somewhat different than the cortex primarily the activity of superoxide dismutase being decreased. However, it was confirmed that NO donors/metabolites primarily increase the oxidative load on the cell which results in damage to cellular macromolecules, particularly the membrane. When a fish oil-enriched diet was given along with NO donors/metabolites treatment, it prevented/retarded NO donors/metabolites-induced alterations in various biochemical parameters and enzyme activities most likely due to their incorporation in cellular membranes and antioxidant properties. Dietary n–3 PUFA enriched fish oil to a larger extent prevented NO donors/metabolites induced nephrotoxicity parameters by enhancing nutrition/energy metabolism and phosphate transport capacity, by strengthening antioxidant defense mechanism and by altering membrane organization/fluidity/permeability. The n–3 PUFA-enriched fish oil diet leads to an enhancement in the metabolic processes. The results also suggest that n–3 PUFA strengthen the biological antioxidant defense system thereby reducing oxidative/nitrosative damage induced by NO donors/metabolites (Fig. 28.1).

It is apparent that n–3 PUFA is a source of a wide range of neutraceuticals that are digested, absorbed, and metabolized and that they exert their effects at the cellular level. Fish oil enriched in n–3 PUFA provides a dietary source of biologically active components that have been shown to be copreventative and cotherapeutic in a wide variety of ailments. Based on observations and already known numerous health benefits, it can be said that n–3 PUFA enriched-fish oil may provide a cushion for a prolonged therapeutic option against drug/chemical-induced nephropathy without harmful side effects.

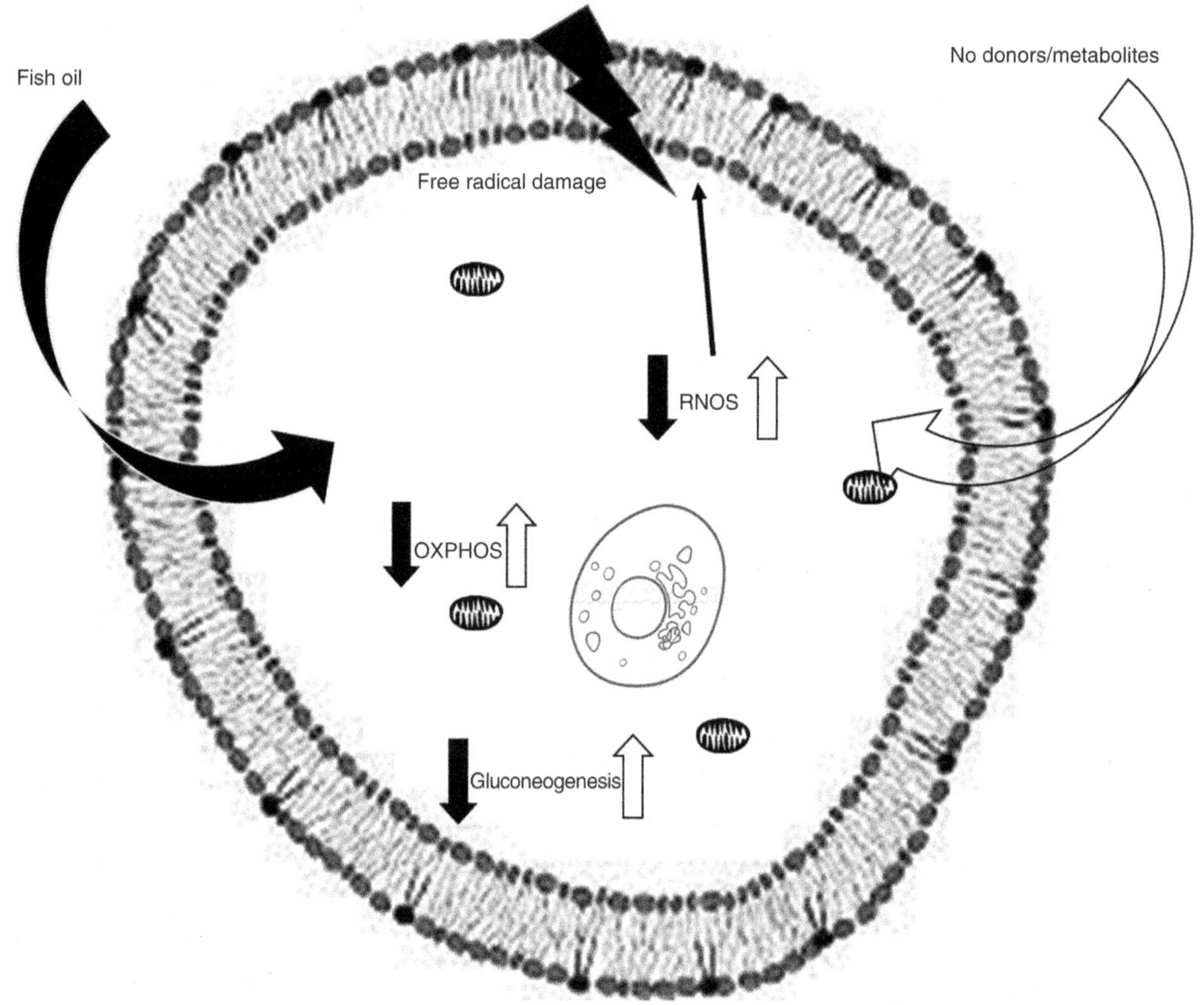

FIGURE 28.1 **Fish oil protects against nitric oxide donor/metabolites mediated damage: NO donors/metabolites (*hollow arrows*) produce reactive nitrogen oxygen species (RNOS) that damages the membrane and perturbs the cellular metabolic machinery.** Fish oil (*solid arrows*) on the other hand ameliorates the toxic effects of NO donors/metabolites primarily by reducing RNOS mediated damage to the membranes and other organelles.

SUMMARY AND CONCLUSION

As summarized in Figs. 28.1 and 28.2, the present biochemical studies clearly demonstrate that long-term administration of nitric oxide donor/metabolites and GM/CP/UN elicited deleterious nephrotoxic effects by causing major damage to mitochondria, lysosomes, and in particular to BBM of renal proximal tubules as reflected by a significant decrease in the activities of their specific biomarker enzymes, confirming morphologic and/or toxicogenomic observations that showed these organelles as prime targets. These drugs and chemicals, in general, seem to enhance the glycolytic enzyme LDH in the kidney in order to increase energy dependence on anaerobic glycolysis due to drug-induced mitochondrial dysfunction and depressed TCA cycle enzymes. A significant decrease in G6Pase and FBPase activities (gluconeogenic enzymes) also appeared to be due to mitochondrial damage. The decrease/increase in the activities of various enzymes by GM/CPUN/SNP/SNT/ARG might be due to suppression/induction of their synthesis as microsomes are reported to be possible targets. The toxicant induced decrease of serum phosphate and renal Pi transport suggests a decrease in energy metabolism as well.

The nephrotoxic and other adverse effects appeared to be mediated at least in part due to GM/CP/UN/SNP/SNT/ARG elicited oxidative damage as evident by enhanced LPO and suppressed antioxidant enzymes. Although these pharmaceutical agents and chemicals are different structures and exert different physiological effects by different mechanisms, they appear to have similar nephrotoxic effects. However, they seem to be different models of ARF as GM is known to affect early whereas CP affects late proximal tubule in the kidney. UN/SNP appears to affect pars recta similar to CP.

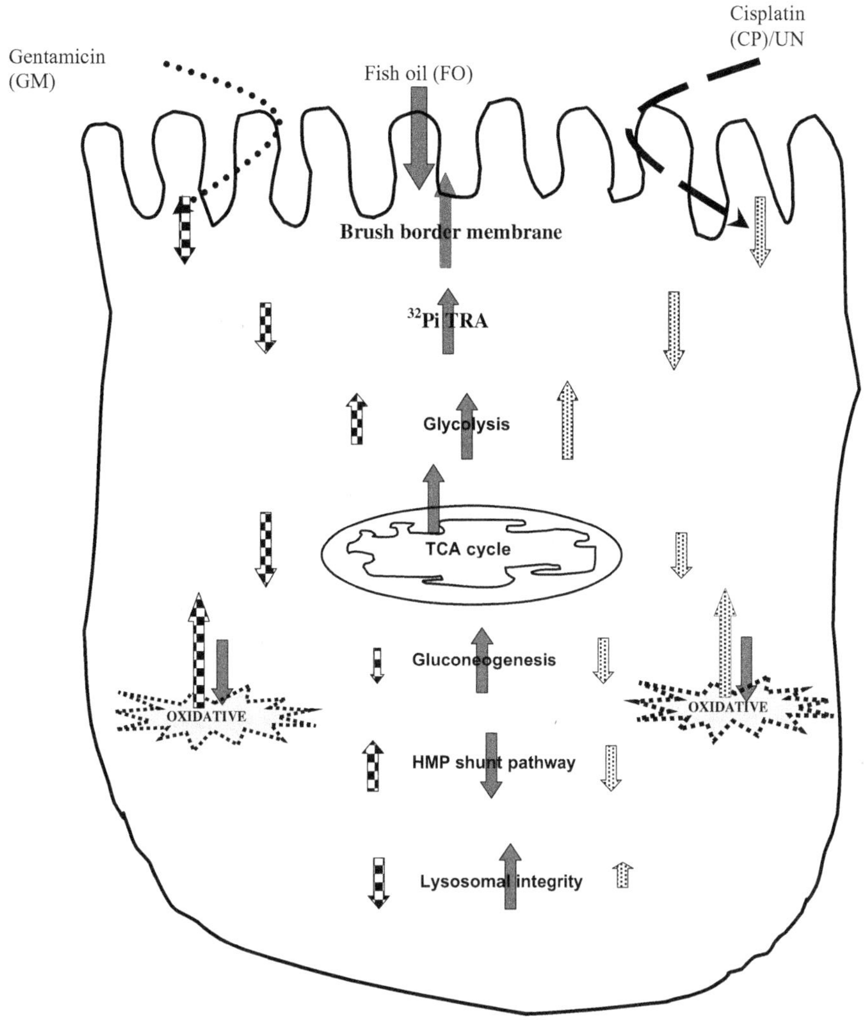

FIGURE 28.2 **A summarized schematic representation of the effect of GM/CP/UN on the enzymes of carbohydrate metabolism and on the overall membrane integrity of the BBM and the protection conferred by FO administration.**

In contrast, FO-diet enriched in n–3 fatty acids with toxicant induced alterations in the activities of various enzymes of carbohydrate metabolism, BBM, and oxidative stress. This is due to the fact that dietary n–3 PUFA is incorporated in cellular membranes and changes their fatty acid compositions that affect membrane organization, fluidity, permeability, and functions. FO appears to accelerate repair and/or regeneration of injured BBM and other cellular organelles as evident by increased activities of certain BBM and metabolic enzymes. Most importantly, by enhancing endogenous antioxidant defense mechanism FO provided protection from GM/CP/UN nitric oxide donors/metabolites induced free radical attack and reduced lipid peroxidation and enhanced the activity of antioxidant enzymes (Fig. 28.2). FO and n–3 fatty acids (PUFA) target cell cycle regulation/cell signaling which may also underlie its protective effects. Since FO has been known to possess antibacterial, antihypertensive, and anticarcinogenic properties along with other known health benefits, it would be able to maximize the clinical use of these drugs in exerting their physiological effects due to its intrinsic biochemical properties.

Taken together, our present and past studies clearly demonstrate that diet has pivotal role in maintaining health and expression/prevention of disease. Dietary supplementation with omega-3 polyunsaturated fatty acids-enriched fish oil/green tea, sources of biologically active components provide an important option in the management of various diseases and drug induced toxicities with additive benefits and without harmful side effects. We suggest that to remain healthy and be protected from various diseases and environmental contaminants, one should eat fish or FO supplement frequently, a few kernels of walnuts, a snack of flaxseeds, and a few cups of green tea.

Abbreviations

ACPase Acid phosphatase
ALP Alkaline phosphatase
ARG Arginine
ATP Adenosine 5′-triphosphate
BBM Brush border membrane
BBMV Brush border membrane vesicles
BUN Blood urea nitrogen
DHA Docosahexanoic acid
EPA Eicosapentanoic acid
FBPase Fructose,1,6,bisphosphatase
FO Fish oil
G6Pase Glucose-6-phosphatase
G6PDH Glucose-6-phosphate dehydrogenase
GGTase γ-Glutamyl transferase
GM Gentamicin
GT Green tea
HK Hexokinase
HMP Hexose monophosphate
LAP Leucine aminopeptidase
LCn3 Long chain omega-3 fatty acids
LDH Lactate dehydrogenase
LPO Lipid peroxidation
MDH Malate dehydrogenase
ME Malic enzyme
n-3 Omega-3
Pi Inorganic phosphate
PUFA Polyunsaturated fatty acids
ROS Reactive oxygen species
SOD Superoxide dismutase
SNP Sodium nitroprusside
SNT Sodium nitrite
TCA Tricarboxylic acid cycle
w/v Weight/volume

References

Abdel-Gayoum, A.A., Ali, B.H., Abdel-Razig, A.A., Bashir, A.A., Ghywarsha, K., 1994. Effect of gentamicin-induced nephrotoxicity on some carbohydrate metabolic pathways in the rat renal cortex. Archiv. Toxicol. 68, 643–647.

Abdel-Gayoum, A.A., Bashir, A.A., El-Fakhri, M.M., 1995. Effect of fish oil and sunflower oil supplementations on gentamicin induced nephrotoxicity in rat. Human Experiment. Toxicol. 14, 884–888.

Ali, B.H., 1995. Gentamicin nephrotoxicity in humans and animals: some recent research. General Pharmacol. 26, 1477–1487.

Ali, B.H., 2003. Agents ameliorating or augmenting experimental gentamicin nephrotoxicity: some recent research. Food Chem. Toxicol. 41, 1447–1452.

Ali, B.H., 2004. The effect of Nigella sativa oil on gentamicin nephrotoxicity in rats. Am. J. Clin. Med. 32, 49–55.

Ali, B.H., Al-Moundhri, S.M., 2006. Agents ameliorating or augmenting the nephrotoxicity of cisplatin and other platinum compounds: A review of some recent research. Food Chem. Toxicol. 44, 1173–1183.

Ali, B.H., Bashir, A.A., 1994. Effect of fish oil treatment on gentamicin nephrotoxicity in rats. Annal. Nutr. Metab. 38, 336–339.

Amin, R.P., Vickers, A.E., Sistare, Frank, et al.,2004. Identification of putative gene-based markers of renal toxicity. Environ. Health Perspectiv. 112, 465–479.

Andreassi, M.G., Picano, E., Del Ry, S., Botto, N., Colombo, M.G., Giannessi, D., Lubrano, V., Vassalle, C., Biagin, A., 2001. Chronic long term nitrate therapy: possible cytogenetic effect in humans? Mutagenesis 16, 517–521.

Anti, M., Arm Clau, F., Marra, G., et al.,1994. Effects of different doses of fish oil on rectal cell proliferation in patients with sporadic colonic adenomas. Gastroenterology 107, 1892–1894.

Arany, I., Safirstein, R., 2003. Cisplatin nephrotoxicity. Seminar Nephrol. 23, 460–464.

Asaka, M., Takeda, H., Sugiyama, T., Kato, M., 1997. What role does *Helicobacter pylori* play in gastric cancer? Gastroenterology 113, S56–S60.

Baggio, B., Budakovic, A., Priante, G., Gambaro, G., Manzato, E., Khan, S., 2002. Dietary fatty acid supplementation modulates the urinary excretion of calcium and oxalate in the rat. Insight into calcium lithogenesis. Nephron 91, 486–491.

Banday, A.A., Farooq, N., Priyamvada, S., Yusufi, A.N.K., Khan, F., 2008a. Time dependent effects of gentamicin on the enzymes of carbohydrate metabolism, brush border membrane and oxidative stress in rat kidney tissues. Life Sci. 82, 450–459.

Banday, A.A., Priyamvada, S., Farooq, N., Yusufi, A.N.K., Khan, F., 2008b. Effect of uranyl nitrate on enzymes of carbohydrate metabolism and brush border membrane in different kidney tissues. Food Chem. Toxicol. 46, 2080–2088, 2009b.

Bang, H.O., Dyerberg, J., Hjoorne, N., 1976. The composition of food consumed by Greenland Eskimos. Acta Medica Scandinavia 200, 69–73.

Barbier, O., Jacquillet, G., Tauc, M., Cougnan, M., Poujeol, P., 2005. Effect of heavy metals ion, and handling by kidney. Nephron Physiol. 99, 105–110.

Barbosa, D.S., Cecchini, R., El Kadri, M.Z., Rodriguez, M.A., Burini, R.C., Dichi, I., 2003. Decreased oxidative stress in patients with ulcerative colitis supplemented with fish oil omega-3 fatty acids. Nutrition 19, 837–842.

Belles, M., Linares, V., Luisa Albina, M., Sirvent, J., Sanchez, D.J., Domingo, J.L., 2007. Melatonin reduces uranium-induced nephrotoxicity in rats. J. Pineal Res. 43, 87–95.

Bem, H., Bou-Rabee, F., 2004. Environmental and health consequences of depleted uranium use in the 1991Gulf war. Environ. Int. 30, 123–134.

Bhattacharya, A., Ghosal, S., Bhattacharya, S.K., 2006. Effect of fish oil on offensive and defensive factors in gastric ulceration in rats. Prostagland. Leukotr. Essent. Fatty Acid. 74, 109–116.

Blantz, R.C., 1975. The mechanism of acute renal failure after uranyl nitrate. J. Clin. Investig. 55, 621–635.

Bosshard, E., Zimmerli, B., Schalatter, C., 1992. Uranium in diet: risk assessment of its nephro- and radiotoxicity. Chemosphere 24, 309–321.

Bourre, J.M., 2005. Where to find omega-3 fatty acids and how feeding animals with diet enriched in omega-3 fatty acids to increase nutritional value of derived products for human: what is actually useful? J. Nutr. Health Aging 9, 232–242.

Brown, G.C., Borutaite, V., 2002. Nitric oxide inhibition of mitochondrial respiration and its role in cell death. Free Radical Biol. Med. 33, 1440–1450.

Burr, G.O., Burr, M.M., 1930. The nature and role of the fatty acids essential in nutrition. J. Biol. Chem. 86, 587–621.

Carmichael, A.J., Steel-Goodwin, L., Gray, B., Arroyo, C.M., 1993. Reactions of reactive oxygen species studied by EPR and spin trapping. Free Radical Res. Commun. 19, S1–S16.

Carrie, I., Clement, M., De Javel, D., Frances, H., Bourre, J.M., 1999. Learning deficits in first generation OF1 mice deficient in (n-3) polyunsaturated fatty acids do not result from visual alteration. Neurosci. Letters 266, 69–72.

Carrillo-Tripp, M., Feller, S.E., 2005. Evidence for a mechanism by which omega-3 polyunsaturated lipids may affect membrane protein function. Biochemistry 44, 10164–10169.

Chang, B., Nishikawa, M., Sato, E., Utsumi, K., Inoue, M., 2002. L-Carnitine inhibits cisplatin-induced injury of the kidney and small intestine. Archive. Biochem. Biophys. 405, 55–64.

Cohen, S.M., Lippard, S.J., 2001. Cisplatin: from DNA damage to cancer chemotherapy. Progress Nucleic Acid Res. Molecul. Biol. 67, 93–130.

Coux, G., Trurumper, L., Elias, M.M., 2001. Cortical Na^+-K^+ ATPase activity, abundance and distribution after in vivo renal ischemia without reperfusion in rats. Nephron 89, 82–89.

Culotta, E., Koshland, D.E., 1992. NO news is good news. Science 258, 1862–1865.

Cuzzocrea, S., Mazzon, E., Dugo, L., Serraino, I., Di Paola, R., Britti, D., De Sarro, A., et al.,2002. A role for superoxide in gentamicin mediated nephropathy in rats. Eur. J. Pharmacol. 450, 67–76.

De Caterina, R., Craven, P.A., 1993. Eicosanoid in the pathogenesis of the functional and structural alterations of the kidney in diabetes. Am. J. Kidney Dis. 22, 727–735.

De Caterina, R., Endres, S., Kristensen, S.D., Schmidt, E.B., 1994. n-3 fatty acids and renal diseases. Am. J. Kidney Dis. 24, 397–415.

Deckelbaum, R.J., Worgall, T.S., Seo, T., 2006. n-3 fatty acids and gene expression. Am. J. Clin. Nutr. 83, 1520S–1524S.

Devipriya, S., Shyamaladevi, C.S., 1999. Protective effect of quercetin in cisplatin-induced cell injury in the rat kidney. Ind. J. Pharmacol. 31, 422–426.

Dobyan, D.C., Levi, J., Jacobs, C., Kosek, J., Weiner, M.W., 1980. Mechanism of cisplatinum nephrotoxicity: II. Morphologic observations. J. Pharmacol. Experiment. Therapeutics 213, 551–556.

Domingo, J.L., De La Torre, A., Belles, M., Mayayo, E., Llobet, J.M., Corbella, J., 1997. Comparative effect of the chelators sodium 4,5-dihydroxybenzene-1,3-disulfonate (Tiron) and diethylenetriaminicpentacetic acid (DTPA) on acute uranium nephrotoxicity in rats. Toxicology 118, 49–59.

Donadio, J.V., 2001. The emerging role of omega-3 polyunsaturated fatty acids in the management of patients with IgA nephropathy. J. Renal Nutr. 11, 122–128.

Donadio, Jr., J.V., Larson, T.S., Bergstralh, E.J., Grande, J.P., 2001. A randomized trial of high-dose compared with low-dose omega-3 fatty acids in severe IgA nephropathy. J. Am. Soc. Nephrol. 12, 791–799.

Doughman, S.D., Krupanidhi, S., Sanjeevi, C.B., 2007. Omega-3 fatty acids for nutrition and medicine: considering microalgae oil as a vegetarian source of EPA and DHA. Curr. Diabetes Rev. 3, 198–203.

Dublineau, I., Grandcolas, L., Grison, S., Baudelin, C., Paquet, F., Voisin, P., Aigueperse, J., Gourmelon, P., 2007. Modifications of inflammatory pathways in rat intestine following chronic ingestion of depleted uranium. Toxicol. Sci. 98, 458–468.

Duncan, C., Dougall, H., Johnston, P., Green, S., Brogan, R., Liefert, C., Smith, L., Gloden, M., Benjamin, N., 1995. Chemical generation of nitric oxide in the mouth from the enterosalivary circulation of dietary nitrate. Nature Med. 1, 546–551.

Durakoviae, A., 1999. Medical effects of internal contamination with uranium. Curr. Med. J. 40, 1–17.

Dyerberg, J., Bang, H.O., Hjorne, N., 1975. Fatty acid composition of the plasma lipids in Greenland Eskimos. Am. J. Clin. Nutr. 28, 958–966.

Fatima, S., Yusufi, A.N.K., Mahmood, R., 2004. Effect of cisplatin on renal brush border membrane enzymes and phosphate transport. Human Experiment. Toxicol. 23, 547–554.

Fatima, S., Arivarasu, N.A., Banday, A.A., Yusufi, A.N.K., Mahmood, R., 2005. Effect of potassium dichromate on renal brush border membrane enzymes and phosphate transport in rats. Human Experiment. Toxicol. 24, 631–638.

Feldmann, G., 1997. Liver apoptosis. J. Hepatol. 26, 1–11.

Gamoh, S., Hashimoto, M., Sugioka, K., Hossain, M.S., Hatta, N., Misawa, Y., Masumura, S., 1999. Chronic administration of docosahexaenoic acid improves reference memory –related learning ability in young rats. Neuroscience 93, 237–241.

Ger, J., Kao, H., Shih, T.S., Deng, J.F., 1996. Fatal toxic methemoglobinemia due to occupational exposure to methyl nitrite. Clin. Med. J. 57, S78.

Gilman, A.P., Villeneuve, D.C., Secours, V.E., Yagminas, A.P., Tracyl, B.L., Quinn, J.M., Valli, V.E., Yagminas, A.P., Tracy, B.L., Quinn, J.M., Valli, V.E., Wiles, R.J., Moss, M.A., 1998. Uranyl nitrate: 28-day and 91-day toxicity studies in the Sprague-Dawley rat. Toxicol. Sci. 41, 117–128.

Goldman, M., Yaari, A., Doshnitzki, Z., Cohen-Luria, R., Moran, A., 2006. Nephrotoxicity of uranyl acetate: effect on rat kidney brush border membrane vesicles. Archiv. Toxicol. 80, 387–393.

Gonzales, R., Romay, C., Borrego, A., Hernande, F., Zamor, Z., Rojas, E., 2005. Lipid peroxides and antioxidant enzymes in cispaltin chronic nephrotoxicity in rats. Mediators Inflam. 3, 139–143.
Gross, S.S., Wolin, M.S., 1995. Nitric oxide: Pathophysiological mechanisms. Ann. Rev. Physiol. 57, 737–769.
Guéguen, Y., Souidi, M., Baudelin, C., Dudoignon, N., Grison, S., Dublineau, I., Marquette, C., Voisin, P., Gourmelon, P., Aigueperse, J., 2006. Short-term hepatic effects of depleted uranium on xenobiotic and bile acid metabolizing cytochrome P450 enzymes in the rat. Archiv. Toxicol. 80, 187–195.
Haley, D.P., 1982. Morphologic changes in uranyl nitrate-induced acute renal failure in saline- and water-drinking rats. Laboratory Investig. 46, 196–208.
Haley, D.P., Bulger, R.E., Dobyan, D.C., 1982. The long term effects of uranyl nitrate on the structure and function of the rat kidney. Virchows Archiv. B 41, 181–192.
Hamid, J.W., 2012. Uranyl nitrate induce histological changes in the kidney. Int. J. Eng. Technol. 12, 9–13.
Hibbeln, J., 1998. Fish consumption and major depression. Lancet 351, 1213.
Hill, M.J., 1991. Nitrates and nitrites in food and water in relation to human disease. Nitrates Nitrites Food Water, 163–193.
Kacew, S., Bergeron, M.G., 1990. Pathogenic factors in aminoglycoside- induced nephrotoxicity. Toxicol. Letters 51, 241–259.
Kakar, P., Watson, T., Gregory, Y.H., 2008. New approaches to therapy with omega-3 fatty acids. Curr. Atheroscler. Rep. 10, 79–87.
Katakura, M., Hashimoto, M., Inoue, T., Al Mamun, A., Tanabe, Y., Iwamoto, R., Arita, M., Tsuchikura, S., Shido, O., 2014. Omega-3 fatty acids protect renal functions by increasing docosahexaenoic acid-derived metabolite levels in SHR.Cg-Lepr(cp)/NDmcr rats, a metabolic syndrome model. Molecules 19 (3), 3247–3263.
Kato, A., Hishida, A., Nakajima, T., 1994. Effects of oxygen free radical scavengers on uranium-induced acute renal failure in rats. Free Radical Biol. Med. 16, 855–859.
Kaur, M., Kaur, J., Ojha, S., Mahmood, A., 1996. Dietary fat effects on brush border membrane composition and enzyme activities in rat intestine. Ann. Nutr. Metabol. 40, 269–276.
Khan, N., Mukhtar, H., 2007. Tea polyphenols for health promotion. Life Sci. 81, 519–533.
Khan, S.A., Priyamvada, S., Khan, S., Khan, M.W., Yusufi, A.N.K., 2009a. Protective effect of green tea extract on gentamicin-induced nephrotoxicity and oxidative stress in kidney and other rat tissues. Pharmacol. Res. 59, 254–262.
Khan, S.A., Priyamvada, S., Khan, M.W., Khan, S., Farooq, N., Yusufi, A.N.K., 2009b. Studies on the protective effect of green tea against cisplatin induced nephrotoxicity. Pharmacol. Res. 60, 382–391.
Khan, S., Priyamvada, S., Khan, S.A., Khan, M.W., Farooq, N., Khan, F., Yusufi, A.N.K., 2009c. Effect of trichloroethylene (TCE) toxicity on the enzymes of carbohydrate metabolism, BBM, and oxidative stress in kidney and other rat tissues. Food Chem. Toxicol. 47, 1562–1568.
Khan, M.W., Priyamvada, S., Khan, S.A., Khan, S., Naqshbandi, A., Yusufi, A.N.K., 2012a. Protective effect of ω-3 polyunsaturated fatty acids (PUFA) on Sodium nitroprusside induced nephrotoxicity and oxidative damage in rat kidney. Human Experiment. Toxicol. 31, 1035–1049.
Khan, M.W., Priyamvada, S., Khan, S.A., Khan, S., Naqshbandi, A., Yusufi, A.N.K., 2012b. Protective effect of ω-3 polyunsaturated fatty acids (PUFA) on L-arginine induced nephrotoxicity and oxidative damage in rat kidney. Human Experiment. Toxicol. 10, 1022–1034.
Khan, M.W., Arivarasu, N.A., Priyamvada, S., Khan, S.A., Khan, S., Yusufi, A.N.K., 2013. Studies on the protective effect of polyunsaturated fatty acids on sodium nitrite induced nephrotoxicity in rats. J. Function. Foods 2, 956–967.
Khan, S.A., Priyamvada, S., Khan, S., Khan, M.W., Agharia, E.R., Yusufi, A.N.K., 2015. Protective effect of green tea extract on Gentamicin induced gastro- and hepatotoxicity in rats. Int. Res. J. Chem. 8, 52–72.
Khundmiri, S.J., Asghar, M., Banday, A.A., Khan, F., Salim, S., Levi, M., Yusufi, A.N.K., 2004. Effect of ischemia and reperfusion on enzymes of carbohydrate metabolism in rat kidney. J. Nephrol. 17, 377–383.
Khundmiri, S.J., Asghar, M., Banday, A.A., Khan, F., Salim, S., Levi, M., Yusufi, A.N.K., 2005. Effect of reperfusion on sodium dependent phosphate transport in renal brush border membranes. Biochim. Biophys. Acta 1716, 19–28.
Kramer, J.A., Pettit, S.D., Amin, R.P., et al.,2004. Overview of the application of transcription profiling using selected nephrotoxicants for toxicology assessment. Environment. Health Perspect. 112, 460–464.
Kromann, N., Green, A., 1980. Epidemiological studies in the Upernavik District, Greenland. Acta Med. Scandinavia 208, 401–406.
Kuhlmann, K., Burkhardt, G., Kohler, H., 1997. Insights into potential cellular mechanisms of cisplatin nephrotoxicity and their clinical application. Nephrol. Dialysis Transplant 12, 2478–2480.
Kurttio, P., Auvinem, A., Salonem, L., Saha, H., Pekkanem, J., Makelainem, I., Vaisanen, S.B., Pentilla, I.M., Komulainen, H., 2002. Renal effects of uranium in drinking water. Environment. Health Perspect. 110, 337–342.
Lang, H., Liu, C., 1997. Apoptosis and hair cell degeneration in the vestibular sensory epithelia of the guinea pig following gentamicin insult. Hear Res. 111, 177–184.
Larsson, S., Kulin, M., Ingelman-Sundberg, M., Wolk, A., 2004. Dietary long chain n-3 fatty acids for the prevention of cancer. Am. Soc. Clin. Nutr. 79, 935–945.
Laurent, G., Kishore, B.K., Tulkens, P.M., 1990. Aminoglycoside induced renal phospholipidosis and nephrotoxicity. Biochem. Pharmacol. 40, 2383–2392.
Leaf, A., 2008. Historical overview of n-3 fatty acids and coronary heart disease. Am. J. Clin. Nutr. 87, 1978S–1980S.
Leibbrandt, M.E.I., Grushenka, H.I.W., Metz, A.L., Ozobia, A.A., Haskins, J.R., 1995. Critical subcellular targets of cisplatin and related platinum analogs in rat renal proximal tubule cells. Kidney Int. 48, 761–770.
Lin, W., Xue, H., Liu, S., He, Y., Fu, J., Zhou, Z., 1998. Genotoxicity of nitric oxide produced from sodium nitroprusside. Mutation Res. 413, 121–127.
Lundberg, J.O., Govoni, M., 2004. Inorganic nitrate is a possible source for systemic generation of nitric oxide. Free Radical Biol. Med. 37, 395–400.
Lundberg, J.O., Weitzberg, E., Gladwin, M.T., 2008. The nitrate-nitrite-nitric oxide pathway in physiology and therapeutics. Nature 7, 156–167.
Magee, P.H., Barnes, J.M., 1956. The production of malignant primary hepatic tumors in the rat by feeding dimethylnitrosamine. Br. J. Cancer 10, 114–122.
Mahmood, I., Waters, D.H., 1994. A comparative study of uranyl nitrate and cisplatin-induced renal failure in rat. Eur. J. Drug Metabol. Pharmacokinet. 19, 327–336.

Maletic, S.D., Dragicevic-Djokovic, L.J.M., Zikic, R.V., Stajn, A.S., Milenkovic, P., Kostic, M.M., 2000. Effects of nitric oxide donors on energy metabolism of rat erythrocytes, Journal of Environmental Pathology. Toxicol. Oncol. 19, 383–390.

Markman, M., 2003. Toxicities of the platinum antineoplastic agents. Experiment. Opin. Drug Safety 2, 597–607.

Martinez, A.B., Mandalunis, P.M., Bozal, C.B., Cabrini, R.L., Ubios, A.M., 2003. Renal function in mice poisoned with oral uranium and treated with ethane-1-hydroxy-1, 1-bisphosphonate (EHBP). Health Phys. 85, 343–347.

McDonald-Taylor, C.K., Singh, A., Gilman, A., 1997. Uranyl nitrate-induced proximal tubule alterations in rabbits: a quantitative analysis. Toxicol. Pathol. 25, 381–389.

McKeage, M.J., 1995. Comparative adverse effect profiles of platinum drugs. Drug Safety 13, 228–244.

Mingeot-Leclercq, M., Tulkens, P.M., 1999a. Aminoglycoside nephrotoxicity. Antimicrobial Agents Chemother. 43, 1003–1101.

Mingeot-Leclercq, M., Tulkens, P.M., 1999b. Aminoglycosides: activity and resistance. Antimicrob. Agents Chemother. 43, 727–737.

Montori, V.M., Wollan, P.C., Farmer, A., Dinneen, S.F., 2000. Fish oil supplementation in type 2 diabetes. Diabetes Care 23, 1407–1415.

Mostad, I.L., Bjerve, K.S., Bjorgass, M.R., Lydersen, S., Grill, V., 2006. Effects of n-3 fatty acids in subjects with type 2 diabetes: reduction of insulin sensitivity and time dependent alteration from carbohydrate to fat metabolism. Am. J. Clin. Nutr. 84, 540–550.

Nagai, J., Takano, M., 2004. Molecular aspects of renal handling of aminoglycosides and strategies for preventing nephrotoxicity. Drug Metabol. Pharmacokinet. 19, 159–170.

Naqshbandi, A., Khan, M.W., Rizwan, S., Rehman, S.U., Khan, F., 2012. Studies on the protective effect of dietary fish oil on cisplatin induced nephrotoxicity in rats. Food Chem. Toxicol. 50, 265–273.

Neuringer, M., 2000. Infant vision and retinal function in studies of dietary long-chain polyunsaturated fatty acids: methods, results, and implications. Am. J. Clin. Nutr. 71, 256S–267S.

Pedraza-Chaverri, J., Maldonado, P.D., Medina-Campos, O.N., Olivares-Corichi, I.M., Grandos-Silvestre, M., Hernandez-Pando, R., Ibarra-Rubio, M.E., 2000. Garlic ameliorates gentamicin nephrotoxicity: relation to antioxidants. Free Radical Biol. Med. 29, 602–611.

Pedraza-Chaverrí, J., González-Orozco, A.E., Maldonado, P.D., Barrera, D., Medina-Campos, O.N., Hernández-Pando, R., 2003. Diallyl disulfide ameliorates gentamicin-induced oxidative stress and nephropathy in rats. Eur. J. Pharmacol. 473, 71–78.

Periyakaruppan, A., Kumar, F., Sarkar, S., Sharma, C.S., Ramesh, G.T., 2007. Uranium induces oxidative stress in lung epithelial cells. Archiv. Toxicol. 81, 389–395.

Priyamvada, S., Priyadarshini, M., Arivarasu, N.A., Farooq, N., Khan, S., Khan, S.A., Khan, M.W., Yusufi, A.N.K., 2008. Studies on the protective effect of dietary fish oil on gentamicin-induced nephrotoxicity and oxidative damage in rat kidney. Prostagland. Leukotr. Essent. Fatty Acid. 78, 369–381.

Priyamvada, S., Khan, S.A., Khan, M.W., Khan, S., Farooq, N., Yusufi, A.N.K., 2010. Studies on the protective effect of dietary fish oil on uranyl nitrate-induced nephrotoxicity and oxidative damage in rat kidney. Prostagland. Leukotr. Essent. Fatty Acid. 82, 35–44.

Sampson, J.B., Ye, Y., Rosen, H., Beckman, J.S., 1998. Myeloperoxidase and horseradish catalyze tyrosine nitration in proteins from nitrite and hydrogen peroxide. Archiv. Biochem. Biophys. 356, 207–213.

Sanchez, D.Z., Belles, M., Albina, M.L., Sirvent, J.J., Domingo, J.L., 2001. Nephrotoxicity of simultaneous exposure to mercury and uranium in comparison to individual effects of these metals in rats. Biol. Trace Element Res. 84, 139–154.

Santos, N.A., Catao, C.S., Martins, N.M., Curti, C., Bianchi, M.L., Santos, A.C., 2007. Cisplatin induced nephrotoxicity is associated with oxidative stress, redox state unbalance, impairment of energetic metabolism and apoptosis in rat kidney mitochondria. Archiv. Toxicol. 81, 495–504.

Shahid, S., Rizwan, S., Khan, M.W., Khan, S.A., Naqshbandi, A., Yusufi, A.N.K., 2014. Studies on the effect of sodium arsenate on the enzymes of carbohydrate metabolism, brush border membrane, and oxidative stressing the rat kidney. Environment. Toxicol. Pharmacol. 37, 592–599.

Siddiqui, R.A., Jenski, L.J., Harvey, K.A., Wiesehan, J.D., Stillwell, W., Zaloga, G.P., 2003. Cell-cycle arrest in Jurkat Leukaemic cells: a possible role for docosahexaenoic acid. Biochem. J. 371, 621–629.

Simmons, Jr., C.F., Boqusky, R.T., Humes, H.D., 1980. Inhibitory effect of GM on renal mitochondrial oxidative phosphorylation. J. Pharmacol. Experiment. Therapeutics 214, 709–715.

Simopoulos, A.P., 1991. Omega-3 fatty acids in health and disease and in growth and development. Am. J. Clin. Nutr. 54, 438–463.

Simopoulos, A.P., 2000. Human requirement for n-3 polyunsaturated fatty acids. Poultry Sci. 79, 961–970.

Small, M.F., 2002. The happy fat. New Scientist 24, 34–37, August.

Spencer, J.M., Whiteman, M., Jenner, A., Halliwell, B., 2000. Nitrite-induced deamination and hypochlorite-induced oxidation of DNA in intact human respiratory tract epithelial cells. Free Radic. Biol. Med. 28 (7), 1039–1050.

Sun, J., Aoki, K., Wang, W., Guo, A., Misumi, J., 2006. Sodium nitrite-induced cytotoxicity in cultured human gastric epithelial cells. Toxicol. In Vitro 20, 1133–1138.

Sundin, D.P., Sandoval, R., Molitoris, B.A., 2001. Gentamicin inhibits renal protein and phospholipid metabolism in rats: implications involving intracellular trafficking. J. Am. Soc. Nephrol. 12, 114–123.

Taguchi, T., Nazneen, A., Abid, M.R., Razzaque, M.S., 2005. Cisplatin-associated nephrotoxicity and pathological events. Contribution Nephrol. 148, 107–121.

Tannenbaum, S.R., Frett, D., Young, V.R., Land, P.D., Bruce, W.R., 1978. Nitrite and nitrate are formed by endogenous synthesis in the human intestine. Science 200, 1487–1489.

Taulan, M., Paquet, F., Maubert, C., Delissen, O., Demaille, J., Romey, M.C., 2004. Renal toxicogenomic response to chronic uranyl nitrate insult in mice. Environ. Health Perspect. 112, 1628–1635.

Thakkar, R.R., Wang, O.L., Zerouga, M., Stillwell, W., Haq, A., Kissling, R., et al.,2000. Docosahexaenoic acid reverses cyclosporin-A induced changes in membrane structure and function. Biochim. Biophys. Acta 1474, 183–195.

Townsend, D.M., Deng, M., Zhang, L., Lapus, M.G., Hanigan, M.H., 2003. Metabolism of cisplatin to a nephrotoxin in proximal tubule cells. J. Am. Soc. Nephrol. 14, 1–10.

Walker, P.D., Barri, Y., Shah, S.V., 1999. Oxidant mechanisms on gentamicin nephrotoxicity. Renal Failure 21, 433–442.

Ward, J.M., Fauvie, K.A., 1976. The Nephrotoxic Effects of Cis-Diamminedichloroplatinum II in Male F344 rats. Toxicol. Appl. Pharmacol. 38, 535–547.

Watkins, B.A., Hannon, K., Ferruzzi, M., Li, Y., 2007. Dietary PUFA and flavonoids as deterrents for environmental pollutants. J. Nutr. Biochem. 18, 196–205.

Weiner, M.W., Jacobs, C., 1983. Mechanism of cisplatin nephrotoxicity. Federation Proc. 42, 2974–2978.

Xi, S., Chen, L.H., 2000. Effects of dietary fish oil on tissue glutathione and antioxidant defense enzymes in mice with murine AIDS. Nutr. Res. 20, 1287–1299.

Yusufi, A.N.K., Siddiqi, M., 1974. studies on the hypolipidemic and hypocholesterolemic effect of 3-hydroxy-3-methylglutaric acid in rabbits. Atherosclerosis 20, 517–526.

Yusufi, A.N.K., Murayama, N., Gapstur, S.M., Szczepanska-Konkel, M., Dousa, T.P., 1994. Differential properties of brush border membrane vesicles from early and late proximal tubules of rat kidney. Biochim. Biophys. Acta 1191, 117–132.

Yusufi, A.N.K., Cheng, J., Thompson, M.A., Walker, H.J., Gray, C.E., Warner, G.M., Grande, J.P., 2003. Differential effects of low-dose docosahexaenoic acid and eicosapentaenoic acid on the regulation of mitogenic signaling pathways in mesangial cells. J. Laboratory Clin. Med. 141, 318–329.

Zamaria, N., 2004. Alteration of polyunsaturated fatty acid status and metabolism in health and disease. Reproductive Nutr. Dev. 44, 273–282.

Zhang, J.G., Lindup, W.E., 1993. Role of mitochondria in cisplatin-induced oxidative damage exhibited by rat renal cortical slices. Biochem. Pharmacol. 45, 2215–2222.

PART IV

UNIQUE SOURCES

CHAPTER

29

Seafood Proteins and Human Health

R. Tahergorabi*, J. Jaczynski**

*Department of Family and Consumer Sciences, North Carolina Agricultural and Technical State University, Greensboro, North Carolina, United States; **Division of Animal and Nutritional Sciences, West Virginia University, Morgantown, West Virginia, United States

INTRODUCTION

Unlike carbohydrate and fat, the human body does not generally store protein in stores other than muscle mass and does not preferentially use it as a source of energy. Dietary protein of adequate quality must be provided to humans as a part of balanced nutrient intake. Proteins from different dietary sources vary in quality as well as quantity. Protein consists of building blocks called amino acids (AAs), which are linked together in different patterns to form specific proteins with different functional activities and structural characteristics, thus protein serves different physiological roles in humans. A high quality protein, also known as a complete protein, contains all of the nine essential amino acids (EAAs) in adequate quantity to support human health. A low quality or incomplete protein, on the other hand, is either missing one or more of the EAAs or they are present in insufficient quantity. Complete proteins typically come from animal sources such as beef, poultry, fish, eggs, dairy, etc., whereas incomplete proteins generally include plant sources such as legumes, grains, nuts, and vegetables. Not only do proteins provide structure to the human body by being the main component of organs and tissues, but proteins also have many physiologically important activities in the body such as enzymatic and hormonal. Proteins also function as transport biomolecules such as hemoglobin in the blood. Inadequate protein or AA intake causes diminished content of protein in cells and organs, which in turn leads to deterioration in the capacity of cells to carry out their normal functions. In extreme cases, this may lead to increased morbidity and eventually death.

Seafood is the only dietary source of animal protein that is still provided in significant amounts through capture of wild aquatic species; whereas seafood aquaculture is a counterpart for farming of terrestrial animals for food. Seafood is an excellent source of high quality protein that contains sufficient amounts of EAAs required to support human health. Not only are all EAAs provided in sufficient quantity, but seafood protein is also easily digestible and absorbable, making it highly bioavailable (Sánchez-Alonso et al., 2007). Therefore, seafood protein has a high biological value (Venugopal, 2009; Tou et al., 2007). The high nutritional quality and overall health benefits of seafood protein is very important for consumers and their acceptability of seafood products (Schwarz et al., 1998). For this reason, dietary recommendations to the public from multiple, reputable health authorities indicate that seafood should be an integral component of a healthy diet, particularly as it can replace other protein-rich food products that tend to be high in saturated fat and dietary cholesterol (Venugopal, 2009).

SEAFOOD PROTEIN

Following water, protein is the second most prevalent component of seafood muscle tissue which is the source of dietary seafood protein. The protein content of finfish muscle tissue is typically 17–22%. Generally, marine fish have slightly higher protein and lower moisture content than freshwater fish. The protein content in shellfish (crustaceans and mollusks) varies among species, but typically is as follows: shrimp 17–22%, scallop 12–20%, squid 15–18%, crab 18–22%, lobster 16–26%, krill 12–15%, and mussel and oyster 6–18% (USDA Agricultural Research Service National Nutrient Database, 2015; Tou et al., 2007).

Fish and Fish Oil in Health and Disease Prevention. http://dx.doi.org/10.1016/B978-0-12-802844-5.00029-4

Two muscle types are present in seafood. They can be visually differentiated as striated muscle characterized by transverse stripes and smooth muscle that lacks the striation, and thus, has a smooth appearance. Striated muscle is the main component in finfish muscle, while smooth muscle is typical of molluscan muscle tissue. Finfish muscle is divided further into white and dark muscle. The dark muscle lies alongside the fish body and under the skin. The white muscle of finfish is the main source of seafood protein in human diet. White muscle protein can be further classified into three major groups according to their water solubility characteristics, that is, myofibrillar, sarcoplasmic, and stroma proteins which account for connective tissue including collagen (Connell, 1970a,b).

The content of myofibrillar proteins in fish is typically 65–75% of total muscle protein, while sarcoplasmic proteins (water soluble proteins including enzymes and other regulatory proteins) are 20–35%. Myosin is the major component of myofibrillar proteins and it does not dissolve in water under typical physiological conditions. Myosin constitutes 50–58% of fish myofibrillar proteins. Even though there is a slight difference in the AA composition between various species, myosin found in vertebrates such as rabbit, chicken, cod, and tilapia are considered generally similar (Skaara and Regenstein, 1990; Konasu and Yamaguchi, 1982). As compared with terrestrial food animals, fish muscle contains much less of stroma proteins (connective tissue including collagen), only about 3%, except in sharks, rays, and skates, which may contain up to 10% of stroma proteins. Stroma proteins are highly insoluble in water.

All proteins, including seafood muscle proteins, are chains of AAs bonded together into a long and structurally complex biomolecule. There are about 20 naturally occurring AAs and 9 of them are EAAs. The EAAs are particularly important in human nutrition because humans do not have a physiological capability (ie, biochemical pathway) to synthesize them de novo. Therefore, the only way to provide EAAs to humans is through adequate dietary intake. The EAAs are: histidine, phenylalanine, valine, threonine, tryptophan, leucine, isoleucine, methionine, and lysine. All nine EAAs are required for efficient protein synthesis in humans. If the diet is insufficient in any EAA, the overall rate of protein synthesis will be limited by the least abundant EAA. The EAA that limits protein synthesis; that is, does not allow protein synthesis to proceed at its full speed in humans is called a limiting EAA. Two of the nine EAAs, lysine and methionine, are often limiting EAAs in food systems. Lysine and methionine are typically found in high concentrations in seafood proteins (Taskaya et al., 2009; Chen et al., 2007). This is in contrast to, for example, plant-derived proteins that often contain lower amounts of these two limiting EAAs. In addition, shrimp, lobster, crab, squid, and other shellfish generally contain larger amounts of arginine, glutamic acid, glycine, and alanine than finfish (Konasu and Yamaguchi, 1982).

Unlike carbohydrate and lipid, protein is the only nutrient that provides nitrogen. However, animals including seafood, normally have low quantities of nitrogen-containing compounds in their muscle that are not proteins. They are collectively called nonprotein nitrogen compounds. These compounds present in seafood muscle tissue include free AAs, small peptides, trimethylamine oxide (TMAO), trimethylamine (TMA), creatine, creatinine, and nucleotides. TMAO is important in aquatic animals because it is an osmoprotectant responsible for maintaining their fluid volume and balance at a cellular level in an aquatic environment. This is mainly why the nonprotein nitrogen content of seafood muscle is normally higher than that of terrestrial animals. Demersal fish generally contain larger quantities of TMAO than pelagic fish, while TMAO content in mollusks is low and levels are relatively insignificant in freshwater fish species; although some species, such as Nile perch, contain a greater amount of TMAO. Following fish death TMAO degrades to TMA under unfavorable storage condition, which is responsible for the typical "fishy" odor.

NUTRITIONAL VALUE OF SEAFOOD PROTEINS IN HUMAN HEALTH

The nutritional value of seafood muscle proteins is relatively high because of their favorable EAA content (Connell, 1970a,b). Although marine fish tend to have slightly higher protein content, there are no significant differences in the AA composition of freshwater and marine fish. However, certain marine fish such as mackerel and tuna may be exceptionally rich in the EAA, histidine. As compared with red meat, fish proteins are considered nutritionally equivalent or slightly superior. Fish proteins are easily broken down in human gastrointestinal tract by proteolytic (ie, protein digesting) enzymes, resulting in their digestibility exceeding 90%. The in vivo digestibility of proteins from raw finfish and shellfish meat is in the range of 90–98% and 85%, respectively. The enhanced digestibility of seafood as compared to dietary protein derived from terrestrial animals is largely due to the absence of strong collagenous fibers and tendons as well as lower content of stroma proteins (mainly connective tissue) in seafood, which are common in terrestrial animals.

Protein efficiency ratio (PER) is often used in human nutrition as an index of protein quality which is defined as body weight gained per protein weight consumed (Gigliotti et al., 2008). Since the human body utilizes protein from different sources with different efficiency in terms of incorporating the protein into the body, the PER makes it easy to compare the quality of protein from different dietary sources. The PER of fish muscle protein is slightly above that of casein, the major milk protein. Casein is commonly used in human nutrition for comparison purposes. The net protein utilization (NPU) reflects the ratio of AAs used to synthesize protein in the human body to AAs consumed (Gigliotti et al., 2008). Therefore, NPU is a good indicator of EAAs content in a protein source. The NPU for fish muscle protein is 83 as compared with 80 and 100 for red meat and egg proteins, respectively (Skaara and Regenstein, 1990). Egg protein is considered a standard for protein nutritional quality and it is often used for comparison purposes. Friedman (1996) provided a comprehensive comparison of various indices of nutritional quality for dietary proteins from different sources, including seafood.

Fish muscle proteins have been used in several different commercial applications likely due to their good technological functionalities and nutritional value. As an example of a commercial application, fish protein concentrates and isolates or their hydrolyzates have been used as a protein supplement in food systems. Specifically, the relatively low nutritional value of cereal proteins can be increased when combined with fish protein concentrates and isolates. A 3% addition of fish protein concentrate to wheat flour with protein content of 10.4% increased its protein content, resulting in concurrent increase of NPU from 50 to 67 (Frokjaer, 1994). Another example is a commercial collagen hydrolysate from fish, *Peptan F*. It has been found to enhance protein quality and flavor characteristics of beverages (Pszczola, 2004).

The development of successful new food applications is typically a result of health benefits associated with those food applications. The potential health benefits are usually determined in animal studies. One such example related to fish protein was the animal feeding study conducted by Wergedah et al. (2004). This study suggested that fish protein has cardio-protective benefits. Obese zucker rats were subjected to a dietary treatment with fish protein, resulting in improved markers for cardiovascular health including reduced plasma cholesterol level, increased high density lipoprotein (HDL) content, and favorably altered fatty acid composition in plasma, liver, and triglycerol-rich lipoproteins.

The later section discusses some of the health effects of seafood protein in diet-related chronic human diseases. However, vast majority of published studies relate the health benefits of seafood consumption to its fatty acid content, while the literature about the effect of seafood protein on human health is scarce.

Seafood Protein and Cardiovascular Health

Cardiovascular disease (CVD) has continually been the number one cause of death in the United States since 1919 (American Heart Association, 2009). Therefore, addressing this significant public health issue, particularly diet-driven CVD, with an appropriate dietary intervention is a pressing need. A recent metaanalyses indicated that frequent dietary intake of fish is associated with reduced risk of coronary death and ischemic stroke (He et al., 2004a, 2004b). Similarly, Hu et al. (1999) found that replacing red meat with fish in human diet is associated with a significantly decreased risk of coronary heart disease (CHD). Compared with red meat, white meat from fish contains similar amounts of protein but substantially greater concentrations of n–3 polyunsaturated fatty acids (n–3 PUFAs) as well as reduced concentrations of saturated fat and cholesterol. Although cardiovascular benefits associated with fish consumption are most likely attributable to n–3 PUFAs, other nutrients, including protein have beneficial effects. Traditionally, studies aimed at health benefits associated with seafood consumption have been focused on n–3 PUFAs. However, a more holistic research approach is recommended. Seafood is a complex mixture of various nutrients, including protein and n–3 PUFAs. These nutrients likely have complex interactions in humans when ingested in whole foods such as seafood. This could be a basis for human health benefits beyond those associated only with n–3 PUFAs that have been well-documented in scientific literature.

Seafood Protein and Obesity

Among macronutrients, protein has a stronger effect on satiety and satiation than equivalent quantities of energy from carbohydrate or fat (Benelam, 2009). Weight loss diets containing higher protein levels seem to be more effective in reducing appetite; and therefore, result in diminished ad libitum food intake compared to diets with low protein content (Benelam, 2009). Fish is a protein-rich food with a relatively low energy density, particularly white fish when compared to oil-rich fish. Therefore, as a part of a balanced diet, fish contributes to increased satiety and satiation. A small number of studies have investigated the satiating effects of fish protein compared with protein derived from other animals. One crossover study with 23 normal weight young men (20–32 years) found that a protein-rich (40% of energy) fish-based lunch meal compared with a beef-based lunch meal led to a significantly decreased energy intake (2765 vs 3080 kJ; $p < 0.01$; Borzoei et al., 2006). Both meals were isocaloric (ie, provided the same amount of food energy) and in order to reduce dietary bias they were also similar in taste and appearance. A very small crossover study with six normal-weight young men (17–25 years) investigated the effects of protein on satiety and post-prandial response. The dietary treatments were low in fat (<2%) and consisted of lean steak, chicken breast with skin removed, and fish. The authors found that satiety was significantly greater after the fish meal compared with the steak or chicken counterparts. The satiety produced by the fish meal also declined more slowly than that of the other two meals. The greater effect of the fish meal on satiety was correlated with two putative satiety signals, serotoninergic activity due to differences in the postprandial ratio of tryptophan to large neutral AAs and longer digestibility as determined by longer time to reach peak concentration of plasma AAs after the fish meal (Uhe et al., 1992).

In summary, dietary patterns that include seafood as a part of balanced diet have been associated with a lower risk of over weight and obesity. However, prospective studies do not suggest that seafood intake per se has a significant or directly beneficial effect on waist circumference.

Seafood Protein and Colorectal Cancer

Data from prospective cohort studies suggest there may be protection associated with seafood consumption against colorectal cancer (CRC), although the evidence is too inconsistent to draw any firm conclusions at this point (Geelen et al., 2007). Data from case–control studies show a stronger correlation, but these studies are typically heterogeneous, which has been argued as less appropriate to study effects of diet on cancer (Wu et al., 2012). It is possible that the protective effects observed may be due to other dietary factors such as lower intake of red meat in people whose diet is abundant in seafood.

SEAFOOD PROCESSING BY-PRODUCTS AS A SOURCE OF MUSCLE PROTEINS

Seafood processing by-products (frames, heads, viscera, etc.) generally account for 60%–70% of the total fish weight after commercial filleting. The by-products contain highly nutritious seafood muscle proteins and oil rich in n-3 PUFAs that are of comparable quality to the proteins and oil in the primary products such as fish fillets at the time of processing. The proteins and oil can be recovered from the by-products through a relatively novel processing technology called isoelectric solubilization/precipitation (ISP) (Gehring et al., 2011). The ISP processing relies on the isoelectric point (pI) of muscle proteins. The pI of a protein is a pH at which the net (ie, overall) electrostatic charge of the protein is zero. The pI is a protein fundamental property and different proteins have different pI. When a protein is at its pI, the protein is least water soluble or it simply precipitates. The pI of seafood muscle proteins is generally at pH of 5.50. The ISP-recovered protein isolates may subsequently be used in the development of human food products and dietary supplements.

The main component of seafood muscle, myofibrillar proteins tend to aggregate in solutions due to weak intermolecular bonds (Undeland et al., 2003). Depending on the solution acidity/alkalinity, however, the charge normally present on protein residues shifts, resulting in protein water solubility or insolubility (Fig. 29.1). The charge shift can be considered as an "on" or "off" switch yielding conditions that are or are not favorable for protein solubility, respectively.

In general, there are five steps in recovering proteins and lipids from seafood processing by-products with ISP (Fig. 29.2). The first step is to homogenize by-products in water at a 1:6 ratio (by-products:water, wt/wt) in order to provide a reaction medium and increase the available surface area for the subsequent protein solubilization reaction.

In the second step, muscle proteins are dissolved under either acidic or alkaline conditions. As the pH moves further away from the pI, fish muscle proteins assume a more negative or positive surface charge for alkaline or acidic conditions, respectively (Fig. 29.1). This charge shift results in protein–protein electrostatic repulsion, which weakens the protein–protein hydrophobic interactions with a simultaneous increase of protein–water electrostatic interactions. Ultimately, these changes lead to protein solubility in water. When the proteins begin interacting with water, a drastic increase of viscosity occurs, but the viscosity drops as soon as proteins are dissolved. Solubilization of muscle proteins is ascribed to protonation of aspartyl and glutamyl (p*Ka* = 3.8 and 4.2, respectively) residues at acidic pH and deprotonation of lysyl, tyrosyl, and cysteinyl (p*Ka* = 9.5–10.5, 9.1–10.8, and 9.1–10.8, respectively) residues

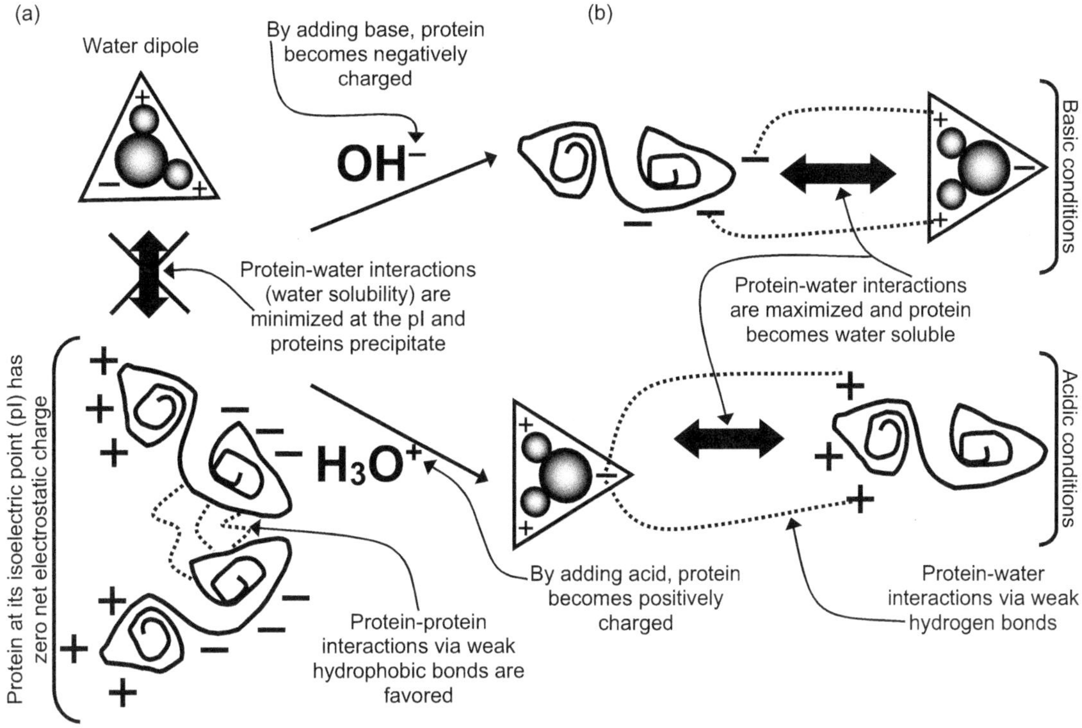

FIGURE 29.1 A protein at its isoelectric point (pI) has a zero net electrostatic charge. (a) At its pI, protein-water interactions are at its minimum, while protein-protein interactions via weak hydrophobic bonds are at its maximum, causing protein precipitation. (b) Protein-water interactions prevail under acidic or basic conditions far from the pI, resulting in protein solubility in water. *Source: Adapted from Gehring et al. (2011).*

at alkaline pH. The accumulation of a net positive or negative charge causes electrostatic repulsion and an increased hydrodynamic volume due to expansion and swelling (Undeland et al., 2003).

While the muscle proteins are dissolved in water, the third step, separation, is applied. Typically, centrifugation separates the solution for light, medium, and heavy fractions containing fish oil, dissolved muscle proteins, and impurities (bones, scale, skin, insoluble proteins, etc.), respectively. While the hydrophobic triglycerides are fairly easy to separate from the solution, the membrane phospholipids are relatively persistent because they are amphiphilic. Greater than 50% of the membrane phospholipids are retained with the dissolved proteins after the third step. Although membrane phospholipids are present in smaller amounts in the seafood muscle than triglycerides, the membrane phospholipids contribute more to rancidity. Therefore, it is desirable to remove as much lipid as possible during the separation step. The third step results in separation of crude seafood oil that is rich in n–3 PUFAs which can be further processed for numerous food and nonfood applications. The heavy fraction is rich in minerals such as Ca, Mg, and P; and therefore, can be a main ingredient in the development of animal feeds and value-added pet foods (Chen et al., 2007).

The medium fraction, containing dissolved seafood muscle proteins is recovered and subjected to the second pH adjustment in the fourth step. The pH is adjusted to the average pI of the seafood muscle proteins (pH 5.50). At pH 5.50, muscle proteins precipitate due to increased protein–protein hydrophobic interactions and decreased protein–water interactions as well as decreased protein–protein electrostatic repulsion. Similar to the first pH adjustment in the second step, as the proteins gradually stop interacting with water, the viscosity increases significantly. This viscosity issue can be overcome by continuous maintenance of the pH at 5.50 (Torres et al., 2007). In the fifth step, the precipitated seafood muscle proteins are separated from the process water, typically by centrifugation. The process water can be recycled in the first step if a continuous system is used (Torres et al., 2007).

The muscle proteins retain their gel-forming ability; and therefore, can be used as a functional and major ingredient in human food products such as surimi seafood (commonly referred to as crab-flavored seafood). Processors should keep in mind that similar to surimi and other muscle foods products, ISP protein isolates should include cryoprotectants for frozen storage in order to preserve protein functionality. ISP protein with high functionality has been isolated from various aquatic species at bench-top and pilot-plant levels in batch systems (Undeland et al., 2003; Mireles DeWitt et al., 2007). Chen et al. (2007) proposed and tested an ISP system working in a continuous mode of operation to isolate functional protein from krill, whole fish, and seafood processing by-products.

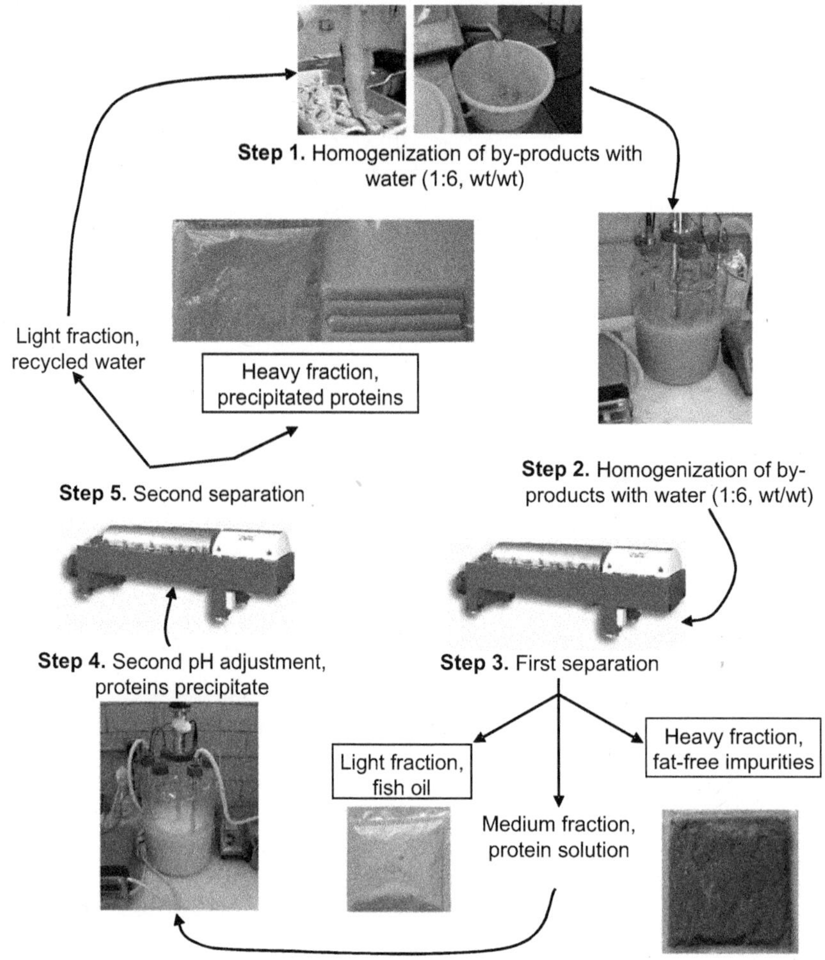

FIGURE 29.2 **Diagram of the isoelectric solubilization/precipitation technology with concurrent oil separation proposed for fish processing by-products.** *Source: Adapted from Tahergorabi et al. (2011).*

Amino Acid Profile of ISP-Recovered Proteins and their Health Benefits

Nutritional quality of a novel protein source is typically based on the amount of EAAs present in that protein source. As shown in Table 29.1, generally alkaline conditions during ISP of seafood by-products resulted in a greater EAA concentration than acidic conditions (Chen et al., 2007; Taskaya et al., 2009). EAAs in the ISP protein were also compared to the initial material prior to ISP processing, as well as generally recognized standards for protein nutritional quality such as whole egg and the values recommended by FAO/WHO/UNU for adults and infants (Connell, 1970b). When protein is subjected to extreme pH conditions, it undergoes hydrolysis releasing AAs due to pH-induced proteolysis. The differences in AA composition resulting from different pH conditions during ISP was probably due to different levels of proteolysis occurring at alkaline and acidic conditions. Table 29.1 suggests that less proteolysis occurred at alkaline pH. The hydrophilic AAs such as such as lysine and threonine released due to proteolysis are water soluble. This is most likely why the hydrophilic AAs were retained to a lesser degree in the ISP protein isolated at acidic conditions, resulting in slightly higher nutritional quality of the ISP protein isolate from alkaline conditions.

In human nutrition, lysine is recognized as a limiting EAA. Therefore, lysine content in a protein source is of critical importance. Chen et al. (2007, 2009) and Taskaya et al. (2009) demonstrated that the ISP protein isolated from seafood by-products had a similar or higher content of lysine than whole egg depending on which seafood species was processed with ISP. The ISP protein isolated from seafood has a biological value (BV) that is higher than that of soybean protein concentrate and comparable to that of milk protein, casein (Gigliotti et al., 2008). In summary, the ISP protein isolated from aquatic resourced have a higher, similar, and lower nutritional quality when compared to soybean, milk, and egg proteins; respectively.

Gigliotti et al. (2008) determined several key parameters of protein nutritional quality for krill protein concentrate (KPC) isolated with ISP and subsequently compared them to casein. As shown in Table 29.2, KPC compares favorably

TABLE 29.1 Essential Amino Acid (EAA) Content (mg/g) in Fish Processing By-products and in the Protein Recovered from Fish Processing By-products by Solubilization at Different pH and Precipitation at pH = 5.5 as Compared to the Reference Protein of Whole Egg and the Recommended Values for Adults and Infants

Essential amino acids	Protein recovered from fish processing by-products at different treatments (pH value; mg/g protein)						Fish processing by-products (mg/g protein)	Whole egg (mg/g protein)	FAO/WHO/ UNU 1985 Adults (infants) (mg/g protein)
	2.0	2.5	3.0	12.0	12.5	13.0			
Isoleucine	38.91 ± 0.50b	36.31 ± 0.20c	39.52 ± 0.75b	42.11 ± 0.36a	41.49 ± 0.43a	42.81 ± 0.28a	18.27 ± 0.64d	63	13 (46)
Leucine	65.51 ± 0.08c	60.47 ± 0.20d	65.89 ± 0.31c	69.50 ± 0.00b	69.08 ± 0.32b	71.02 ± 0.37a	30.57 ± 0.86e	88	19 (93)
Lysine	73.61 ± 0.40c	66.96 ± 0.23d	73.38 ± 0.35c	76.34 ± 0.24b	76.28 ± 0.39b	78.35 ± 0.42a	35.13 ± 0.95e	70	16 (66)
Methionine	26.30 ± 0.50a	22.40 ± 0.15b	25.53 ± 0.04a	26.21 ± 0.54a	26.14 ± 0.67a	26.21 ± 0.37a	14.27 ± 0.23c	56[a]	17 (42)[a]
Phenylalanine	33.94 ± 0.35d	30.96 ± 0.48e	34.17 ± 0.13cd	35.48 ± 0.43b	35.06 ± 0.12bc	36.79 ± 0.07a	16.27 ± 0.44f	98[b]	19 (72)[b]
Threonine	36.85 ± 0.78c	34.25 ± 0.33d	36.77 ± 0.60c	38.38 ± 0.84bc	39.00 ± 0.36ab	40.59 ± 0.18a	18.33 ± 0.26e	49	9 (43)
Tryptophan	10.24 ± 0.20c	9.25 ± 0.38d	9.02 ± 0.15d	11.00 ± 0.21ab	10.65 ± 0.28bc	11.55 ± 0.14a	5.27 ± 0.22e	16	5 (17)
Valine	46.48 ± 0.84c	42.88 ± 0.26d	47.01 ± 0.83c	49.93 ± 0.35ab	48.87 ± 0.45b	50.83 ± 0.24a	22.23 ± 0.68e	72	13 (55)
Histidine	21.25 ± 0.20c	19.03 ± 0.13d	21.02 ± 0.15c	22.61 ± 0.12b	22.47 ± 0.18b	23.44 ± 0.12a	11.73 ± 0.23e	24	16 (26)

Data are presented as mean values ± standard error of means. Values shown with different letters are significantly different within rows at $p < 0.05$.

[a] *Methionine + Cysteine.*

[b] *Phenylalanine + Tyrosine.*

Adapted from Chen et al. (2007).

TABLE 29.2 Nutritional Quality of Krill Protein Concentrate (KPC) Isolated with ISP at Alkaline Conditions

Protein quality measurement	Casein	KPC
Digestibility (%)	93.3 ± 2.0	93.2 ± 1.0
PDCAAS	1	1
PER (g body wt/g protein)	1.57 ± 0.05	1.44 ± 0.15
Final body weight (g)	235.4 ± 5.8	241.8 ± 3.4
Total body weight gain (g/4 weeks)	73.3 ± 3.0	80.0 ± 3.5
Total food intake (g)	451.1 ± 11.5	462.7 ± 11.6
Feed efficiency (g body wt/g food intake)	0.16 ± 0.005	0.17 ± 0.009

KPC, krill protein concentrate; *PDCAAS*, protein digestion corrected amino acid score; *PER*, protein efficiency ratio.
Adapted from Gigliotti et al. (2008).

with casein. In addition, KPC and casein in the study by Gigliotti and coworkers, equally supported growth of experimental rats. Therefore, KPC isolated with ISP is a complete protein. However, changes in dietary protein may mediate pathological conditions such as renal disease initiated by nephrocalcinosis due to mineral deposition in kidneys. Thus, not only is nutritional quality of a new protein important, but also its safety needs to be assessed. This is why in a follow-up study using experimental rats fed KPC, Gigliotti et al. (2011) determined that the rats deposited much less calcium and phosphorus in the kidneys as compared to rats on the casein diet. Histological evaluation of the renal tissue showed a decreased mineralization in experimental rats fed KPC as compared to casein. Based on histological examination, rats fed KPC did not exhibit microtubular calcium deposits in kidneys unlike rats on the casein diet. Therefore, the ISP KPC seems safe for consumption. In fact, the ISP KPC may offer some renal health benefits by decreasing development of nephrocalcinosis, and thus, kidney stones. However, more comprehensive and long-term research is needed to determine the safety and quality of the ISP seafood protein.

CONCLUSION

It is well established that seafood is an excellent source of a large variety of nutrients including high quality protein. Due to its high nutrient content, including protein, seafood consumption can make a significant contribution to fulfill human dietary needs for indispensable nutrients. The high content of a large variety of nutrients compared to its balanced energetic value means that seafood fits into low energy diets designed for weight management and other chronic diet-driven conditions such as cardiovascular disease. Further, seafood processing by-products, underutilized aquatic species such as krill or nuisance fish like carp, provide a valuable source of dietary protein that could be recovered with novel processing technologies such as isoelectric solubilization/precipitation.

References

American Heart Association, 2009. Heart disease and stroke statistics–2009 update. https://my.americanheart.org/professional/General/Heart-Stroke-2009-Statistical-Update_UCM_423920_Article.jsp

Benelam, B., 2009. Satiation, satiety and their effects on eating behaviour. Nutr. Bull. 34, 126–173.

Borzoei, S., Neovius, M., Barkeling, B., et al., 2006. A comparison of effects of fish and beef protein on satiety in normal weight men. Eur. J. Clin. Nutr. 60, 897–902.

Chen, Y.C., Tou, J.C., Jaczynski, J., 2007. Amino acid, fatty acid, and mineral profiles of materials recovered from rainbow trout (*Oncorhynchus mykiss*) processing by-products using isoelectric solubilization/precipitation. J. Food Sci. 72 (9), C527–C535.

Chen, Y.C., Tou, J.C., Jaczynski, J., 2009. Amino acid and mineral composition of protein and other components and their recovery yields from whole Antarctic krill (*Euphausia superba*) using isoelectric solubilization/precipitation. J. Food Sci. 74 (2), H31–H39.

Connell, J.J., 1970a. In: Lawrie, R.A. (Ed.), Proteins as Human Food. AVI Publisher, Westport, CT.

Connell, J.J., 1970b. In: Lawrie, R.A. (Ed.), Proteins as Human Food. AVI Publisher, Westport, CT, FAO/WHO/UNU expert consultation; World Health Organization Technical Report Series 724; Geneva, Switzerland.

Friedman, M., 1996. Nutritional value of proteins from different food sources. A review. J. Agricultural Food Chem. 44 (1), 6–29.

Frokjaer, S., 1994. Use of hydrolyzates for protein supplementation. Food Technol. 48 (10), 86.

Geelen, A., Schouten, J., Kamphuis, C., et al., 2007. Fish consumption, n-3 fatty acids, and colorectal cancer: a meta-analysis of prospective cohort studies. Am. J. Epidemiol. 166, 1116–1125.

Gehring, C.K., Gigliotti, J.C., Moritz, J.S., Tou, J.C., Jaczynski, J., 2011. Functional and nutritional characteristics of proteins and lipids recovered by isoelectric processing of fish by-products and low-value fish: A review. Food Chem. 124 (2), 422–431.

Gigliotti, J.C., Jaczynski, J., Tou, J.C., 2008. Determination of the nutritional value, protein quality and safety of krill protein concentrate isolated using an isoelectric solubilization/precipitation technique. Food Chem. 111 (1), 209–214.

Gigliotti, J.C., Smith, A.L., Jaczynski, J., Tou, J.C., 2011. Consumption of krill protein concentrate prevents early renal injury and nephrocalcinosis in female Sprague-Dawley rats. Urol. Res. 39 (1), 59–67.

He, K., Song, Y., Daviglus, M.L., et al., 2004a. Accumulated evidence on fish consumption and coronary heart disease mortality: a meta-analysis of cohort studies. Circulation 109, 2705–2711.

He, K., Song, Y., Daviglus, M.L., et al., 2004b. Fish consumption and incidence of stroke: a meta-analysis of cohort studies. Stroke 35, 1538–1542.

Hu, F.B., Stampfer, M.J., Manson, J.E., et al., 1999. Dietary saturated fats and their food sources in relation to the risk of coronary heart disease in women. Am. J. Clin. Nutr. 70, 1001–1008.

Konasu, S., Yamaguchi, K., 1982. In: Martin, R.E. et al., (Ed.), Chemistry and biochemistry of marine food products. AVI Publisher, Westport, CT, pp. 367–404.

Mireles DeWitt, C.A., Nabors, R.L., Kleinholz, C.W., 2007. Pilot plant scale production of protein from catfish treated by acid solubilization/ isoelectric precipitation. J. Food Sci. 72, E351–E355.

Pszczola, D.E., 2004. Dawning of the age of proteins. Food Technol. 58 (2), 56.

Sánchez-Alonso, I., Jiménez-Escrig, A., Saura-Calixto, F., Borderías, A.J., 2007. Effect of grape antioxidant dietary fiber on the prevention of lipid oxidation in minced fish: evaluation by different methodologies. Food Chem. 101, 372–378.

Schwarz, F.J., Kirchgessner, M., Deuringer, U., 1998. Studies on the methionine requirement of carp (*Cyprinus carpio* L.). Aquaculture 161, 121–129.

Skaara, T., Regenstein, J.M., 1990. Structure and composition of fish muscle. J. Muscle Foods 1, 269.

Tahergorabi, R., Hosseini, S.V., Jaczynski, J., 2011. Seafood Proteins. In: Phillips, G.O., Williams, P.A. (Eds.), Handbook of Food Proteins. Woodhead Publishing Ltd, Cambridge, pp. 116–149.

Taskaya, L., Chen, Y.C., Beamer, S., Tou, J.C., Jaczynski, J., 2009. Compositional characteristics of materials recovered from whole gutted silver carp (*Hypophthalmichthys molitrix*) using isoelectric solubilization/precipitation. J. Agricultural Food Chem. 57 (10), 4259–4266.

Torres, J.A., Chen, Y.C., Rodrigo-Garcia, J., Jaczynski, J., 2007. Recovery of byproducts from seafood processing streams. In: Shahidi, F. (Ed.), Maximising the Value Of Marine By-Products. CRC Press, Boca Raton, USA, pp. 65–90.

Tou, J.C., Jaczynski, J., Chen, Y.C., 2007. Krill for human consumption: nutritional value and potential health benefits. Nutr. Rev. 65 (2), 63–77.

Uhe, A., Collier, G., O'Dea, K., 1992. A comparison of the effects of beef, chicken and fish protein on satiety and amino acid profiles in lean male subjects. J. Nutr. 122, 467–472.

Undeland, I., Kelleher, S.D., Hultin, H.O., McClements, J., Thongraung, C., 2003. Consistency and solubility changes in herring (*Clupea harengus*) light muscle homogenates as a function of pH. J. Agricultural Food Chem. 51, 3992–3998.

United States Department of Agriculture Agricultural Research Service National Nutrient Database for Standard Reference, Release 28. 2015. http://ndb.nal.usda.gov/ndb/search

Venugopal, V., 2009. Marine products for healthcare: Functional and bioactive nutraceutical compounds from the ocean. CRC Press (Taylor & Francis Group), Boca Raton, FL.

Wergedah, H., et al., 2004. Fish protein hydrolysate reduces plasma cholesterol, increases the proportion of HDL-cholesterol and lowers acyl-coA-cholesterol acyltransferase activity in liver of zucker rats. J. Nutr. 134, 1320.

Wu, S., Feng, B., Li, K., et al., 2012. Fish consumption and colorectal cancer risk in humans: a systematic review and meta-analysis. Am. J. Med. 125, 551–559.

CHAPTER

30

Metabolic Effects of Krill Oil

S.M. *Ulven*

Department of Nutrition, University of Oslo, Oslo, Norway

INTRODUCTION TO KRILL OIL

The beneficial health effects of fish are well documented. For individuals who do not like fish or for other reasons do not include fish in their diet, use of nutritional supplements is recommended. This has led to increased demand for products containing marine n–3 polyunsaturated fatty acids (PUFAs). Since fish is a limited resource, there is a growing interest for exploiting alternative n–3 PUFA sources. Antarctic krill (*Euphausia superba*) has been considered as a new alternative, sustainable source of long chain n–3 PUFA (Kwantes and Grundmann, 2015). Krill are small shrimp-like crustaceans found in all oceans and serve as a major food source for much of the larger marine life. Krill is by far the most dominant member of the Antarctic zooplankton community in terms of biomass. Krill survive the cold environment due to the high content of the long chain PUFA, including eicosapentaenoic acid (C20;5, n–3) and docosahexaenoic acid (C22;6, n–3), attached to their cell membranes via phospholipids mainly phosphatidylcholine (Tou et al., 2007). More than 80% of EPA and DHA in krill oil is found in this form (Burri and Johnsen, 2015). Krill oil extracted from krill contains 30–65% of the fatty acids bound to phospholipids, which is in contrast to fish oil where fatty acids are bound to triglycerides. Krill oil also contains antioxidants such as astaxanthin and vitamins A and E (Tou et al., 2007). While it has been claimed that the bioavailability of EPA and DHA from krill oil versus fish oil differ due to the form of these fatty acids, phospholipid bound versus triglyceride bound, respectively, it has been difficult to compare the bioavailability due to different doses of oil and the amount of EPA and DHA used in the experiments. It is therefore still unclear if krill oil has a better bioavailability of EPA and DHA compared to fish oil (Salem and Kuratko, 2014).

Krill oil is found to be Generally Recognized as Safe (GRAS) by the American Food and Drug Administration (FDA) and obtained a Novel Food status from the European Union. Krill oil has been used as a supplement in several human studies and so far the reported side effects of krill oil are generally limited to mild gastrointestinal distress, similar to intake of fish oil and control oils, and krill oil is described as being mostly well tolerated (Kwantes and Grundmann, 2015). Krill oil is a relatively new marine n–3 supplement and the numbers of studies are therefore limited compared to the large number of fish oil studies being performed. More studies will be needed to document the health benefits of krill oil before firm conclusions can be drawn. In this chapter, the results from human and animal studies that look at the effects of krill oil on blood lipids, inflammation, glucose tolerance and insulin sensitivity, body weight, and the levels of plasma endocannabinoids are described in order to show the evidence so far of the metabolic health effects of krill oil.

METABOLIC HEALTH EFFECTS OF KRILL OIL

Effects on Blood Lipids

Human Studies

Dyslipidemia is a major risk factor for cardiovascular disease. The effects of krill oil on blood lipids have been investigated in a limited number of studies performed in patients or healthy subjects with normal lipid serum levels or lipid disturbances. In most of these studies, the effect of krill oil is compared with fish oil. One of the first

Fish and Fish Oil in Health and Disease Prevention. http://dx.doi.org/10.1016/B978-0-12-802844-5.00030-0

studies that investigated the effect of krill oil on blood lipids reported a large reduction in blood triglycerides, total cholesterol, and LDL-cholesterol, and an increase in HDL cholesterol (Bunea et al., 2004). This was a multicenter, randomized, double-blind and placebo controlled study where 120 patients diagnosed with mildly high to very high blood cholesterol (193.9–347.9 mg/dL) and triglyceride levels (203.8–354.4 mg/dL) were treated for 12 weeks with krill oil (Neptune, Neptune Technologies and Biosources, Canada), fish oil, or placebo (Bunea et al., 2004). The krill oil group was divided into two subgroups to receive a high dose or a low dose of krill oil, and these subgroups were further subdivided based on body mass index (BMI). In total four groups received krill oil, and the high dose group received 2 or 3 g of krill oil per day, dependent on BMI and the low dose group received 1 or 1.5 g of krill oil per day, dependent on BMI. The fish oil group received 3 g of fish oil (containing 540 mg of EPA and 360 mg of DHA). The placebo group was given a 3 g daily dose of microcrystalline cellulose. Total cholesterol, LDL cholesterol, and triglycerides were reduced in all groups receiving krill oil and fish oil. Both krill oil groups reduced total cholesterol by 13–18%, and this effect was larger than the effect seen in the fish oil group, which had a 6% reduction in total cholesterol. In contrast, subjects in the placebo group increased mean total cholesterol level by 9%. Both krill oil groups reduced LDL cholesterol by 32–39%, while the fish oil had a reduction in LDL cholesterol by 5% (not significant) and the placebo group had an increase of 13%. Also HDL cholesterol was increased in the krill oil groups, from 43–60%, depending on dose. In the fish oil group and the placebo group, the HDL cholesterol increased by 4%, but it was only a significant change in the fish oil group. The triglyceride levels were significantly reduced by 27% in the high dose krill oil groups. In the low dose krill oil groups, triglyceride levels were reduced by 11–12%, but these changes were not significantly changed from baseline. In the fish oil group, the triglyceride levels were reduced by 3%, and in the placebo group, the reduction was 10% (not significant changes in both groups).

In later studies, these large effects on blood lipids have still not been confirmed. Krill oil reduced serum triglyceride levels, but had no effect on fasting serum total cholesterol, LDL cholesterol, and HDL cholesterol in a study with healthy subjects with borderline or high triglycerides (Berge et al., 2014). This was shown in a 12 week, double-blind, randomized, multicenter, placebo controlled study performed in the United States (Berge et al., 2014). In total, 300 healthy men and women (21–79 years) with borderline high or high fasting serum triglyceride levels (150–499 mg/dL) were included in the study. They were randomized into five different groups receiving either krill oil [four different doses 0.05, 1, 2, or 4 g/day (Aker BioMarine, Norway) or 4 g olive oil (placebo; Ruiz-Canela e Hijos, Spain)]. The daily dose of EPA + DHA in the krill oil groups corresponded to 100, 200, 400, and 800 mg. After 6 weeks, subjects receiving 1, 2, and 4 g krill oil per day showed significantly reduced serum triglyceride levels compared to baseline, but after 12 weeks, this reduction was not statistically significant. When data from all subjects receiving krill oil was pooled, there was a significant 10.2% reduction in serum triglyceride levels after 12 weeks compared to placebo. Total cholesterol, LDL cholesterol, and HDL cholesterol were unchanged at both 6 and 12 weeks compared to baseline in all five groups.

To the contrary, no effect of krill oil on plasma triglyceride levels and HDL cholesterol were observed in three human studies including healthy subjects with normal or slightly elevated total blood cholesterol and/or triglycerides (Maki et al., 2009; Ramprasath et al., 2013; Ulven et al., 2011). Two of the studies also did not observe any effect of krill oil on total cholesterol and LDL cholesterol (Maki et al., 2009; Ulven et al., 2011), while in one of the studies, an increase in total cholesterol and LDL cholesterol was observed (Ramprasath et al., 2013). In the study by Maki and coworkers, a 4 week, randomized, double-blind, controlled, parallel designed study was performed at two clinical research sites in the United States (Maki et al., 2009). In total 76 healthy men and women (35–64 years) were included in the study and these were randomized into three groups receiving 2 g per day of either krill oil (Superba, Aker Biomarine, Norway), menhaden oil (Omega-Pure, US), or olive oil (control). The daily dose of EPA and DHA was 216 mg EPA and 90 mg DHA in the krill oil group and 212 mg EPA and 176 mg DHA in the menhaden group. In this study, no effects of krill oil or fish oil on plasma total cholesterol, LDL cholesterol, HDL cholesterol, and triglyceride levels were observed (Maki et al., 2009). This was also the conclusion in the study by Ulven and coworkers, who performed a 7 week, open label, single centre, randomized, parallel designed study in Norway (Ulven et al., 2011). In total 113 healthy men and women with normal or slightly elevated total blood cholesterol and/or triglyceride levels were randomized into three groups receiving 3 g of krill oil (Superba, Aker BioMarine, Norway) or 1.8 g fish oil (Peter Møller AS, Norway) per day, or a control group who did not receive any supplement. The daily dose was 348 mg EPA and 195 mg DHA in the krill oil group and 450 mg EPA and 414 mg DHA in the fish oil group. However, a significant increase in serum LDL cholesterol was observed within the fish oil group, and a significant increase in the HDL cholesterol/TG ratio was observed within the krill oil group (Ulven et al., 2011).

In 2013, Ramprasath and coworkers, reported data from a 4 week, double blind, randomized, placebo controlled, crossover designed study performed in Canada (Ramprasath et al., 2013). In total 24 healthy men and women (18–49 years) were included in the study and they received either 3 g of krill oil (K-REAL, Enzymotec) or fish oil (Napro Pharma, Norway) or corn oil (control) in a random order with 8 week wash-out in between each treatment. The daily dose was 493 mg EPA and 284 mg DHA in the krill oil group and 404 mg EPA and 260 mg DHA in the fish oil group (Ramprasath et al., 2013; Salem and Kuratko, 2014). They also confirmed that the change in serum triglyceride levels and HDL cholesterol were not different between treatment groups. However, they did show that the serum levels of total cholesterol and LDL cholesterol increased, both after intake of krill oil and fish oil compared with control (Ramprasath et al., 2013).

One study has shown that krill powder, which contains 34% proteins in addition to krill oil (61.8%), reduced plasma triglyceride levels in mildly obese men (Berge et al., 2013). This was a single center, open label pilot study performed in Germany. In total 12 mildly obese men (BMI 30–35, 30–55 years) were given 4 g krill powder (Aker BioMarine, Norway) daily for 24 weeks. The daily dose was 268 mg EPA and 132 mg DHA. In addition, six subjects were included as controls and received no treatment. Plasma total cholesterol, LDL cholesterol, and HDL cholesterol were not changed within the krill powder group after 12 and 24 weeks. Plasma triglyceride levels were reduced by 22.5% and 20.6% after 12 and 24 weeks within the group, respectively, however the reduction was only significant after 24 weeks. No changes occurred in the control group (Berge et al., 2013).

Since the numbers of human studies are limited and the results of the effects of krill oil in blood lipids are not unambiguous due to limitations in study design, it is too early to make any firm conclusions on the role of krill oil on blood lipids. Thus, the impact of krill oil on triglycerides and lipoproteins is not fully elucidated, and available data indicate only modest or no effects in the study populations that have been examined. It seems like subjects with borderline or high triglyceride levels are the group of subjects that can best benefit from krill oil supplementation but further studies need to confirm this.

Animal Studies

The effect of krill in animal studies has been recently reviewed (Burri and Johnsen, 2015). Krill oil supplementation significantly reduced plasma triglyceride levels and total cholesterol in normolipidemic male Wistar rats, fed a standard diet supplemented with 2.5% fish oil (Lysi, Iceland) or 2.5% krill oil (Aker BioMarine, Norway) for 6 weeks compared to controls (olive oil) (Ferramosca et al., 2012b). Krill oil supplementation with different doses (from 0 to 200 g/L krill oil) also significantly reduced serum levels of triglycerides, total cholesterol, and LDL cholesterol after 4 weeks of treatment in high fat diet fed Sprague-Dawley rats with hyperlipidemia (Zhu et al., 2008). The highest doses of krill oil could also increase HDL cholesterol (Zhu et al., 2008). In another study, 2.5% krill oil (Aker BioMarine, Norway) supplementation for 12 weeks prevented hypertriglyceridemia induced by high fat diet in Sprague-Dawley rats (Ferramosca et al., 2012a). These data are in line with a study by Li and coworkers, who fed Wistar rats with a high cholesterol diet for 4 weeks to establish hyperlipidemia (Li et al., 2013). The rats were supplemented with different doses of whole krill oil (extracted from krill powder, Liaoning Province Dalian Ocean Fishery Group of Corporations, China) and phospholipid type krill oil for 4 weeks together with the high cholesterol diet. Krill oil supplementation (50 mg krill oil/kg body weight, 200 mg krill oil/kg body weight, and 400 mg krill oil/kg body weight) significantly reduced plasma triglycerides and plasma LDL cholesterol compared to baseline. The phospholipid type krill oil seemed to have a more pronounced effect (Li et al., 2013). Also hTNF-α mice fed a high fat diet for 6 weeks and supplemented with either 5.8% krill oil (Aker BioMarine, Norway) or 2.9% fish oil (EPAX, Norway) of similar doses of EPA and DHA, found that krill oil, and not fish oil, significantly decreased plasma triglycerides by 19% suggesting that krill oil is more effective than fish oil in lowering plasma triglycerides (Vigerust et al., 2013). Total plasma cholesterol, free cholesterol, and HDL cholesterol were significantly reduced in both groups compared to controls (Vigerust et al., 2013).

In contrast, animal experiments have shown that krill oil supplementation had no effect on triglycerides or even increased triglycerides after supplementation (Batetta et al., 2009; Burri et al., 2011; Tandy et al., 2009; Tillander et al., 2014). High fat fed mice supplemented with 1.25, 2.5, and 5% krill oil (Superba, Aker BioMarine, Norway) for 8 weeks showed no influence on serum triglycerides compared to mice not supplemented with krill oil. However, 1.25, 2.5, and 5% krill oil supplementation significantly reduced serum cholesterol compared to mice not supplemented with krill oil (Tandy et al., 2009). Zucker rats (an obese rat model) supplemented with krill oil or fish oil for 4 weeks increased plasma triglyceride levels by 30% compared to the controls (Batetta et al., 2009). In this experiment, the Zucker rats were supplemented with krill oil (Superba, Aker BioMarine, Norway) and fish oil (GC Rieber Oils, Norway) with balanced levels of EPA and DHA, corresponding to 1.8 g/day of EPA and DHA in an 8.4-MJ/day diet in humans. Krill oil and fish oil led to 75% lower plasma LDL cholesterol levels compared to controls (soybean oil), whereas HDL cholesterol did not differ among the groups (Batetta et al., 2009). Tillander and coworkers, fed mice a high fat diet with 5.7% krill oil (Superba, Aker Biomarine, Norway) for 6 weeks and found no effect of krill oil on plasma cholesterol and plasma triglycerides (Tillander et al., 2014). These data are in agreement with the study by Burri and coworkers, who fed lean mice for 12 weeks with 1.1% fish oil (GC Rieber Oil AS, Norway) or 1.5% krill oil (Superba, Aker BioMarine ASA, Norway) or control oil (4% soybean oil) and did not see any changes in plasma cholesterol and plasma triglycerides in any of the groups (Burri et al., 2011).

In general, most of these studies show that krill oil reduces triglyceride levels, but the effect on lipids differs between experiments due to the dose of krill oil, the amount of EPA and DHA, and duration of the experiment, and the type of animal models.

Inflammation and Oxidative Stress

Human Studies

Few studies have investigated the effect of krill oil on inflammation in human trials. In one study, the effect of Neptune krill oil on inflammation and arthritic symptoms was evaluated a primary outcome (Deutsch, 2007). In this study, 90 patients with confirmed diagnosis of cardiovascular disease and/or rheumatoid arthritis and/or osteoarthritis, all with increased levels of C-reactive protein (CRP) (> 1.0 mg/dL), received either 300 mg krill oil or placebo daily for 30 days in a randomized, double blind, placebo controlled study with a crossover design. CRP was measured as an indicator of systemic inflammation (Deutsch, 2007). To determine arthritic symptoms, patients were asked to complete the Western Ontario and McMaster Universities (WOMAC) assessment questionnaire. The level of serum CRP and the three WOMAC scores (pain, stiffness, and functional impairment) were measured at baseline, and after 7, 14, and 30 days. The krill oil group showed a decrease in the level of CRP and the three WOMAC scores compared to placebo at all time points (Deutsch, 2007).

In two of the human trials mentioned above describing effects of krill oil on lipoproteins and triglyceride levels, inflammatory markers and oxidative stress markers were part of the secondary outcome analysis (Maki et al., 2009; Ulven et al., 2011). No effect of krill oil on plasma high sensitive CRP (hsCRP) and urine F2-isoprostanes, which is a marker of oxidative stress, was observed in the study by Maki and coworkers, who conducted a 4 week, randomized, double blind controlled study where 76 healthy subjects with a mean BMI of about 32 were randomized into three groups receiving 2 g per day of either krill oil, menhaden oil, or olive oil (Maki et al., 2009). No statistically significant differences in urine F2-isoprotanes and serum levels of hsCRP between the study groups were reported by Ulven and coworkers, who performed a 7 week, open label, single center, randomized, parallel designed study with 113 healthy men and women with mean BMI of 24 who were randomized into three groups receiving 3 g of krill oil or 1.8 g fish oil per day, or a control group (Ulven et al., 2011). Since these markers were not the primary outcome of the studies, the lack of effects may be due to lack of power to detect changes on these markers in these two studies. More studies are needed before conclusions can be made if krill oil affects inflammation and oxidative stress.

Animal Studies

In the arthritis-induced mice model, krill oil (Aker BioMarine, Norway), and fish oil (GC Rieber Oils, Norway), with balanced levels of EPA and DHA, corresponding to 1.8 g/day of EPA and DHA in an 8.4-MJ/day diet in humans, significantly reduced clinical arthritis score and hind paw swelling compared to controls (Ierna et al., 2010). Mice fed the krill oil also had lower infiltration of inflammatory cells into the joint and lower synovial layer hyperplasia when compared to control. Krill oil did not modulate the levels of serum cytokines (Ierna et al., 2010).

Krill oil also reduced inflammation in an experimental model of ulcerative colitis in rats (Grimstad et al., 2012). Male rats received 5% krill oil for 30 days. Acute colitis was induced by dextran sulfate sodium from day 23 and disease activity index was assessed after 7 days of colitis induction (day 30) (Grimstad et al., 2012). One of the main findings was that the colon length was preserved in the rats supplemented with krill oil, while it was shortened, as a result from edema and inflammation in the colonial mucosa, in the rats induced with colitis compared to controls. Prostaglandin E3 was significantly increased by krill oil, while cytokines (TNFα and IL-1β) and histological combined scores tended to be lower after krill oil supplementation. Krill oil supplementation significantly reduced oxidative stress markers in the distal colon (Grimstad et al., 2012).

Obesity is associated with low grade chronic inflammation and transgenic mice expressing human TNFα in a mouse model represents an appropriate model to investigate lipid-induced inflammation. hTNFα transgenic mice fed with a high fat diet for 6 weeks supplemented with either 5.8% krill oil or 2.9% fish oil or controls (soya oil) did not substantially differ in levels of proinflammatory cytokines (between treatments groups), but krill oil tended to decrease MCP-1 in mesenteric adipose tissue (Vigerust et al., 2013).

Zucker rats supplemented with krill oil and fish oil with balanced level of EPA and DHA did not influence plasma proinflammatory (TNFα, IL-6, IL-1β), antiinflammatory cytokines (IL-10 and TGFβ), and CRP compared to controls (Batetta et al., 2009). However, in macrophages incubated for 24 h in the presence of lipopolysaccharide (LPS), the TNFα secretion was significantly lower in fish oil- and krill oil-supplemented rats compared to controls. This observation may suggest that the increased incorporation of EPA and DHA in the cell membrane due to krill oil and fish oil supplementation could reduce the inflammatory response caused by LPS. The plasma levels of IL-1β, IL-6, and IL-10 however, did not differ among the three groups following LPS stimulation (Batetta et al., 2009). In another animal experiment, 1.25, 2.5, and 5% krill oil supplementation for 8 weeks significantly reduced TNFα compared to high fat fed mice without krill oil supplementation (Tandy et al., 2009).

Krill oil supplementation has also been shown to reduce oxidative damage. Reactive oxygen species (ROS) may modify cellular proteins and lipids, which may cause pathologies leading to diseases. Oxidative damage of lipids caused by ROS can be measured by analyzing the levels of lipid peroxides (LPO). In Sprague–Dawley rats fed a high fat diet, the increase in LPO was reversed by supplementing the rats with 2.5% krill oil for 12 weeks (Ferramosca et al., 2012).

These animal studies show that krill oil may dampen inflammation in chronic inflammatory diseases such as arthritis and colitis, but very limited studies have been performed. Obesity-induced inflammation models also suggest that krill oil may reduce inflammation. More studies are needed before any conclusions on the role of krill oil on inflammation and oxidative stress can be made.

Body Weight and Endocannabinoids

Human Studies

Plasma endocannabinoids have been suggested to be involved in the regulation of the homeostasis of body composition by regulating food intake and energy expenditure. A limited number of studies have looked at the effect of krill oil on plasma endocannabinoids, and the results are not unambiguous. Intake of krill oil has been shown to reduce the level of the plasma endocannabinoid called 2-arachidonoylglycerol (2-AG) in obese subjects, but not in overweight subjects (Banni et al., 2011). In a 4 week, randomized, double blind, controlled, parallel designed trial that was conducted in two centers in the United States, the effects of 2 g/day of krill oil (Superba, Aker BioMarine, Norway) or menhaden oil (Omega-Pure, US) on plasma endocannabinoids were investigated (Banni et al., 2011). A third group received 2 g/day of olive oil and served as a control group. It included 63 healthy overweight and obese men and women (35–64 years) with waist circumference of 102 cm, or greater (men) or 88 cm or greater (women). In the krill oil group, the daily dose was 216 mg EPA and 90 mg DHA, and in the menhaden oil group daily dose was 212 mg EPA and 178 mg DHA (Banni et al., 2011). There were no changes in BMI and waist circumference in any of the groups. Intake of krill oil, but not menhaden oil or olive oil, significantly decreased 2-arachidonoylglycerol (2-AG) in obese subjects, but not in overweight subjects. There was no effect of any of the oils on arachidonoylethanolamine (AEA; Banni et al., 2011). One study has investigated the effect of krill powder on plasma endocannabinoids (Berge et al., 2013). This pilot study included 12 mildly obese men who were given 4 g krill powder daily for 24 weeks. The daily dose was 268 mg EPA and 132 mg DHA. The waist/hip ratio was reduced by 2.9%, which was a significant change within the group after 24 weeks, but body weight did not change. The levels of 2-AG were not changed after 12 and 24 weeks compared to baseline, but there was a significant 59% and 84% decrease in plasma AEA levels at 12 and 24 weeks, respectively within the krill powder group (Berge et al., 2013). The preliminary results need to be confirmed in future long term, randomized, controlled studies before firm conclusions can be drawn.

Animal Studies

Animal studies have confirmed a possible effect of krill oil on reducing the plasma levels of endocannabinoids. Supplementation of both krill oil and fish oil to Zucker rats for 4 weeks, led to a reduction in AEA levels in visceral adipose tissue compared to controls. The levels of 2-AG were also significantly lower in the krill oil fed rats compared to controls in visceral adipose tissue (Batetta et al., 2009). In this experiment, Zucker rats were treated with krill oil (Superba, Aker BioMarine) and fish oil (GC Rieber Oils) with balanced levels of EPA and DHA, corresponding to 1.8 g/day of EPA and DHA in an 8.4-MJ/day diet in humans (Batetta et al., 2009). The levels of endocannabinoids in subcutaneous adipose tissue did not differ in any of the groups. Krill oil also reduced the levels of endocannabinoids in liver and heart, and krill oil seemed to have a more pronounced inhibitory effect on the endocannabinoid system compared to fish oil (Batetta et al., 2009). Krill oil supplementation did not influence the body weight of the animals. These data are in accordance with the human study by Banni et al. (2011).

In a study with high fat fed mice for 8 weeks, increasing doses of krill oil reduced the levels of endocannabinoids and its precursors in all tissues except the liver in a dose-dependent manner (Piscitelli et al., 2011). There was no effect on body weight by krill oil in this study. That is in line with previous studies (Tandy et al., 2009; Tillander et al., 2014), but in contrast to others who have showed that krill oil reduces body weight in obesity models (Ferramosca et al., 2012; Zhu et al., 2008) and in high cholesterol fed rats (Li et al., 2013).

Thus, these limited animal studies support the findings that krill oil has a positive effect on plasma levels of endocannabinoids. If krill oil truly has an effect on body weight or not still needs to be confirmed in future studies.

Blood Pressure, Glucose Homeostasis and Insulin Sensitivity

Human Studies

In all of the above mentioned human studies, the effect of krill oil on blood pressure, glucose homeostasis, and insulin sensitivity have not been the primary outcome of the trials, but these metabolic health markers have been measured in some of the studies. No effect of krill oil on systolic and diastolic blood pressure has been observed (Albert et al., 2015; Berge et al., 2014; Maki et al., 2009; Ramprasath et al., 2013). Furthermore, Maki and coworkers, reported that krill oil had no effect on measures of glucose homeostasis (HOMA-IR, insulin, and glucose) compared to controls among healthy subjects with mean BMI of about 32 (Maki et al., 2009). This is in accordance with the results of Berge and coworkers, who reported no effect of krill powder on insulin and glucose levels in mildly obese men (Berge et al., 2013). Banni and coworkers, also reported no effect of krill oil on these markers in overweight and obese subjects (Banni et al., 2011). Since these markers were not the primary outcome in any of these studies, the lack of effects may be due to lack of power to detect changes on these markers in these studies. In contrast, krill oil reduced blood glucose levels compared to baseline, whereas placebo treatment resulted in a nonsignificant increase compared to baseline (Bunea et al., 2004).

In a recent randomized, double blind, controlled crossover trial with 47 healthy overweight men (BMI 25-30) in New Zealand, a mixture of krill oil (88%, Nutrizeal, New Zealand) and salmon oil (12%, Nutrizeal, New Zealand) resulted in decreased insulin sensitivity after 8 week supplementation, compared to controls (canola oil; Albert et al., 2015). The daily dose was 230 mg EPA and 154 mg DHA in the krill and salmon oil group. In this study, the primary outcome was insulin sensitivity measured with a 75 g oral-glucose tolerance test by using the Matsuda method measuring glucose and insulin at 0, 30, 60, 90, and 120 min. In addition, the oral disposition index (a measure of β cell function corrected for insulin sensitivity) and the HOMA-IR was calculated. There were no significant differences between control group and the krill and salmon oil group in the secondary outcomes including 24 h ambulatory blood pressure, hsCRP, and lipids. There was a trend of an increase in apolipoprotein B and carotid intima–media thickness in the krill and salmon oil group compared to controls (Albert et al., 2015). The results show that overweight adults may exacerbate risk of diabetes and cardiovascular disease due to reduced insulin sensitivity if supplemented with a mixture of krill oil and salmon oil. These results are of concern, and need be confirmed in future studies before conclusions can be drawn.

Animal Studies

Obese New Zealand white rabbits were supplemented with krill oil (Aker BioMarine, Norway) and fish oil (Aker BioMarine, Norway) giving a daily dose of 600 mg n–3 PUFA for 60 days (Ivanova et al., 2014). Both krill oil and fish oil significantly reduced fasting glucose and insulin levels compared to controls. After an intravenous glucose tolerance test, glucose concentration after 60 min in the krill oil group returned to baseline, which was significantly lower when compared to controls, while no difference in insulin levels between the groups was observed after 60 min. No significant differences in the HOMA–IR between groups were observed, but it tended to be higher in in nonsupplemented animals compared to the krill oil and fish oil supplemented animals. Also the HOMA β-cell index was higher in nonsupplemented animals (Ivanova et al., 2014). Thus, these results indicate the krill oil and fish oil improves glucose tolerance and improves insulin sensitivity and secretion. Supplementation of 2.5% krill oil for 12 weeks in Sprague–Dawley rats fed a high fat diet counteracted the hyperglycemic effects of a high fat diet by normalizing the plasma glucose level and preventing an increase in the plasma insulin levels (Ferramosca et al., 2012). In another study, high fat fed mice supplemented with 5% krill oil for 8 weeks also significantly reduced serum glucose levels compared to high fat fed mice without krill oil supplementation (Tandy et al., 2009). However, the insulin levels and HOMA–IR were not significantly changed by krill oil supplementation (Tandy et al., 2009). No effect on insulin levels was observed in lean mice fed with 1.1% fish oil or 1.5% krill oil or control oil for 12 weeks (Burri et al., 2011). Thus, in obese rodent models, krill oil seems to improve fasting glucose levels, but the effect of krill oil on insulin sensitivity is less clear.

References

Albert, B.B., Derraik, J.G., Brennan, C.M., Biggs, J.B., Garg, M.L., Cameron-Smith, D., Hofman, P.L., Cutfield, W.S., 2015. Supplementation with a blend of krill and salmon oil is associated with increased metabolic risk in overweight men. Am. J. Clin. Nutr. 102, 49–57.

Banni, S., Carta, G., Murru, E., Cordeddu, L., Giordano, E., Sirigu, A.R., Berge, K., Vik, H., Maki, K.C., Di Marzo, V., Griinari, M., 2011. Krill oil significantly decreases 2-arachidonoylglycerol plasma levels in obese subjects. Nutr. Metab. (London) 8, 7.

Batetta, B., Griinari, M., Carta, G., Murru, E., Ligresti, A., Cordeddu, L., Giordano, E., Sanna, F., Bisogno, T., Uda, S., Collu, M., Bruheim, I., Di Marzo, V., Banni, S., 2009. Endocannabinoids may mediate the ability of (n-3) fatty acids to reduce ectopic fat and inflammatory mediators in obese Zucker rats. J. Nutr. 139, 1495–1501.

Berge, K., Musa-Veloso, K., Harwood, M., Hoem, N., Burri, L., 2014. Krill oil supplementation lowers serum triglycerides without increasing low-density lipoprotein cholesterol in adults with borderline high or high triglyceride levels. Nutr. Res. 34, 126–133.

Berge, K., Piscitelli, F., Hoem, N., Silvestri, C., Meyer, I., Banni, S., Di Marzo, V., 2013. Chronic treatment with krill powder reduces plasma triglyceride and anandamide levels in mildly obese men. Lipids Health Dis. 12, 78.

Bunea, R., El Farrah, K., Deutsch, L., 2004. Evaluation of the effects of Neptune Krill Oil on the clinical course of hyperlipidemia. Altern. Med. Rev. 9, 420–428.

Burri, L., Berge, K., Wibrand, K., Berge, R.K., Barger, J.L., 2011. Differential effects of krill oil and fish oil on the hepatic transcriptome in mice. Front. Genet. 2, 45.

Burri, L., Johnsen, L., 2015. Krill products: an overview of animal studies. Nutrients 7, 3300–3321.

Deutsch, L., 2007. Evaluation of the effect of Neptune Krill Oil on chronic inflammation and arthritic symptoms. J. Am. Coll. Nutr. 26, 39–48.

Ferramosca, A., Conte, A., Burri, L., Berge, K., De Nuccio, F., Giudetti, A.M., Zara, V., 2012a. A krill oil supplemented diet suppresses hepatic steatosis in high-fat fed rats. PLoS One 7, e38797.

Ferramosca, A., Conte, L., Zara, V., 2012b. A krill oil supplemented diet reduces the activities of the mitochondrial tricarboxylate carrier and of the cytosolic lipogenic enzymes in rats. J. Anim. Physiol. Anim. Nutr. (Berlin) 96, 295–306.

Grimstad, T., Bjorndal, B., Cacabelos, D., Aasprong, O.G., Janssen, E.A., Omdal, R., Svardal, A., Hausken, T., Bohov, P., Portero-Otin, M., Pamplona, R., Berge, R.K., 2012. Dietary supplementation of krill oil attenuates inflammation and oxidative stress in experimental ulcerative colitis in rats. Scand. J. Gastroenterol. 47, 49–58.

Ierna, M., Kerr, A., Scales, H., Berge, K., Griinari, M., 2010. Supplementation of diet with krill oil protects against experimental rheumatoid arthritis. BMC Musculoskelet. Disord. 11, 136.

Ivanova, Z., Bjorndal, B., Grigorova, N., Roussenov, A., Vachkova, E., Berge, K., Burri, L., Berge, R., Stanilova, S., Milanova, A., Penchev, G., Vik, R., Petrov, V., Georgieva, T.M., Bivolraski, B., Georgiev, I.P., 2014. Effect of fish and krill oil supplementation on glucose tolerance in rabbits with experimentally induced obesity. Eur. J. Nutr. 54 (7), 1055–1067.

Kwantes, J.M., Grundmann, O., 2015. A brief review of krill oil history, research, and the commercial market. J. Diet Suppl. 12, 23–35.

Li, D.M., Zhou, D.Y., Zhu, B.W., Chi, Y.L., Sun, L.M., Dong, X.P., Qin, L., Qiao, W.Z., Murata, Y., 2013. Effects of krill oil intake on plasma cholesterol and glucose levels in rats fed a high-cholesterol diet. J. Sci. Food Agric. 93, 2669–2675.

Maki, K.C., Reeves, M.S., Farmer, M., Griinari, M., Berge, K., Vik, H., Hubacher, R., Rains, T.M., 2009. Krill oil supplementation increases plasma concentrations of eicosapentaenoic and docosahexaenoic acids in overweight and obese men and women. Nutr. Res. 29, 609–615.

Piscitelli, F., Carta, G., Bisogno, T., Murru, E., Cordeddu, L., Berge, K., Tandy, S., Cohn, J.S., Griinari, M., Banni, S., Di Marzo, V., 2011. Effect of dietary krill oil supplementation on the endocannabinoidome of metabolically relevant tissues from high-fat-fed mice. Nutr. Metab. (London) 8, 51.

Ramprasath, V.R., Eyal, I., Zchut, S., Jones, P.J., 2013. Enhanced increase of omega-3 index in healthy individuals with response to 4-week n-3 fatty acid supplementation from krill oil versus fish oil. Lipids Health Dis. 12, 178.

Salem, Jr., N., Kuratko, C.N., 2014. A reexamination of krill oil bioavailability studies. Lipids Health Dis. 13, 137.

Tandy, S., Chung, R.W., Wat, E., Kamili, A., Berge, K., Griinari, M., Cohn, J.S., 2009. Dietary krill oil supplementation reduces hepatic steatosis, glycemia, and hypercholesterolemia in high-fat-fed mice. J. Agric. Food Chem. 57, 9339–9345.

Tillander, V., Bjorndal, B., Burri, L., Bohov, P., Skorve, J., Berge, R.K., Alexson, S.E., 2014. Fish oil and krill oil supplementations differentially regulate lipid catabolic and synthetic pathways in mice. Nutr. Metab. (London) 11, 20.

Tou, J.C., Jaczynski, J., Chen, Y.C., 2007. Krill for human consumption: nutritional value and potential health benefits. Nutr. Rev. 65, 63–77.

Ulven, S.M., Kirkhus, B., Lamglait, A., Basu, S., Elind, E., Haider, T., Berge, K., Vik, H., Pedersen, J.I., 2011. Metabolic effects of krill oil are essentially similar to those of fish oil but at lower dose of EPA and DHA, in healthy volunteers. Lipids 46, 37–46.

Vigerust, N.F., Bjorndal, B., Bohov, P., Brattelid, T., Svardal, A., Berge, R.K., 2013. Krill oil versus fish oil in modulation of inflammation and lipid metabolism in mice transgenic for TNF-alpha. Eur. J. Nutr. 52, 1315–1325.

Zhu, J.J., Shi, J.H., Qian, W.B., Cai, Z.Z., Li, D., 2008. Effects of krill oil on serum lipids of hyperlipidemic rats and human SW480 cells. Lipids Health Dis. 7, 30.

CHAPTER

31

Risks and Possible Health Effects of Raw Fish Intake

A. Daschner

Allergy Department, Health Research Institute, University Hospital La Princesa, Madrid, Spain

BACKGROUND

Early epidemiological studies have associated health benefits with fish consumption, initially by a reduced risk of coronary heart disease. Further studies in several fields of epidemiology, nutrition or immunology have searched for the causes of the nutritional benefits of fish and seafood. These have been found to be due to the presence not only of n-3 PUFA, but also of proteins of high nutritional value, minerals, such as calcium, selenium, iron, zinc, vitamins, such as B3, B6, E, and D (Sidhu, 2003), the free amino acid taurine, and possibly also of bioactive peptides (Ryan et al., 2011).

Discussion of the nutritive and functional properties of fish and seafood components is out of the scope of this chapter and is presented elsewhere in the text. However, direct studies on health benefits of specifically consuming *raw* fish are lacking. When presented in scientific or popular press are described in relation to general intake of food, independent on whether it is eaten raw or cooked. Therefore, an indirect means of evaluation can be performed assessing the possible drawbacks on postulated healthy nutrients by the different processing and cooking methods.

Cooking itself is associated with human evolution, and the first evidence of fire use can be related to the first cooking methods. The precise date when cooking was adopted is unknown, although brain development and digestive tract shrinking, estimated to have evolved up to about 1.8 million years ago, is related to the switch to a more energetically rich diet by cooking of starch foods (Carmody et al., 2011; Wrangham, 2013). Otherwise, it is the inclusion of fish or other lacustrine foods, which could have provided a means of initiating and sustaining cerebral cortex growth in the evolution of early modern humans (Broadhurst et al., 1998).

Humans employ a variety of novel food-processing techniques that improve food quality in various ways, not only by elevating energy density but also reducing toxins (Wrangham and Conklin-Brittain, 2003). Cooking as a means of processing food produces an intricate series of physical and chemical changes. We don't know the real purpose of first cooking, but natural selection surely helped not only in ameliorating the digestibility of certain nutrients, but also in preventing the deterioration by microorganisms and the acquisition of parasites. This allowed for further increases in the shelf life of acquired food. Additional human cultural signatures are seen in the attributes of preferences for color, texture, flavor or taste. These have caused the development of a variety of processing and cooking methods.

Cooking can have both beneficial and detrimental effects on the nutrient content of foods. It is able to improve sensory quality, but undesirable changes can be the loss of nutritive quality due to changes in the fatty acid profile and degradation of heat susceptible vitamins. Although there is growing awareness that the degree of processing food may affect general health, raw fish eating can be considered a cultural and culinary phenomenon, and nearly all around the world different raw fish dishes are served (Table 31.1). Local dishes are out of the scope of this chapter, but clearly cooking or processing methods have diversified and specialties such as sushi, sashimi (Japanese), or carpaccio (Italian) are spreading throughout the world.

Fish and Fish Oil in Health and Disease Prevention. http://dx.doi.org/10.1016/B978-0-12-802844-5.00031-2

TABLE 31.1 Most Popular Raw Fish Dishes on a Worldwide Scale

Speciality	Country of origin	Description
Anchovies in vinegar sauce	Spain/Italy	Marinated in vinegar, garlic and parsley (olive oil)
Carpaccio	Italy	Thinly sliced marinated swordfish or tuna
Ceviche	Peru	Marinated raw fish (citrus juices, aji, chilli peppers)
Gravlax	Scandinavia	Raw salmon, lightly cured in salt, sugar, dill, mustard. Sometimes fermented
Maatjes herring	Netherlands/Germany	Herring soaked in a mild preserving liquid
Rollmops	Germany	Pickled herring fillets (and onion gherkin)
Sashimi	Japan	Thinly sliced raw fish and seafood. Accompanied by soy sauce and wasabi
Sushi	Japan	Cooked (vinegared) rice, often prepared with raw seafood

HEALTH EFFECTS OF RAW FISH INTAKE

Introduction

Pre-agricultural diets are increasingly acknowledged as templates for healthy diets (Lindeberg, 2010). In these, health benefits have been demonstrated by increasing protein intake from meat, fish, and shellfish (O'Dea, 1984). Early epidemiological evidence demonstrated some populations to be protected from cardiovascular disease (Raatz et al., 2013) and a diet rich in fish and seafood has been the main way to provide a sufficiently high intake of n–3 PUFA. Otherwise, the possible contributions from other beneficial substances of marine food is warranted (Elvevoll et al., 2008) as is the fact that Eskimo and Japanese diets include frequently minimally processed marine food and eating habits. Japanese enjoy the longest life expectancy in the world. But the possible positive health effect of raw fish eating habits has not been sufficiently studied in epidemiological and comparative studies to make an associative link.

Several institutions and health agencies worldwide provide nutritional guidelines with specific recommendations on fish intake (Raatz et al., 2013). Recommendations are based on benefit-risk assessment. Standard tables of food compositions are mostly based on raw material. But during cooking and other forms of fish processing, nutrients with beneficial effects may be altered, destroyed or lowered. Consumption of fish as a source of n–3 PUFA has been demonstrated to be superior to the use of n–3 oil supplements (Elvevoll et al., 2006; Raatz et al., 2013; Visioli et al., 2003). Likewise, cooking methods compared to raw fish eating could have significant impact on the bioavailability not only of n–3 PUFA, but also of other nutrients. In addition, other concerns exist regarding to the possibility that cooking of fish could lead to the formation of potentially deleterious compounds, such as lipid oxidation products (Raatz et al., 2011). A further concern is that frying or grilling of fish products might generate low ppb levels of mutagenic/carcinogenic heterocyclic amines. Some of them are formed via the Maillard reaction from creatine, free amino acids and monosaccharides, compounds naturally occurring in protein-rich foods of animal origin (Skog et al., 1998).

There are a variety of studies addressing the influence of cooking on different fish components. The results are highly variable due to the variety of cooking methods, different fish species, and of distinct analytical methods used. Further, inconsistent findings could be due to different composition of raw material when comparing aquacultured or wild captured fish, as well as the known effect of season, capture zone, and other factors on nutrient content, especially fatty acid content (Lund, 2013). Additional complicating factors include some studies highlight the proximate composition, others only specific fatty acids, minerals of vitamins, and only a few studies are concerned with the possible bioavailability of the studied nutrients. Some epidemiologic evidence shows clinical outcome to be associated with cooking methods. Thus, only boiled and baked, but not fried fish and fish sandwiches were associated with a lower incidence of ischemic heart disease (Mozaffarian et al., 2003). These differences have been explained by low resistance of LC PUFAs to high cooking temperatures (Marangoni and Poli, 2013).

Some of the necessary points of interest for the analysis of health effects of raw versus cooked fish and seafood are summarized below.

Fatty Acid Composition

Most studies address those long chain omega-3 fatty acids which have been postulated to exert beneficial health effects. These PUFA are more susceptible to oxidation during heating than mono- or saturated fatty acids. In a digestion model, total lipid bio-accessibility showed a decrease to 70–80% in boiled and grilled meagre (*Argyrosomus regius*), with respect to raw fish and less in roasted fish (Afonso et al., 2015). Similar tendencies have also been detected when analyzing EPA and DHA.

Some studies show that in some kinds of fish (*Salmonidae*) n–3 PUFA levels remain unchanged after boiling, roasting or are only slightly reduced after frying (Gladyshev et al., 2006). EPA and DHA of cultivated meagre (*A. regius*) displayed identical profiles in raw or boiled samples (Costa et al., 2013). Baked salmon (*Salmo salar*) showed unaffected long chain n–3 PUFA content (Raatz et al., 2011, 2013). Another study assessed frying, broiling and baking of Chinook salmon (*Oncorhynchus tshawytscha*), common carp (*Cyprinus carpio carpio*) and lake trout (*Salvelinus namaycush*) without any appreciable changes in EPA and DHA or total n–3 FA, but slight reduction of DHA in walleye (*Sander vitreus*; Neff et al., 2014).

Wild and farmed sea bream (*Sparus aurata*) showed decreased levels of n–3 PUFA after steaming, grilling and frying in corn or sunflower oil, but increased n–6 PUFA, thus limiting the benefits of the high n–3 PUFA in raw fish (Mnari Bhouri et al., 2010). Deep frying may more importantly alter the fatty acid content of fish. Absorption of oil seems primarily responsible for the sometimes dramatic increase of some fatty acids, such as linoleic acid when fish is fried (Musaiger and R, 2011). Depending on the composition of the frying oils, PUFA levels generally rise due to absorption of oil during the frying process (Musaiger and R, 2011).

Interestingly, LC PUFA losses during cooking depend on the initial fat content of the species. In white species of fish, the main presence of fatty acids in phospholipids make them vulnerable to oxidation and losses during cooking were 28% for pollock (*Theragra chalcogramma*) and 8% for cod (*Gadus morhua*); however no significant fatty acid changes could be measured for oily Atlantic salmon (*S. salar*; James et al., 2009). Interestingly it has been hypothesized that high levels of natural antioxidants evolved as adaptation in to ecological niches in some species making PUFA less vulnerable to oxidation by heat treatment (Gladyshev et al., 2006).

Some studies indirectly address nutritional quality indices. Atherogenic and thrombogenic indices decreased after frying of a variety of frozen shellfish in sunflower oil and claimed to be beneficial from a nutritional point of view (Czech et al., 2015). Boiling, grilling or roasting of meagre (*Argyrosomus regius*) showed important changes in fatty acid composition, but without affecting atherogenic and thrombogenic indices (Costa et al., 2013). One study showed an increase of n–3/n–6 fatty acid ratio in canola oil fried silver catfish (*Rhamdia quelen*; Weber et al., 2008).

LC PUFA, EPA, and DHA serum incorporation after an 8 weeks trial from cooked salmon fillets was higher compared with smoked salmon, but did not reach statistical significance (Elvevoll et al., 2006).

Another concern is the possible production of *trans*-FAs through cooking (Hunter and Applewhite, 1991; Li et al., 2013). Boiling and baking of silver catfish (*Rhamdia quelen*) increased thiobarbituric acid reactive substances, a measure used in oxidation studies (Weber et al., 2008). Grilling of anchovies causes formation of potentially hazardous lipid oxidation products (Turhan et al., 2011). Conversely, baking of salmon lead to a decrease in most n–3 and n–6 lipid oxidation products (Raatz et al., 2011).

Generally, the evidence seems to indicate that taking into account the species and cooking methods, reduction of EPA and DHA or other LC PUFA cannot be ruled out especially after frying. Changes in the n–3/n–6 as well as saturated/polyunsaturated fatty acid could be negatively affected by some cooking methods.

Taurine and Bioactive Peptides

Taurine has been postulated to have antioxidant and osmoregulatory functions and to be an important membrane stabilizer (Huxtable, 1992). The synthesis rate of taurine in humans is low and is even fortified in infant formula. High content is found in invertebrates, such as mussels and scallops and overall the content is significantly higher in fish than in meat. Taurine is a reliable biomarker of fish intake and uptake from marine sources was shown to be higher in Japanese than in a Mediterranean population (Yamori et al., 2009). Overall, thermal processing seems to reduce significantly taurine content of seafood. Boiling removes taurine up to 70%, possibly by leaching into the boiling water (Larsen et al., 2007).

Bioactive peptides can originate from fish and some of them have been found to exert antihypertensive, antibacterial, anticoagulant, antiinflammatory, or antioxidant activities. Examples are ACE inhibitory peptides found in various fish and shellfish species. However, the possible and real physiological effect in vivo is dependent on the bioavailability of the peptides (Ryan et al., 2011).

Vitamins

A fish portion of 200 g may provide the recommended daily intake of vitamins D, B6, and B12 (Oehlenschläger, 2012), but this depends on the species of fish, its fat content, or the parts eaten. There are great differences depending on whether fish originates from wild capture or aquaculture. For the last, different cultivation approaches yield variable quantities of these vitamins (Lund, 2013). Thus, fish as a whole dietary source is unlikely to provide the recommended daily doses (Lu et al., 2007).

The vitamin A and D content of baked and microwaved fish did not change with respect to raw for kutum roach (*Rutilus frisiikutum*, family Cyprinidae), but significant reductions were found for frying and boiling (Hosseini et al., 2014). In another study, when frying salmon in vegetable oil, approximately 50% vitamin D3 was recovered (Lu et al., 2007). The vitamin B12 of round herrings (*Etrumeus teres*) decreases on the order of 50% by grilling, frying, steaming, and microwaving (Nishioka et al., 2011).

Few studies directly address the health effects of popular raw fish dishes. One study calculated that five portions of sushi with 20 g of seawater sashimi toppings would supply the recommended daily allowance of vitamin B6 (Do and Yagi, 2012). This is important, as losses of Vitamin B have been estimated to be 10%–70% with different cooking methods, and specifically around 30% for Vitamin B6 by boiling and braising (Bognar, 1998). Vitamin E lipid soluble and stability in fish muscle to microwave cooking was observed (Polat et al., 2013).

Generally, vitamin C is very low or absent in fish or seafood. Interestingly, the Eskimo practice of eating their food (mainly fish) in the raw, frozen, or lightly cooked state was a critical factor in preserving the small amounts of vitamin C necessary to prevent scurvy (less than 10 mg per day; Draper, 1977).

Minerals

Depending on the species and origin, fish provides a well balanced supply of minerals in a readily usable form and includes important ones such as iodine, selenium, calcium, and phosphorus. But other minerals such as magnesium, zinc, and manganese are found in lesser quantities (Hosseini et al., 2014). Plasma selenium has been found to correlate with the number of high selenium fish meals consumed per month (Hagmar et al., 1998). Different cooking practices have been shown to reduce selenium content by 36–46% in fish (Bratakos et al., 1988). Content of other minerals (ash) is reduced by 25–50% when fish is prepared by boiling or steaming (Bognar, 1998).

Boiling and microwave caused significant reduction of trace elements (Hosseini Farahabadi et al., 2006), while magnesium, iron, and potassium levels were reduced in boiled and roasted samples (Costa et al., 2013). Different cooking methods such as boiling, grilling or baking of farmed or wild sea bream (*Sparus aurata*) caused important losses of minerals, such as magnesium, calcium, potassium and zinc, but frying yielded the most losses (Mnari et al., 2012).

Other

There is a concern that freezing and defrosting the fish could ruin the texture and overall culinary quality of fish. While degradation by formation of ice crystals and rupture of membranes are effects of freezing, undesirable modifications in taurine or other low molecular weight compounds seem not to be significant for freezing of less than 6 months for raw mullet (*Mugil* spp.) or fish roe (Piras et al., 2014). Although a recent randomized double-blind trial did not find freezing to ruin sushi's taste, individuals who consume raw fish more than once a week were excluded from the analysis, which could bias the conclusions (Iwata et al., 2015). It is possible that people who like raw fish dishes, such as sushi and sashimi, would prefer never-frozen far better than previously frozen fish.

Additional practical issues are processes, such as "warmholding" or "coldholding", with the risk of deterioration of heat-labile components of fish. Warmholding has been shown to produce differences in the content of fatty acids after frying compared to immediately cooked fish (Candela et al., 1997).

HEALTH RISKS OF RAW FISH INTAKE

Introduction

As is the case for other food items, fish is normally submitted to a culinary treatment to make it more digestible and microbiologically safe, and also to enhance its sensory attributes. However, to preserve fishery products for a long storage life, traditional preserving methods have been applied throughout history. These include salting, drying, smoking, or fermenting. Of note traditional fish preparation could be protecting against auto-oxidation during the preparation process (Montano et al., 2001). Frequently these evolved specialties are consumed without further cooking. Whereas these methods cause changes in the water activity, pH and other antibacterial activities by for example, the salt and smoke components, these processes still maintain a potential risk for parasites, and also histamine poisoning. Increased risk may also be due to changes in the originally evolved methodologies over the years (Köse, 2010).

Risk of Parasites in Raw Fish

Fish and seafood product-borne parasitic diseases include primarily those caused by cestodes, trematodes, nematodes and recently also Myxosporidia. These diseases are caused by an infection following ingestion of viable parasites. They are sometimes accompanied by an allergic (hypersensitivity) reaction against parasite antigens for nematodes of the family *Anisakidae*. Human fishery product-borne parasitic infections have originally been limited to populations living in low- and middle-income countries, but due to commercial and cultural globalization, the geographical limits and populations at risk are expanding (Chai et al., 2005). The World Health Organization has estimated that the number of people currently infected with fish-borne clinically significant trematodes exceeds 40 million (World Health Organization, 2004), but worldwide the number of people at risk, including those in developed countries, is more than half a billion. Awareness of the public health significance of these diseases is increasing due to intensification of aquaculture, cultural traditions, as well as increasing tendencies to eat raw or minimally processed fishery products (World Health Organization, 1995, 2004). A further emerging health concern is the recognition of allergic reactions associated to *Anisakis* spp., which could have important deleterious effects on the implementation of a healthy diet. Therefore, a special emphasis on this topic will be given in this chapter.

Trematodes

Within the more than 100 fish-borne trematode species infecting humans, Clonorchiasis and Opisthorchiasis are the most important for human illnesses. These parasitic diseases are produced by trematodes infecting freshwater fish and shrimp in wide areas of the world, such as Europe, North America, and Asia and can be sources of human infection. People get infected if they eat raw or undercooked freshwater and sometimes brackish water fish (or rarely shrimps), containing active metacercariae (Chai et al., 2005). Examples of culinary risk factors in specific regions are consumption of: rice gruel with slices of raw freshwater fish in southern China and Hong Kong; slices of raw freshwater fish with red pepper sauce in Korea; half roasted or undercooked fish in Guangdong Province; raw shrimps in Fujian Province in China; 'Koi pla' dish consisting of raw fish flesh chopped with garlic, lemon juice, fish sauce, chili, roasted ground rice, and local vegetables in north-eastern Thailand and Laos, (*Opisthorchis viverrini*) (EFSA, 2010). The transmission of fish-borne trematodiases is generally associated to focal areas where the first (snail species) and second intermediate (freshwater fish) hosts coexist and humans (final host together with carnivores, human pets and birds) eat raw fish dishes. But emerging patterns of infection have been recently caused by the increased consumption elsewhere of regional fish dishes such as sushi, sashimi, ceviche, carpaccio based on raw or minimally processed fish, due to the growth in the international trade in fish and fish products, and the development of aquaculture (World Health Organization, 2011). The recirculation of waste material including human and animal manure is conducive for the life cycle of fish-borne zoonotic trematodes (Hung et al., 2013). In fact, the future impact of these parasite group is associated with growing aquaculture in Asia, providing nearly 90% of freshwater production (World Health Organization, 2004).

The number of people currently infected with liver flukes (family Opisthorchiidae) exceeds 40 million and unknown millions are infected with intestinal flukes (Chai et al., 2009; World Health Organization, 1995, 2004) but it is estimated that more than 700 million are at risk of infection (Petney et al., 2013; World Health Organization, 1995).

Clonorchis sinensis (Chinese liver fluke) is acquired by eating parasitized raw freshwater fish. Endemic areas are several countries of East Asia, with an estimated number of infected people of 7–10 million (Crompton, 1999). Other causative agents are *Opisthorchis viverrini*, *Opisthorchis felineus* and several minor species, for example, *Metorchis conjunctus* (Hung et al., 2013). Serious complications of liver fluke infection include cholangitis, choledocholithisais, pancreatitis or even cholangiocarcinoma.

In contrast to the high morbidity of the described liver flukes, intestinal trematodes (especially *Heterophyes* spp. and *Echinostoma* spp.) are more common, and in fact are the most common parasitic infections in humans and animals. About 70 species of intestinal food-borne zoonotic trematodes have been reported to infect people (Yu, 1994) and around 30 of these are transmitted through intake of raw or undercooked fish (Chai et al., 2009). These trematodes are associated with less mortality, but still pose health concerns due to morbidity, food safety and quality issues.

The lung fluke *Paragonimus westermani* is mainly from Asia and infection occurs via intake of raw or undercooked freshwater crustaceans (mainly crabs and crayfish) in which live larvae (metacercariae) are present. This infection is also known in other areas of the world due to immigration or returning travelers, or the presence of other indigenous species, such as *Paragonimus kellicotti* in areas of the United States, Africa, South America, and Europe (Diaz, 2013; EFSA, 2010). If patients complain of unexplained fever, cough, hemoptysis, pleural effusions, and eosinophilia with a history of previous intake of raw or undercooked crustaceans, diagnostic evaluation should be performed to rule out lung fluke.

Cestodes

Diphyllobothrium spp. are widely distributed tapeworms in fish, mammal and bird hosts (Dick et al., 2001) and are generally associated with intermediate and definitive hosts living in cold water habitats. *D. latum* and *D. nihonkaiense* exploit freshwater copepods as their first intermediate host. The infective form is the second larval stage, called plerocercoid larva in freshwater fish. However, in contrast to *D. latum*, which uses freshwater fish such as perch, char, and pike as the second intermediate host, *D. nihonkaiense* uses anadromous fish, *Oncorhynchus* spp., such as *O. masou* (masu salmon), *O. gorbuscha* (pink salmon), and *O. keta* (chum salmon), which migrate in the holoarctic region (Ando et al., 2001). Globally, the incidence of Diphyllobothriasis has declined over the last decades, particularly in North America (Dick et al., 2001). It was reported to be a common infection in Far-Eastern Russia (Muratov, 1990) and is frequently reported in Japan with a recent resurge of cases (Arizono et al., 2009) and other Far East Asian countries. In Europe the incidence has declined except in Switzerland, Sweden, Finland, and Estonia (Dupouy-Camet and Peduzzi, 2004; EFSA, 2010). Consumption of raw or insufficiently cooked or marinated fish containing larval plerocercoids is the main source of infection with *Diphyllobothrium* for humans. Wild-caught fish prepared in a variety of ways such as for sushi, sashimi, carpaccio, or ceviche may pose a high risk of exposure (Deardorff et al., 1991; Kuchta et al., 2013; Scholz et al., 2009). Wild pacific salmon caught in spring has been associated with infection by *D. nihonkaiense* in Japan. It has been emphasized that the epidemiology of this tapeworm has changed drastically from rural to urban areas because of the rapid expansion of the transport system for fresh fish meeting the demand for seafood in healthy diets (Arizono et al., 2009). Cases of infection with *D. nihonkaiense* have been reported after consumption of imported Pacific salmon (Go et al., 2015).

Diphyllobothrium tapeworms can live for several years in the human small intestine and reach a length of more than 15 meters. Symptoms generally do not cause severe problems, although abdominal discomfort (abdominal pain, diarrhea), weight loss and asthenia are seen. Megaloblastic anemia can be due to vitamin B-12 deficiency in prolonged infestation (Bonsdorff, 1977). However, human *Diphyllobothriasis* is generally a mild illness, normally not reported in epidemiologic surveys.

Nematodes

Anisakidae

Anisakis are parasites of the genera *Anisakis, Pseudoterranova, Hysterothylacium. Anisakis simplex, Anisakis pegreffi* and *Pseudoterranova decipiens* are of major public health interest. In contrast to most other fish-borne parasite hazards acquired with intake of freshwater seafood, *Anisakids* are parasites associated with marine fish. Although *Anisakis* infection associated disease has been described for several decades, mainly from raw-fish eating Dutch and Japanese populations, from the mid 90's clinically overt allergic reactions have been associated with this parasite and have produced a world-wide concern on this cosmopolitan parasite. Interest in this parasite has extended to several disciplines, not only in the field of fisheries, parasitology, food safety, but also to several specialties in medicine, with new interest in the fields of Allergy and Immunology. Up to 20% of published papers on *Anisakis* are associated with analysis of allergic phenomena in the last years (Fig. 31.1).

Whereas other health hazards related to parasites are often geographically limited and if of international concern relates to fast transportation systems, import, and returning travelers, *Anisakis* can be detected in a vast array of fish and cephalopods and have a worldwide distribution. Within these, *A. simplex* commonly occurs

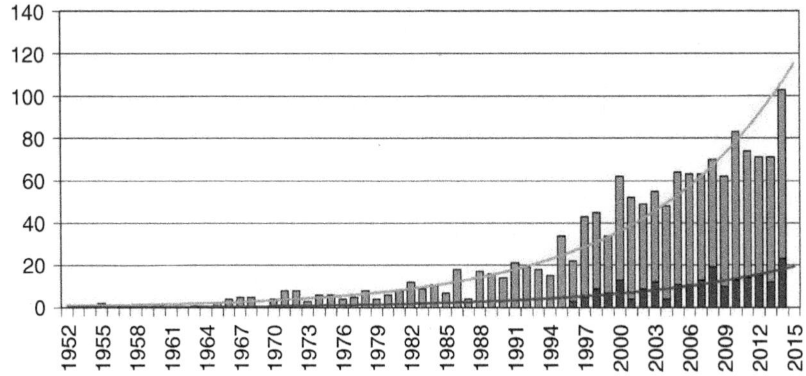

FIGURE 31.1 **Web of Science based annual publications about *Anisakis*.** Grey bars denote the number of all published papers with searchterm "*Anisakis*" and red bars Boolean search for "*Anisakis* and Allergy".

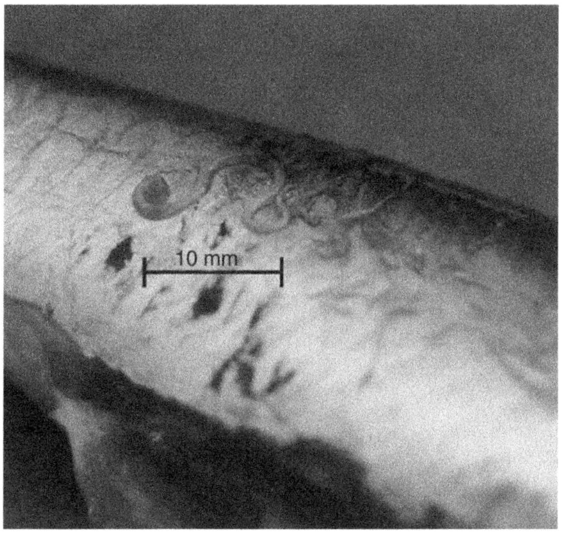

FIGURE 31.2 *Anisakis* sp. on a raw anchovy.

in various ecologically and economically important fish species such as herring, mackerel, blue whiting, cod and monkfish (EFSA, 2010). Therefore, there is emerging and continuous concern of food safety institutions on *Anisakis* as a fish-borne parasite. As will be detailed below, not only are classical *Anisakis* induced digestive or extraintestinal complaints associated with raw fish eating habits, but also emerging *Anisakis* associated allergic phenomena.

Classical Diseases In 1960 van Thiel identified the third stage larva of *Anisakis* in surgical laparotomies and the term anisakiasis as a clinical entity has been used since then. Raw fish eating in form of lightly salted pickled herring (therefore also called herring worm) was the source of acquisition of this parasite by the patients. In 1968, Dutch legislation, that required freezing of fish before further processing, led to a dramatic decrease of anisakiasis cases. Meanwhile the first case of anisakiasis in Japan was described in 1965 (Asami et al., 1965). Since then, Japan has had the most cases of the different forms of anisakiasis with more than 1000 cases yearly. Anisakiasis is beginning to be described also in other countries as well, like in the United States (Kliks, 1983; Oshima, 1987).

Clinical forms can be classified as gastric, intestinal or extra-intestinal anisakiasis depending on the location (Smith and Wootten, 1978). Acute gastric anisakiasis is the most commonly reported form, followed by acute intestinal anisakiasis. Most human cases of anisakiasis likely go unreported, without causing any symptoms or clinical signs. In acute cases, patients complain of epigastric pain, nauseas and vomiting. These symptoms occur mainly within hours of the intake of the suspected meal and are produced by the local inflammatory reaction when the worm penetrates the gastric mucosa. Emergency treatment includes gastroscopic extraction of the live penetrating larva. Acute intestinal infection which appears one to seven days after consuming infected fish has less specific abdominal symptoms and is accompanied by fever and diarrhea and/or constipation.

Chronic anisakiasis is caused by granuloma formation as an immunologic response against the foreign body and can last from weeks to years. In some rare cases the larva reaches extraintestinal locations, such as peritoneum or pleura. Of note, most chronic cases of anisakiasis are diagnosed after surgical removal of the affected zone, because *Anisakis* larvae do not survive longer than a few days in the human host (Fig. 31.2).

Emerging Diseases Japanese authors already described urticaria as one of the possible symptoms accompanying gastric anisakiasis (Asaishi et al., 1980; Kasuya et al., 1990). In fact, abdominal symptoms had already been attributed to be an "allergic" response, because of specific IgE production in these patients, but by 1995 anaphylaxis was interpreted to be due to *Anisakis* allergy. By 2000, it is well established that acute allergic symptoms, such as urticaria, angioedema, or anaphylaxis are produced by the live third stage larva of *Anisakis*. This emerging entity is called gastroallergic anisakiasis (Daschner et al., 1998; Daschner et al., 2000; López-Serrano et al., 2000). Some authors postulate acute allergic reactions to be also possible when sensitized patients enter in contact with allergen alone from killed parasite, but the relative epidemiological impact of the described clinical descriptions is unknown (EFSA, 2010).

Further, no challenge test has been shown to be positive in sensitized patients when they were administered inactivated *Anisakis* larvae or excretory-secretory proteins (Alonso et al., 1999; Baeza et al., 2004).

Gastro-allergic anisakiasis (GAA) was initially described for *A. simplex*, but a recent study showed this entity also to be produced by *A. pegreffi* (Mattiucci et al., 2013). This is an acute IgE-mediated generalized reaction with cutaneous (urticarial-angioedema), and/or respiratory (rhinitis and asthma), and typically abdominal symptoms like nausea, vomiting or epigastric pain. But gastric symptoms in this clinical picture remain often mild or even absent.

A series of papers addressing allergic phenomena has been published from different countries since the late 90's. Although it seems that there is a real increase in larval *Anisakis* populations, the rise in reporting gastro-allergic anisakiasis can at least in part be accounted for by awareness and knowledge of this entity due to the peculiar clinical characteristics. Allergic symptoms can begin up to 24 h and more after the intake of the infected fish contrary to true food-allergic reactions (Daschner et al., 2012; Daschner et al., 2002).

Further studies in the field of immunology have shown the production of various isotypes of immunoglobulins and polyclonal stimulation of these immunoglobulins which are a typical characteristics of an immune response against a living parasite (Cuéllar et al., 2013; Daschner et al., 1999; Daschner et al., 2002).

The fact that *Anisakis* and humans did not coevolve explains that humans are only an accidental host of *Anisakis*, and therefore this larva does not survive more than a few days in humans. This fact is probably responsible for the high prevalence of allergic phenomena associated with this nematode.

Anisakis sensitization associated chronic urticaria has also been associated with the larva. Sensitization (presence of specific IgE against *Anisakis*) has to be interpreted as a sign of a previous acute parasitism. In this scenario, the parasitic episode often goes clinically unidentified, but due to still unknown causes sensitized patients have a higher risk of suffering chronic urticaria (Daschner et al., 2013; Daschner and Pascual, 2005; López-Sáez et al., 2003; Ventura et al., 2013). The presence of anti-*Anisakis* IgE antibodies in frequent fish-eaters was postulated to be associated with the chronic reaction, but a prospective clinical study showed that patients, who followed a diet without fish had a worse prognosis (Daschner et al., 2013). As improvement of chronic urticaria was associated with higher ratios of anti-/proinflammatory cytokines and previous higher oily fish intake was also associated with improvement, it was concluded that intrinsic fish-intake associated benefits were more important than the possible sensitization status in these patients (Daschner et al., 2013).

Prevention Preventive measures for anisakiasis have been implemented in different regions due to the risk of acute parasitism with *Anisakis*. Interestingly, epidemiological studies show that fish consumption per se is not the main risk factor for sensitization. Regions with very high fish consumption, such as Norway or Galicia (North-west Spain) have a very low prevalence of population-based IgE antibodies against *Anisakis* (Lin et al., 2014; Valiñas et al., 2001). Here, no raw fish eating habits exist or awareness of previous freezing has been adopted. But in Japan, with its sushi and sashimi eating habits, Spain and Italy, where anchovies in vinegar sauce are eaten, high prevalence of sensitization has been shown as well as the higher probability of digestive or gastro-allergic anisakiasis (Consortium, 2011; Daschner et al., 1998; Kimura et al., 1999; Puente et al., 2008).

There is more information available on the resistance to physical and chemical treatments by *Anisakis* than for other fish parasites. It is now clear that traditional processing methods are not sufficient to kill *Anisakis*. Importantly, freezing at −20°C for not less than 24, preferably 48 h or heat treatment at >60°C at the core of the fishery products for at least 1 min are recommendations of the European Food Safety agency, which takes into account also the emerging allergic phenomena (EFSA, 2010). Similar recommendations are posted elsewhere.

Gnathostoma

Infection with the nematode *Gnathostoma* spp. (Gnathostomiasis) can result from eating raw or partly cooked freshwater fish. *Gnathostoma spinigerum* is accidentally ingested in the larval third stage of this helminth. Most disease related to *Gnathostoma* was reported from Southeast Asia, but is now considered an emerging disease in Central and South America, especially Mexico, where it is suspected to be acquired by eating ceviche (Martínez-Cruz et al., 1989). International travel, immigration patterns and returning travelers results in increasing notification of this disease in other parts of the world (Moore et al., 2003). Larvae cannot mature to its adult form in humans and clinical symptoms are elicited by the migrating larvae, which produces an inflammatory reaction. Nonspecific visceral symptoms as well as cutaneous symptoms, such as intermittent subcutaneous swellings and urticaria can occur. Rare complications of the central nervous system may cause eosinophilic encephalitis, subarachnoid hemorrhage, myelitis or radiculitis (Herman and Chiodini, 2009). Importantly, the median time from onset of symptoms to diagnosis can be as long as 12 months in nonendemic countries (Moore et al., 2003).

Myxosporean Parasites

Kudoa spp. are myxosporean parasites of sea fishes. They have a worldwide distribution, and infect a wide range of host species. A major concern is that species are responsible for causing economic losses to the fisheries sector by causing postmortem myoliquefaction. *K. septempunctata* has recently been shown to be a causative agent of previously unidentified food poisoning when eating olive flounder (*Paralichthys olivaceus*) in Japan (Harada et al., 2012; Kawai et al., 2012). This food-borne disease is typically associated with the intake of traditional sushi or sashimi, prepared using raw flounder muscle tissue containing more than 10,000 spores of *K. septempunctata* per gram (Kawai et al., 2012). Since 2003, outbreaks of unidentified food-borne illness associated with raw fish intake have increased and this myxosporean is implicated as the etiological agent, thus showing the pathogenic potential of *Kudoa* spores (Kawai et al., 2012). This resulted in the suspicion that other *Kudoa* species could be pathogenic for humans. Further studies showed other species, such as *K. neothunni* in Pacific bluefin and an adult yellowfin tuna have also been suspected to be responsible for food borne outbreaks (Abe and Maehara, 2013). Clinical symptoms include self-limiting, but intense diarrhea and emesis 2–20 h after ingestion of raw parasitized fish (Kawai et al., 2012). International trade of aquacultured fish has already caused this parasite to be detected in imported fish from Korea (Matsukane et al., 2010).

In one study, anti-*Kudoa* spp. IgE antibodies were observed in patients with allergic reactions after fish consumption (Martínez de Velasco et al., 2007). In experimental models, oral administration of pseudocysts to mice induced specific IgE antibodies. These IgE responses confirm the possible allergenic nature of some of the parasite components (Martínez de Velasco et al., 2008).

Risk of Bacterial Pathogens in Raw Fish

Most outbreaks occur after ingestion of inadequately heat-treated fish dishes or products contaminated after or during their processing. Most gastroenteritis episodes are self limiting and sources of infection include raw or undercooked fish-meals.

Species like *Listeria vibrio* have been isolated from sea or coastal waters (Novotny et al., 2004). Fish are carriers of bacteria which can be pathogenic, such as *Salmonella* spp., *Clostridia* spp. or pathogenic *Staphylococcus* spp., and are able to contaminate through mishandling (Köse, 2010). Examples of some species associated with specific processing techniques are: the risk of *Clostridium botulinum* in smoked fish (Kapchunka; Telzak et al., 1990), outbreaks of listeriosis associated with vacuum-packed gravlax and cold-smoked fish (Tham et al., 2000) or *Staphylococcus aureus* detected during the process of drying and smoking of eels in Alaska (Eklund et al., 2004). The required safety precautions of the use of very fresh fish handled in hygienic conditions and chilling the product to 2°C reduces the risk of foodborne illness from fish products.

Scombroid Poisoning

Scombroid poisoning or histamine fish poisoning results when biogenic amines are formed in large quantities by bacterial decarboxylation of histidine, especially of scombroid fish, such as bonito, tuna, and mackerel with high levels of this amino acid. It can also be produced with nonscombroid fatty and migrating fish species. Several bacteria are involved and most seem to be derived from postcatching contamination. Histamine forming bacteria exist on the gills and in the gut of these fish. Histidine decarboxylase responsible for the generation of histamine and bacteria can be inactivated by cooking.

Freezing is also able to inactivate bacteria. However, once the enzyme histidine decarboxylase has been formed, it can continue to produce histamine in the fish even if the bacteria are not active (Köse, 2010). Histamine that has already been formed is not destroyed by cooking, while bacteria may rapidly reactivate after thawing.

If the histamine is ingested in large quantities, it may cause an anaphylactoid reaction with a variety of symptoms from moderate to severe to life-threating.

Further Considerations

Traditional fish products applying ancient methods of preservation originally developed to allow for a long storage life. These methods include fermenting, drying or smoking which limit the growth of bacteria, and frequently are consumed without further cooking. Further elaboration evolved to gain acceptance because of specific taste and aroma.

Of note, brining and pickling may reduce the parasite hazard, but it does not eliminate it. Species that normally have a parasite hazard as a result of consuming infected prey normally do not have the same parasite hazard when raised only on pelleted feed in aquaculture. In one study addressing farmed Atlantic salmon, individual fish with clear signs of poor performance over time and abnormal appearance showed infection by *A. simplex* and *Hysterothylacium aduncum*, but these runts are not processed for human consumption. Otherwise no nematodes were found in the musculature or viscera of harvest quality salmon specimen (Mo et al., 2014).

In some countries it seems that fish consumption is reduced because of fears about mercury or chemical contaminants. Further, increased awareness of parasite infection, especially *Anisakis* spp., may result in reduced fish consumption, even when it has been demonstrated that only live parasites are able to elicit disease. For the case of raw fish consumption, proper food preparation by adequate freezing prior to consumption is sufficient for inactivation of parasites.

CONCLUSIONS

It is possible that evolutionary pressure has gone hand in hand with traditional processing of fish. With respect to raw fish preparations, the addition of traditional spices or salting would have been sufficient to kill the bacterial pathogens which cause acute illness. In this scenario symptoms would have been associated with food, especially when affecting several communities and could have led to adopting adequate processing techniques. Most parasites which produce chronic disease are resistant to these techniques. In the special case of *Anisakis*, clinical peculiarities make it difficult to diagnosis in many cases.

According to FAO, it is necessary to assess the health benefits and risks associated with the consumption of fish and balance them in order to enjoy the benefits while minimizing the risks (FAO, 2010, 2014). The risk of consuming potentially contaminated foods has recently received greater attention than the benefits of eating them. This holds for both chemical contamination as well as parasite infection (FAO, 2010, 2014). In fact, as an example, the benefits are likely to be at least 100-fold greater than the estimates of harm, when analyzing prenatal cognitive development, coronary heart disease mortality, and stroke with respect to the possible harm of MeHg compared to the benefit of high n–3 fish intake. Although high compliance with recommended fish consumption patterns can improve public health, unintended shifts in consumption can lead to public health losses (Cohen et al., 2005).

Fish is often not included in the diet. One should be aware of the opportunity given by the world-wide expansion of raw fish eating habits and restaurants which offer raw fish specialties, not only from the culinary viewpoint, but also as a means of partially satisfying essential nutritional necessities. Proper handling of raw fish prior to its intake has been shown to be sufficient to inactivate possible parasite hazards. Further studies should focus on comparative nutritional end-effects of raw versus cooked fish and seafood preparations. It is clear that there is a broad array of health risks associated with raw fish eating habits. These risks can easily be prevented by regulatory means and even at the consumer level by freezing of fish prior to consumption Scientific evidence provides evidence of adequate preparation techniques for raw fish consumption not only on a private, but also commercial basis. These effective methods for preventing disease risk from consuming raw fish should therefore be instituted.

Abbreviations

n–3 PUFA omega-3 polyunsaturated fatty acids
n–6 PUFA omega-3 polyunsaturated fatty acids
LC PUFA long chain polyunsaturated fatty acids
EPA Eicosapentaenoic acid
DHA Docosahexaenoic acid

References

Abe, N., Maehara, T., 2013. Molecular characterization of kudoid parasites (Myxozoa: Multivalvulida) from somatic muscles of Pacific bluefin (*Thunnus orientalis*) and yellowfin (*T. albacores*) tuna. Acta Parasitol. 58, 226–230.

Afonso, C., Costa, S., Cardoso, C., Bandarra, N.M., Batista, I., Coelho, I., Castanheira, I., Nunes, M.L., 2015. Evaluation of the risk/benefit associated to the consumption of raw and cooked farmed meagre based on the bioaccessibility of selenium, eicosapentaenoic acid and docosahexaenoic acid, total mercury, and methylmercury determined by an in vitro digestion model. Food Chem. 170, 249–256.

Alonso, A., Moreno-Ancillo, A., Daschner, A., López-Serrano, M., 1999. Dietary assessment in five cases of allergic reactions due to gastroallergic anisakiasis. Allergy 54, 517–520.

Ando, K., Ishikura, K., Nakakugi, T., Shimono, Y., Tamai, T., Sugawa, M., Limviroj, W., Chinzei, Y., 2001. Five cases of *Diphyllobothrium nihonkaiense* infection with discovery of plerocercoids from an infective source, *Oncorhynchus masou* ishikawae. J. Parasitol. 87, 96–100.

Arizono, N., Yamada, M., Nakamura-Uchiyama, F., Ohnishi, K., 2009. Diphyllobothriasis associated with eating raw pacific salmon. Emerg. Infect. Dis. 15, 866–870.

Asaishi, K., Nishino, C., Totsuka, M., Hayasaka, H., Suzuki, T., 1980. Studies on the etiologic mechanism of anisakiasis. –2. Epidemiologic study of inhabitants and questionaire survey in Japan. Gastroenterol. Japan 15, 128–134.

Asami, K., Watanuki, T., Sakai, H., Imano, H., Okamoto, R., 1965. Two cases of stomach granuloma caused by Anisakis-like larval nematodes in Japan. Am. J. Trop. Med. Hyg. 14, 119–123.

Baeza, M., Rodríguez, A., Matheu, V., Rubio, M., Tornero, P., de Barrio, M., Herrero, T., Santaolalla, M., Zubeldia, J., 2004. Characterization of allergens secreted by Anisakis simplex parasite: clinical relevance in comparison with somatic allergens. Clin. Exp. Allergy 34, 296–302.

Bognar, A., 1998. Comparative study of frying to other cooking techniques influence on the nutritive value. Grasas. Y. Aceites. 49, 250–260.

Bonsdorff, B.v., 1977. Diphyllobothriasis in man. Academic Press, London; New York.

Bratakos, M.S., Zafiropoulos, T.F., Siskos, P.A., Ioannou, P.V., 1988. Selenium losses on cooking Greek foods. Int. J. Food Sci. Technol. 23, 585–590.

Broadhurst, C.L., Cunnane, S.C., Crawford, M.A., 1998. Rift Valley lake fish and shellfish provided brain-specific nutrition for early Homo. Br. J. Nutr. 79, 3–21.

Candela, M., Astiasaran, I., Bello, J., 1997. Effects of frying and warmholding on fatty acids and cholesterol of sole (*Solea solea*), codfish (*Gadus morrhua*) and hake (*Merluccius merluccius*). Food Chem. 58, 227–231.

Carmody, R.N., Weintraub, G.S., Wrangham, R.W., 2011. Energetic consequences of thermal and nonthermal food processing. Proc. Natl. Acad. Sci. USA 108, 19199–19203.

Chai, J., Darwin Murrell, K., Lymbery, A., 2005. Fish-borne parasitic zoonoses: status and issues. Int. J. Parasitol. 35, 1233–1254.

Chai, J.Y., Shin, E.H., Lee, S.H., Rim, H.J., 2009. Foodborne intestinal flukes in Southeast Asia. Kor. J. Parasitol. 47 (Suppl.), S69–102.

Cohen, J.T., Bellinger, D.C., Connor, W.E., Kris-Etherton, P.M., Lawrence, R.S., Savitz, D.A., Shaywitz, B.A., Teutsch, S.M., Gray, G.M., 2005. A quantitative risk-benefit analysis of changes in population fish consumption. Am. J. Prev. Med. 29, 325–334.

Consortium, A.-I.A., 2011. Anisakis hypersensitivity in Italy: prevalence and clinical features: a multicenter study. Allergy 66, 1563–1569.

Costa, S., Afonso, C., Bandarra, N.M., Gueifão, S., Castanheira, I., Carvalho, M.L., Cardoso, C., Nunes, M.L., 2013. The emerging farmed fish species meagre (*Argyrosomus regius*): how culinary treatment affects nutrients and contaminants concentration and associated benefit-risk balance. Food Chem. Toxicol. 60, 277–285.

Crompton, D.W., 1999. How much human helminthiasis is there in the world? J. Parasitol. 85, 397–403.

Cuéllar, C., Valls, A., de Frutos, C., Rodero, M., Daschner, A., 2013. Avidity studies in anisakis simplex-associated allergic diseases. J. Allergy (Cairo) 2013, 106781.

Czech, A., Grela, E.R., Ognik, K., 2015. Effect of frying on nutrients content and fatty acid composition of muscles of selected freezing seafoods. J. Food Nutr. Res. 3, 9–14.

Daschner, A., Alonso-Gómez, A., Caballero, T., Barranco, P., Suarez-De-Parga, J.M., López-Serrano, M.C., 1998. Gastric anisakiasis: an underestimated cause of acute urticaria and angio-oedema? Br. J. Dermatol. 139, 822–828.

Daschner, A., Alonso-Gómez, A., Caballero, T., Suarez-De-Parga, J., López-Serrano, M., 1999. Usefulness of early serial measurement of specific and total immunoglobulin E in the diagnosis of gastro-allergic anisakiasis. Clin. Exp. Allergy 29, 1260–1264.

Daschner, A., Alonso-Gómez, A., Cabañas, R., Suarez-de-Parga, J., López-Serrano, M., 2000. Gastroallergic anisakiasis: borderline between food allergy and parasitic disease-clinical and allergologic evaluation of 20 patients with confirmed acute parasitism by *Anisakis simplex*. J. Allergy Clin. Immunol. 105, 176–181.

Daschner, A., Cuéllar, C., Rodero, M., 2012. The Anisakis allergy debate: does an evolutionary approach help? Trends Parasitol. 28, 9–15.

Daschner, A., Cuéllar, C., Sánchez-Pastor, S., Pascual, C., Martín-Esteban, M., 2002. Gastro-allergic anisakiasis as a consequence of simultaneous primary and secondary immune response. Parasite Immunol. 24, 243–251.

Daschner, A., Fernández-Fígares, V., Valls, A., de Frutos, C., Rodero, M., Ubeira, F.M., Cuéllar, C., 2013. Different fish-eating habits and cytokine production in chronic urticaria with and without sensitization against the fish-parasite anisakis simplex. Allergol. Int. 62, 191–201.

Daschner, A., Pascual, C., 2005. Anisakis simplex: sensitization and clinical allergy. Curr. Opin. Aller. Clin. Immunol. 5, 281–285.

Deardorff, T., Kayes, S., Fukumura, T., 1991. Human anisakiasis transmitted by marine food products. Hawaii Med. J. 50, 9–16.

Diaz, J.H., 2013. Paragonimiasis acquired in the United States: native and nonnative species. Clin. Microbiol. Rev. 26, 493–504.

Dick, T.A., Nelson, P.A., Choudhury, A., 2001. Diphyllobothriasis: update on human cases, foci, patterns and sources of human infections and future considerations. Southeast Asian J. Trop. Med. Public Health 32 (Suppl. 2), 59–76.

Do, H.T., Yagi, T., 2012. Individual vitamin B6 contents in selected Japanese sushi toppings. Int. J. Food. Sci. Nutr. 63, 246–249.

Draper, H.H., 1977. The aboriginal Eskimo diet in modernperspectiv. Am. Anthrop. 79, 309–316.

Dupouy-Camet, J., Peduzzi, R., 2004. Current situation of human diphyllobothriasis inEurope. Euro. Surveill. 9, 31–35.

EFSA, 2010. Scientific opinion on risk assessment of parasites in fishery products. EFSA J., 1543–1634.

Eklund, M.W., Peterson, M.E., Poysky, F.T., Paranjpye, R.N., Pelroy, G.A., 2004. Control of bacterial pathogens during processing of cold-smoked and dried salmon strips. J. Food Prot. 67, 347–351.

Elvevoll, E.O., Barstad, H., Breimo, E.S., Brox, J., Eilertsen, K.E., Lund, T., Olsen, J.O., Osterud, B., 2006. Enhanced incorporation of n-3 fatty acids from fish compared with fish oils. Lipids 41, 1109–1114.

Elvevoll, E.O., Eilertsen, K.E., Brox, J., Dragnes, B.T., Falkenberg, P., Olsen, J.O., Kirkhus, B., Lamglait, A., Østerud, B., 2008. Seafood diets: hypolipidemic and antiatherogenic effects of taurine and n-3 fatty acids. Atherosclerosis 200, 396–402.

FAO, 2010. The State of World Fisheries and Aquaculture 2010 (SOFIA). Food and Agriculture Organization of the United Nations, Rome.

FAO, 2014. The State of World Fisheries and Aquaculture.

Gladyshev, G., Nn, S., Ga, G., Sm, D., Gs, K., 2006. Effect of way of cooking on content of essential polyunsaturated fatty acids in muscle tissue of humpback salmon (*Oncorhynchus gorbuscha*). Food Chem. 96, 446–451.

Go, Y.B., Lee, E.H., Cho, J., Choi, S., Chai, J.Y., 2015. *Diphyllobothrium nihonkaiense* infections in a family. Kor. J. Parasitol. 53, 109–112.

Hagmar, L., Persson-Moschos, M., Akesson, B., Schütz, A., 1998. Plasma levels of selenium, selenoprotein P and glutathione peroxidase and their correlations to fish intake and serum levels of thyrotropin and thyroid hormones: a study on Latvian fish consumers. Eur. J. Clin. Nutr. 52, 796–800.

Harada, T., Kawai, T., Jinnai, M., Ohnishi, T., Sugita-Konishi, Y., Kumeda, Y., 2012. Detection of *Kudoa septempunctata* 18S ribosomal DNA in patient fecal samples from novel food-borne outbreaks caused by consumption of raw olive flounder (*Paralichthys olivaceus*). J. Clin. Microbiol. 50, 2964–2968.

Herman, J.S., Chiodini, P.L., 2009. Gnathostomiasis, another emerging imported disease. Clin. Microbiol. Rev. 22, 484–492.

Hosseini Farahabadi, S., Tavakkol-Afshari, J., Ganjali, R., Rafatpanah, H., Ghaffari, J., Farid-Hosseini, R., 2006. Association between the polymorphism of TGF-beta1 gene promoter (-509C > T) and idiopathic chronic urticaria. Iran J. Allergy Asthma Immunol. 5, 109–113.

Hosseini, H., Mahmoudzadeh, M., Rezaei, M., Mahmoudzadeh, L., Khaksar, R., Khosroshahi, N.K., Babakhani, A., 2014. Effect of different cooking methods on minerals, vitamins and nutritional quality indices of kutum roach (*Rutilus frisii kutum*). Food Chem. 148, 86–91.

Hung, N.M., Madsen, H., Fried, B., 2013. Global status of fish-borne zoonotic trematodiasis in humans. Acta Parasitol. 58, 231–258.

Hunter, J.E., Applewhite, T.H., 1991. Reassessment of trans fatty acid availability in the US diet. Am. J. Clin. Nutr. 54, 363–369.

Huxtable, R.J., 1992. Physiological actions of taurine. Physiol. Rev. 72, 101–163.

Iwata, K., Fukuchi, T., Yoshimura, K., 2015. Is the quality of sushi ruined by freezing raw fish and squid? A randomized double-blind trial with sensory evaluation using discrimination testing. Clin. Infect. Dis.

James, M.V.P., Flint, K.D., Ruxton, C.H.S., 2009. Cooking losses of long-chain n–3 fatty acid in seafood commonly eaten in the UK. Proc. Nutr. Soc., E106.

Kasuya, S., Hamano, H., Izumi, S., 1990. Mackerel-induced urticaria and Anisakis. Lancet 335, 665.

Kawai, T., Sekizuka, T., Yahata, Y., Kuroda, M., Kumeda, Y., Iijima, Y., Kamata, Y., Sugita-Konishi, Y., Ohnishi, T., 2012. Identification of *Kudoa septempunctata* as the causative agent of novel food poisoning outbreaks in Japan by consumption of *Paralichthys olivaceus* in raw fish. Clin. Infect. Dis. 54, 1046–1052.

Kimura, S., Takagi, Y., Gomi, K., 1999. IgE response to Anisakis compared to seafood. Allergy 54, 1225–1226.

Kliks, M., 1983. Anisakiasis in the western United States: four new case reports from California. Am. J. Trop. Med. Hyg. 32, 526–532.

Kuchta, R., Brabec, J., Kubáčková, P., Scholz, T., 2013. Tapeworm *Diphyllobothrium dendriticum* (Cestoda)—neglected or emerging human parasite? PLoS Negl. Trop. Dis. 7, e2535.

Köse, E., 2010. Evaluation of seafood safety health hazards for traditional fish products: preventive measures and monitoring issues. Turk. J. Fisheries Aquat. Sci. 10, 139–160.

Larsen, R., Stormo, S.K., Dragnes, B.T., Elvevoll, E.O., 2007. Losses of taurine, creatine, glycine and alanine from cod (*Gadus morhua* L.) fillet during processing. J. Food Comp. Anal. 20, 396–402.

Li, J., Xun, P., Zamora, D., Sood, A., Liu, K., Daviglus, M., Iribarren, C., Jacobs, D., Shikany, J.M., He, K., 2013. Intakes of long-chain omega-3 (n–3) PUFAs and fish in relation to incidence of asthma among American young adults: the CARDIA study. Am. J. Clin. Nutr. 97, 173–178.

Lin, A.H., Nepstad, I., Florvaag, E., Egaas, E., Van Do, T., 2014. An extended study of seroprevalence of anti-*Anisakis simplex* IgE antibodies in Norwegian blood donors. Scand. J. Immunol. 79, 61–67.

Lindeberg, S., 2010. Food and western disease: health and nutrition from an evolutionary perspective. Wiley-Blackwell, Oxford; Ames, Iowa.

Lu, Z., Chen, T.C., Zhang, A., Persons, K.S., Kohn, N., Berkowitz, R., Martinello, S., Holick, M.F., 2007. An evaluation of the vitamin D3 content in fish: Is the vitamin D content adequate to satisfy the dietary requirement for vitamin D? J. Steroid Biochem. Mol. Biol. 103, 642–644.

Lund, E.K., 2013. Health benefits of seafood; is it just the fatty acids? Food Chem. 140, 413–420.

López-Serrano, M., Gomez, A., Daschner, A., Moreno-Ancillo, A., de Parga, J., Caballero, M., Barranco, P., Cabañas, R., 2000. Gastroallergic anisakiasis: findings in 22 patients. J. Gastroenterol. Hepatol. 15, 503–506.

López-Sáez, M., Zubeldia, J., Caloto, M., Olalde, S., Pelta, R., Rubio, M., Baeza, M., 2003. Is Anisakis simplex responsible for chronic urticaria? Allergy Asthma Proc. 24, 339–345.

Marangoni, F., Poli, A., 2013. n–3 fatty acids: functional differences between food intake, oral supplementation and drug treatments. Int. J. Cardiol. 170, S12–S15.

Martínez de Velasco, G., Rodero, M., Chivato, T., Cuéllar, C., 2007. Seroprevalence of anti-*Kudoa* sp. (Myxosporea: Multivalvulida) antibodies in a Spanish population. Parasitol. Res. 100, 1205–1211.

Martínez de Velasco, G., Rodero, M., Cuéllar, C., Chivato, T., Mateos, J.M., Laguna, R., 2008. Skin prick test of *Kudoa* sp. Antigens in patients with gastrointestinal and/or allergic symptoms related to fish ingestion. Parasitol. Res. 103, 713–715.

Martínez-Cruz, J.M., Bravo-Zamudio, R., Aranda-Patraca, A., Martínez-Marañón, R., 1989. Gnathostomiasis in Mexico. Salud. Publica. Mex. 31, 541–549.

Matsukane, Y., Sato, H., Tanaka, S., Kamata, Y., Sugita-Konishi, Y., 2010. *Kudoa septempunctata* n. sp. (Myxosporea: Multivalvulida) from an aquacultured olive flounder (*Paralichthys olivaceus*) imported from Korea. Parasitol. Res. 107, 865–872.

Mattiucci, S., Fazii, P., De Rosa, A., Paoletti, M., Megna, A.S., Glielmo, A., De Angelis, M., Costa, A., Meucci, C., Calvaruso, V., Sorrentini, I., Palma, G., Bruschi, F., Nascetti, G., 2013. Anisakiasis and gastroallergic reactions associated with *Anisakis pegreffii* infection. Italy Emerg. Infect. Dis. 19, 496–499.

Mnari, B.A., Zaghbib, S.F., Dhibi, M., Harzallah, H.J., Dabbou, S., El Cafsi, M., Hammami, M., Chaouch, A., 2012. Effects of different cooking methods on the mineral contents of wild and farmed sea bream (*Sparus aurata*). Int. J. Food Sci. Technol. 47, 1964–1969.

Mnari Bhouri, A., Jrah Harzallah, H., Dhibi, M., Bouhlel, I., Hammami, M., Chaouch, A., 2010. Nutritional fatty acid quality of raw and cooked farmed and wild sea bream (*Sparus aurata*). J Agric. Food Chem. 58, 507–512.

Mo, A., Gahr, A., Hansen, H., Hoel, H., Oaland, O. T.T. P., 2014. Presence of *Anisakis simplex* (Rudolphi, 1809 det. Krabbe, 1878) and *Hysterothylacium aduncum* (Rudolphi, 1802) (Nematoda; Anisakidae) in runts of farmed Atlantic salmon, *Salmo salar* L. J. Fish Dis., 37, pp. 135–140.

Montano, N., Gavino, G., Gavino, V.C., 2001. Polyunsaturated fatty acid contents of some traditional fish and shrimp paste condiments of the Philippines. Food Chem. 75, 155–158.

Moore, D.A., McCroddan, J., Dekumyoy, P., Chiodini, P.L., 2003. Gnathostomiasis: an emerging imported disease. Emerg. Infect. Dis. 9, 647–650.

Mozaffarian, D., Lemaitre, R.N., Kuller, L.H., Burke, G.L., Tracy, R.P., Siscovick, D.S., Study, C.H., 2003. Cardiac benefits of fish consumption may depend on the type of fish meal consumed: the cardiovascular health study. Circulation 107, 1372–1377.

Muratov, I.V., 1990. *Diphyllobothriasis* in the far east of the USSR. Med. Parazitol. (Mosk.), 54–58.

Musaiger, A.O., R., D.S., 2011. Fatty acid profile of raw and cooked fish consumed in Bahrain. Afr. J. Food Sci. 5, pp. 213–218.

Neff, M.R., Bhavsar, S.P., Braekevelt, E., Arts, M.T., 2014. Effects of different cooking methods on fatty acid profiles in four freshwater fishes from the Laurentian Great Lakes region. Food Chem. 164, 544–550.

Nishioka, M., Kanosue, F., Yabuta, Y., Watanabe, F., 2011. Loss of vitamin B(12) in fish (round herring) meats during various cooking treatments. J. Nutr. Sci. Vitaminol. (Tokyo) 57, 432–436.

Novotny, L., Dvorska, L., Lorencova, A., Beran, V., Pavlik, I., 2004. Fish: a potential source of bacterial pathogens for human beings. Vet. Med. Czech. 49, 343–358.
O'Dea, K., 1984. Marked improvement in carbohydrate and lipid metabolism in diabetic Australian aborigines after temporary reversion to traditional lifestyle. Diabetes 33, 596–603.
Oehlenschläger, J., 2012. Seafood: nutritional benefits and risk aspects. Int. J. Vitam. Nutr. Res. 82, 168–176.
Oshima, T., 1987. Anisakiasis—is the sushi bar guilty? Parasitol. Today 3, 44–48.
Petney, T.N., Andrews, R.H., Saijuntha, W., Wenz-Mücke, A., Sithithaworn, P., 2013. The zoonotic, fish-borne liver flukes *Clonorchis sinensis*, *Opisthorchis felineus*, and *Opisthorchis viverrini*. Int. J. Parasitol. 43, 1031–1046.
Piras, C., Scano, P., Locci, E., Sanna, R., Marincola, F.C., 2014. Analysing the effects of frozen storage and processing on the metabolite profile of raw mullet roes using ^{1}H NMR spectroscopy. Food Chem. 159, 71–79.
Polat, A., Ozogul, Y., Kuley, E., Ozogul, F., Ozyurt, G., Simsek, A., 2013. Tocopherol content of commercial fish species as affected by microwave cooking. J. Food Biochem. 37, 381–387.
Puente, P., Anadón, A., Rodero, M., Romarís, F., Ubeira, F., Cuéllar, C., 2008. Anisakis simplex: the high prevalence in Madrid (Spain) and its relation with fish consumption. Exp. Parasitol. 118, 271–274.
Raatz, S.K., Golovko, M.Y., Brose, S.A., Rosenberger, T.A., Burr, G.S., Wolters, W.R., Picklo, Sr., M.J., 2011. Baking reduces prostaglandin, resolvin, and hydroxy-fatty acid content of farm-raised Atlantic salmon (*Salmo salar*). J. Agric. Food Chem. 59, 11278–11286.
Raatz, S.K., Silverstein, J.T., Jahns, L., Picklo, M.J., 2013. Issues of fish consumption for cardiovascular disease risk reduction. Nutrients 5, 1081–1097.
Ryan, J.T., Ross, R.P., Bolton, D., Fitzgerald, G.F., Stanton, C., 2011. Bioactive peptides from muscle sources: meat and fish. Nutrients 3, 765–791.
Scholz, T., Garcia, H.H., Kuchta, R., Wicht, B., 2009. Update on the human broad tapeworm (genus *Diphyllobothrium*), including clinical relevance. Clin. Microbiol. Rev. 22, 146–160.
Sidhu, K.S., 2003. Health benefits and potential risks related to consumption of fish or fish oil. Regul. Toxicol. Pharmacol. 38, 336–344.
Skog, K.I., Johansson, M.A., Jägerstad, M.I., 1998. Carcinogenic heterocyclic amines in model systems and cooked foods: a review on formation, occurrence and intake. Food Chem. Toxicol. 36, 879–896.
Smith, J., Wootten, R., 1978. Anisakis and anisakiasis. Adv. Parasitol. 16, 93–163.
Telzak, E.E., Bell, E.P., Kautter, D.A., Crowell, L., Budnick, L.D., Morse, D.L., Schultz, S., 1990. An international outbreak of type E botulism due to uneviscerated fish. J. Infect. Dis. 161, 340–342.
Tham, W., Ericsson, H., Loncarevic, S., Unnerstad, H., Danielsson-Tham, M.L., 2000. Lessons from an outbreak of listeriosis related to vacuum-packed gravad and cold-smoked fish. Int. J. Food Microbiol. 62, 173–175.
Turhan, S., Ustun, N., S., T., T., 2011. Lipid quality of annchovy (*Engraulis encrasicholus*) fillets affected by different cooking methods. Int. J. Foof. Prop. 14, pp 1358–1365.
Valiñas, B., Lorenzo, S., Eiras, A., Figueiras, A., Sanmartín, M., Ubeira, F., 2001. Prevalence of and risk factors for IgE sensitization to Anisakis simplex in a Spanish population. Allergy 56, 667–671.
Ventura, M.T., Napolitano, S., Menga, R., Cecere, R., Asero, R., 2013. Anisakis simplex hypersensitivity is associated with chronic urticaria in endemic areas. Int. Arch. Allergy Immunol. 160, 297–300.
Visioli, F., Risé, P., Barassi, M.C., Marangoni, F., Galli, C., 2003. Dietary intake of fish vs. formulations leads to higher plasma concentrations of n-3 fatty acids. Lipids 38, 415–418.
Weber, J., Bochi, V.C., Ribeiro, C.P., Victorio, A.d.M., Emanuelli, T., 2008. Effect of different cooking methods on the oxidation, proximate and fatty acid composition of silver catfish (*Rhamdia quelen*) fillets. Food Chem. 106, 140–146.
World Health Organization, 1995. Control of foodborne trematode infections. WHO Technical Report Series Number 849.
World Health Organization, 2004. Report of Joint WHO/FAO workshop on foodborne trematode infections in Asia, Ha Noi, Vietnam 26-28 Nov. 2002.
World Health Organization, 2011. Report of the WHO Expert Consultation on Foodborne Trematode Infections and Taeniasis/Cysticercosis. Vientiane, Lao People's Democratic Republic 2009.
Wrangham, R., 2013. The evolution of human nutrition. Curr. Biol. 23, R354–355.
Wrangham, R., Conklin-Brittain, N., 2003. Cooking as a biological trait. Comp. Biochem. Physiol. A 136, 35–46.
Yamori, Y., Liu, L., Mori, M., Sagara, M., Murakami, S., Nara, Y., Mizushima, S., 2009. Taurine as the nutritional factor for the longevity of the Japanese revealed by a world-wide epidemiological survey. Adv. Exp. Med. Biol. 643, 13–25.
Yu, S.-H., 1994. Epidemiology and morbidity of food-borne intestinal trematode infections. World Health Organization, Geneva.

Index

H

I

J

K

N

O

P